Basic Sciences for Core Medical Training and the MRCP

OXFORD
UNIVERSITY PRESS

Great Clarendon Street, Oxford, OX2 6DP,
United Kingdom

Oxford University Press is a department of the University of Oxford.
It furthers the University's objective of excellence in research, scholarship,
and education by publishing worldwide. Oxford is a registered trade mark of
Oxford University Press in the UK and in certain other countries

Impression: 1

Published in the United States of America by Oxford University Press
198 Madison Avenue, New York, NY 10016, United States of America

British Library Cataloguing in Publication Data

Data available

Library of Congress Control Number: 2015949661

ISBN 978–0–19–959967–7

Printed in Great Britain by Ashford Colour Press Ltd, Gosport, Hampshire

Foreword

I was honoured and delighted to be asked by Neil and Robert to write a foreword to this book. Honoured because two great scientists who have co-edited an excellent book asked me to do so, but delighted because I thus read the book, including chapters relevant to specialities other than my own, which is something I might otherwise not have done. It is so easy to forget some basic principles and so often they transcend disciplines. However, when starting one's career the task can seem insurmountable and breaking principles down and applying them to one system at a time produces more manageable challenges.

We live in changing times. Access to information is now almost instantaneous. Rote learning of facts may never have been appropriate but is even less sensible now. However, the ability to use knowledge to solve problems remains of paramount importance and, as medicine becomes more complex, the scientific underpinning of the practice of medicine is of increasing rather than lessening importance. As the provision of healthcare is shared with more fellow health professionals a doctor's especial responsibilities for diagnosis, prescribing and the explanation of risk can only be done adequately with such an underlying understanding. During a 40-year professional career new diseases and new interventions will bring new challenges to all, but a sound understanding of the science of health and disease makes such challenges easier to tackle. Unfortunately current assessment methods can appear to involve rather bland assessment of competency in discrete domains rather than necessarily assessing overall ability to solve the often complex challenges of modern medicine. Published data suggests that performance in postgraduate examinations does vary between graduates from different medical schools and this is more likely to reflect basic educational experience within those schools than academic qualifications on entry to medicine.

Students and trainees appreciate the importance of basic science but sometimes their inquisitiveness and thirst for a better understanding only comes later in their training when they try to disentangle what is going on in difficult clinical cases. It is almost impossible to understand why a pregnant lady has an increased heart rate and a quiet heart murmur without understanding the normal physiological response to pregnancy, and one will not be able to differentiate between normality and abnormality without such understanding. Similarly, an understanding of the variability in carbohydrate metabolism and insulin kinetics between individuals is essential if we are to truly offer personalized prescribing for those with diabetes, and why one intervention is preferred to another in complex cardiac rhythm disturbances necessitates a firm understanding of electrophysiology. Understanding mechanisms is thus crucial—mechanisms in health, mechanisms giving rise to disease, and mechanisms by which medication can cure or ameliorate the underlying disorders.

A system approach can thus be justified as a basis for our learning but such an approach needs to also respect the importance of the science of population health, epidemiology, genetics, statistics, and clinical pharmacology and this fusion of approaches is particularly well done in *Basic Sciences for Core Medical Training and the MRCP*.

Martyn R Partridge
Professor of Respiratory Medicine
Imperial College London

Preface

Medical education, like medical science, is constantly evolving. Traditional courses often start by focusing on the basic sciences such as physiology, cell biology, biochemistry, and anatomy, studying each in isolation. However, medical school teaching is moving to a more systems based approach, often based around the clinical specialties. From the first year of study, students may learn about the basic science, pathology, diagnosis, and treatments related to a particular specialty whilst also seeing patients in the clinical setting. Old-style textbooks, which focus on a particular medical science, are therefore not always ideal for this structure for learning. Similarly post-graduate medical examinations, such as those for Membership of the Royal College of Physicians (MRCP) in the UK, require a detailed knowledge of core medical science, and yet examine it in a way that focuses on its relevance to clinical practice.

This concise text provides an up-to-date and easily readable explanation of the relevant basic science behind each of the medical specialties. The text is often presented in bullet point format with simple concise explanations. It makes extensive use of tables, lists, and diagrams, with each chapter also containing multiple-choice questions aimed at consolidating the material covered and highlighting topics that are frequently examined. No book of this length covering such a wide area can be completely comprehensive. For the busy junior doctor or medical student, we hope it will provide a coherent starting point for improving their understanding of medical science before turning to other texts that focus more on pathology, diagnosis, and management.

Although we have structured the chapters around the syllabus for the MRCP (UK) Part 1 examination, we hope that the specialty-based approach makes it a useful text for undergraduate medical education and other post-graduate examinations, such as the US Medical Licensing Examinations.

Neil Herring
Robert Wilkins
Oxford 2015

Acknowledgements

We are particularly grateful to our contributing authors: Dr Hussein Al-Mossawi, Dr Sophie Anwar, Dr Chris Duncan, Dr Brad Hillier, Dr James Kolasinski, Dr David McCartney, Dr Niki Meston, Dr Joel Meyer, Dr Michal Rolinski, and Dr Susanne Hodgson.

We are also grateful to our medical consultant colleagues for their valuable critique and advice. In particular: Dr Sue Burge, Dr Niki Karavitaki, Dr Annabel Nichols, Prof Chris Pugh, and Dr John Reynolds.

Dedication

This book is dedicated to our late fathers, our teachers, and the students we have taught.

Contents

Contributors

Dr Hussein Al-Mossawi
Department of Rheumatology,
Southmead Hospital,
Bristol, UK

Dr Sophie Anwar
The Oxford Clinic,
Littlemore Mental Health Centre,
Oxford, UK

Dr Christopher J. A. Duncan
Department of Infection & Tropical Medicine,
Royal Victoria Infirmary,
University of Newcastle,
Newcastle-Upon-Tyne, UK

Prof Neil Herring
Oxford Heart Centre, John Radcliffe Hospital,
Department of Physiology, Anatomy and Genetics,
University of Oxford,
Oxford, UK

Dr Bradley Hillier
Shaftesbury Clinic, South West London Forensic Psychiatry Service,
Springfield University Hospital, London, UK

Dr James Kolasinski
Oxford Centre for fMRI of the Brain,
University of Oxford, UK

Dr David McCartney
Nuffied Department of Primary Care Health Sciences,
University of Oxford, UK

Dr Niki Meston
Department of Newborn Screening,
St Helier Hospital,
Carshalton, UK

Dr Joel Meyer
Centre for Clinical Vaccinology and Tropical Medicine,
Churchill Hospital,
University of Oxford, UK

Dr Michal Rolinski
Nuffield Department of Clinical Neurosciences,
University of Oxford, UK

Dr Susanne H. Hodgson
The Jenner Institue,
University of Oxford, UK

Prof Robert Wilkins
Department of Physiology, Anatomy and Genetics,
University of Oxford,
Oxford, UK

Abbreviations

A adenine
ABC ATP-binding cassette
Abs antibodies
ACh acetylcholine
ACP acyl carrier protein
ACPA anti-cyclic citrullinated peptide
ACTH adrenocorticotrophic hormone
ADCC antibody-dependent cellular cytotoxicity
ADH alcohol dehydrogenase
ADH anti-diuretic hormone
ADP adenosine diphosphate
AE1 anion-exchanger isoform 1
AF atrial fibrillation
AFC antibody-forming cell
AFP α-foetoprotein
ALA amino laevulinic acid
ALDH aldehyde dehydrogenase
AMP adenosine monophosphate
AMPK AMP-activated protein kinase
ANA anti-nuclear antibody
ANCA anti-neutrophil cytoplasmic antibodies
APC antigen-presenting cell
ARDS acute respiratory distress syndrome
ARR absolute risk reduction
ATP adenine triphosphate
AV atrioventricular
BCG Bacille Calmette–Guerin
BCR B-cell receptor
BM body mass
BNP brain type natriuretic peptide
BP blood pressure
BPAD bipolar affective disorder
C cytosine
cAMP cyclic adenosine monophosphate
cART combination antiretroviral therapy
CBT cognitive behavioural therapy
cDNA complementary DNA
CE condensing enzyme
CEA carcinoembryonic antigen
CER control event rate
CFTR cystic fibrosis transmembrane conductance regulator
CGD chronic granulomatous disease
CI confidence interval
CML chronic myeloid leukaemia
CMV cytomegalovirus
CNS central nervous system
COPD chronic obstructive pulmonary disease
CPAP continuous positive airway pressure
CPT I carnitine palmitoyltransferase I
CR complement receptors
CRH corticotrophin-releasing hormone
CSF cerebrospinal fluid
CStF colony-stimulating factor
CTL cytotoxic T lymphocytes
CVA cerebrovascular accidents
CVID common variable immunodeficiency
CXR chest X-ray
DA dopaminergic
DAF Decay activating factor
DAMP Damage-associated molecular patterns
DCT distal convoluted tubule
DF degrees of freedom
DHEA dehydroepiandrosterone
DI diabetes insipidus
DIC disseminated intravascular coagulation
DKA diabetic ketoacidosis
DM diabetes mellitis
DMD Duchenne muscular dystrophy
DNA deoxyribonucleic acid
DPPC dipalmitoylphosphatidylcholine
Ds-DNA anti-double-stranded DNA
DST dexamthasone suppression test
DVT deep vein thrombosis
EBV Epstein–Barr virus
ECG electrocardiogram
ECL enterochromaffin-like
ECT electroconvulsive therapy
EEG electroencephalographic
EER experimental event rate
EGF 1 epidermal growth factor 1
EGPA eosinophillic granulomatosis with polyangiitis
ELISA enzyme-linked immunosorbent assay
ER endoplasmic reticulum
ERV expiratory reserve volume
ESBL extended beta lactam
ESR erythrocyte sedimentation rate
FA fatty acid

FAD	flavin adenine dinucleotide
FAS	fatty acid synthase
FBC	full blood count
FcR	Fc receptors
FGFR	fibroblast growth factor receptor
FMN	flavin mononucleotide
fMRI	functional magnetic resonance imaging
FRC	functional residual capacity
FSH	follicle-stimulating hormone
G	guanine
G6PD	glucose-6-phosphate dehydrogenase deficiency
GAD	glutamic acid dehydrogenase
GALT	galactose-1-phosphate uridyl transferase
GCA	giant cell arteritis
GFR	glomerular filtration rate
GH	growth hormone
GHRH	growth hormone-releasing hormone
GI	gastrointestinal
GLP	glucagon like peptide
GM-CStF	granulocyte-macrophage colony stimulating factor
gp	glycoprotein
GPA	granulomatosis with polyangiitis
GR	glucocorticoid receptors
GvHD	graft versus host disease
HAPE	high altitude pulmonary oedema
Hb	haemoglobin
HbF	foetal haemoglobin
HbS	sickle haemoglobin
HBsAg	hepatitis B surface antigen
HIT	heparin-induced thrombocytopenia
HIV	human immunodeficiency virus
HLA	human leucocyte antigen
HP	hydrostatic pressure
HPA	hypothalamic–pituitary–adrenal
HTT	Huntington
HVA	homovanillic acid
IA2	islet-associated antigen 2
IC	immune complex
ICAM	intercellular adhesion molecules
IGf	impaired fasting glucose
IGF	insulin-like growth factor
IGF-1	insulin-like growth factor 1
IGRA	IFNγ release assays
IGt	impaired glucose tolerance
il-3	interleukin 3
im	intramuscular
IPEX	immune dysregulation, polyendicrinopathy, enteropathy, X-linked syndrome
IRIS	immune reconstitution inflammatory syndrome
IRS	insulin-receptor substrate
IRV	inspiratory reserve volume
ITP	immune thrombocytopenic purpura
iv	intravenous
KIRs	killer immunoglobulin-like receptors
LEKTI	lympho-epithelial Kazal-type-related inhibitor
LFA	leucocyte functional antigen
LFT	liver function test
LGN	lateral geniculate nucleus
LH	luteinizing hormone
LIP	lymphocytic interstitial pneumonitis
LTOT	long-term oxygen therapy
MAO-A	monoamine oxidase-A
MCAD	medium chain acyl CoA dehydrogenase
MCP	Membrane cofactor protein
MELAS	mitochondrial encephalomyopathy, lactic acidosis, and stroke-like episodes
MEN 1	multiple endocrine neoplasia type 1
MEN	multiple endocrine neoplasia
MHC	major histocompatibility complex
MLCK	myosin light chain kinase
MMC	migrating motor complexes
MODY	maturity onset diabetes of the young
MPA	microscopic polyangiitis
MPO	myeloperoxidase
MRI	magnetic resonance imaging
mRNA	messenger RNA
MRSA	methicillin-resistant *Staphylococcus aureus*
NA	noradrenergic
NAD	nicotinamide adenine dinucleotide
NADPH	nicotinamide adenine dinucleotide phosphate
NCC	Na^+-Cl^- cotransporter
NK	natural killer
NMS	neuroleptic malignant syndrome
NNH	number needed to harm
NNRTI	non-nucleotide reverse transcriptase inhibitor
NNT	number needed to treat
NPV	negative predictive value
NRTI	nucleotide reverse transcriptase inhibitor
NSAID	non-steroidal anti-inflammatory drug
NSIP	non-specific interstitial pneumonia
OA	osteoarthritis
OI	opportunistic infections
OTC	ornithine transcarbamoylase
PAF	platelet-activating factor
PAH	para-aminohippurate
PAI	plasminogen activator inhibitor
PAMP	Pathogen-associated molecular patterns
PBG	porphobilinogen
PBP	penicillin-binding proteins
PCD	passive cell death
PCI	percutaneous coronary intervention
PCP	phenylcyclidine
PCR	polymerase chain reaction
PDGF	platelet-derived growth factor
PE	pulmonary embolism
PEER	patient expected event rate
PEP	phosphoenol pyruvate
PET	positron emission tomography
PKD	polycystic kidney disease
PKU	phenylketonuria
PMR	polymyalgia rheumatic
PNS	peripheral nervous system
po	by mouth
POMC	proopiomelanocortin
PPAR	peroxisome proliferator activated receptors
PPV	positive predictive value

PR3	proteinase 3
PRL	prolactin
PRR	pattern recognition receptors
RA	rheumatoid arthritis
RCT	randomized controlled trials
RER	rough endoplasmic reticulum
RFLP	restriction fragment length polymorphism
Rh	Rhesus factor
RNA	ribonucleic acid
ROC	receiver operating characteristic
RPF	renal plasma flow
RR	relative risk
rRNA	ribosomal RNA
RRR	relative risk reduction
RTA	renal tubular acidosis
sc	subcutaneous
SCID	severe combined immunodeficiency
SD	standard deviation
SEM	standard error of the mean
SIADH	syndrome of inappropriate ADH
SIRS	systemic inflammatory response syndrome
SLE	systemic lupus erythematosus
SNR	single nucleotide polymorphism
snRNA	small nuclear RNA
SSRI	selective serotonin re-uptake inhibitor
STR	short tandem repeat
T	thymine
TB	tuberculosis
TBG	thyroxine-binding globulin
TCA	tricarboxylic acid/Krebs cycle
TCA	tricyclic antidepressant
TCR	T-cell receptors
TD	T-cell dependent
TF	transcription factor
TFT	thyroid function test
TGFß	transforming growth factor beta
TI	T-cell independent
TIBC	total iron binding capacity
TLC	total lung capacity
TLR	toll-like receptors
tMRS	transcranial magnetic resonance stimulation
TPMT	thiopurine methyltransferase
TRH	thyrotrophin-releasing hormone
tRNA	transfer RNA
TSC	tuberous sclerosis complex
TSH	thyroid-stimulating hormone
TST	tuberculin skin test
TTP	thrombotic thrombocytopenic purpura
TV	tidal volume
TXA2	thromboxane A2
U	uracil
U&E	urea & electrolytes
VC	vital capacity
VEGF	vascular endothelial growth factor
VLCFA	very long chain fatty acids
VNTR	variable number tandem repeat
vWF	von Willebrand factor
VZV	*Varicella zoster* virus
WBC	white blood count
WCC	white cell count

CHAPTER 1

Genetics

The structure and function of genes

Genes and nucleotides

Genes are inherited units of information that determine phenotype. They are stretches of the nucleic acid DNA, a polymer of nucleotides, which encode proteins. The sequence of nucleotides determines the amino acid sequence of the protein and, hence, its function. With 22 homologous chromosomes, each gene is represented twice in the genome (alleles).

The *nucleotides* (also termed bases) are formed from a nitrogenous base (the purines guanine [G] and cytosine [C] and the pyrimidines adenine [A] and thymine [T]), deoxyribose, and a phosphate group. (In RNA, the sugar is ribose, and T is replaced by uracil [U].) Nucleic acids display polarity with a 5′ end at which a phosphate group is attached to C5 of the sugar and a 3′ end at which a hydroxyl group is attached to C3 of the sugar.

DNA strands associate as pairs and run in an antiparallel fashion, with the 3′ end of one associating with the 5′ end of the other in a double helix arrangement. There is base pairing—G with C and A with T. Amino acids are coded by a three base pair sequence, called a codon (Table 1.1).

Table 1.1 The genetic code

5′ base	Middle base				3′ base
	U	C	A	G	
U	UUU Phe	UCU Ser	UAU Tyr	UGU Cys	U
	UUC Phe	UCC Ser	UAC Tyr	UGC Cys	C
	UUA Leu	UCA Ser	UAA Stop*	UGA Stop*	A
	UUG Leu	UCG Ser	UAG Stop*	UGG Trp	G
C	CUU Leu	CCU Pro	CAU His	CGU Arg	U
	CUC Leu	CCC Pro	CAC His	CGC Arg	C
	CUA Leu	CCA Pro	CAA Gln	CGA Arg	A
	CUG Leu	CCG Pro	CAG Gln	CGG Arg	G
A	AUU Ile	ACU Thr	AAU Asn	AGU Ser	U
	AUC Ile	ACC Thr	AAC Asn	AGC Ser	C
	AUA Ile	ACA Thr	AAA Lys	AGA Arg	A
	AUG Met†	ACG Thr	AAG Lys	AGG Arg	G
G	GUU Val	GCU Ala	GAU Asp	GGU Gly	U
	GUC Val	GCC Ala	GAC Asp	GGC Gly	C
	GUA Val	GCA Ala	GAA Glu	GGA Gly	A
	GUG Val	GCG Ala	GAG Glu	GGG Gly	G

*Stop codons have no amino acids assigned to them.

†The AUG codon is the initiation codon as well as that for other methionine residues.

BOX 1.1 MUTATIONS

- *Point mutations* in genes, in which a single nucleotide is changed, will change the amino acid encoded (unless the new codon encodes the same amino acid as the original one). Whether this change has an impact on protein function depends on the precise amino acid substitution that has occurred and how the original amino acid influenced the protein's function. Some point mutations will generate stop codon sequences (non-sense mutations).
- *Mis-sense* or *frame shift-mutations*, in which there is insertion or deletion of bases, can significantly disrupt amino acid coding and are liable to result in proteins of considerably altered structure that cannot replicate the wild type protein function. Insertion or deletion of (multiples of) three bases will result in insertion or deletion of amino acids from the protein sequence. The impact of these changes on protein function will again be dependent on the nature of the amino acids added or removed. The ΔF_{508} phenotype of CFTR arises from removal of three bases from the DNA sequence that leads to loss of phenylalanine at amino acid 508 and results in a failure to traffic the protein to the plasma membrane.
- *Dynamic mutations* are typically triplet sequences repeated many times, the number of which expands with each successive generation. The probability of expression of a mutant phenotype is a function of the number of copies of the mutation and becomes apparent when a threshold level of repeats is reached (for example, Huntington's disease). The resultant trinucleotide repeat disease presents at a younger age and with increasingly severe phenotype with each successive generation (the phenomenon of 'anticipation')

Mutations in regulatory elements (promoter or repressor regions) result in inappropriate levels of gene expression, while mutations at a splice site (the point at which introns are excised from transcribed RNA to unite exons) can result in frame shifts or the loss of an exon or retention of an intron.

There are 4^3 potential triplet sequences, so some amino acids are encoded by more than one codon (redundancy). The sequence AUG is the start codon for all proteins, while TAG, TGA, and TAA are stop codons. The start and stop codons define the 'open reading frame'.

Exons

Genes comprise exons (highly conserved sequences of DNA that encode proteins), introns (poorly-conserved longer sequences of unclear function that are spliced out during processing of mRNA and regulatory elements. Of the ~3.2×10^9 base pairs in the human genome, exons (on average around 145 base pairs in length) make up only about 1.5% of the total DNA. There are around 30,000 genes, with around nine exons per gene

Sequences of DNA may be present as a single copy (almost 50% of the genome, comprising introns and regulatory elements), or repeated to varying degrees (10^3–10^6 times). Inverted repeat sequences of around 200 bases pairs allow DNA to form hairpin structures.

Mutations in exons (changes in the base sequence) have effects of varying magnitude, depending on the nature of the mutation. When there is an impact, the most common outcome is a loss of function of the encoded protein, although some gain of function mutations also exist (for example, constitutive activation of membrane receptors; see Box 1.1).

Gene expression

Gene expression requires transcription of the open reading frame to produce pre-mRNA, which is processed before its translation generates a protein. Other RNA variants involved in mRNA translation (ribosomal RNA (rRNA), transfer RNA (tRNA), and small nuclear RNA (snRNA)) are also transcribed, but not themselves translated. *Transcription* progresses in three stages—initiation, elongation, and termination.

Initiation

During initiation, the transcription factor TFIID (transcription factor II D) binds through its TBP subunit to the TATA box (a core promoter sequence in DNA, located 30 base pairs upstream from the transcription start site). Binding of TFIID initiates the formation of an initiation complex as other TFII variants and RNA polymerase II bind (Fig. 1.1). One of the transcription factors, TFIIH, exhibits helicase activity, and acts to separate DNA strands. The initiation complex also interacts with activators and repressors that modulate the basal rate of transcription.

Elongation

This can proceed without a primer and occurs in the 5′→3′ direction. The polymerase progresses along the template (non-coding 3′→5′) strand of DNA catalysing the formation of phosphodiester bonds between the ribose sugars of nucleotides. As for DNA, purine (adenine, guanine)–pyrimidine (thymine, cytosine) pairing occurs, except that uracil, rather than thymine is incorporated into the RNA strand when adenine arises in the DNA template sequence. A single polymerase progresses undirectionally along the DNA template and transcribes the complete RNA strand. In contrast to DNA replication, proof-reading of the transcribed RNA sequence does not take place.

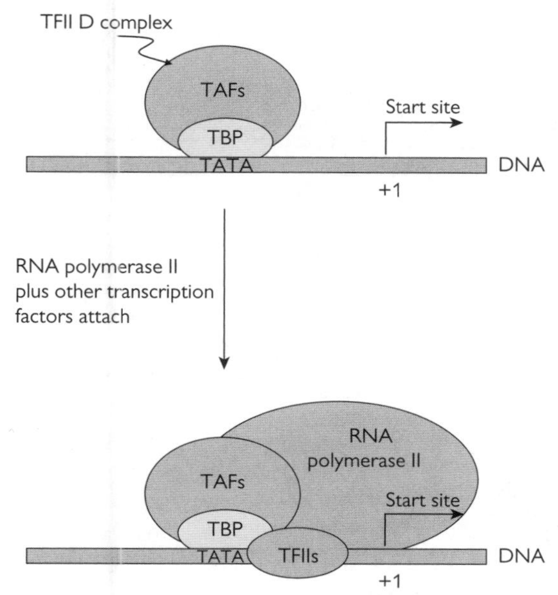

Fig. 1.1 Diagrammatic representation of the components of the basal initiation complex.

Reproduced from R Wilkins et al., *Oxford Handbook of Medical Sciences*, Second Edition, 2011, Figure 3.2, p. 193, by permission of Oxford University Press.

Termination

Termination occurs when the polymerase encounters a GC-rich sequence in the template that is followed by a poly-A sequence. A GC-rich sequence in the counterpart RNA is generated, which self-associates to form a hairpin loop. The poly-U sequence that follows the loop in the RNA strand forms only weak associations with the poly-A sequence in the DNA template. This destabilizes the DNA–RNA duplex and the polymerase disengages. The duplex unravels and DNA strands reunite as a double helix. In Rho-dependent termination, Rho factor (an ATP-dependent RNA helicase) binds to the RNA strand at C-rich, G-poor regions and progresses along the sequence. When it encounters the polymerase, it disrupts the polymerase–DNA–RNA complex to terminate transcription. Polymerase I catalyses transcription of rRNA (except the 5S subunit), while polymerase III catalyses the transcription of the 5S subunit of rRNA, tRNA, and snRNA.

Regulation of expression

Although many genes are expressed constitutively (typically housekeeping genes, such as β-actin) regulation of expression also occurs. This is achieved primarily through regulation of transcription, although expression is also regulated through changes in the processing, translation, and degradation of mRNA. Sequence-specific transcription factors (encoded by *trans-acting elements*) bind to *cis-regulatory (response) elements* within DNA. These elements are typically up to 12 base pairs long. The CAAT and GC boxes lie within around 100 base pairs of the origin of transcription and increase the activity of the TATA box. Other elements may be several hundreds or even thousands of base pairs away from the start site of the gene. Trans-acting factors may be activators, which bind enhancer elements, or repressors, which bind silencer elements. The combined activity of trans-acting factors on different regulatory elements determines the timing, pattern, and level of expression. Transcription factors comprise a DNA-binding domain and a trans-activating domain that can interact with co-regulators or with the initiation complex (directly, or via adapter proteins). Transcription factors can combine to form homomeric (for example, CREB) or hetero-multimeric (for example, c-Fos/Jun) complexes and may also possess a signal sensing (ligand binding) domain responsive to external signals (for example, the steroid hormone receptor family). Physiological signals can exert effects on gene expression by increasing expression or activity of transcription factors, often by the generation of intracellular second messengers (for example, cyclic adenosine monophosphate (cAMP), Ca^{2+}). The activity of transcription factors is commonly modulated by phosphorylation by protein kinases.

Processing of pre-mRNA

Processing of pre-mRNA to yield mature mRNA occurs as transcription proceeds (Fig. 1.2). Shortly after transcription is initiated, a transferase catalyses the formation of a 5′–5′ triphosphate bond between a modified guanine residue (7-methylguanylate) and the 5′ end of the RNA. The *5′ cap* that results facilitates ribosomal recognition of mRNA and protects against RNase activity. In addition, an endonuclease acts around 30 base pairs downstream from a consensus sequence at the 3′ end to cleave RNA. The addition of up to 250 adenosine residues at the cleaved 3′ end by a polymerase (polyadenylation) creates a *poly(A) tail* that also protects against degradation. Introns are removed from pre-mRNA by splicing at specific recognition sites (GU nucleotide sequence at the 5′ site, AG nucleotide sequence at the 3′ site) by a complex of snRNA and proteins called a spliceosome. The sequence of the mature mRNA represents that of the exons alone. Alternative splicing, in which different combinations of exons are combined, generates distinct mRNA sequences that encode different protein isoforms. The mRNA sequence can also be edited by deamination of C to U (for example, deamination of C to U in a CAA sequence in the apolipoprotein *B* gene in the intestine generates a UAA stop codon, resulting in apo B48, rather than apoB100 found in the liver). Deamination of A to I (inosine) also occurs, with I acting as G in subsequent translation.

mRNA translation

After processing is complete, mRNA translocates from the nucleus to the cytoplasm through pores for translation, which takes place on ribosomes (Fig. 1.3). mRNA encoding proteins that will enter the secretory pathway, be targeted to membranes or reside in organelles, is translated on ribosomes that

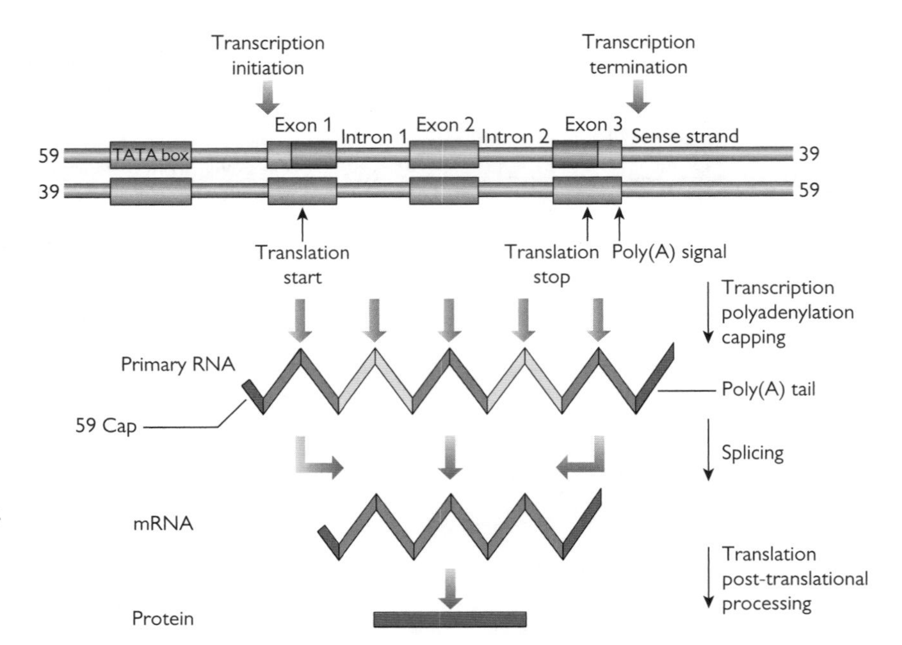

Fig. 1.2 Transcription, post-transcriptional processing, translation, and post-translational processing.

Reproduced from R Wilkins et al., *Oxford Handbook of Medical Sciences*, Second Edition, 2011, Figure 3.3, p. 195, by permission of Oxford University Press.

associate with the cytoplasmic face of rough endoplasmic reticulum (RER). Ribosome association with the RER membrane takes place once protein synthesis is under way and a hydrophobic signal sequence that facilitates the passage of the newly-synthesized protein into or across the RER membrane has been detected. Signal sequences are typically cleaved in the RER lumen. Translation of mRNA encoding cytoplasmic proteins takes place on free ribosomes. Ribosomes comprise two subunits, a small 40S subunit and a large 60S subunit, each a complex of rRNA molecules (18S in the 40S subunit, 5S, 5.8S, and 23S in the 60S subunit) and proteins.

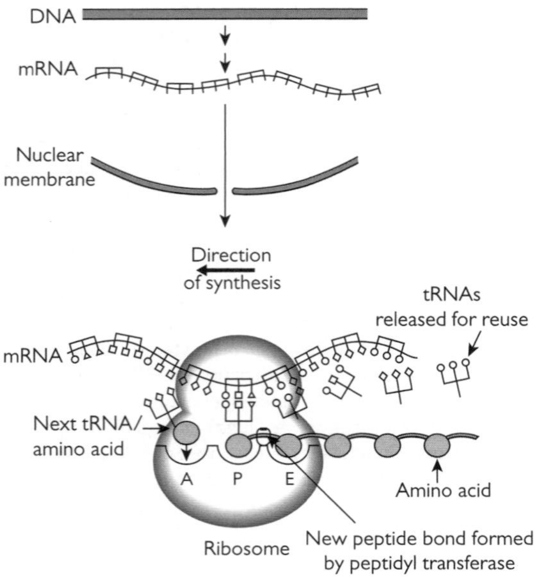

Fig. 1.3 Representation of the way in which genetic information is translated into protein.

Reproduced from R Wilkins et al., *Oxford Handbook of Medical Sciences*, Second Edition, 2011, Figure 3.4, p. 197, by permission of Oxford University Press.

mRNA is translated in the 5′→3′ direction, with protein synthesis proceeding from the N- to the C-terminus. Translation progresses in four stages.

- In *initiation*, the 40S and 60S subunits dissociate and initiation factor proteins bind to the 40S subunit. One of the initiation factors is a GTP-binding protein that recognizes a specific tRNA (Met-tRNA) required for initiation. The 40S subunit associates with the 5′ cap of the mRNA and identifies the start codon (typically the most proximal AUG) that always codes for methionine. Once the start codon has been identified, the initiation factors are released from the 40S subunit, which can then associate once more with the 60S subunit. The 80S ribosome complex so formed possesses three binding sites for tRNA: A, P and E. The A site is the point of association for incoming aminoacyl-tRNA, which pairs codons with the appropriate amino acid (except for the first methionine: Met-tRNA binds at the P site).
- Peptidyl transferase catalyses the formation of a peptide bond between the amino acid at the A site and the polypeptide at the P site (*elongation*). The uncharged tRNA at the P site transfers to the E (exit) site, freeing the P site.
- *Translocation* of the peptidyl-tRNA from the A site to the P site follows. The tRNA at the E site dissociates and the liberated A site accepts the next aminoacyl-tRNA. Elongation factors are responsible for the selection of the cognate aminoacyl-tRNA and translocation of the peptidyl-tRNA.

BOX 1.2 INHIBITING GENE EXPRESSION AT THE LEVEL OF mRNA TRANSLATION

Antisense oligonucleotides

These can be delivered using liposomes. They bind mRNA to inhibit the expression of genes at the protein level. Inhibition of the exon-splicing enhancer sequence within the dystrophin gene (which impairs accurate splicing of pre-mRNA to mRNA) using antisense oligonucleotides can be used to generate in-frame mutations which offset the out-of-frame mutations causing Duchenne muscular dystrophy and result in the milder Becker phenotype.

RNA interference

This involves the delivery of double-stranded RNA in the form of a drug or through a plasmid or viral vector. The RNA is degraded to form *short interfering RNA* (siRNA), which activates endogenous RNA-induced silencing complexes. In turn, these activate RNase, which degrade endogenous mRNA molecules containing sequences homologous to the siRNA.

- Codon-by-codon migration along the RNA is repeated until a stop codon is encountered, which binds release factors that trigger ribosome dissociation and release of the polypeptide chain (*termination*). Protein synthesis can be inhibited by purine and pyrimidine analogues (mercaptopurine and 5-fluorouracil); some antibiotics act as specific inhibitors of bacterial RNA polymerase (for example, rifampicin).

Gene expression can also be inhibited by targeting mRNA translation as summarized in Box 1.2.

Recombinant DNA technology

Recombinant DNA technology has a variety of applications, including the identification, mapping and sequencing of genes, the investigation of gene expression and the generation of recombinant proteins, such as recombinant insulin and recombinant factor VIII.

Cloning

Molecular *cloning* is used to develop recombinant DNA (rDNA), which contains sequences that originate from more than one source. Sequences from foreign sources can be combined with host sequences that drive replication of the foreign material when introduced into the host. The source material is a collection of restriction fragments of DNA, which are generated using *restriction endonucleases* (for example, *Eco*R1). Alternatively, complementary DNA (cDNA), synthesized from mRNA using reverse transcriptase, can be employed.

Cloning requires the exploitation of *vectors*, which are derived from bacterial plasmids or bacteriophages, small circular molecules of double-stranded DNA that can replicate autonomously. The 'sticky ends' of host and foreign DNA generated by treatment with a restriction endonuclease are covalently linked by a *DNA ligase*. Vectors include elements for the replication of the parental DNA and its insert in the host, along with sequences facilitating insertion of foreign DNA. The vector is transformed into the recipient bacterial cell, within which it replicates. Vectors typically include a gene conferring antibiotic resistance, which can be used as a screening tool for successful DNA transfer. Colonies of transgenic cells (clones) containing specific DNA sequence insertions can be selected for subsequent culture using nucleic acid hybridization. Manipulation of the foreign gene to include sequences that permit mRNA translation (promoter sequence, initiation, and termination signals) is often necessary.

A genomic DNA library is a collection of clones that contain between them the entire genome of an organism. (Reverse transcription of mRNA from a specific tissue or cell population produces a cDNA library that represents the genes undergoing transcription at the point at which the mRNA was extracted.)

Polymerase chain reaction

The *polymerase chain reaction* (PCR) is an alternative to *in vivo* vector-based cloning (Fig. 1.4). It can be performed using limited quantities of DNA, but relies on prior knowledge of the DNA sequence of the fragment to be amplified. Short single-strand oligonucleotide primers (around 20 base pairs in length) that are complementary to sequences flanking the target are generated. Heat denaturation of double-stranded DNA produces single-stranded templates, to which the primers are annealed. Using the template, the primer is extended by a heat-stable DNA polymerase (Taq polymerase) to produce a complementary strand. Repeated cycles (typically up to 35) of heat denaturation and primer annealing generate millions of copies of the target DNA. Variations in PCR product sizes can reveal deletion and insertion mutations. *Real-time PCR* allows the simultaneous detection and quantification of a DNA molecule and selection of mutant DNA. It employs fluorescence reporter molecules, the emission from which increases as the reaction proceeds. These molecules may be dyes that bind to double-stranded DNA, or sequence specific probes that contain a fluorophore and a quencher that are separated during amplification. PCR is used to detect DNA from infectious organisms (human immunodeficiency virus (HIV), methicillin-resistant *Staphylococcus aureus* (MRSA)) and chromosomal translocations associated with malignancies.

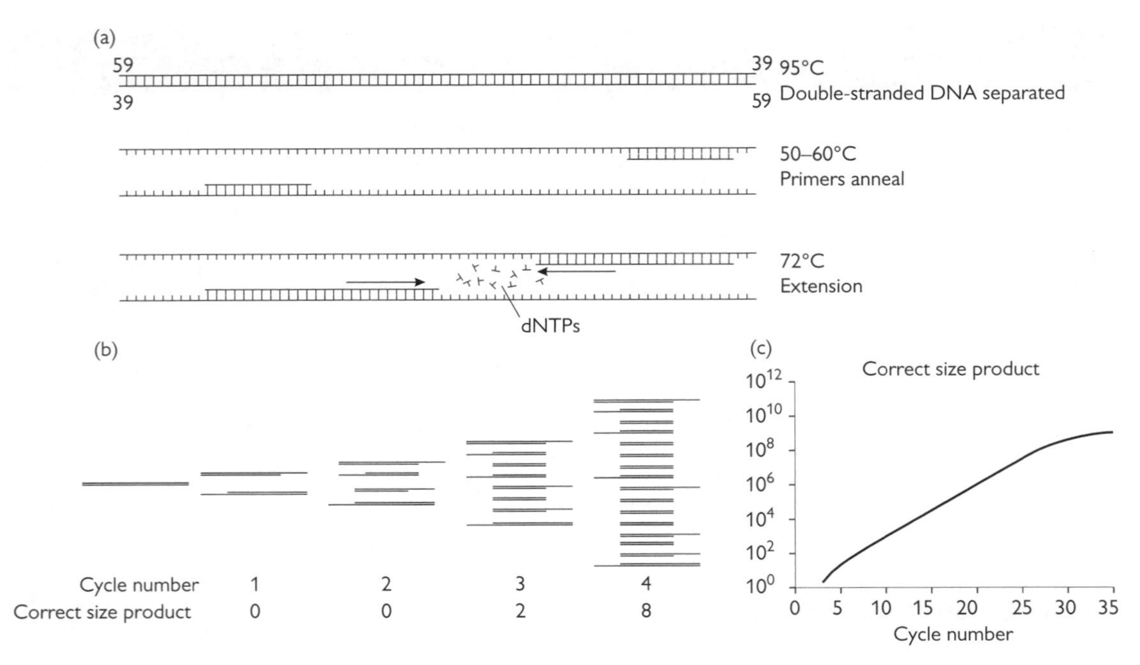

Fig. 1.4 Principles of PCR. (a) The three stages of the PCR cycle. (b) There is exponential amplification of the region of interest, whereas longer PCR products undergo linear amplification. Thus after several cycles the correct sized product predominates. (c) There is a linear region of amplification, followed by non-linear region as reagents are exhausted. Classical PCR is non-quantitative and usually analysed by electrophoresis on an agarose gel and visualization by ethidium bromide staining.

DNA analysis

A variety of techniques have been developed for DNA analysis.

Probe hybridization

This makes use of short single-stranded DNA sequences that are labelled with radioisotope (^{32}P), a chemiluminescent substrate or a fluorescent molecule (for example, fluorescein).

- In *Southern blotting* (developed by Edwin Southern), restriction fragments of DNA are generated by exposure to a restriction endonuclease and separated by electrophoresis (Fig. 1.5, Box 1.3). The fractionated DNA is denatured by alkali to yield single strands, which are transferred ('blotted') onto a nitrocellulose filter. The single stranded ^{32}P-labelled probe for the DNA of interest hybridizes with the complementary sequence on the filter and the binding can be visualized by autoradiography.
- *Northern blotting* employs similar principles to probe mRNA transcripts and, like Western blotting, is named in acknowledgment of Southern's technique.
- *DNA microarray* ('DNA chip') is another technology based on the Southern methodology. Thousands of spots of short nucleotide probes are attached to a slide and hybridization of fluorescently labelled DNA analysed. Microarrays can be used to assess expression of a large number of genes or to screen DNA for specific mutations.

DNA sequencing

This is performed using the di-deoxy-DNA (Sanger) method. A sequence complementary to a single-stranded (denatured) DNA template is synthesized from a primer by DNA polymerase. Di-deoxy-nucleotides, which lack the hydroxyl group through which the phosphodiester bond to the subsequent nucleotide is formed, are included in the reaction mix along with normal nucleotides. When the di-deoxy variant is incorporated into the DNA, its extension is terminated. A population of fragments of differing lengths is generated, which can be separated by electrophoresis. Labelling the di-deoxy-nucleotide with a radioactive or fluorescent label allows identification of the terminal nucleotide in each of the DNA sequences.

Pre-natal screening

Pre-natal screening for genetic diseases can be undertaken through amniocentesis, chorionic villus sampling, magnetic

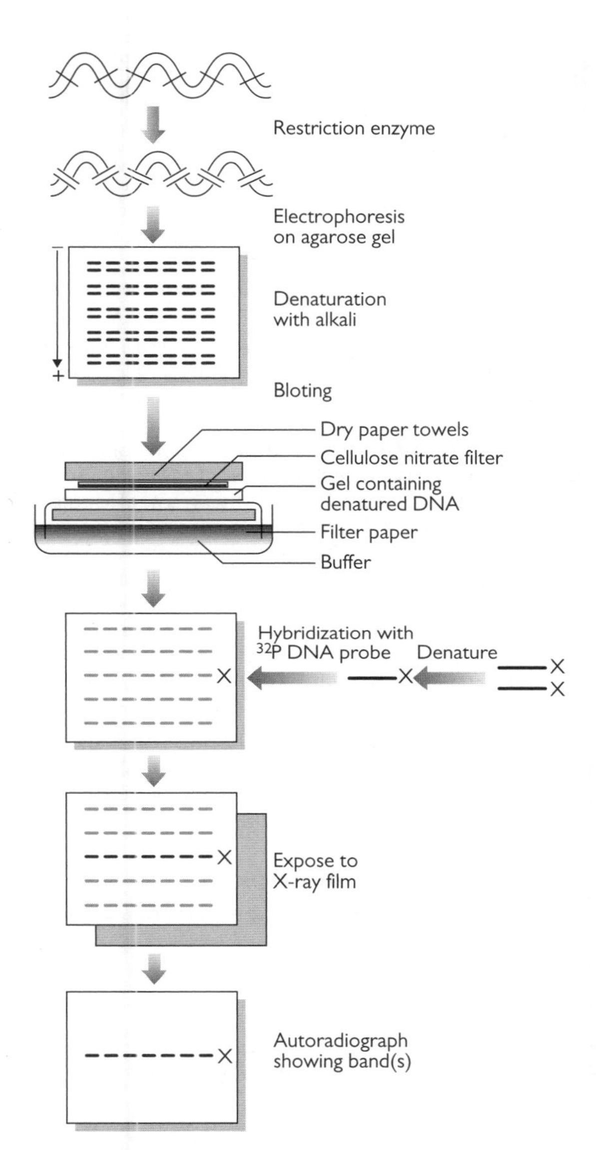

Fig. 1.5 Diagram of the Southern blot technique showing site fractionation of the DNA fragments by gel electrophoresis, denaturation of the double-stranded DNA to become single-stranded, and transfer to a nitrocellulose filter.

This figure was published in *Emery's Elements of Medical Genetics, Eleventh Edition*, Mueller RF and Young ID, Copyright Elsevier 2003.

resonance imaging (MRI), ultrasonography fetoscopy, radiography and by the sampling of fetal blood from the umbilical cord (cordiocentesis) and analysis of maternal serum. For example, neural tube defects can be diagnoses through screening of maternal serum and amniotic fluid for α-fetoprotein (AFP). Reduced levels of AFP and oestriol, in combination with elevated levels of human chorionic gonadotrophin in maternal fluid (the 'triple test') and ultrasonographic observation of nuchal translucency, can identify pregnancies with Down syndrome. Amniocentesis and chorionic villus sampling are also employed to detect cystic fibrosis and thalassemia.

BOX 1.3 DNA ANALYSIS

Restriction fragment length polymorphism (RFLP)

Polymorphism of restriction sites results in variation in the size of restriction fragments. RFLP analysis can be used to detect gene mutations and in linkage studies of genetic disease (in which the tendency for alleles that lie close to each on a chromosome to be inherited together during meiosis is exploited to identify the location of a gene causing a disease phenotype). Fragment length polymorphism can also arise when there are *variable number tandem repeats* (VNTR), where a variable number of identical adjacent sequence patterns results in variations in DNA length between the restriction sites. VNTR analysis can be used for matching identification and inheritance.

Minisatellites

Minisatellites are VNTR of 10–60 nucleotides containing a core sequence of GGGCAGGAXG (where X can be any nucleotide). There are over 1000 microsatellites, which can contain several-hundred tandem repeats, within the human genome; their profile is very polymorphic, giving rise to the 'genetic fingerprint' of an individual. Microsatellites are shorter sequences (short tandem repeat; STR) of 2–4 base pairs repeated up to 100 times, which act as markers of genetic disease.

Single nucleotide polymorphism

Variation in the DNA sequence of a single nucleotide gives rise to a single nucleotide polymorphism (SNP). The majority of SNPs lie in non-coding DNA and, given the redundancy within the genetic code, even those that are found within exons do not necessarily have an impact upon the sequence of the protein encoded by the gene. Most of the millions of SNPs that exist, therefore, have no deleterious effects; they can, however, influence the susceptibility to disease and responses to drugs and toxins. Linkage studies of SNPs are used to map disease loci and assess genes associated with susceptibility to disease.

Post-natal screening

Post-natal screening for thalassemia and sickle cell disease involves electropheretic analysis of haemoglobin. Screening for congenital hypothyroidism is performed by measurements of serum thyroxine and thyroid-stimulating hormone levels. Tay–Sachs disease (hexosaminidase A deficiency) is diagnosed through serum assay tests, while phenylketonuria and galactosaemia can be detected by variants of the Guthrie bacterial inhibition assay. Raised levels of serum immunoreactive trypsin is indicative of cystic fibrosis.

Genetic disease

Genetic disease is the result of abnormalities in genes or chromosomes, which can be heritable or arise during meiosis (see Chapter 2). Chromosome abnormalities include trisomy, monosomy, deletion, inversion and translocation. Diseases can arise from mutations in a single gene (Box 1.1) or be polygenic, the result of the combination of many genes and environmental factors (for example, heart disease).

Single gene disorders

These demonstrate Mendelian inheritance and can be:

- *Autosomal dominant:* an effect is apparent even when a normal gene is present on the corresponding allele of the homologous chromosome. These disorders are inherited when one parent is affected and there is a 50% chance that their offspring will be affected.
- *Autosomal recessive:* an effect is only apparent when the mutation is present in both alleles. These disorders are inherited from unaffected parents (carriers) who both possess one copy of the mutated gene and there is, therefore, a 25% chance that their offspring will be affected.
- *X-linked:* the mutation is in a gene that resides on the X chromosome. X-linked disorders can be dominant or recessive. The chances of the offspring being affected depend upon whether the father or the mother has the mutated gene.
  - *X-linked dominant disorders*—the condition is more common in women; all daughters of an affected father will be affected, whereas sons will not; half of the offspring (male or female) of an affected mother are affected.
  - *X-linked recessive disorders*—the condition is more common in men (homozygous females are rare); all of the female offspring of an affected male will be carriers; half of the male offspring of a female carrier are affected, while half of the female offspring of a female carrier are themselves carriers.
- *Y-linked:* although rare are inevitably passed from father to son.
- *Genetic imprinting:* Genetic disease can also arise from "imprinting", or silencing of a copy of the gene from a particular parent, such that only the other copy of the gene is expressed. Examples of this are the reciprocally inherited Prader-Willi syndrome and Angelman syndrome. Both syndromes are associated with loss of the chromosomal region 15q11-13 (band 11 of the long arm of chromosome 15). This region contains the paternally expressed genes SNRPN and NDN and the maternally expressed gene UBE3A. Paternal inheritance of a deletion of this region is associated with Prader-Willi syndrome (characterized by hypotonia, obesity, and hypogonadism). Maternal inheritance of the same deletion is associated with Angelman syndrome (characterized by epilepsy, tremors, and a smiling facial expression).

In contrast, a polymorphism represents multiple versions of the sequence of a gene within a population, resulting in different phenotypes that are not necessarily deleterious (for example, the ABO blood type antigens).

Common genetic diseases

Table 1.2 summarizes the genetic basis and presentation of commonly examined genetic diseases.

Table 1.2 Examples of genetic diseases

Disease	Gene/Protein	Common mutation	Effect	Clinical presentation
Autosomal dominant				
von Willebrand disease type 1	*VWF*: 12p13.3: von Willebrand factor	Various reported: nonsense mutations, missense mutations, and small deletions (frameshift)	Reduction in blood concentration of VWF	Typically mild presentation. Post-surgical bleeding, bruising, and menorrhagia in some patients
Neurofibromatosis type 1	*NF1*: 17q11.2 neurofibromin 1	Various nonsense mutations leading to production of curtailed neurofibromin protein	Aberrant intracellular Ras signalling due to loss of NF1 tumour suppressor function	Café au lait skin spots, axillary and inguinal freckling, cutaneous neurofibromas, iris Lisch nodules. Central nervous system (CNS) tumours less commonly
Autosomal dominant polycystic kidney disease (PKD)	*PKD-1*: 16p13.3: polycystin-1	Various non-conservative missense mutations	Disrupted intracellular calcium signalling; aberrant renal tubule development; growth of fluid-filled renal cysts	Hypertension, cardiac valve defects, liver cysts, kidney stones, aortic aneurysms, end-stage renal disease

Table 1.2 Examples of genetic diseases (*continued*)

Disease	Gene/Protein	Common mutation	Effect	Clinical presentation
Tuberous sclerosis complex (TSC)	*TSC1*: 9q34: hamartin	Commonly small insertions or deletions	Disrupted function of hamartin-tuberin tumour-suppressor action	Benign tumour growth in brain, kidneys, heart, eyes, lungs, and skin. Seizures, mental retardation, behaviour problems
Gilbert's syndrome	*UGT1A1*: 2q37: bilirubin-UDP-glucuronyltransferase (UGT)	Missense mutation in coding region. Also recessive form caused by promoter mutation	Inability of hepatocytes to process bilirubin	Mild hyperbilirubinaemia, which worsens with stress, dehydration, vigorous exercise and fasting
Achondroplasia	*FGFR3*: 4p16.3: Fibroblast growth factor receptor (FGFR)	Missense point mutation: G380R	Overactive *FGFR3*: disturbance of bone growth	Short stature, particularly short upper arms and legs, apnoea, obesity, recurrent ear infections, kyphosis/lordosis
Huntington's disease	*Htt*: 4p16.3: Huntington (HTT) protein	CAG triplet expansion coding polyglutamine tract 40–50 repeats: adult onset >60 repeats: juvenile onset	HTT protein and cleavage fragments are neurotoxic. Striatal neurodegeneration and progressive global brain atrophy	Reduced motor coordination and subtle disturbance in mood and behaviour. Progressive chorea and psychiatric disturbance
Autosomal recessive				
Phenylketonuria	*Pah*: 12q22: phenylalanine hydroxylase (PAH)	Missense point mutation: R408W	Inability to metabolize dietary phenylalanine due to complete or near complete lack of PAH enzyme function	Toxic build-up of phenylalanine leads to disrupted neurological development, skin abnormalities, and epilepsy and movement disorders
Cystic fibrosis	*CFTR*: 7q31.2: Cystic fibrosis transmembrane conductance regulator (CFTR)	ΔF508: loss of phenylalanine at position 508	Defective apical epithelial chloride channel CFTR protein degraded via cellular quality control mechanisms	Aberrant mucociliary clearance; recurrent respiratory infection; gastrointestinal (GI) and endocrine dysfunction; infertility
Glycogen storage disease type I	*G6PC*: 17q21: glucose-6-phosphatase catalytic subunit SLC37A4: 11q23.3: glucose-6-phosphate transporter	Mainly missense/nonsense mutations	Inability to break down glucose-6-phosphate into glucose, leading to excessive glycogen and fat production for intracellular storage. Build-up damages tissues, especially kidneys and liver	Presents at 3–4 months. Hypoglycaemia, seizures, lactic acidosis, hyperuricaemia, hyperlipidaemia, enlarged liver/kidneys, xanthomas, diarrhoea. Short stature and thin arms/legs
Recessive/dominant forms				
Alpha-1 antitrypsin deficiency	*Serpina1*: 14q32.1: alpha-1 antiproteinase	Various non-conservative missense mutations	Deficient or dysfunctional alpha-1 antiproteinase leading to lung damage due to excessive exposure to neutrophil elastase	Stimulation of immune responses in the lungs and ensuing neutrophil elastase production can lead to early onset emphysema and COPD
Sickle cell anaemia	*Hbb*: 11p15.5: Haemoglobin-beta	Missense point mutation: E6V	Production of abnormal Hb subunits, which accumulate to produce long, rigid complexes, leading to sickling of erythrocytes	Anaemia due to haemolysis of sickle-cells. Vaso-occlusive crisis and splenic sequestration crisis due to reduced deformity of RBCs and aggregation in small vessels

(*continued*)

Table 1.2 Examples of genetic diseases (*continued*)

Disease	Gene/Protein	Common mutation	Effect	Clinical presentation
Trinucleotide repeat				
Fragile X syndrome	5'UTR of *Fmr1*: Xq27.3	CGG triplet expansion extending into Fmr1 promoter. > 200 repeats symptomatic	*Transcriptional silencing of FMR1 protein:* regulator of translation and synaptic plasticity in the CNS	*Males:* moderate–severe mental retardation, characteristic facial features, large testes. *Females:* milder learning disability; 50% penetrant
Myotonic dystrophy	3'UTR of *Dmpk* and promoter of *Dmahp*: 19q13.3	CTG triplet expansion. *50–80 repeats:* asymptomatic. *40–160 repeats:* mild disease. *65–1200 repeats:* adult onset. *500–2500 repeats:* congenital	Broad splicing defects due to transcription factor sequestration by triplet expansion in mRNA	Myotonia, posterior iridescent cataracts, cardiomyopathy/ conduction defects, abnormal glucose tolerance, hypogamma-globulinaemia
Huntington's disease	*As above*			
X-linked recessive				
Ornithine transcarbamylase deficiency	*OTC*: Xq21.1: ornithine transcarbamylase			
Duchenne muscular dystrophy (DMD)	*Dmd* gene: Xp21.2: dystrophin	Large deletions	*Absent protein product:* disrupting coupling of skeletal muscle fibre, cytoskeleton, and basal lamina, leading to structural instability	*Neuromuscular degenerative disorder:* onset at 3–5 years with progression to wheelchair use at around 12 years and eventual respiratory failure
Haemophilia A	*F8*: Xq28: Coagulation Factor VIII	Commonly large inversion. Point mutations and small insertions/deletions reported	Ineffective clotting cascade	Excessive bleeding, difficult to control and achieve haemostasis
Haemophilia B	*F9*: Xq27.1: Coagulation Factor IX	Point mutations and small insertions/ deletions		
X-linked dominant				
Alport syndrome	*COL4A5*: Xq22: Collagen type IV alpha 5 (80% cases)	Mainly missense mutations	Reduces ability of collagen chain to associate with other chains of the same kind. Kidney, inner ear, and eye basement membrane defects leading to scarring	Sensorineural hearing loss in late childhood. Nephritis leading to end stage renal disease. Anterior lenticonus and retinal abnormalities
Fragile X syndrome	*As above*			
Trisomies/monosomies				
Down Syndrome	Trisomy of chromosome 21	Meiotic non-dysjunction event or Robertsonian translocation	Additional copies of genes on chromosome 21	Intellectual disability, hypotonia, cardiac defects, gastroesophageal reflux, underactive thyroid, auditory and visual defects, predisposition to leukaemias

Table 1.2 Examples of genetic diseases (*continued*)

Disease	Gene/Protein	Common mutation	Effect	Clinical presentation
Edwards Syndrome	Trisomy 18	Three copies of chromosome 18. 5% mosaicism, but only some cells affected (disease severity varies accordingly)	Additional copies of genes on chromosome 18 in cells disrupts normal development	Heart and other major organ developmental defects. Microcephaly, small, abnormally shaped mouth and jaw. Clenched fist with overlapping fingers. 5–10% survive beyond 1 year; severe intellectual disability
Patau Syndrome	Trisomy 13	Three copies of chromosome 13	Additional copies of genes on chromosome 13 in cells disrupts normal development	Heart defects and CNS abnormalities; microphthalmia; cleft lip and cleft palate, hypotonia. 5–10% survive beyond 1 year
Cri-du-chat syndrome	Monosomy of the end of short arm of chromosome 5 (5p)	Size of deletion varies, proportional to disease severity	Loss of specific genes in region of 5p deleted leads to disease presentation. *CTNND2* gene specifically implicated in CNS effects	Hypotonia in infancy, low birth weight, microcephaly, intellectual disability, delayed development, hypertelorism, low set ears, rounded face. Increased incidence of heart defects
Klinefelter Syndrome	Trisomy: 47, XXY	Additional copy of X chromosome in cells of affected males	Additional copies genes on the X chromosome disrupt male sexual development, including reduced testosterone production	*In children:* learning disabilities; low testosterone during puberty leads to gynecomastia, reduced body hair, infertility. *Adults:* taller stature and increased risk of breast cancer/systemic lupus erythematosus (SLE)
Turner syndrome	Monosomy of X chromosome in females: 45 X	Missing copy of X chromosome in cells of affected females	Missing genetic material affects pre and post-natal development. Short stature homeobox (*SHOX*) gene loss associated with defects in bone development and growth	Short stature. Ovarian hypofunction or premature ovarian failure. Infertility. Many do not undergo puberty at all. Webbed neck and lymphoedema seen in some patients. Increased incidence of heart defects
Mitochondrial disorders				
MELAS: mitochondrial encephalomyopathy, lactic acidosis, and stroke-like episodes	MT-TL1 in 80% of cases	Commonly A3243G, but various reported	*Defect in mitochondrial tRNA:* $tRNA^{Leu(UUR)}$ leading to disrupted mitochondrial energy metabolism function	*In childhood:* muscle weakness, recurrent headaches, vomiting, and seizures. Stroke-like episodes before 40 years of age leading to hemiparesis, altered consciousness, vision abnormalities, seizures, and migraine. Progressive reduction in motor abilities and dementia. Recurrent lactic acidosis
Kearns–Sayre syndrome	Various mitochondrial genes	Commonly large deletion of ~5000bp, leading to loss of 12 mitochondrial genes	Impaired function at every level of oxidative phosphorylation	Progressive external ophthalmoplegia, ptosis, pigmentary retinopathy. In some patients, cardiac conduction defects, ataxia, raised cerebrospinal fluid (CSF) protein

(*continued*)

Table 1.2 Examples of genetic diseases (*continued*)

Disease	Gene/Protein	Common mutation	Effect	Clinical presentation
Leber's hereditary optic neuropathy	Various mitochondrial genes	Various. Some individuals with certain mutations/deletions are affected, whilst others are not. Manifests more commonly in males than females	Defects in oxidative phosphorylation pathway leads to death of optic nerve cells. The specific effect of this defect on the optic nerve remains unclear	Typical onset in adolescence or early adulthood. Progressive loss of visual acuity/colour vision in both eyes simultaneously or sequentially over a period of weeks or months. Vision loss is profound and permanent

Multiple choice questions

1. Genetic anticipation:

A. Is not seen with Huntingdon's disease.
B. Is characteristic of neurofibromatosis type 2.
C. Results from amplification of triplet repeats within genes.
D. Occurs in cystic fibrosis.
E. Refers to early diagnosis because of improved awareness.

2. Which one of the following statements regarding gene expression is correct?

A. Mutation in the DNA sequence encoding a gene always result in changes to the amino acid sequence of the resulting protein.
B. The majority of cellular RNA is mRNA.
C. The addition of a poly(A) tail targets mRNA for degradation.
D. Introns are not transcribed into mRNA.
E. RNA polymerase II gives rise to protein encoding mRNA.

3. The polymerase chain reaction:

A. Occurs at 45°C.
B. Is of low sensitivity, but high specificity.
C. Produces multiple copies of mRNA.
D. Requires oligonucleotide primers.
E. Cannot be used to detect genetic polymorphisms.

4. Which of the following conditions is not a chromosomal trisomy?

A. Downs syndrome.
B. Turner syndrome.
C. Edwards syndrome.
D. Klinefelter syndrome.
E. Patau syndrome.

5. Which of the following genetic diseases is due to a chromosomal translocation?

A. Chronic myeloid leukaemia (CML).
B. Wolf–Hirschhorn syndrome.
C. Fragile X syndrome.
D. Cri du chat syndrome.
E. Pallister–Killian syndrome.

6. If the prevalence of carrying a ΔF508 carrier in the *CFTR* gene is 1 in 25, what is the probability that a couple without cystic fibrosis will have will have offspring with cystic fibrosis?

A. 1 in 100.
B. 1 in 2500.
C. 1 in 10,000.
D. 1 in 25,000.
E. 1 in 100,000.

7. Which of the following conditions follow a recessive pattern of inheritance?

A. Duchene muscular dystrophy.
B. Alport's syndrome.
C. Adult polycystic kidney disease.
D. von Hippel–Lindau.
E. Acute intermittent porphyria.

8. Which of the following conditions have an X-linked pattern of inheritance?

A. Cystic fibrosis.
B. sickle cell disease.
C. Fabry's disease.
D. Tuberous sclerosis.
E. Retinoblastoma.

9. **All of the following genetic diseases directly involve the kidney except:**

A. Alport's syndrome.
B. Fabry's disease.
C. von Hippel–Lindau.
D. Fanconi anaemia.
E. Turner syndrome.

10. **Genetic imprinting:**

A. Is an inheritance process that follows classical Mendelian inheritance.
B. Occurs such that only imprinted alleles are expressed.
C. Involves an alteration in the genetic sequence of one allele in order to achieve mono-allelic gene expression.
D. Is a mechanism of control of gene expression unique to mammals.
E. Deletion of paternal copies of imprinted genes on chromosome 15 can cause Prader–Willi.

For answers, please see Appendix: Answers to multiple choice questions, page 313.

CHAPTER 2

Cellular, molecular, and membrane biology

Cell structure

The plasma membrane (Fig. 2.1) envelops the cell and comprises a fluid mosaic of proteins embedded in a lipid bilayer. The proteins are present in varying proportions and can be variably glycosylated.

Bipolar phospholipids (for example, phosphatidylcholine and phosphatidylserine) constitute most of the lipid, and possess a charged head group and two uncharged hydrophobic tails. The polar heads face the aqueous extra- and intracellular milieu, while the intramembranous tails can be kinked due to the presence of double bonds. Phospholipids are formed from fatty acids, glycerol, phosphate, and a fourth variable species. Cholesterol dovetails between phospholipids to confer membrane fluidity, which facilitates the lateral diffusion of proteins in the bilayer. An

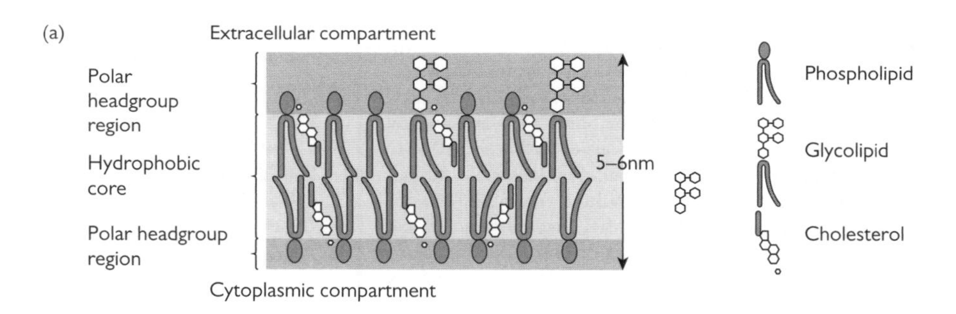

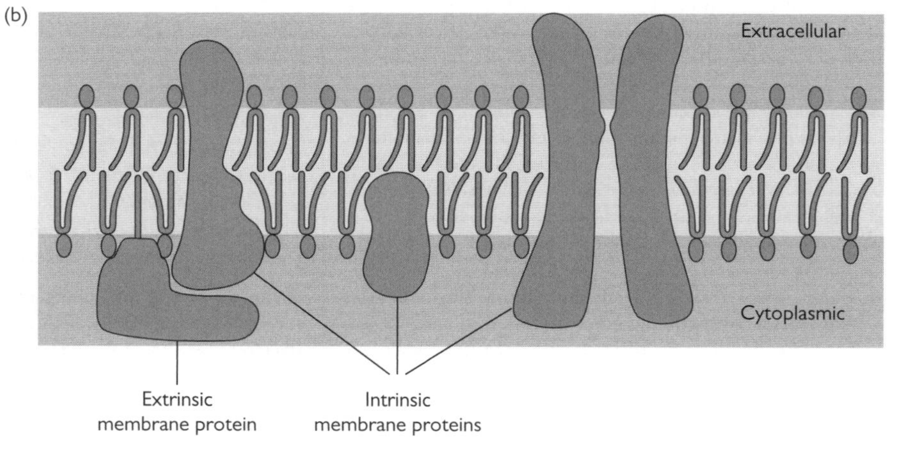

Fig. 2.1 The structure of the plasma membrane: (a) the basic arrangement of the lipid layer; (b) a simplified model showing the arrangement of some of the membrane proteins.

Reproduced from R Wilkins et al., *Oxford Handbook of Medical Sciences, Second Edition*, 2011, Figure 1.28, p. 45, by permission of Oxford University Press.

asymmetric distribution of phospholipids, with greater proportions of phosphatidylserine in the internal membrane leaflet is maintained by a flippase (an ABC protein) and helps to define cell shape and align proteins.

Proteins may be integral or extrinsic. Integral proteins include receptors (coupled to signalling cascades or acting as pores), enzymes, solute transport pathways, and adhesion molecules. Polytopic proteins completely cross the membrane and can possess a single membrane span of around 25 hydrophobic amino acids arranged as an α helix or multiple spans. Monotopic proteins only partially cross the membrane and can be linked to phospholipids by oligosaccharides (glycosylated phosphatidyl inositol or GPI anchors). Proteins may exist as homomers or heteromers and can be assembled with other proteins in platforms of the bilayer called lipid rafts. Extrinsic proteins include cytoskeletal components or G proteins and can form non-covalent bonds with integral proteins.

Organelles

Within the cell, membranes also define a number of intracellular inclusions, or organelles—a distinguishing feature of eukaryotic cells—including the nucleus, mitochondria, the endoplasmic reticulum (ER), Golgi apparatus, lysosomes, and endosomes. 90% of fluid mosaic membrane resides within the cell.

- *The nucleus* possesses a double membrane that envelopes chromosomes and nucleoli (aggregates of protein and nucleic acids, responsible for assembly of ribosomes), and is characterized by pores that facilitate the exchange of macromolecules (nucleotides, mRNA) with the cytoplasm. The two membranes define the perinuclear space and the inner membrane displays a network of scaffold proteins called lamins that maintain shape. There are 22 homologous pairs of chromosomes along with a pair of sex chromosomes, visible when maximally condensed during cell division, but otherwise packaged with proteins as heterochromatin and euchromatin. The less dense euchromatin mostly contains genes under active transcription. In female cells, a darkly stained mass of chromatin—the Barr body—represents the inactive X chromosome.
- *Mitochondria* also possess a double membrane, the inner bilayer of which has many folds, called cristae, to increase its surface area. The space between the membranes is called the intercristal space, while that inside the inner membrane is the matrix space. The four enzymes that perform oxidative phosphorylation reside in the inner membrane.
- *Endoplasmic reticulum* is defined by a single bilayer that forms interconnected tubular structures called cisternae. ER may be rough or smooth depending on whether ribosomes (complexes of RNA and protein that catalyse translation of proteins, and confer a studded appearance) are bound to the ER membrane. RER is found adjacent to the nucleus and its membrane is continuous with the outer membrane of the nucleus. (In muscle cells, smooth ER is called the sarcoplasmic reticulum.) Ribosome association with the ER is dynamic, only occurring when synthesis of proteins destined for secretion or insertion into the plasma membrane gets underway. Secretory proteins are synthesized directly into the lumen of the rough ER, membrane proteins are inserted into the ER membrane.
- *The Golgi apparatus* is defined by a single bilayer arranged as a stack of flattened disc-shaped cisternae; those nearest the nucleus constitute the *cis*-Golgi, while those furthest away are the *trans*-Golgi and are associated with a series of interconnected tubules and vesicles called the trans-Golgi network. Proteins synthesized in the RER are transferred to the Golgi apparatus in vesicles that fuse with the *cis* face. After modification (for example, glycosylation), they exit at the *trans* face in vesicles that fuse with the trans-Golgi network where they are sorted for delivery. Vesicles from the trans-Golgi network fuse to the plasma membrane, releasing their contents to the extracellular surroundings. Proteins synthesized on free ribosomes are released to cytoplasm or enter the nucleus through nuclear pores (Fig. 2.2).
- *Lysosomes* are acidic single bilayer structures containing hydrolase enzymes.
- *Endosomes* are membrane vacuoles containing proteins that have been internalized by receptor-mediated endocytosis to be translocated between the plasma membrane, Golgi apparatus, and lysosomes.
- *Proteasomes* are non-membrane bound organelles that degrade proteins targeted by ubiquitylation.

Cytoskeletal filaments

Cytoskeletal filaments are proteins that contribute to cell shape and maintain cell stability. Three types of filament are found:

- Microfilaments, made of linear polymers of actin, which attach to myosin and confer cell motility.
- Intermediate filaments, α-helical scaffold structures (for example, vimentin) that bear tension.
- Microtubules, hollow tubes of α- and β-tubulins, which can traffic intracellular inclusions.

Arranged as nine triplet sets, microtubules form the centriole; arranged as nine doublet sets surrounding two other microtubules, they form cilia and flagella.

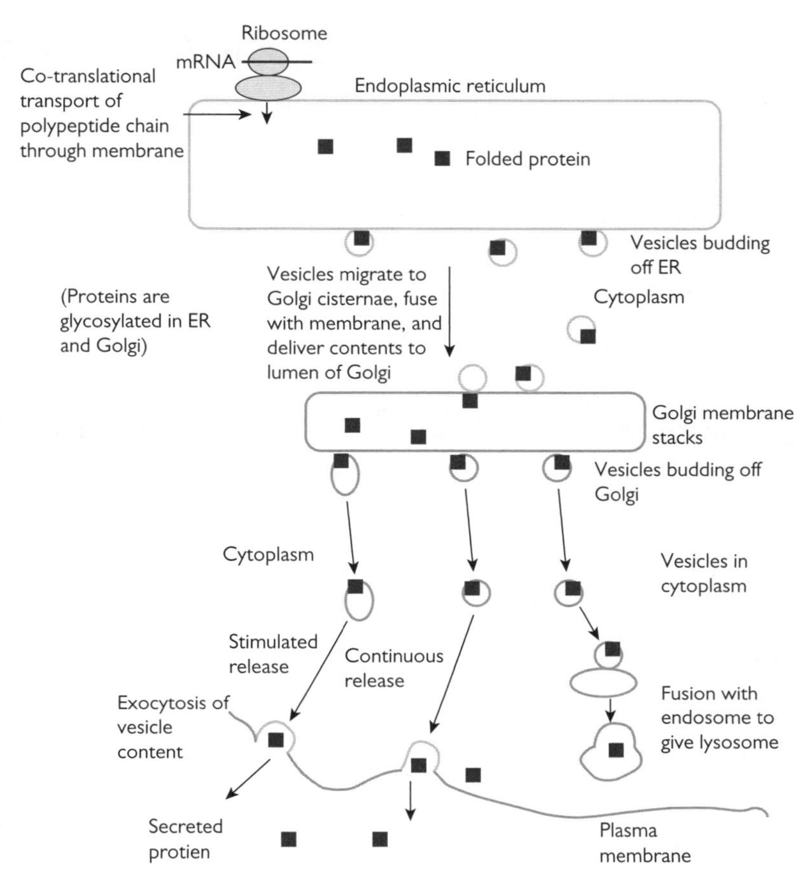

Fig. 2.2 Overview of protein trafficking: how proteins are secreted from cells and how enzymes are delivered to lysosomes.

Reproduced from R Wilkins et al., *Oxford Handbook of Medical Sciences, Second Edition*, 2011, Figure 1.34, p. 67, by permission of Oxford University Press.

Cell division

The cell cycle (Fig. 2.3) is a sequence of events that results in the replication of a cell. Cell division replaces cells lost through apoptosis or maturation (for example, epithelial cells) and augments cell numbers in response to various stimuli (for example, elevated hormone levels, see Box 2.1).

Cell division comprises an interphase, during which there is cell growth and nutrient accumulation followed by replication of DNA, and a *mitosis* (M) phase when cell division occurs. Interphase can be divided into three distinct phases: G1, S, and G2. In the variable length G1 phase (where G denotes gap), biosynthetic activities are elevated to lay the foundations for the subsequent DNA replication in the S (synthesis) phase (Box 2.2). The cycle can be arrested between G1 and S at the G1 restriction checkpoint by modulation of cyclin-dependent kinase activity (for example, by retinoblastoma protein, RB1) if environmental conditions do not favour cell division. By the end of the short-lasting S phase, DNA replication is complete and two duplicates of each chromosome (chromatids) exist, bound together at the centromere by cohesins.

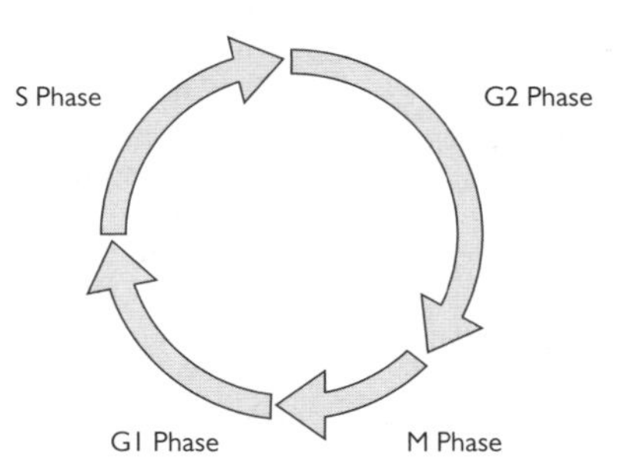

Fig. 2.3 Schematic diagram of the cell cycle.

Reproduced from R Wilkins et al., *Oxford Handbook of Medical Sciences, Second Edition*, 2011, Figure 1.36, p. 71, by permission of Oxford University Press.

BOX 2.1 APOPTOSIS

Apoptosis is genetically regulated (programmed) cell death. It is distinct from necrosis, which is the death of a number of neighbouring cells that arises in response to an external factor such as infection or ischaemia.

Apoptosis is controlled by a variety of signals, which include glucocorticoid hormones, cytokines, toxins, heat, radiation, and hypoxia. Apoptotic cells are characterized by cell shrinkage and rounding, condensation of chromatin, DNA fragmentation, and the appearance of membrane buds (blebs). Cells fragment into vesicles called apoptotic bodies that are phagocytosed by other cells.

A family of enzymes, the caspases, which target intracellular proteins (for example, in the nuclear lamina), typically mediate apoptosis. Pro-apoptotic proteins (for example, p53) induce caspase activity, in part by inducing mitochondrial pores, through which activators are released.

Apoptosis is a physiological, beneficial process for cell turnover, embryonic development, and immunological function. Inappropriate levels of apoptosis are, however, associated with disease. Excess apoptosis is associated with HIV progression and neurodegenerative diseases, while insufficient apoptosis can cause malignancy.

BOX 2.2 REPLICATION OF DNA

Replication of DNA before cell division is a semi-conservative process (Fig. 2.4). DNA helicase unwinds the helical double strand of DNA, assisted by DNA gyrase (a topoisomerase), which relieves the torsional strain that would otherwise occur. A replication fork is created, with leading (3′→5′) and lagging (5′→3′) strand templates that are stabilized by single-stranded DNA binding proteins.
A newly-synthesized 5′→3′ strand is generated from the leading strand by DNA polymerase III. The polymerase extends a short (~10 nucleotides) RNA primer synthesized by RNA primase, pairing A with T and C with G.
The RNA primer is removed by an endonuclease, RNase H, and replaced by DNA synthesized by DNA polymerase I. The orientation of the lagging strand runs counter to the working direction of DNA polymerase, so it must be copied in small sections. Primase generates RNA primers that are lengthened by polymerase III into Okazaki fragments (1000 nucleotides). RNase H and polymerase I again act to replace RNA with DNA. The fragments are united by DNA ligase. Polymerase I also has a proof-reading role—it possesses exonuclease activity, which allows it to remove mismatched nucleotides at the 3′ terminus of the DNA chain before polymerization continues. An endonuclease can cleave damaged DNA chains (for example, following exposure to ultraviolet light), allowing polymerase I to synthesize a new stretch of DNA to replace that excised by its exonuclease activity. The new and original segments are united by DNA ligase.

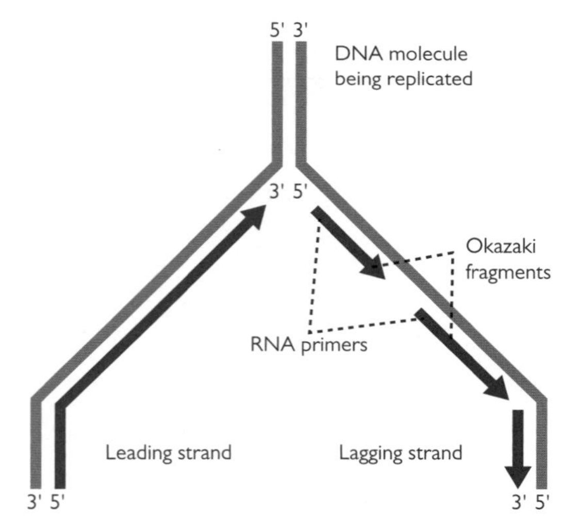

Fig. 2.4 Diagram of a replicative fork. The leading strand is synthesized continuously, while the lagging strand is synthesized as a series of short (Okazaki) fragments.

Reproduced from R Wilkins et al., *Oxford Handbook of Medical Sciences, Second Edition*, 2011, Figure 1.33, p. 65, by permission of Oxford University Press.

The G2 phase

In the G2 phase that follows the S phase, biosynthetic activity is, again, high as the cell synthesizes proteins, such as microtubules, required for the mitotic process that will follow. The G2 checkpoint marks the end of interphase after which cells enter the M phase. The transition is arrested if DNA is damaged or replication is incomplete (by damaging DNA, radiotherapy and some chemotherapeutic agents arrest cell proliferation at this checkpoint).

The M phase

The M phase (comprising around 10% of the cell cycle duration) is divided into four phases on the basis of chromosome morphology and is the part during which nuclear division occurs (Fig. 2.5). Chromatin first condenses to reveal discrete chromosomes (prophase), after which the nuclear membrane disintegrates as the chromosomes align on the equator of the nuclear spindle (metaphase). The spindle is a fusiform structure composed of clusters of microtubules radiating from two centrioles at the poles of the cell. Centromeres attach to the microtubules at kinetochores with the mitotic spindle checkpoint ensuring that all chromosomes are attached. Once the checkpoint is passed, cohesins uniting chromatids are cleaved to liberate separate

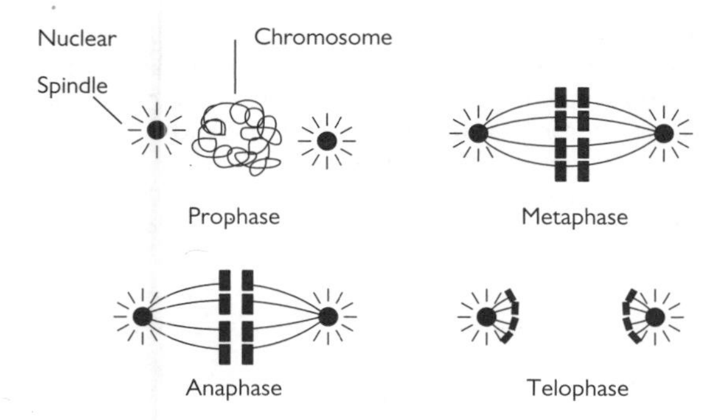

Fig. 2.5 Diagrams of the subprocess within the M (mitotic) phase of the cell cycle.

Reproduced from R Wilkins et al., *Oxford Handbook of Medical Sciences, Second Edition*, 2011, Figure 1.37, p. 71, by permission of Oxford University Press.

chromosomes that are drawn towards the centrioles by microtubule rearrangement (anaphase). Chromosomes now form tight clusters at the cell poles, the nuclear membrane is reformed and chromosome condensation is reversed to yield chromatin (telophase). Cytokinesis follows, in which the cell membrane is constricted to form a cleavage furrow by a contractile ring of cytoskeletal filaments. The ring progressively constricts until a residual midbody is formed, which is then cleaved to produce two separate diploid daughter cells. Some chemotherapeutic agents act by destabilizing microtubules of the nuclear spindle.

Cells can exit the cell cycle from the G_1 phase and enter the G_0 (resting) phase. Quiescent cells may remain in the G_0 phase for variable periods of time before re-entering the G_1 phase; neurons persist in the G_0 phase, although re-entry and failure to pass the G_2 checkpoint may contribute to Alzheimer's disease. Senescent cells permanently enter the G_0 phase. Growth factors—endocrine, paracrine, or autocrine mediators—bind to membrane receptors and initiate intracellular signalling cascades that activate transcription regulation factors. Transcription of cyclins and cyclin-dependent kinases, which regulate the transitions out of gap (G) phases, ensues. Anti-VEGF (vascular endothelial growth factor) therapies inhibit the proliferation of blood vessels in the retina causing macular degeneration, while recombinant granulocyte colony-stimulating factor (G-CStF) and granulocyte macrophage colony-stimulating factor (GM-CStF) therapies are used in the treatment of acute myeloid leukaemia and aplastic anaemia. Elevated levels insulin-like growth factor (IGF-1) provide a reliable diagnostic test for acromegaly.

In *meiosis*, cell division of diploid cells results in four genetically distinct haploid cells (rather than two identical diploid cells as occurs in mitosis), thereby ensuring that genetic diversity is achieved (Fig. 2.6). DNA is first replicated to produce paired chromatids, joined at the centromere.

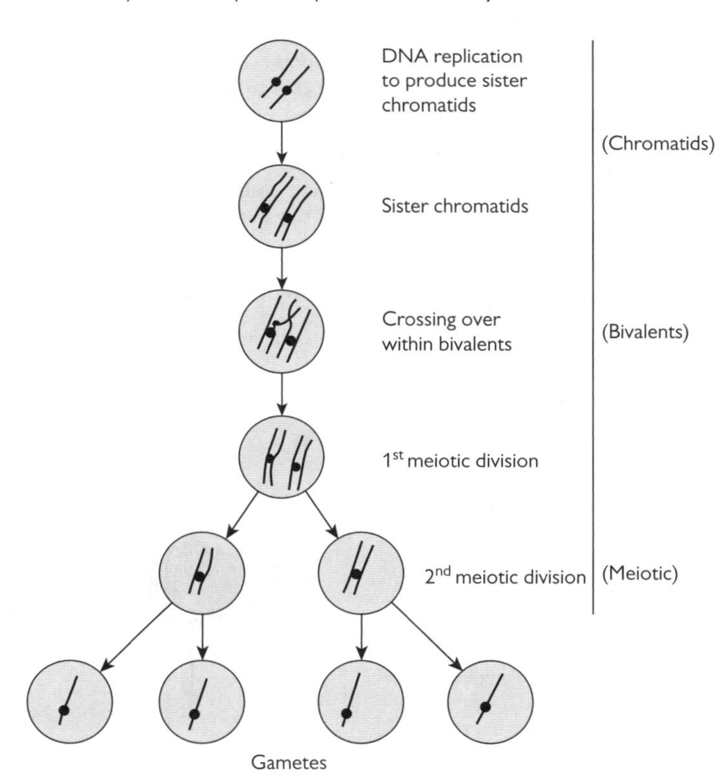

Fig. 2.6 The process of genetic recombination and segregation during meiosis.

Reproduced from R Wilkins et al., *Oxford Handbook of Medical Sciences, Second Edition*, 2011, Figure 1.38, p. 77, by permission of Oxford University Press.

The maternal and paternal homologues then unite to form bivalents and there is genetic recombination as crossing over of segments of the chromosomes occurs. Bivalents align at the mitotic spindle and cell division (meiosis I) results in two daughter cells, containing a haploid number of chromosomes (each of which is a chromatid pair). A second round of cell division (meiosis II) segregates each chromatid into a separate cell: four haploid gametes result. Failure to separate bivalents or chromatids during the first and second divisions (non-disjunction) results in gametes with two copies of a chromosome and gametes devoid of the chromosome (aneuploidy). Fertilization of a diploid gamete results in trisomy (for example, Down's syndrome); fertilization of the gamete lacking the chromosome results in monosomy.

Ions and organic solutes

Ions and organic solutes dissolved in water account for 70% of cytosolic volume, with macromolecules making up the remainder. The cytosol is markedly different in composition from the extracellular fluid, notably in terms of the distribution of Na^+, K^+ and Cl^- ions (Table 2.1).

The plasma membrane separates the two compartments and maintains these differences in composition. Small, non-polar species (for example, O_2) can diffuse passively across the lipid bilayer. Membrane proteins allow the passage of other solutes—the activity of these proteins dictates intracellular composition.

Ions can diffuse passively down electrochemical gradients across the membrane through water-filled protein pores. These *channels*, which can be selective for the ions that they convey, can be constitutively permeable (leak channels) or gated by membrane potential changes, ligand-binding (directly or to an associated G-protein linked receptor) and mechanical deformation. In most cells, aquaporin channels render the plasma membrane highly permeable to water, such that osmotic gradients cannot be sustained.

In addition to channels, a number of *carrier proteins* mediate trans-membrane fluxes of ions and other solutes (Fig. 2.7). Carriers bind their substrate and undergo a conformation change to deliver it to the opposite side of the plasma membrane. Carrier-mediated transport is consequently slower and can saturate. During each cycle of conformation change, carriers may transport one species (uniport) or transport more than one species in the same direction (symport) or in opposite directions (antiport).

Carrier-mediated transport

Carrier-mediated transport may be passive or active. In the case of *passive transport* (for example, glucose transport by GLUT), substrates move down gradients

Table 2.1 Composition of extracellular and intracellular fluids

	Extracellular fluid	Intracellular fluid
Osmolarity	290 mOsm	290 mOsm
pH	7.35–7.45	7.1
$[Na^+]$	135–145 mM	5–15 mM
$[K^+]$	3.5–5 mM	120 mM
Ca^{2+}	2.12–2.62 mM	1–2 mM (100 nM free)
Cl^-	95–115 mM	20–50 mM
HCO_3^-	22–26 mM	15 mM

Corrected $[Ca^{2+}]$, mM = measured $[Ca^{2+}]$, mM + [(40 − [albumin, g l^{-1}]) × 0.02].

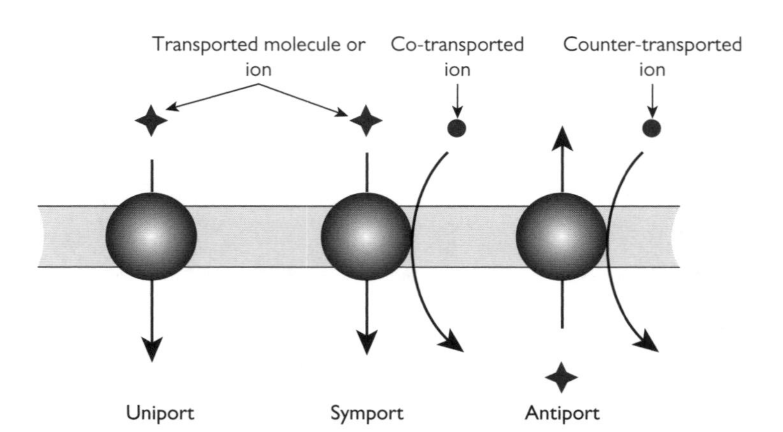

Fig. 2.7 The main types of carrier proteins employed by mammalian cells.

Reproduced from R Wilkins et al., *Oxford Handbook of Medical Sciences, Second Edition*, 2011, Figure 1.38, p. 77, by permission of Oxford University Press.

across the membrane until equilibrium is achieved. (For uncharged solutes, equilibrium represents equalization of concentrations; however, for charged solutes, the equilibrium distribution is influenced both by concentration and membrane potential.)

In the case of *active transport*, substrates are accumulated on one side of the membrane at levels above the equilibrium distribution. The conformational changes by which solutes are moved against their electrochemical gradients are energized by ATP hydrolysis, either directly (primary active transport, for example, the Na^+, K^+-ATPase) or indirectly, using a gradient established by a primary process (secondary active transport, for example, Na^+-glucose cotransport by SGLT). Primary active transport proteins are also found on membranes of intracellular inclusions (for example, Ca^{2+}-ATPase in ER and mitochondria, and H^+-ATPase of lysosomes).

Distribution of Na^+ and K^+ ions

The most striking difference between the cytosol and its surroundings is the distribution of Na^+ and K^+ ions, maintained by the Na^+, K^+-ATPase. Diffusion of ions through leak channels down electrochemical gradients established by the ATPase establishes the resting membrane potential, while the opening of gated channels alters Na^+ and K^+ fluxes, and is the basis of electrical excitability in nerve and muscle. The gradients are also exploited to energize secondary active transport. The cytosolic level of Cl^- ions varies between cell types, although it is always lower than that of K^+. Cl^- ion uptake by Na^+-driven active processes is opposed by passive efflux through channels. Although positively charged ions outnumber negatively charged ones, the high levels of negatively charged macromolecules inside the cell ensures that, as is the case in the extracellular fluid, there is bulk electroneutrality in the cytosol.

Ca^{2+} levels

Ca^{2+} levels are kept low in cells by sequestration in intracellular organelles by Ca^{2+}-ATPases and extrusion across the plasma membrane by ATPases and by a secondary active transporter, Na^+–Ca^{2+} exchange. Although Ca^{2+} is toxic to cells, the low baseline level permits its use as an intracellular messenger when it is mobilized from intracellular stores, such as the ER.

H^+ ions

H^+ ions are highly reactive with proteins, eliciting conformational changes that alter their function. Cell metabolism and inward leak of H^+ ions attracted by the negative inside membrane potential, subjects cells to constant acid loading. Cytosolic pH is maintained close to neutrality by the extrusion of H^+ ions by ATPases and the secondary active transporter Na^+–H^+ exchanger, or by influx of HCO_3^- on other carriers.

Osmolyte content

Changes in intracellular osmolyte content, such as might be associated with metabolic activity or uptake of nutrients, causes water to move by osmosis through aquaporins, eliciting changes in cytosolic volume. Cells constrain these changes by opening channels and altering the activity of carriers so as to lose or gain solutes and hence water.

Cell signalling

Cells are exposed to a diverse array of autocrine, endocrine, neurocrine, and paracrine chemical mediators, which can be peptides, steroids, nucleotides, and gases that bind membrane or cytosolic receptors to modulate cellular function (Fig. 2.8).

On binding, the mediator (or ligand) induces a conformational change in the binding protein. For ionotropic receptors (for example, the nicotinic acetylcholine (Ach) receptor), ligand binding induces the opening of a channel pathway within the protein that conveys cations across the plasma membrane.

Catalytic receptors

These are either enzymes themselves or are associated with enzyme complexes. They are activated upon ligand (often growth factor) binding, and phosphorylate proteins to alter their conformation and modulate their function. (Phosphorylation is reversed by phosphatase activity.) Receptor occupancy can induce serine-threonine kinase, tyrosine kinase activity, or guanylyl cyclase activity. Guanylyl cyclase converts GTP to cGMP, which in turn activates the serine-threonine kinase protein kinase G (guanylyl cyclase also exists as a soluble, cytosolic form that can be directly activated by binding of ligands such as NO.) Kinase activity initiated by catalytic receptors often leads to phosphorylation cascades (for example, tyrosine kinases phosphorylate MAP kinases, which then phosphorylate transcription factors).

G-protein coupled receptors

These are linked to heterotrimeric ($\alpha\beta\gamma$ subunit) complexes called guanosine-5′-triphosphate (GTP) -binding proteins, that split when GTP binds following a conformational change induced by receptor occupancy (Fig. 2.9). The trimer is reformed when GTP hydrolysis occurs after the ligand has dissociated from the receptor. α subunit association can subsequently stimulate (G_s, G_q) or inhibit (G_i) the activity of enzymes that generate intracellular second messengers.

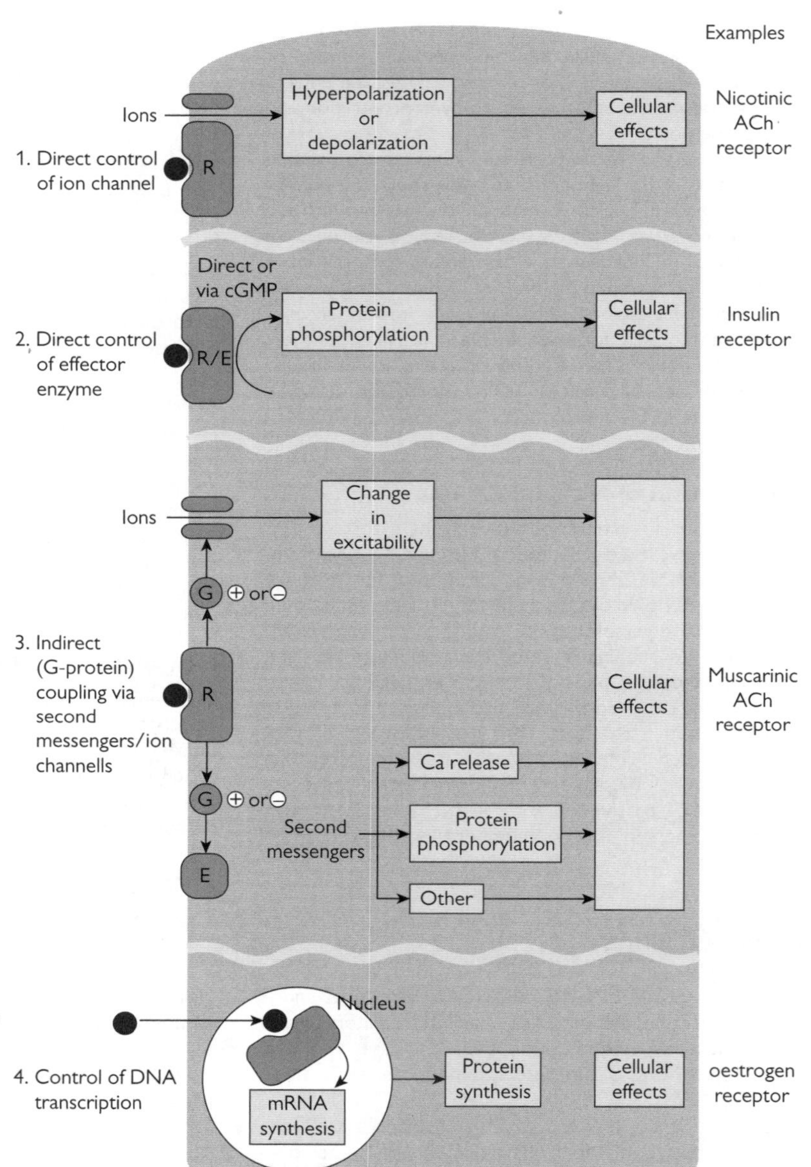

Fig. 2.8 The principal ways in which chemical signals affect their target cells. Examples of each type of coupling are shown. (R = receptor; E = enzyme; G = G-protein; + indicates increased activity; – indicates decreased activity.)

- *Adenylyl cyclase* converts ATP to cAMP, which in turn activates the serine-threonine kinase protein kinase A. Phosphorylation of target proteins to alter their conformation and, hence, function ensues. Exemplified by noradrenaline occupancy of β-adrenoreceptors in the heart to elicit positive inotropic actions.
- *Phospholipase C* converts membrane phosphatidyl inositol to IP3 and diacyl-glycerol (DAG). IP_3 liberates Ca^{2+} from the ER, by binding to an ionotropic receptor. Ca^{2+} binds to transduction proteins such as calmodulin to activate serine-threonine kinases. DAG remains in the membrane and also activates protein kinase C. It is exemplified by angiotensin II occupancy of AT_1 receptors to activate myosin light chain kinase and cause smooth muscle contraction.
- *Phospholipase A_2* converts membrane phospholipids to arachidonic acid, a precursor for the eicosanoids that

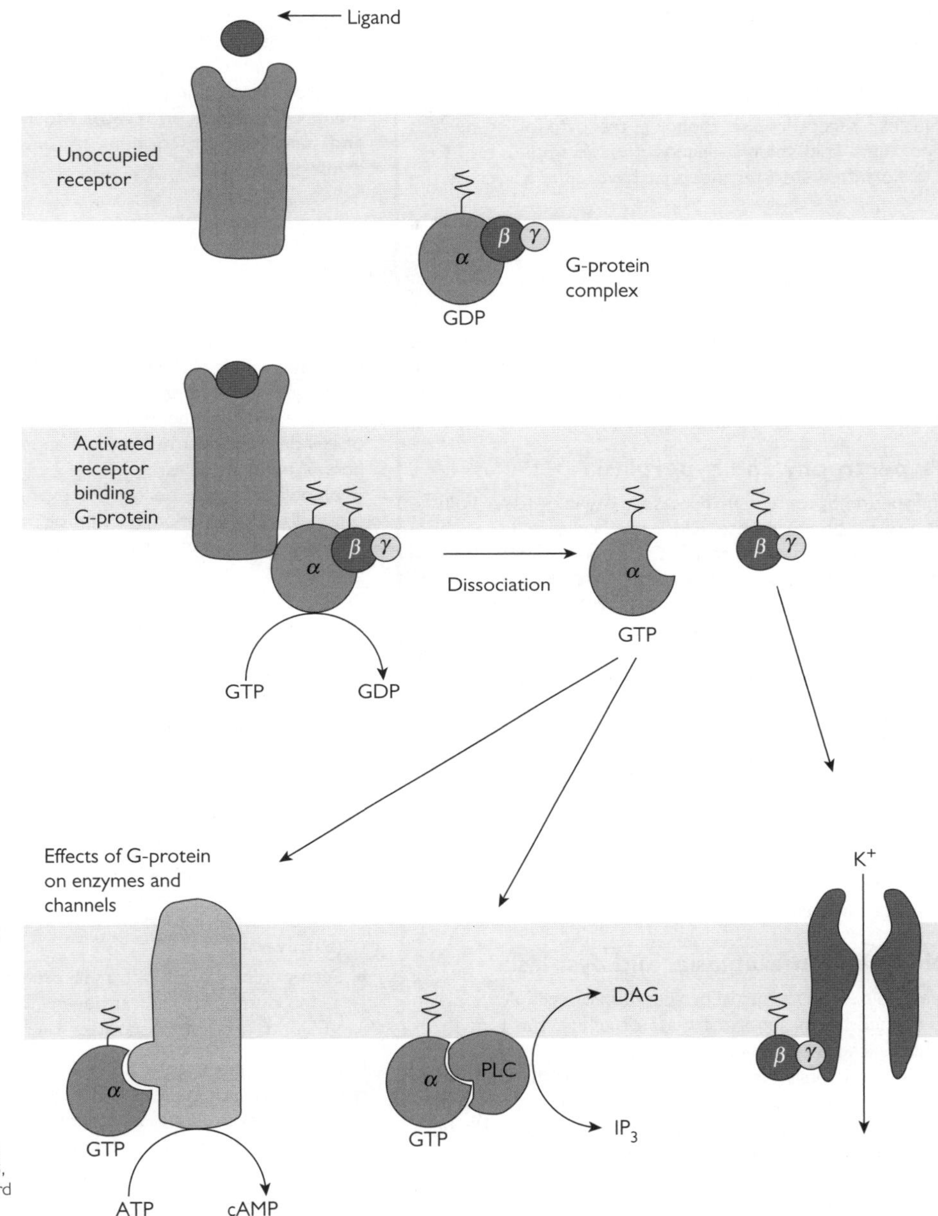

Fig. 2.9
Receptor activation of heterotrimeric G-proteins leads to activation of enzymes and ion channels.

Reproduced from R Wilkins et al., *Oxford Handbook of Medical Sciences, Second Edition*, 2011, Figure 1.31, p. 53, by permission of Oxford University Press.

inter alia mediate inflammatory responses and act as messengers in the central nervous system. Cycloxygenase generates prostanoids (prostaglandins, prostacyclins, thromboxanes); 5-lypoxygenase generates leukotrienes. Exemplified by serotonin occupancy of 5-HT2 receptors to modulate neurotransmitter release.

G proteins can also couple directly to ion channels (for example, β-adrenoreceptor gating of L-type Ca^{2+} channels in the heart is mediated by direct interaction of the Gα subunit).

Ras family

The Ras family is a collection of small G proteins, similar in structure to the α subunit, which coordinate kinase cascades between the cell membrane and nucleus to regulate cell growth. Mutations in *ras* create oncogenes that can cause constitutive activation of Ras and malignant transformation of the cell.

Nuclear receptors

Nuclear receptors are found in the cytosol or nucleus and bind lipid-soluble ligands (for example, the steroid hormone aldosterone) that have diffused across the plasma or nuclear membrane. Receptors in the cytosol are translocated to the nucleus when chaperone heat shock proteins dissociate upon ligand binding. In the nucleus, receptor–ligand complexes bind hormone response elements (sequences of DNA within a gene promoter) and act as transcription factors to regulate gene transcription.

Cell growth

Cell growth is a term that is typically employed to describe an increase in organ or tissue volume that arises from an increase in the number of constituent cells, although an increase in individual cell size can also occur.

Hypertrophy and hyperplasia

In *hypertrophy* there is an increase in organ or tissue volume as a result of an increase in individual cell size, usually arising from increased demands. Common examples include skeletal muscle hypertrophy in response to strength training and cardiac ventricular hypertrophy in response to aortic valve stenosis. In contrast, *hyperplasia* represents an increase in organ or tissue volume that results from increased numbers of cells and is a physiological response to an altered stimulus. Examples include hyperplasia of the adrenal cortex in Cushing's disease (elevated ACTH), benign prostatic hyperplasia (ill-defined cause) and skin callouses (skin thickening arising from keratinocyte accumulation secondary to repeated friction or pressure). Hypertrophy and hyperplasia can occur in combination (for example, hormone-induced changes in the uterus during pregnancy) and can lead to obstruction of adjacent tissues or infarction.

Neoplasia, metaplasia, and dysplasia

Neoplasia is the abnormal proliferation of cells. A neoplasm is defined as an abnormal mass of tissue, the growth of which exceeds and is uncoordinated with that of the normal tissues, and persists in the same excessive manner after cessation of the stimulus that evoked the change. Neoplasia is often preceded by metaplasia or dysplasia (although these do not necessarily always result in neoplasia). In *metaplasia*, there is the reversible transformation of one differentiated cell type to another in response to environmental stress. Examples include the replacement of cuboidal columnar epithelial cells with squamous epithelial cells in the airways of smokers and the replacement of squamous epithelial cells with columnar epithelial cells in the oesophagus with excess acid reflux (Barrett's oesophagus). In *dysplasia*, there is an abnormality of development with high numbers of immature cells that are variable in size, irregularly shaped, and excessively pigmented. There is also a very high degree of cell division, illustrated by the appearance of large numbers of mitotic bodies.

Neoplasia can be benign (for example, uterine fibroids), pre-malignant (carcinoma *in situ*) or malignant (invasive carcinoma). *Carcinoma* in situ describes a pronounced (high grade) dysplasia in which cells have not penetrated the basement membrane to invade surrounding tissues. In *malignant carcinoma*, cells have invaded surrounding tissues and can migrate to distant sites in the body (commonly bone, brain, liver and lung) through lymphatic vessels, the vasculature and body cavities.

This *metastasis* requires a number of cellular activities, including:

- Altered expression of cell adhesion molecules to allow detachment from neighbouring cells.
- Secretion of enzymes (collagenases, matrix metalloproteinases) and acquisition of cell motility to facilitate invasion into surrounding tissues, lymphatic and blood vessels (intravasation) and the destination tissue (extravasation).
- Secretion of growth factors to promote cell proliferation at the destination and angiogenic factors (for example, VEGF) to promote vascularization of the tumour.

Mutations in genes that control the cell cycle are associated with neoplasia. Examples include a gain or function mutation in the oncogene *RAS* (*RAS* mutations are found in about 25% of human tumours) and deletion mutations in the tumour suppressor genes *RB1* and *TP53*. Failure of DNA repair mechanisms produces a replication error (mutator) phenotype also leads to neoplasia (for example, deficiency of the DNA mismatch repair proteins MSH1 and 2). The genes associated with neoplasia that are commonly examined are summarized in Table 2.2.

Table 2.2 Genes associated with cancer

Gene	Function	Associated cancer
Oncogenes		
BRAF	Serine-threonine kinase signalling pathway	Colorectal; lung adenocarcinoma; melanoma
HER2	Epidermal growth factor receptor	Breast
MYC	Transcription factor	Breast; colorectal; melanoma; prostate
RAS	MAP/ERK signalling pathway	Pancreatic; colon; lung adenocarcinoma; thyroid
VEGF	Angiogenesis	Metastatic breast, colorectal cancer
Tumour suppressor genes ('Gatekeeper' genes)		
APC	Cell attachment and signalling	Colorectal; medulloblastoma
ATM	Cell cycle arrest, apoptosis	Breast; leukaemia; lymphoma
RB	Cell cycle arrest	Retinoblastoma; cervical
TP53	Cell cycle arrest, apoptosis	Bladder; breast; lung
VHL	Mitosis, angiogenesis	Kidney
'Caretaker' genes		
BRCA1, 2	DNA mismatch repair	Breast
MLH1, MSH1, 2	DNA break, mismatch repair	Colorectal; uterus
XPA	Nucleotide excision	Lung, skin

Multiple choice questions

1. Which of the following is a tumour suppressor gene?

A. *VEGF.*
B. *RET.*
C. *RAS.*
D. *BCR-Abl (Philadelphia translocation)*_
E. *VHL.*

2. Concerning the plasma membrane, which of the following statement is incorrect?

A. The plasma membrane contains a fluid mosaic of proteins in a lipid bilayer.
B. Phospholipids contain a charged tail and hydrophobic head.
C. The asymmetric distribution of phospholipids between the cytosolic and extracellular face is maintained by an enzyme called 'flippase'.
D. Carbon dioxide can diffuse readily across the plasma membrane.
E. Polytopic proteins completely cross the membrane.

3. Which of the following is a non-membrane bound organelle, which degrades proteins targeted by ubiquitylation?

A. Endosomes.
B. Lysosomes.
C. Proteasomes.
D. Endoplasmic reticulum.
E. Golgi apparatus.

4. During which phase of the cell cycle does DNA replication occur?

A. G0.
B. G1.
C. S.
D. G2.
E. M.

5. Which of the following enzymes has a 'proofreading' role to remove unmatched nucleotides during DNA replication?

A. RNA primase.
B. DNA ligase.
C. DNA helicase.
D. DNA gyrase.
E. DNA polymerase 1.

6. A 40-year-old woman with a history of depression and recurrent kidney stones has the following blood results: haemoglobin (Hb) = 13 g/dL, white cell count (WCC) = 12 × 109/L, calcium (uncorrected) = 2.60 mmol/L, albumin = 30 g/L, urea = 15 mmol/L, creatinine = 120 µmol/L. The most likely type of kidney stones are:

A. Uric acid stones.
B. Cysteine stones.
C. Struvite stones.
D. Calcium oxalate stones.
E. Cholesterol stones.

7. Which of the following hormones binds to receptors that are ligand gated ion channels?

A. Acetylcholine.
B. Norepinephrine.
C. Histamine.
D. Dopamine.
E. Nitric oxide.

8. Lipid synthesis mainly occurs in which organelle?

A. Rough endoplasmic reticulum.
B. Smooth endoplasmic reticulum.
C. Sarcoplasmic reticulum.
D. Lysosomes.
E. Proteosomes.

9. A physiological increase in organ size as a result of an increase in cell number is known as:

A. Neoplasia.
B. Metaplasia.
C. Dysplasia.
D. Hyperplasia.
E. Hypertrophy.

10. Genetically regulated cell death is known as:

A. Apoptosis.
B. Meiosis.
C. Necrosis.
D. Auxotophy.
E. Metaplasia.

For answers, please see Appendix: Answers to multiple choice questions, page 313.

CHAPTER 3

Biochemistry and metabolism

General principles

'Biochemistry is the science concerned with the various molecules that occur in living cells and organisms and with their chemical reactions. Anything more than a superficial comprehension of life—in all its diverse manifestations—demands a knowledge of biochemistry' (definition from *Harper's Biochemistry* 25th edn). Despite the overwhelming temptation and importance of biochemistry in all processes essential to life, the aim of this chapter is not to turn you into a biochemist, but to provide you with an overview and explanatory expansions, where relevant, into subjects often featured in the MRCP exam.

In its considerable extent, the subject of Biochemistry can easily lapse into complicated metabolic pathways, but outside a few medical specialities, including Chemical Pathology, these are less relevant in everyday medical knowledge and will therefore be generally omitted in detail, unless essential. A working understanding of biochemical processes can, however, provide a useful and frequently employed insight into physiology, pathology, and therapeutic interventions, and hopefully the almost ubiquitous clinical relevance of this subject can be demonstrated within this chapter.

The staple dietary components of any particular organism are a major factor in deciding the activity of various metabolic pathways necessary to extract usable energy from food. In the case of ruminants, the main dietary component of cellulose is processed into short chain simple fatty acids, such as ethanoic acid (2 carbon atoms), propanoic acid (3C), and butanoic acid (4C) with alternative metabolic pathways seeking to efficiently extract maximum energy from these available materials. In humans, three main food groups are involved—protein is digested to amino acids, fat to fatty acids and glycerol, and carbohydrate to glucose and other simple sugars, dependent on composition. Therefore, the processes and integration of metabolism revolve around these main substrates. Acetyl residues in the form of acetyl CoA, a 2-carbon ester of CoA containing pantothenic acid (vitamin B5), are the common end product in carbohydrate, fat, and protein metabolism. The linking of these three pathways by production of a common end-product allows integration of several different energy sources to provide an uninterrupted supply during a wide variety of activities and situations.

The basic processes occurring in the body can be broadly divided into *catabolic* reactions, where energy is released from a molecule during degradation, often involving the oxidation of fuel molecules, and *anabolic* reactions ultimately leading to the synthesis of new molecules. Metabolism can be defined as the combination of these two processes. The basic format of a biochemical reaction involves the conversion of substance A to substance B, either generating or requiring energy, and potentially other substances, such as cofactors, electron carriers, vitamins, etc. These reactions generally occur at a rate too slow to support life unless they are accelerated/catalysed by the action of a protein known as an enzyme (see Fig. 3.1).

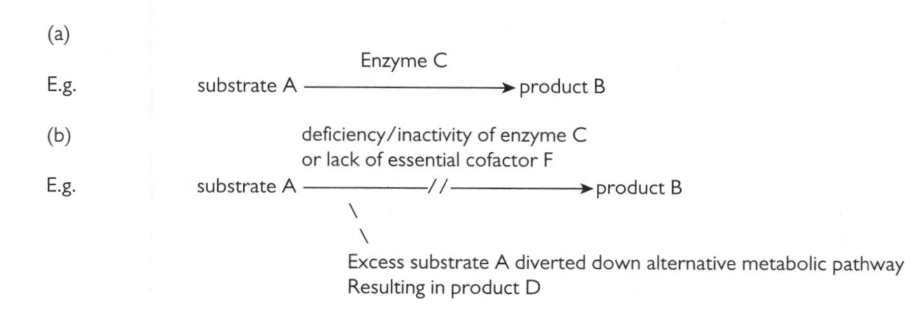

Fig. 3.1 (a) Basic enzymatic reaction; (b) Inborn error of metabolism affecting enzyme C.

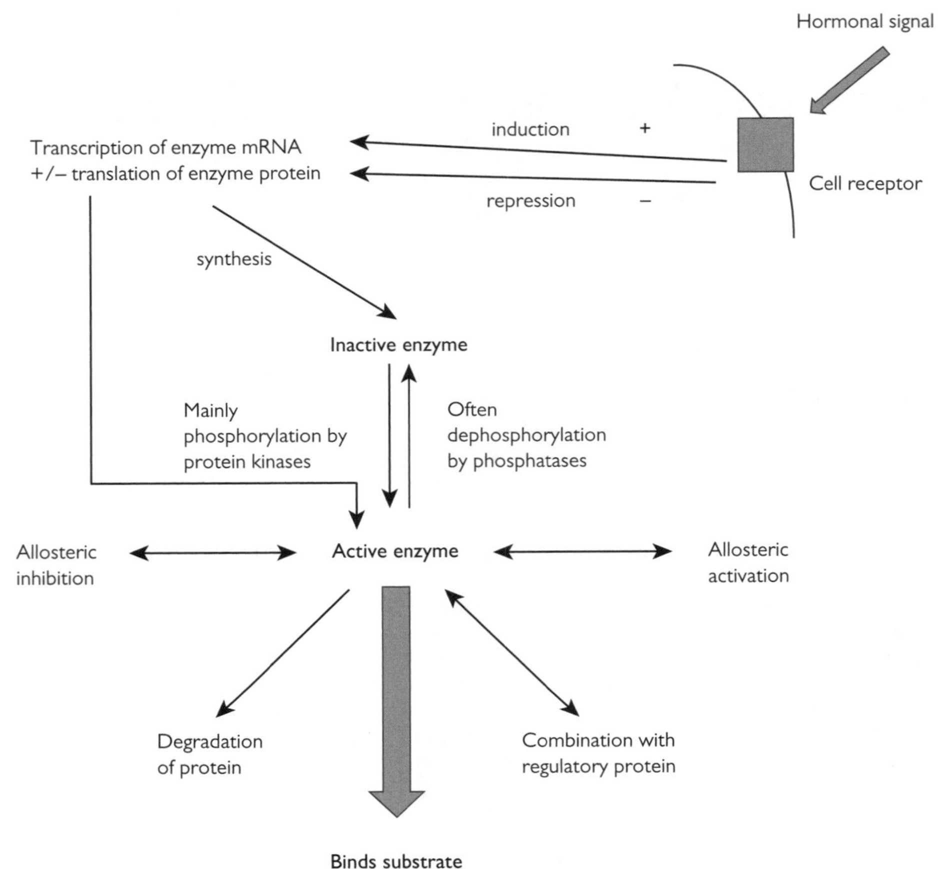

Fig. 3.2 Regulation of enzyme activity.

The human body's health, growth, and development is fundamentally hinged on the action of thousands of enzymes, without which important processes would fail, resulting in an accumulation of substrate A (which may then be converted to an alternative harmful product D) and a deficiency of product B (which may be also be essential for normal cell function). The speed of the catalytic process may also be slowed significantly by lack of an essential cofactor or vitamin required for the successful conversion process, despite having all the essential substrates, enzyme, and energy available.

Many pathological conditions can be defined by an abnormality in the speed, efficiency, or timing of a fundamental reaction, or by the abnormal conversion of excess substrates produced by the alterations described previously.

Fig. 3.2 summarizes methods by which enzyme activity can be regulated.

Clinical biochemistry pathology examples

- *Enzyme malfunction:* cystathionine beta-synthase is the most common enzyme affected in the clinical syndrome of homocystinuria. Children with this autosomal recessive condition appear healthy at birth, but progressive symptoms occur including failure to thrive, developmental delay, and visual problems, which often prompt diagnosis. Additional clinical symptoms and signs include chest deformities, some signs of Marfan's syndrome including long limbs, arachnodactyly, tall, thin build and increased risk of thrombosis. Lack of function of this enzyme prevents conversion of methionine to cysteine (gene locus 21q22), allowing accumulation of homocysteine and methionine in tissues that interferes with collagen cross linkage.
- *Lack of substrate or cofactor:* 25–50% of patients with homocystinuria typically have a milder form, responsive to large doses of pyridoxine (vitamin B6); pyridoxine is the essential cofactor for cystathionine beta synthase action. This clinical form is thought to result from reduced enzyme activity, but retained response to the cofactor activation.
- *Conversion of excess substrate:* in alkaptonuria due to a deficiency of homogentisic acid oxidase the substrate homogentisic acid builds up, and is oxidized and polymerized to the pigmented product alkapton in cartilage. This process is known as ochronosis, and results in visible darkening of ears and often arthritis in later life.

- *Lack of product:* in congenital adrenal hyperplasia due to 21 α-hydroxylase deficiency the clinical features are a result of androgen excess in female patients producing ambiguous genitalia, and lack of cortisol and aldosterone production, seen more so in males where there are no obvious external clinical changes prompting further investigation, resulting in salt wasting crises until diagnosis is made. Both sexes are at risk of Addisonian crisis and require cortisol replacement.

Medical applications of clinical biochemistry

- Analytical clues to a diagnosis suggested by history and clinical examination, e.g. elevated urea and creatinine in a hypotensive and tachycardic elderly woman with a 2-day history of vomiting and diarrhoea.
- *Prognostic information in disease processes:* such as acute pancreatitis (Ranson's criteria or part of the Apache II scoring system).
- *Recurrence of underlying disease process:* such as using tumour marker carcinoembryonic antigen (CEA) elevation prior to surgical intervention for a Dukes B grade colorectal carcinoma, which then returns into the reference interval post-operation. Regular CEA monitoring can then provide an early clue to possible recurrence in an otherwise asymptomatic individual.
- *Pre-symptomatic identification of underlying serious metabolic abnormality:* e.g. sickle cell disorder diagnosed by newborn screening often prior to any onset of symptoms. The clinical course can be significantly altered and improved by simple early-instigated treatment, such as antibiotics and immunizations.
- *Prediction of response to treatment or dose adaptation based on enzyme activity:* e.g. Thiopurine methyltransferase (TPMT) activity prior to azathioprine treatment in inflammatory bowel disorder. This overlaps with the expanding field of pharmacogenomics, where medication choice and dose individualization can be better defined by identification of rate-limiting enzyme activity.
- An overlap with physiology in understanding demands on various energy systems in various extreme physiological and pathological situations:
  - Energy systems utilized in providing for anaerobic respiration in rapid acceleration from rest in short distance sprints.
  - Adequate energy supply in aerobic respiration in long distance and ultra-endurance events, using a combination of carbohydrate and fatty acids supplies to extend energy reserves.
  - Recovery post-exercise by optimization of rapid access carbohydrate and protein supply to skeletal musculature.
  - Extension of carbohydrate deficiency and maximal usage of other energy supplies in pathological situations, such as diabetic ketoacidosis in type 1 diabetes mellitus in relative insulin deficiency.
- In combination with physiology and genetics to increase available treatment options in chronic diseases of major worldwide health burdens, e.g. type 2 diabetes mellitus. Aerobic exercise results in increased glucose transport, independent of insulin activation and increasing GLUT 4 glucose transport. Over a period of training this can result in peripheral tissue, mainly skeletal muscle, and sensitization to insulin action, and so reducing endogenous insulin production requirement. This effect has been repeatedly shown to be more effective than oral medication, such as metformin and can significantly improve glycaemic control prior to the need for instigation for any further medical intervention.

Nutrition

Dietary components are required to maintain life by providing energy to meet a vast range of activities, essential components to allow growth and development, vitamins, and cofactors to maintain enzyme function, etc. Extreme ends of the potential nutritional success spectrum range from *kwashiorkor* (protein deficiency) and *marasmus* (energy deficiency) to obesity in excess. Various vitamin and mineral deficiencies produce a variety of clinical symptoms and signs, dependent on their requirement and function in normal metabolism.

Delivery of required amounts is not the only aspect to maintaining adequate serum and tissue levels; various absorptive processes must be successfully enabled to allow uptake of the specific substance, by transporter, co-transporter, or osmotic gradient, hampered by reduced surface area in conditions such as autoimmune coeliac disease or inflammatory bowel disorders. Some diets contain high concentrations of interfering substances, such as excess copper reducing zinc absorption. Acceptable gut transit time to allow adequate absorption is also a necessity; transit time is reduced, as is the potential to absorb by diarrhoea or hypermotility syndromes.

Macronutrients

The usual human diet can be divided into various constituent groups. Macronutrients are defined as those components comprising the bulk of the diet and providing the main energy supply; carbohydrate, protein, and fat. The metabolism associated with each is individually discussed in subsequent sections.

Micronutrients

Micronutrients are required in far smaller, but still essential amounts. These include *vitamins*, as well as *trace elements* and *minerals* that provide essential cofactors to enzymes.

Vitamins

These are organic nutrients required in very small quantities for essential cellular processes. They cannot usually be synthesized in the body and, therefore, optimal absorption from a varied diet is essential for maintenance of full function. Deficiencies of specific vitamins tend to give rise to well recognized clinical syndromes depending on the individual functionality of the particular micronutrient. Vitamins can be generally divided depending on a lipophilic (fat soluble) or hydrophilic (water soluble) nature, as discussed in the next section.

Water-soluble vitamins

These include the B vitamins and vitamin C. The full list of clinically essential B vitamins is summarized in Table 3.1, along with a brief discussion of their main functions and characteristic features of deficiency.

Table 3.1 Essential B vitamins and their pathophysiology

Vitamin specific name	Functions	Pathology associated with deficiency
B1: thiamine	Functions as a coenzyme (as thiamine pyrophosphate) in the following processes: (i) transketolase reactions in the pentose-phosphate pathway; an alternative pathway for glucose metabolism, not generating ATP, but instead NADPH for use in fatty acid and sterol biosynthesis, and provision of ribose residues for nucleic acid biosynthesis; (ii) oxidative decarboxylation of α-keto-acids, such as α-ketoglutarate, pyruvate and branched chain amino acids	*Beriberi:* peripheral neuropathy, lethargy, anorexia, oedema, and cardiovascular, neurological and muscular degeneration. Wernicke's encephalopathy is a particular risk, especially in thiamine poor diets of alcoholics, and results in irreversible loss of short-term memory function
B2: riboflavin	Essential component of flavoproteins; flavin mononucleotide (FMN) and flavin adenine dinucleotide (FAD), serving as prosthetic groups of oxidoreductase enzymes, required in processes such as amino acid deamination, purine degradation, aldehyde metabolism, fatty acid oxidation and succinate dehydrogenase function in the TCA cycle	Deficiency (ariboflavinosis) is surprisingly non-fatal. Symptoms include angular stomatitis, glossitis, seborrhoea and photophobia. Some rare metabolic diseases have a riboflavin-responsive subtype e.g. a subgroup of individuals with multiple acyl-CoA dehydrogenation deficiency
B3: niacin, nicotinic acid, nicotinamide	Essential component of nicotinamide adenine dinucleotide electron carriers (NAD+ and NADP+) functioning as coenzymes in oxidation-reduction reactions. Dietary tryptophan can be metabolized to niacin to compensate for dietary deficiency	*Pellagra:* dermatitis, diarrhoea and dementia
B5: pantothenic acid	Cofactor of coenzyme A so aiding intermediate metabolism	Failure to thrive in infants
B6: pyridoxine, pyridoxal, pyridoxamine	Cofactor in decarboxylation and deamination reactions (as pyridoxine phosphate)	Pyridoxine responsive anaemia and dermatitis
Biotin	Essential factor in action of 4 carboxylase enzyme playing key roles in intermediary metabolism: propionyl CoA carboxylase, pyruvate carboxylase, β-methylcrotonyl CoA carboxylase, and acetyl CoA carboxylase	Failure to thrive in infants due to biotinidase deficiency. May be complicated by acidosis, hypoglycaemia and hyperammonaemia if propionyl coenzyme A (CoA) carboxylase if affected
B12: cobalamin	Cofactor in nucleic acid synthesis. Require intrinsic factor produced by gastric mucosa to enable absorption of 60% of vitamin B12 in terminal ileum, therefore pernicious anaemia reducing intrinsic factor production or surgical resection of terminal ileum both inevitably result in a degree of deficiency	Megaloblastic anaemia, subacute combined degeneration of the spinal cord, raised homocysteine
Folic acid: pteroylglutamic acid	Purine and pyrimidine metabolism, essential for maturation of red blood cells	Macrocytic anaemia, often seen as a complication of inflammatory bowel disease or intestinal malabsorption syndromes
Vitamin C: ascorbic acid	Acts as a hydrogen carrier and anti-oxidant as well as a function in collagen synthesis	Scurvy, seen in sailors before the 18th century, but also seen today in the elderly with poor diets and may be associated with iron overload, resulting in increased bleeding tendency, poor wound healing, osteoporosis and poor fracture healing, and anaemia

Fat-soluble vitamins

The fat-soluble vitamins are generally stored in the liver and are particularly prone to deficiency in fat-malabsorption syndromes, such as cystic fibrosis and steatorrhoea. Each has more than one active form, but as they are each chemically similar they have been regarded as occurring in one form for the discussion in Table 3.2.

Trace elements

Trace elements or micronutrients are chemical compounds required by living organisms in minute amounts for essential reactions, generally to activate or regulate enzymatic steps. The most important examples include iron, zinc, copper, cobalt, molybdenum, iodine, and selenium (Table 3.3).

Minerals

Minerals in order of abundance in the human body include the seven major minerals calcium, phosphorus, sodium, potassium, and magnesium (Table 3.4).

Water and plasma volume control

This is the most abundant molecule in the body, constituting 40–70% of total body weight, and is the only solvent for the many ions found intra- and extracellularly. Its control depends on assessment of the overall concentration of plasma (heavily influenced by sodium concentration) at the hypothalamus and assessment of plasma volume by blood pressure monitoring at baroreceptors.

Table 3.2 Fat soluble vitamins and their pathophysiology

Vitamin specific name	Functions	Pathology associated with deficiency
Vitamin A: retinol	Produced from carotene precursors found in yellow and green plants, essential for the formation of rhodopsin, a purple retinal pigment required for vision in poor light, and for mucopolysaccharide synthesis, and mucous secretion. Large hepatic stores means deficiency symptoms are late	Night blindness, reduced mucous secretion resulting in drying and potential squamous metaplasia of mucous membranes, follicular keratosis, conjunctival dryness and keratinisation (Bitot's spots), anaemia, and poor skull bone growth
Vitamin D: calciferol	Produced endogenously by exposure to bright sunlight or in diet. Reduced endogenous production in high latitude countries, low sunlight exposure, reduced skin exposure, and skin pigmentation results in increased risk of deficiency. Not actually a vitamin, but a misnamed steroid molecule	Rickets in children and osteomalacia in adults. May also be linked to seasonal affective disorder (low mood in winter), increased cardiovascular disease risk, multiple sclerosis, etc., although evidence currently slim for these latter associations
Vitamin E: α-tocopherol	Anti-oxidant, may be low in abetalipoproteinaemia or hypobetalipoproteinaemia	Haemolysis, possible increased risk of atherosclerosis and retrolental fibroplasia and intraventricular haemorrhage in low birth weight babies
Vitamin K: 2 methyl-1,4-naphthoquinone	Essential for endogenous synthesis of prothrombin and coagulation factors II, VII, IX, and X. can be found in diet or synthesized by ileal bacteria after colonization, from infancy onwards	Bleeding tendency, prolonged prothrombin time. May be used in treatment to reverse the effect of warfarin, which is a vitamin K antagonist

Table 3.3 Dietary trace elements and their pathophysiology

Trace Element	Function	Deficiency associations
Iron	Essential haemoglobin and myoglobin component	Hypochromic microcytic anaemia
Zinc	Catalytic centre of more than 300 enzymes	Poor growth and development in children, poor wound healing and dermatitis, reduced taste, reduced immunity
Copper	Cofactor for important enzymes	Anaemia, hypercholesterolaemia (mainly LDL), bone demineralisation, leukopaenia, etc.
Cobalt	Essential for vitamin B12 activity	No recognized deficiency syndrome in humans
Molybdenum	Present in xanthine oxidase	No recognized deficiency syndrome in humans
Iodine	Incorporated into thyroid hormones	Thyroid enlargement and potential dysfunction
Selenium	Found in selenoproteins, such as glutathione peroxidase	Reduced sperm motility, reduced activation of thyroid hormones

Table 3.4 Minerals and their pathophysiology

Mineral	Function	Deficiency associations
Calcium	Most abundant mineral in the body, mainly in the skeleton	Rickets in childhood; osteomalacia in adults. Soft, weakened, and painful bone and muscular attachments
Phosphorus	Major intracellular ion (a key element of many intracellular structures), and major component of hydroxyapatite, intrinsic to skeletal strength	Reduced peripheral oxygenation in severe reductions, reduced immunity and long-term osteomalacia
Sodium	The most concentrated extracellular ion, carefully regulated by a combination of concentration assessment and blood pressure adjustment. 40% found in bone, 55% in plasma	Tiredness, confusion, muscle cramps, can result in coma
Potassium	Predominantly intracellular ion	Cardiac arrhythmias, reduced neuronal and muscle excitability; long-term affects many organs functions
Magnesium	Required by many enzymes for adequate function	Weakness, tremor, cardiac arrhythmias, potentiates potassium reduction

Water can move between intra- and extracellular spaces across semi-permeable membranes by osmosis, prompted by a difference in concentration between the two compartments. This can rapidly increase extracellular plasma volume if dehydration occurs, but not if bleeding (and loss of iso-osmotic fluid) reduces blood volume without a concentration difference. Reduced plasma volume dose evoke a hormonal response in increased aldosterone production from adrenal glands to promote sodium and water reabsorption from distal renal tubules, but this takes longer to elicit a response.

Oncotic pressure, governed by plasma protein concentration, also influences water distribution. If reduced protein is synthesized or increased losses occur, e.g. renally through nephrotic syndrome, the oncotic pressure to draw water back from the interstitial fluid at the venous end of peripheral capillary beds is reduced. This results in peripheral oedema, usually affecting ankles first due to gravity, unless lying down. This can also be exacerbated by congestive cardiac failure that increases venous pressure, so increasing fluid collection at the peripheries. In all these clinical situations, the actual overall plasma volume is reduced, so invoking further sodium and water reabsorption to try to increase this, but the reduced oncotic pressure cannot maintain the fluid within the circulation. So this secondary hyperaldosteronism response worsens the oedematous situation.

Glucose

Glucose is the most constant energy source present in the circulation by serum concentration, and is a very common carbohydrate substrate in the human diet. Dietary glucose is derived from three main carbohydrate sources:

- *Starch:* pancreatic amylase action hydrolyses to maltose, which is then hydrolysed by maltase (on the brush border of intestinal enterocytes) to 2 glucose molecules per maltose molecule.
- *Lactose:* lactase hydrolyses to glucose and galactose.
- *Sucrose:* hydrolysed by sucrase to glucose and fructose.

Glucose can also be derived from endogenous glycogen breakdown from hepatic or muscle stores (see ' Glycogen synthesis and breakdown overview').

Glycolysis

The process of energy extraction form carbohydrate food sources begins with the conversion of simple glucose to pyruvate down a series of interlinked reactions known as glycolysis (Fig. 3.3). The product of glucose metabolism via these reactions is pyruvate that can then be channelled into a variety of metabolic pathway options. Some cells can only use glucose for energy supply, e.g. red blood cells, due a limited and more simplified intracellular enzyme repertoire. However, the enzymes responsible for glycolysis are ubiquitous in every cell.

Pyruvate most commonly enters the tricarboxylic acid/Kreb's (TCA) cycle for further energy production by electron transfer to the processes of oxidative phosphorylation that ultimately results in adenine triphosphate (ATP) production. ATP is recognized as the most universal basic energy 'currency' within cells and tissues with energy being stored in high-energy phosphate bonds that can be released in a wide variety of different reactions and conditions.

Glycolysis, as the first stage of glucose metabolism, aims to derive energy from oxidation of this substrate. It is a uniquely flexible system where the amount of energy derived depends upon the availability of oxygen, but partial energy extraction can occur in anaerobic/oxygen-depleted situations. This is particularly important in extreme, rapid alterations in skeletal muscle activity where oxygen supply cannot match demand. The effective utilization of the available energy in the resultant 2 × ATP molecules and by-product of lactic acid is particularly well demonstrated by the demands of the 100 m sprint. In the presence of oxygen—aerobic respiration—the product of glycolysis, pyruvate, is converted to acetyl

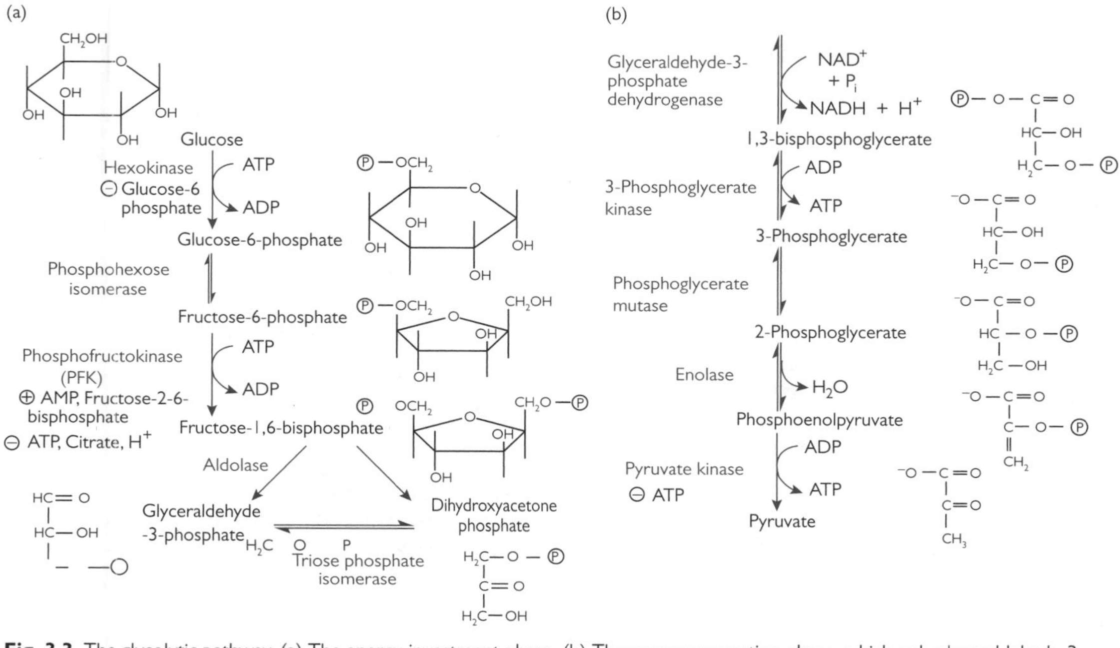

Fig. 3.3 The glycolytic pathway. (a) The energy-investment phase. (b) The energy-generation phase, which only glyceraldehyde-3-phosphate can enter.

CoA, which can enter first the TCA cycle, and then electron transport chain to yield more energy by full oxidation; this complete/aerobic combustion of 1mol of glucose yields approximately 2870 kJ of energy. This is more the picture of metabolism expected in middle distance running, such as the 5-km distance. In longer endurance exercise, to extrapolate this discussion, glucose supplies would not be able to maintain an adequate supply for the demands of, e.g. a 6-hr off-road ultra-marathon, but training encourages earlier and more efficient use of alternative energy supplies. Oxidation of fatty acids (see 'Fatty acid metabolism') becomes far more important in these situations to preserve limited glycogen stores for obligate glucose utilizing cells.

Glycolytic pathway reactions

Glycolysis occurs in the cytoplasm of muscle, fat, and tissues that are not capable of producing their own glucose through gluconeogenesis. The processes can still occur in anaerobic conditions, but the pyruvate in this instance is then converted to lactate, with a reduced energy yield, as there is no continuity with the TCA cycle or oxidative phosphorylation. The net energy yield in glycolysis alone is 2 ATP and 2 NADH per glucose molecule.

Sources of glucose

- *Glycogen:* stored in liver.
- *Galactose feeds in at G6P:* bypassing hexokinase.
- *Fructose from fruit sugar or sucrose (fructose–glucose disaccharide):* bypasses PFK and feeds in at GAP.

Control of glycolysis

There are three rate-limiting steps in glycolysis, regulated by enzymatic control. All these reactions function with large negative free energy conditions.

- *Hexokinase:* phosphorylating enzyme with a high affinity for glucose, whereas the specific liver isoform hexokinase has a low affinity for glucose and is activated by insulin, so hepatic tissue extracts relatively less glucose from the circulation during fasting.
- *Phosphofructokinase:* activated by AMP (in energy depletion), free phosphate (ATP hydrolysis product) and fructose 6-phosphate (substrate). Inhibited by ATP (in energy repletion) and hydrogen ion excess (in extended anaerobic conditions).
- *Pyruvate kinase:* major rate-limiting control point in muscle glycolysis. This is a multi-step reaction requiring K^+ and Mg^{2+} ions for completion, with a large energy release to drive ATP synthesis.

Specific examples of pathology in glycolysis

- *Phosphofructokinase deficiency in muscle* produces Tarui's disease, glycogen storage disorder type VII (see 'Metabolic disorders'). This results in clinical symptoms of energy limitation on muscular activity, reducing exercise tolerance, but there is a lack of lactate build-up on exercise.
- *Pyruvate kinase deficiency in red blood cells* decreases haemoglobin's affinity for oxygen, so preventing effective function of Na^+/K^+ ATPase pump that maintains cellular integrity, so causing haemolytic anaemia by lysis.

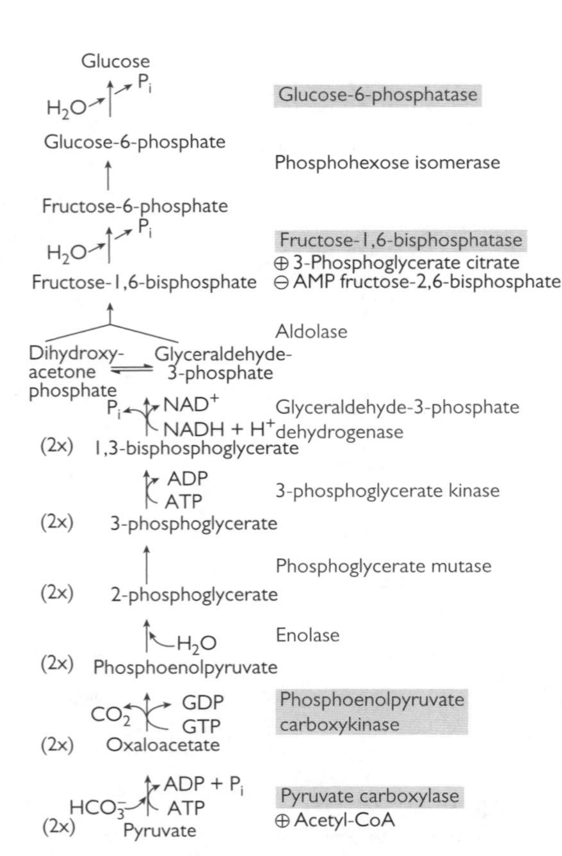

Fig. 3.4 The complete gluconeogenesis pathway from pyruvate to glucose. The highlighted enzymes are not shared with the glycolytic pathway.

Reproduced from R Wilkins et al., *Oxford Handbook of Medical Sciences, Second Edition*, 2011, Figure 2.32, p. 147, by permission of Oxford University Press.

Gluconeogenesis

This is the process where glucose molecules are formed from other substrates such as pyruvate and related 3 and 4C compounds, alanine, and lactate (Fig. 3.4). Whereas glycolysis is a catabolic linear reaction sequence that releases energy from glucose breakdown, gluconeogenesis increases glucose stores for utilization between meals to maintain blood glucose levels for glucose obligate organs and cell populations, such as red blood cells and brain (the latter unless starvation is prolonged). The glucose produced can be stored as glycogen or utilized for energy.

The majority of substrates entering into glycogenesis reactions, occurring mainly in the liver and kidney, are lactate and amino acids. Seven out of the 10 enzymes used for glycolytic conversion of glucose into pyruvate are used in the reverse manner for gluconeogenesis. The glycolytic reactions catalysed by hexokinase, phosphofructokinase, and pyruvate kinase are all associated with large free energy changes, which make their reversal difficult due to very high energy demands, and also explain the rate controlling features of these steps (see Fig. 3.5).

(a) 2 pyruvate + 4ATP + 2GTP + 2NADPH + 2H + $6H_20$

↓

Glucose + 4ADP + 2GDP + 6Pi + $2NAD^+$

(b) Glucose + 2ADP + 2PI + $2NAD^+$

↓

2 Pyruvate + 2ATP +2NADH + $2H^+$ + $2H_20$

Fig. 3.5 (a) Glycogenesis – energy requiring process; (b) glycolysis – energy releasing process.

Gluconeogenic reaction steps

The initial stage of conversion of pyruvate to phosphoenolpyruvate (reverse of pyruvate kinase activity) requires a complicated series of shuttles between the matrix of the mitochondrion and cell cytoplasm.

- 3C conversion of pyruvate to 4C oxaloacetate by pyruvate carboxylase within the mitochondrial matrix (requiring ATP).
- Oxaloacetate cannot leave the mitochondrial matrix without first being converted to 4C malate by malate dehydrogenase.
- Once in the cytoplasm, malate can be converted back to oxaloacetate by cytoplasmic malate dehydrogenase.
- *Phosphoenol pyruvate carboxykinase* then uniquely converts oxaloacetate to phosphoenol pyruvate (PEP)—requiring GTP.
- Reactions then proceed by the exact reverse of glycolytic reactions from PEP to fructose 1,6-bisphosphate.
- Reversal of the highly exergonic phosphofructokinase step requires phosphate cleavage to fructose-6-phosphate by fructose 1,6-bisphosphatase.
- This is then converted to glucose-6-phosphate by phosphoglucose isomerase.
- Then removal of a further phosphate group to produce glucose, by the action of glucose-6-phosphatase.

Control of gluconeogenesis

The main impetus of control of gluconeogenesis and glycolysis is to allow only one process to occur at any one time. There are two separate points of control in this process; the hormone *glycogen* increases the activity of fructose1,6-bisphosphatase, while high levels of *acetyl CoA* (inhibiting pyruvate dehydrogenase and, therefore, inhibit glycolysis) activate pyruvate carboxylase activating gluconeogenesis. Allosteric and covalent modifications at the 3 key enzyme rate-limiting steps also prevent simultaneous activity in the two cycles.

Glycogen synthesis and breakdown overview

Glycogen synthesis

Glycogen is converted into a polymeric form to allow storage and relatively rapid access to maintain blood glucose concentrations inter-prandially. This is primarily stored in the liver and skeletal muscle, and storage in polymeric form prevents significant osmotic/concentration alterations intracellularly despite fluxes of input after meals and output before meals. Generally, body glycogen stores last for 12–24 hr glucose maintenance supply, although this can be reduced considerably by more exertional efforts, such as long distance running. Compared with this, the body's fat stores are far larger, but these can neither be converted into glucose nor metabolized anaerobically if required.

The stages involved in glycogen synthesis are as follows:

Glucose + ATP → glucose 6-phosphate + ADP 1

Hexokinase catalyses this reaction in peripheral tissue, while glucokinase carries out the same role in liver.

Glucose 6-phosphate «» glucose 1-phosphate 2

This step is reversibly catalysed by *phosphoglucomutase*—an enzyme active in both glycogen synthesis and breakdown.

Glucose 1-phosphate + UTP → UDP-glucose + Pi 3

This last step results in the formation of an 'activated glucose' molecule from which the larger branched and granular structure of glycogen can be formed, by action of the action of *glycogen synthase*. This enzyme is unique to the glycogen synthesis process. Each reducing end of a successive glucose molecule (C1) is oxidized to the non-reducing end (C4), and the final residual end is covalently linked to a *glycogenin* protein within the centre of the glycogen core.

Without the action of a branching enzyme to form α1–6 bonds, the molecule that would result would be a straight chain of glucose molecules forming an amylose molecule. With the further complexity of branching at least every 11 residues, the resultant glycogen molecule becomes more tightly packed.

Glycogenolysis/breakdown

Catabolic degradation of glycogen stores relies on the action of three fundamental enzymes: *glycogen phosphorylase*, *debranching enzyme (α-1,6 glucosidase)*, and

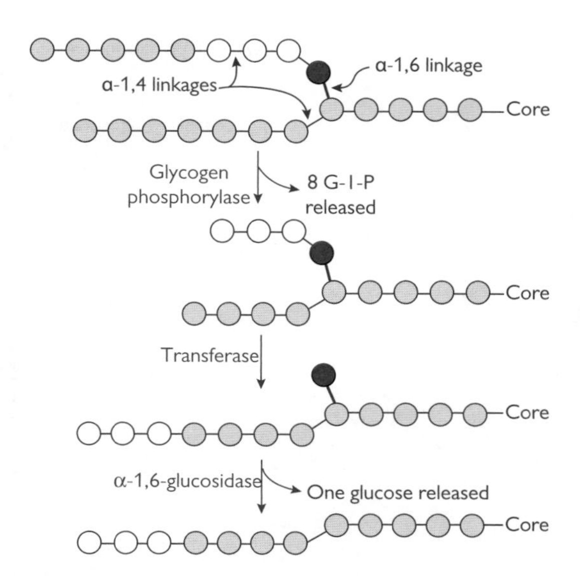

Fig. 3.6 Schematic representation of glycogen breakdown.

Reproduced from R Wilkins et al., *Oxford Handbook of Medical Sciences, Second Edition*, 2011, Figure 2.26, p. 141, by permission of Oxford University Press.

phosphoglucomutase (Fig. 3.6). Glycogen phosphorylase action involves removal of a terminal glucose residue by *phosphorolysis* releasing the glucose as α-d-glucose 1-phosphate, requiring pyridoxal phosphate as an essential cofactor. As opposed to hydrolysis this specific type of reaction preserves some of the energy of the glycosidic bond by using inorganic phosphate to produce a phosphate ester, glucose 1-phosphate. The reaction is limited to non-reducing ends of the glycogen polymer chain, disrupting α1-4 bonds.

Where an α1–6 bond is encountered—these allow closer packing of large amounts of glycogen in a smaller space intracellularly—the debranching enzyme converts this to an α1–4 bond to allow further phosphorolysis. This involves a 2-stage enzymatic conversion by transfer of the last three residues onto a non-reducing end of the glycogen polymer in an α1–4 formation, then hydrolysis of the α1–6 bond. Finally, the glucose 1-phosphate product is converted to glucose 6-phosphate by phosphoglucomutase in a reversible enzymatic step.

The end product of glucose 6-phosphate may then enter the glycolytic pathway to produce energy in the form of ATP, or can be converted to glucose and released into the circulation by the action of glucose 6-phosphatase localized within the endoplasmic reticulum, present in liver and kidney, but not in other tissues.

Defects in the function or activity of glucose 6-phosphate result in hepatomegaly associated with type 1a glycogen storage disorder (von Gierke's disease—). Muscle and

(a) If cell has balanced need for ribose-5-phosphate and NADPH

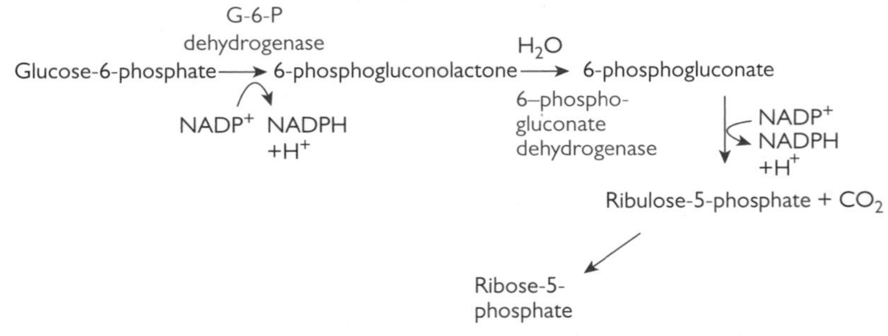

(b) If cell requires more NAPH than ribose-5-phosphate, then the excess ribose-5-phosphate formed in part (a) can be converted into the glycolytic/gluconeogenic intermediate fructose-6-phosphate by the overall reaction

6 ribose-5-phosphate C_5 → 5 fructose-6-phosphate C_6 +Pi

The reaction scheme is shown schematically:

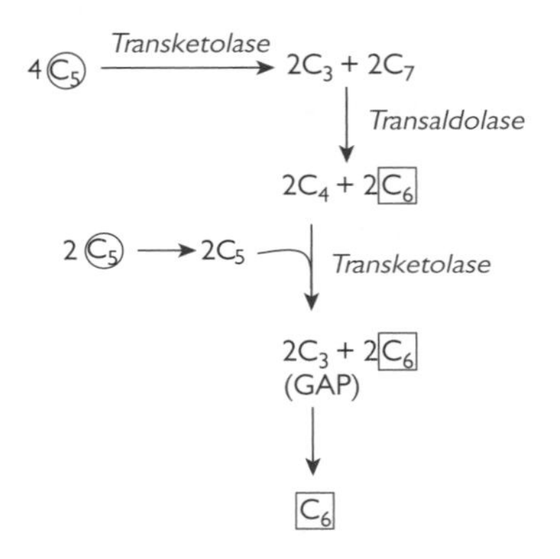

(c) If cell requires moreribose-5-phosphate than NADPH

Glucose-6-phosphate
↓
Fructose-6-phosphate
ATP → ADP, PFK
Fructose-1,6-bisphosphate
Aldolase
Dihydroxyacetone phosphate ⟷ Glyceraldehyde -3-phosphate

(4 molecules) Transketolase/ transaldolase → Ribose-5-phosphate (6 molecules)
(2 molecules)

Fig. 3.7 Pentose phosphate pathway.

Reproduced from R Wilkins et al., *Oxford Handbook of Medical Sciences, Second Edition*, 2011, Figure 2.24, p. 139, by permission of Oxford University Press.

adipose tissue both lack this enzyme, meaning any glucose 6-phosphate gained from glycogen breakdown within these tissues cannot be released into the circulation, and therefore these tissues do not contribute directly to blood glucose concentration maintenance.

Control of glycogenolysis and glycogen synthesis

Cyclic AMP is the key contributor to bilateral control, switching off glycogen synthase, while stimulating increased activity in the glycogen breakdown pathway. Glycogen phosphorylase is activated by cyclic AMP (low energy situations) and inhibited by glucose and ATP (high energy situations) to increase glycogen breakdown when most optimal. Control of both key enzymes is by allosteric inhibitors in a complex interaction.

Pentose-phosphate pathway

The majority of glucose 6-phosphate continues down the glycolytic pathway for energy provision by the processes described previously. However, an alternative fate involves oxidation to produce pentose phosphates, incorporated into RNA, DNA and various coenzymes including ATP, NADH and coenzyme A. This pathway is also known as the *phosphogluconate* or *hexose monophosphate pathway* (Fig. 3.7). A by-product of this pathway is the electron donor NADPH, which acts to maintain glutathione levels to counter the effects of damaging free radicals in some tissues, particularly those with high synthetic rates, such as adrenal glands, liver, lactating mammary gland etc.

Due to their direct exposure to oxygen and therefore free radicals, red blood cells are at a high risk of oxidative damage through this mechanism. By maintaining a high ratio of reduced to oxidized glutathione (NADPH to $NADP^+$), this damage can be prevented. The importance of this mechanism can be seen in the X-linked disorder *glucose-6-phosphate dehydrogenase deficiency* (G6PD), where the very first enzyme in the pentose phosphate pathway is deficient. When a person carrying this enzyme deficiency is exposed to a precipitating factor where highly reactive oxidants are generated as metabolic by-products, such as certain drugs or foods, fava beans, anti-malarial drugs, etc., rapid clinical manifestations of red cell damage resulting in lysis and jaundice can results in 24–48 hr. Interestingly, carrying this enzyme defect seems to imply some reduced susceptibility to malarial infection as well, which may partly explain the high gene frequency, but milder clinical version of G6PD in parts of Africa. The more severe G6PD form seems to be more limited to Mediterranean populations.

TCA cycle

Aerobic respiration, the process generating maximal potential energy for cellular processes from carbohydrate sources in the presence of an adequate oxygen supply, consists of two sequential stages—the TCA cycle (Fig. 3.8) and the electron transport chain/oxidative phosphorylation (Fig. 3.9). The mitochondrial-based TCA provides the most commonly utilized catabolic/breakdown pathway for acetyl CoA integration in metabolism. It is so named due to the formation of a 6 carbon (6C) tricarboxylic compound known as citric acid within a revolving cycle of integrated reactions, the product of each stage feeding into the next reaction step. It is also known as the Krebs cycle, after Sir Hans Krebs who originally identified the constituent reactions in 1937, whilst working in Sheffield before moving his work to Oxford.

The TCA cycle action of catabolizing acetyl CoA residues from multiple dietary sources results in liberation of hydrogen ions carried by hydrogen and electron carriers NAD and FAD as substrates for oxidative phosphorylation. This ultimately results in the production of ATP by a further set of integrated reactions within the mitochondrion, functioning as the main cellular energy substrate. The TCA cycle also has a central role in other processes of intermediary metabolism, including gluconeogenesis, transamination, deamination, and lipogenesis. These reactions occur to varying extents in a variety of tissues, with the liver being the only organ capable of carrying out all of the individual processes in appropriate circumstances.

During each cyclical rotation of the process, a 2 carbon (2C) acetyl CoA compound combines with (4C) oxaloacetate to produce (6C) citrate. The product of each previous reaction then feeds in to become the substrate of the next combination. Each revolution releases 2 × 2C atoms (in the form of CO_2) and $8H^+$ ions (that can then feed onwards into oxidative phosphorylation), until oxaloacetate is regenerated and the cyclical reactions begin again.

Regeneration of one of the primary reactants allows large amounts of acetyl CoA to be processed through the TCA cycle with minimal requirements for additional substrates; the end-point oxaloacetate is then re-used in each subsequent 'turn' of the cycle. As the TCA cycle ultimately feeds hydrogen ions into oxidative phosphorylation reactions to generate ATP/energy, the activity of the TCA cycle within aerobically metabolizing tissues can become frantic, and can accelerate rapidly in response to suddenly increasing demands for energy.

The energy within each ATP (adenosine triphosphate) molecule is stored in the form of a high energy phosphate bond between ADP (adenosine diphosphate) and a further phosphate molecule, which can be released by focused disruption of the bond in a specific and selective cellular process. This bond carries the equivalent of approximately 51.6 kJ/mol. This method of storing energy using high energy phosphate is known as *substrate-level phosphorylation*. However, generating energy via ATP production using NAD-linked dehydrogenase or substrate-level phosphorylation within glycolysis and the TCA cycle yields energy less efficiently then flavoprotein-linked (FAD-linked) dehydrogenase activity within oxidative phosphorylation of the electron-transport chain. Hence, the optimal combination of these processes sequentially to gain the maximum potential energy from ATP stores.

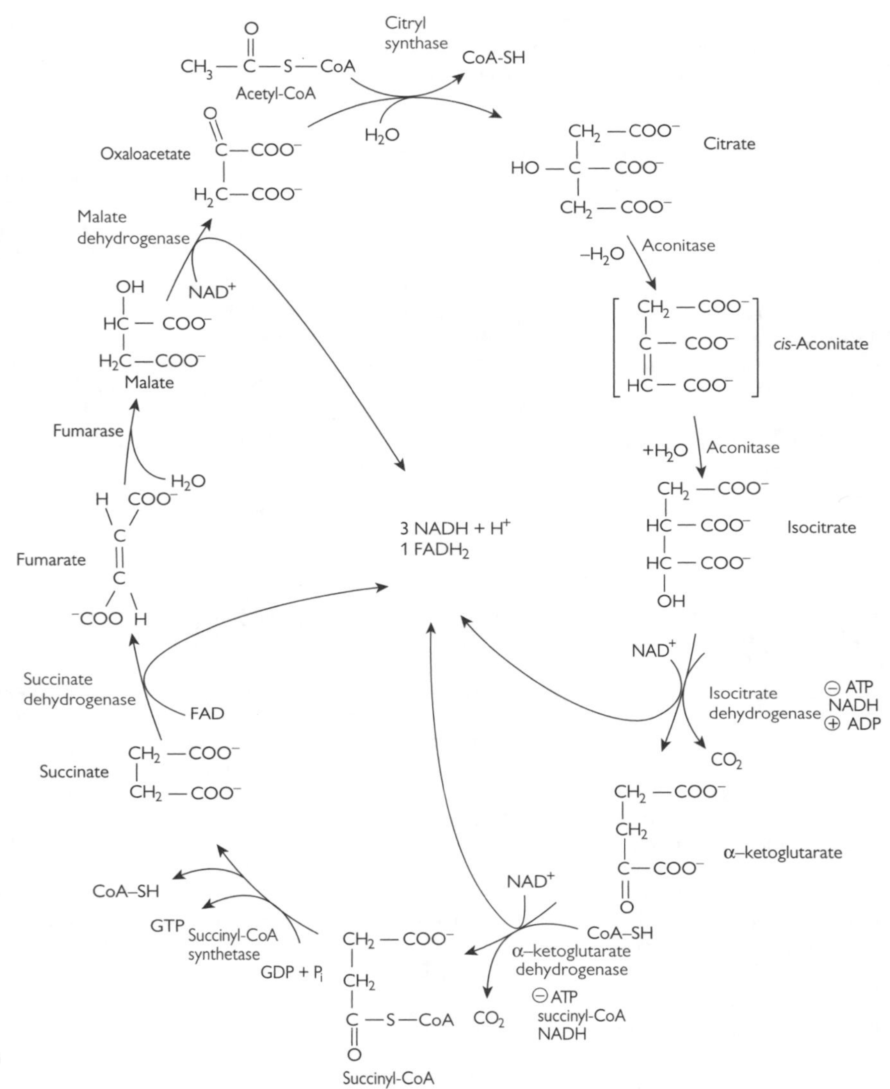

Fig. 3.8 Complete citric acid cycle.

Reproduced from R Wilkins et al., *Oxford Handbook of Medical Sciences, Second Edition*, 2011, Figure 2.6, p. 105, by permission of Oxford University Press.

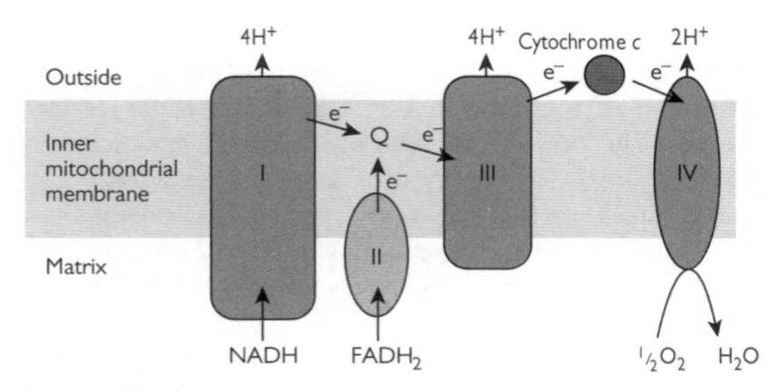

Fig. 3.9 The electron transport chain.

Reproduced from R Wilkins et al., *Oxford Handbook of Medical Sciences, Second Edition*, 2011, Figure 2.8, p. 107, by permission of Oxford University Press.

Control of the TCA cycle

This is initially by the supply of acetyl CoA, derived from pyruvate by glycolysis or from β-oxidation of fatty acids.

The dehydrogenase enzymes involved within the cycle are all dependent on the availability of NAD^+ and FAD, controlled by the activity of the oxidative phosphorylation reactions in the respiratory chain—indirectly controlled itself by ATP production rate and requirement, and supply of ADP, phosphate, and oxygen. Key enzymes, such as *isocitrate dehydrogenase* and *α-ketoglutarate dehydrogenase* are inhibited by abundance of ATP and NADH, while activity is increased by low energy situations of high ADP and AMP availability.

Amino acids

Amino acids, as the components of protein, provide a principal substrate for endogenous protein synthesis, as well as a significant energy source, ideally from the diet after digestion, or less optimally in starvation from muscle breakdown. Twenty different amino acids are combined together by peptide bonds in unique primary structure sequences defined by individual genes during protein construction; the electrostatic charges and various bonds between the constituent amino acids define further folding through secondary, tertiary, and quaternary folding, to produce the final protein shape, so key to function. Protein synthesis and digestion involve very specific set of enzymes, often with a unique set of enzymes reserved for each amino acid's metabolism, so the discussion below necessarily involves generalizations of this process to discuss aspects relevant to energy metabolism.

Amino acids contribute, on average, 10–20% of total daily ATP synthesis by oxidative phosphorylation. This infers that the total body protein of any individual represents a very large potential energy store (skeletal muscle alone contributes around 40% of total body weight). However, proteins have many functions apart from energy storage, such as catalysis to bring the rate of essential cellular reactions to a speed compatible with complex life, structural components of cellular and tissue systems (cytoskeleton; muscle, e.g. actin and myosin filaments, bone proteins, e.g. collagen, etc.) and in functionally indispensable tissues for locomotion and circulation. All this means the protein store that can actually be called on for energy purposes without significant detrimental effects is much more limited.

Digestion of protein

Dietary protein digestion occurs throughout the small intestine, and provides an efficient mechanism for transfer of amino acids into the intestinal enterocytes. The acidic pH of gastric hydrochloric acid activates pepsin, a protease that cleaves internal peptide bonds in close proximity to hydrophobic amino acids, e.g. branched chain amino acids that hide in the interior of protein molecules due to their lipophilic nature. In the duodenum and small intestine, with the elevating pH due to bicarbonate-rich pancreatic enzyme secretions, other proteases become active. All these enzymes are initially secreted in an inactive precursor form, and activation in the most suitable pH conditions cascades further activation of surrounding similar molecules.

Both endopeptidases, including trypsin, chymotrypsin, and elastase—hydrolysing bonds within protein molecules—and exopeptidases, such as carboxypeptidases—releasing terminal amino acid residues—reduce complex dietary proteins to short strings of amino acid chains. These are then further digested by proteases attached to the surface of intestinal cells, allowing active absorption mostly by sodium-linked carriers of 1–3 amino acid oligopeptides. Protein deficiency syndromes can result either from overall deficiency in intake, e.g. in starvation or poor diet, or from a severe pathological reduction in brush border surface area or enterocyte function, e.g. in Crohn's inflammatory bowel disease, or autoimmune coeliac disease.

Protein functions

Enzymes

The half-lives of enzymes vary greatly from about 30 min to 150 hr or longer, dependent on their composition, activity, and function. Integration of proline, glutamate, serine, or threonine within their structure targets these proteins for rapid turnover, while some enzymes, such as cytochromes have half lives up to 50 times longer. Lens proteins are never replaced and haemoglobin proteins last approximately 120 days. Any excess protein beyond that required for incorporation into new proteins is not stored, but becomes rapidly degraded.

Transamination

Metabolic integration: protein exists as both structural and functional elements, and as a free amino acid pool, all of which generally exhibit a high rate of turnover. A fundamental step in amino acid metabolism is transamination, where the nitrogen containing group is transferred from one amino acid to its complementary 2-oxoacid partner, such as alanine (amino acid) and pyruvate (2-oxoacid), aspartate and oxaloacetate, and glutamate and 2-oxoglutarate. These reactions catalysed by transaminases (also known as aminotransferases) allow a wider variety of metabolic integration, such as glutamate and aspartate as intermediary substrates in the TCA cycle. They also increase the variety of amino acids found within the body by allowing endogenous manufacture of further amino acids. Ten amino acids are essential and can only be derived from nutritional intake, but the remaining 10 non-essential amino acids are derived within the body by transamination of a 'carbon skeleton' compound, such as pyruvate (Table 3.5).

Table 3.5 Essential and non-essential amino acids

Essential amino acids	Non-essential amino acids
Histidine	Alanine
Isoleucine	Arginine
Leucine	Asparagine
Lysine	Aspartic acid
Methionine	Cysteine
Phenylalanine	Glutaminic acid
Threonine	Glutamine
Tryptophan	Glycine
Valine	Proline
	Serine
	Tyrosine

Maintenance of glucose inter-prandially

Amino acid circulation is particularly important in maintaining glucose supply in between meals/inter-prandially. Unlike fatty acids, amino acids carbon skeletons can be directly converted into glucose, to preserve glucose supply between meals and in times of starvation. After a period of fasting, such as overnight, the proportion of alanine and glutamine leaving many tissues apart from the liver increases dramatically; these two amino acids provide the best link between protein and carbohydrate metabolism.

The hepatic uptake of these two amino acids increases with elevating hepatic artery concentration. In hepatic tissue, alanine can be used in gluconeogenesis, the rate of which increases with low insulin and high glucagon levels associated with the fasted state. Glutamine is less favoured by hepatocytes, but is removed and metabolized by renal tubular cells, as well as intestinal cells and rapidly dividing cell populations. Here, it may act as a nitrogen donor for synthesis of nucleic acids required for new tissue formation and where it is converted into alanine.

After ingesting a meal and absorption has occurred in the digestive tract, the amino acids reach the portal system and enter the hepatocytes. The composition of amino acids leaving the liver after these processes represents a far greater proportion (about 70%) of branched chain compounds than would be expected to be found in the diet (closer to 20%). These three essential branched chain amino acids valine, leucine, and isoleucine are all preferentially taken up and oxidized by skeletal muscle tissue, while the remaining amino acids are retained by hepatocytes. The presence of a specialized enzyme 2-oxoacid dehydrogenase within muscle allows branched chain amino acids to be oxidized to ATP as an energy source for local tissue metabolism, with the most common end-products of amino group transfer from this process, alanine and glutamine, being released back into the circulation for hepatic, renal tubule, intestinal, or rapidly dividing cell destinations.

Hormonal control of protein turnover

Insulin

Insulin is recognized as an *anabolic* hormone encouraging new protein formation. Insulin's anabolic effect is thought to occur more through preventing breakdown than from stimulating protein synthesis, in physiological quantities. The effect of insulin may best be demonstrated conversely by its lack, and the emaciation of early type 1 diabetes mellitus sufferers before effective insulin replacement was available. Less extreme versions of this massive acceleration of protein degradation can still be seen in newly diagnosed type 1 cases and in the metabolic complication of diabetic ketoacidosis, where relative insulin supply and requirements become unmatched. In these situations protein is broken down to provide glucose as an energy source but remains inaccessible intracellularly without the deficient hormone.

Growth hormone

A further anabolic stimulus lies in growth hormone (GH), which is hepatically-activated to insulin-like growth factor 1 (IGF-1) and acts through the insulin receptor. GH is particularly utilized in growth and development though out childhood, but has a less well defined function in the general adult population; some adults with growth hormone deficiency secondary to pituitary pathology do not appear to gain any obvious symptomatic benefit from replacement. Synthetically manufactured versions of human growth hormone are available to stimulate growth in childhood deficiency or resistance associated with a number of medical conditions, such as Laron dwarfism and Turner syndrome. They have also been compounds abused as an ergogenic drug by some athletes since the late 1980s to increase muscle development, so hoping for illicitly-gained performance improvements. GH seems to be used to mainly increase muscle mass and strength, but the exact effects on athletic performance are difficult to elucidate due to covert use and it commonly being combined with a cocktail of other drugs including anabolic steroids.

Testosterone

Testosterone is also stimulatory to protein and muscle anabolism, and underlies many of the strength differences between the genders; this has also been famously misused in the past in the sports doping arena. However, androgenic (male characteristic) complications produced unfortunate side effects in some of the female athletes forcibly supplemented with testosterone derivatives in decades past. Use of testosterone to aid sporting performance began as early as 776 bc in the original Olympic Games. A far more extreme case of surreptitious abuse is portrayed by the story of Heike Krieger, a shot-putter in the East German team who won gold at the 1985 European Championships, but who was systematically doped with steroids from the age of 16 years. The androgenic effects eventually resulted in gender reassignment surgery in 1997 changing his name to Andreas.

Cortisol

Hormones more specifically active in *protein breakdown* include cortisol and tri-iodothyronine. Cortisol promotes gluconeogenesis from amino acids, glycerol, lactate, etc., glycogenolysis, proteolysis and selective, clinically characteristic lipodystrophy in extreme, and extended over-exposure. In the extreme situation of Cushing's syndrome of cortisol excess muscle breakdown results in many of the characteristic clinical features. These include proximal myopathy (from increased turnover of muscles, particularly the larger limb girdle muscles) affecting mobility especially up and down slopes, and resulting in relatively thin, weakened limbs despite a rotund central trunk; the protein content of the epidermis in the skin is reduced, making underlying capillaries more visible and lending a distinct red hue to facial, axillary, and abdominal skin, and osteoporosis is a longer-term complication from increased bone turnover. The skin also has a reduced ability to withstand damage, in combination with clotting factor alterations leading to increased bruising and poor wound healing due to significant lymphoid tissue involution.

Tri-iodothyronine (T3)

Tri-iodothyronine (T3) is the most active thyroid hormonal product, synthesized from its prohormone thyroxine and has a general regulatory effect, in many tissues in the body, regulating metabolic rate, temperature, heart rate, etc. The exacerbation of such actions in Graves thyrotoxicosis result in tachycardia, weight loss of fat, and muscle bulk, often reduced GI transit time so affecting absorption, elevated temperature, peripheral hyperhidrosis (sweating), etc. By specific stimulation of mRNA polymerases the rate of protein synthesis can increased, but the rate of protein degradation is also accelerated, with the latter exceeding the former in the case of thyrotoxicosis. Excess T3 sensitizes to the effects of adrenaline and other catecholamines that are also released in increased amounts in Graves's disease further exacerbating the generally catalytic nature of the condition.

Protein synthesis

De novo protein synthesis begins with a stimulus to a cell prompting transcription of the specific gene within the nucleus that is then translated to an mRNA template to blueprint protein assembly from a string of available amino acids at the ribosome. This initially produces a dipeptide of the first 2 amino acids combined by a peptide bond, then there is progressive elongation of the polypeptide chain until the protein structure is completed. There follows post-translational modification to varying degrees depending on the construction, function and area of action of the peptide (including trimming, glycosylation, phosphorylation, prosthetic group attachment, etc.), until the protein is ready to be sent to its intracellular destination (e.g. nucleus, lysosome, etc.), stored for future use (e.g. pro-insulin in the β-cells of the Islets of Langerhans in the pancreas), or secreted (e.g. hormones and neurotransmitters).

This process of protein production occurs ubiquitously in all cells, often at huge rates of activities and forms a multitude of different products. However, very small abnormal variations at any stage of the process can result in an abnormal product or complete lack of formation. If this affects the synthesis of an enzyme there may be disastrous effects, even in a one amino acid alteration, as in the case of the first protein synthesis mutation identified in phenylketonuria (PKU). This condition was first described in 1934, then in 1947 the location of the defect within the phenylalanine to tyrosine pathway was discovered, with the specific enzyme activity affected confirmed in 1953. PKU affects the enzyme phenylalanine hydroxylase, which catalyses the breakdown of the amino acid phenylalanine (Phe) to tyrosine. The biochemical result is a build-up of Phe substrate, a diversion of the excess to form phenylpyruvate and neurotoxic substances, and a deficiency of tyrosine, the latter important in the production of the pigment melanin (inadequate supplementation can result in pale hair and skin).

The clinical presentation of a delayed diagnosis combines the features of impaired neurological development, severe learning disability, and seizures, with a characteristic lack of pigment melanin, derived from tyrosine, giving a fairer skin, hair, and eye colour than siblings. Phenylalanine is an essential amino acid derived from the diet. Treatment therefore involves strict and prolonged limitation of Phe derived from foodstuffs, in association with tyrosine and amino acid supplementation.

The diet control used to be relaxed once brain development was complete in late teenage years, and was generally only re-instated in the event of a pregnancy. However, more recent data is available to suggest neurological alterations, such as poor executive functioning, decreased mental processing speed, and psychosocial problems. These subtle alterations that may result in difficulties in forming interpersonal relationships, achieving autonomy and attaining educational goals are often associated with excessive relaxation of Phe restriction.

Since 1970 screening for PKU has been included in the National Newborn Screening Programme in the UK, measuring bloodspot levels of Phe on heel prick blood taken from babies 5–8 days of age. Any elevated levels detected allow rapid referral to a metabolic paediatrician, as early intervention is required to maintain achievable IQ within the normal range.

Protein breakdown: urea cycle

The pathway responsible for conversion of amino nitrogen through ammonia to a relatively non-toxic, water soluble, and renally excretable product is known as the urea cycle (or, more correctly, the ornithine cycle), also first described by Sir Hans Krebs (Fig. 3.10). Amino acids are all essentially a carbohydrate skeleton with a nitrogen group attached. The unique part of amino acid breakdown lies in the removal of the nitrogen group; once removed the carbon skeleton left can be converted to pyruvate, enter the TCA cycle, be used for gluconeogenesis, etc.

Nitrogen is removed from an amino acid within the mitochondrion by transamination and accepted by α-ketoglutarate to produce glutamate and the paired α-keto acid. Oxidative deamination of glutamate by glutamate dehydrogenase produces ammonia and recycles α-ketoglutarate, which can then be used for further nitrogen group removal. Ammonia is toxic, particularly to neural tissue, and is usually removed efficiently by the liver. The neurotoxic effects of a build-up in the general circulation are seen in the 'liver flap' (asterixis) of end-stage liver disease, where the effectiveness of ammonia conversion to a non-toxic substance is impaired. This sign is due to an intermittent neural interruption of sensory input from proprioceptors in elevated arms with hands fully extended, that allows the hands to fall forward into flexion, and then intermittently become replaced in the desired position, simulating a flap action.

Urea cycle reaction details

- Under physiological conditions ammonium ions are joined with ATP and carbon dioxide by carbamoyl phosphate synthetase.
- The resultant carbamoyl phosphate remains within the mitochondrion and is condensed with ornithine to form citrulline by the action of ornithine transcarbamoylase (OTC). The ornithine enters the mitochondrion for this purpose through a specific receptor in the outer mitochondrial membrane, and citrulline leaves by a similar process.

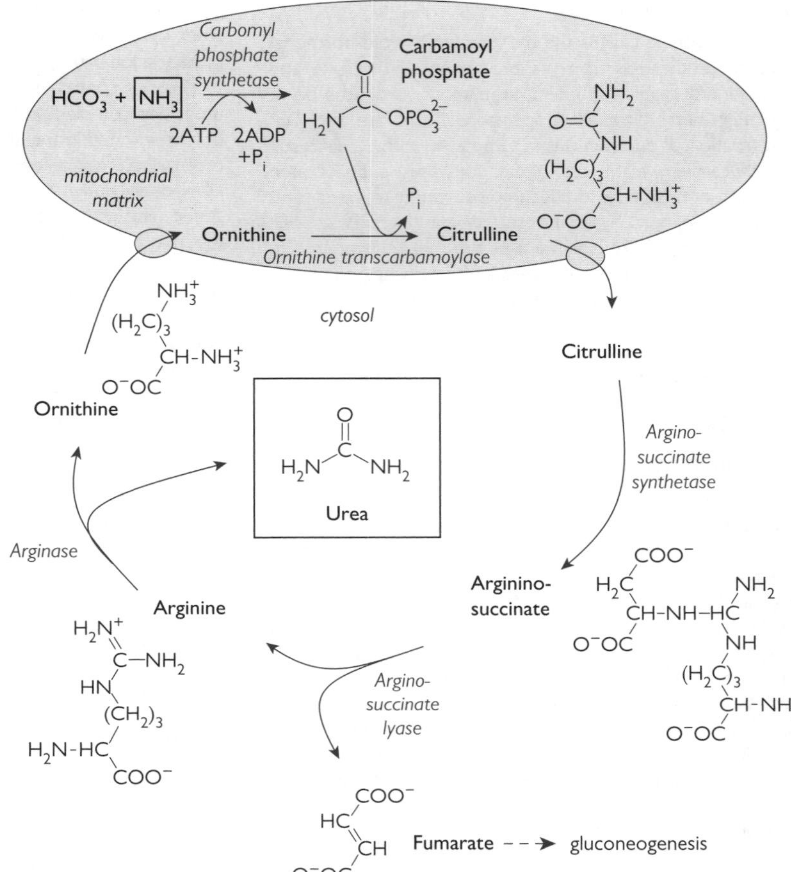

Fig. 3.10 The urea cycle.

Reproduced from R Wilkins et al., *Oxford Handbook of Medical Sciences, Second Edition*, 2011, Figure 2.35, p. 155, by permission of Oxford University Press.

- Citrulline enters the cytosol where it is combined with aspartate to form argininosuccinate.
- This product is divided to form fumarate (which can be converted back to aspartate) and arginine.
- The arginine is hydrolytically cleaved to form ornithine—recycled into the mitochondrion by the specific transporter protein—and releasing urea.

The regulation of this process, which is capable of considerable alterations in activity from the fasting to the fed state, is chiefly governed by allosteric changes in key enzymes, such as CPS I. This enzyme becomes activated by N-acetyl glutamate, a product of acetyl CoA from TCA activity and glutamate, also elevated intracellularly post-prandially. Longer-term elevation in cellular ammonia directly increases transcription of urea cycle enzymes, seen in situations such as extended starvation, where protein breakdown becomes an important energy source.

Urea cycle defects

Metabolic defects of the urea cycle are extremely rare, but the most common affecting approximately 1:80,000 people, is OTC deficiency, which demonstrates the chaos caused by an enzyme block and precursor build-up in an active metabolic process. This condition is an X-linked enzyme deficiency (Xp21.1), where an affected female may complain of protein intolerance or vomiting due to hyperammonaemia after a high protein intake (dependent on the degree of Lyon inactivation of the deficient allele). Excess carbamoyl phosphate caused by the enzyme block overflows into the cytoplasm and is converted to orotate by becoming a substrate for CPS II, usually acting as part of the pyrimidine biosynthetic pathway. The condition is diagnosed by enzyme studies after detection of increase orotic acid excretion in the urine of an affected individual, or prenatally by gene analysis.

An affected male can become severally hyperammonaemic and encephalopathic very rapidly after a protein load. However, there appears to be a wide spectrum of clinical presentation, including intermittent encephalopathic features, chronic progressive neurological decline or the rapidly fatal phenotype. The variation probably reflects the degree of enzyme inhibition. Additionally, use of valproate in OTC deficiency may precipitate acute liver failure. Treatment options include maintenance of a low protein intake, use of sodium benzoate in acute clinical deterioration to divert protein metabolism from the urea cycle to hippurate synthesis, and early use of glucose infusion to prevent increased protein breakdown to provide energy during an intercurrent illness.

Purine metabolism

Purine nucleoside synthesis requires contributing amino acids, including aspartic acid, glycine and glutamine, CO_2, and formyl tetrahydrofolate. The series of reactions involved sequentially adds extra carbon atoms to preformed ribose 5-phosphate. Inhibitors of the process can be used in clinical situations and include structural analogues of folic acid (e.g. methotrexate); trimethoprim selectively inhibits this process in bacteria and mycophenolate—particularly effective in anti-rejection therapy aimed at preventing graft rejection.

Dietary degradation of purine nucleic acids—a ring-shaped structure based on a ribose 5-phosphate molecule—occurs by pancreatic ribonuclease and deoxyribonuclease hydrolytic action, converting to nucleosides and free bases. Intracellular degradation of nucleotides results in the final product uric acid, which is then renally excreted. A late intermediate of this process is hypoxanthine, oxidized to xanthine by xanthine oxidase, then further to uric acid.

Clinical abnormalities associated with abnormalities within this pathway include gout, secondary to increased uric acid production through overload of the system by dietary excess, or secondary to under-excretion due to renal impairment. The uric acid crystals become deposited in joints, provoking a painful inflammatory response. Nodular deposits may also be found in soft tissues producing tophaceous lesions.

Pyrimidine metabolism

Pyrimidines are also ring-shaped molecules, synthesized from glutamine, CO_2, and aspartic acid. Their synthesis requires the production of carbamoyl phosphate, then orotic acid, and finally a pyrimidine ring nucleotide.

Clinical abnormalities associated with abnormalities within this pathway include orotic aciduria, resulting from low activities of enzymes governing the later stages of pyrimidine synthesis, beyond orotic acid formation. Clinical manifestations include poor growth, megaloblastic anaemia, and increased excretion of orotic acid. This can respond to uridine supplementation to reduce orotate excretion.

Unlike the purines, these molecules are degraded to soluble products of ammonia and CO_2.

Fatty acid metabolismt

Fatty acids involve more complicated and prolonged reactions to extract energy compared with sequential glycolysis and oxidative phosphorylation of simple sugars, such as glucose, but they yield proportionally more energy. Fatty acids provide a good source of energy for endurance exercise, especially if the necessary metabolic enzyme systems have been up-regulated by repeated exposure to similar circumstances in distance specific training. Fatty acids yield over twice as much energy per gram as glucose, but the process of energy release involves a more complicated and prolonged series of reactions. Glucose is still the most rapidly accessible energy store for very short notice requirements, such as sprinting, illness response (induced by the action of adrenaline and cortisol, etc.), but adipose tissue holds the key to larger and longer-term energy supply. This is the main site of storage fatty acids in the form of triacylglycerol (TAG) in adipocytes. TAG can be absorbed from the intestine and transported to the liver as chylomicrons, although TAG can also be synthesized by the liver and transported to other tissues as very low density lipoprotein (VLDL).

Fatty acid stores can also be called on to provide more rapid energy in situations where glucose stores are rapidly depleted, energy requirement is suddenly dramatically increased (as in exercise or illness) or utilization of glucose as an energy source becomes impossible, as in type 1 diabetes mellitus where insulin requirement is not met either due to increased need or reduced supply. Fatty acids provide the majority of energy in the fasting state where insulin levels are low, whereas glucose only contributes about 1/3. This mechanism preserves limited glucose stores for important tissues that can only use glucose as an energy source, e.g. red blood cells, or tissues that prioritize glucose, except in longer-term energy deficiency, e.g. brain. Ketone body production is an alternative pathway of fatty acid metabolism in the liver, favoured in situations of starvation.

Fatty acid oxidation

Fatty acid degradation results ultimately in the formation of acetyl CoA, a substrate that can be fed into a number of pathways, including energy generation by TCA cycle or ketone body formation and can also be used as the initial substrate for the biosynthesis of fatty acids. Although these two processes reflect alternate directions, they are not simply the reverse of each other, occurring in distinct areas of the cell and being individually controlled to integrate with current tissue energy requirements. The oxidation of fatty acids to acetyl CoA occurs in mitochondria, and utilizes NAD and FAD coenzymes to generate ATP as an energy currency. This location promotes easy transference of the end product into the TCA cycle for further energy provision. Fatty acid synthesis, however, occurs in the cytosol and sequentially combines acyl residues to form elongating fatty acid derivatives via action of a multi-enzyme complex (fatty acid synthase), incorporating NADP+ as a coenzyme, bicarbonate ions, and requiring ATP as an energy source.

The first stage of β-oxidation of fatty acids involves transport inside the mitochondria (Fig. 3.11). Almost all

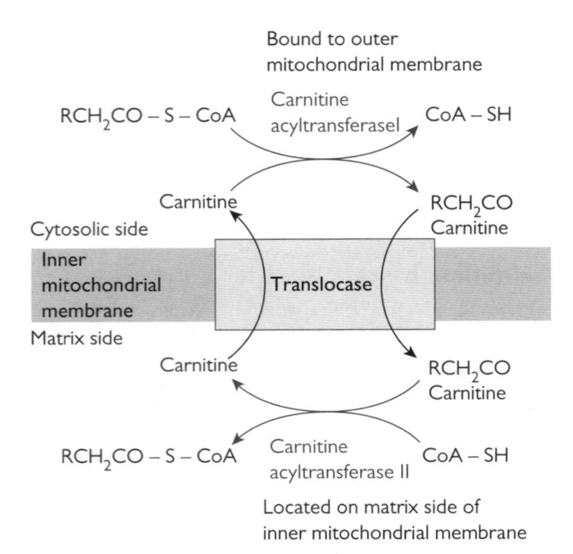

Fig. 3.11 Mechanism of transport of long chain fatty acyl groups into mitochondria where they are oxidized in the mitochondrial matrix.

β-oxidation occurs within mitochondria, apart from very long chain fatty acids (VLCFA's) which are mainly oxidized in peroxisomes. The fatty acids are transported as acyl CoA derivatives, to which the mitochondrial membrane is impermeable to, so they are combined with carnitine to allow transportation. Carnitine attachment to fatty acids is catalysed by the enzyme carnitine palmitoyltransferase I (CPT I), and the carnitine is separated from the acyl CoA molecule and transferred back to the other side of the mitochondrion—recycled—by the action of CPT II.

The remaining stages of β-oxidation consist of four consecutive reactions reducing the length of the fatty acid (FA) and resulting in the production of one molecule of acetyl CoA per cycle of reactions (Fig. 3.12). Each stage is catalysed by a specific enzyme or series of enzymes altered depending on the length of the FA chain being oxidized.

- *Oxidation by acyl CoA dehydrogenase:* this produces reduced flavin adenine dinucleotide (FADH2) acting as a carrier transferring electrons to the oxidative phosphorylation pathway for ATP generation. The other product is an enoyl CoA, which is then transferred to the next stage.
- *Hydration of the double bond* between carbons C2 and C3 of enoyl CoA.
- *Oxidation of this hydrated bond* yields NADH as a further electron transporter.
- *The final cleavage stage* generates acetyl CoA and a shortened acyl CoA chain, the latter then feeds into the next round of β-oxidation; the most common destination for acetyl CoA in most tissues being the TCA cycle.

Ketone body production

Ketone bodies are produced by liver cell conversion of acetyl CoA from fatty acid oxidation. The three main compounds include acetone (non-metabolized volatile by-product, detected on the breath of individuals in excess production, such as diabetic ketoacidosis (DKA)), acetoacetone, and β-hydroxybutyrate (best correlated in point of care monitoring to recovery from DKA on treatment).

- The two metabolically active soluble substances can be transported to peripheral tissue, there converted to acetyl CoA, and so oxidized in the TCA cycle.
- They are produced when there is excess oxidative capacity in the liver, mainly from increased supply of fatty acids when gluconeogenesis is activated, so allowing acetyl CoA to convert to the ketone pathway.
- Used by muscles, renal cortex, and the brain only in longer-term exposure, if the blood level rises sufficiently to spare glucose.

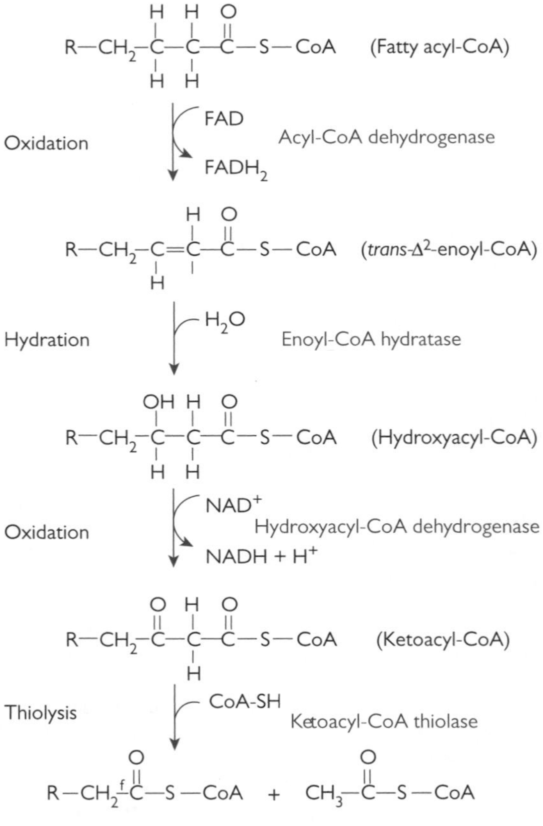

$R{-}CH_2{-}CH_2{-}CH_2{-}C(=O){-}S{-}CoA$ (Fatty acyl-CoA)

Oxidation — FAD → $FADH_2$ — Acyl-CoA dehydrogenase

$R{-}CH_2{-}CH{=}CH{-}C(=O){-}S{-}CoA$ (*trans*-Δ^2-enoyl-CoA)

Hydration — H_2O — Enoyl-CoA hydratase

$R{-}CH_2{-}CH(OH){-}CH_2{-}C(=O){-}S{-}CoA$ (Hydroxyacyl-CoA)

Oxidation — NAD^+ → $NADH + H^+$ — Hydroxyacyl-CoA dehydrogenase

$R{-}CH_2{-}C(=O){-}CH_2{-}C(=O){-}S{-}CoA$ (Ketoacyl-CoA)

Thiolysis — CoA-SH — Ketoacyl-CoA thiolase

$R{-}CH_2{-}C(=O){-}S{-}CoA \; + \; CH_3{-}C(=O){-}S{-}CoA$

Fig. 3.12 One round of the four reactions of β-oxidation by which a fatty acyl-CoA is shortened by two carbon atoms with the production of a molecule of acetyl-CoA.

The clinical difficulties occur in specific situations when ketone bodies are produced in an energy deficit, combined with dehydration. Ketone bodies are acidic substances that can dramatically and rapidly reduce blood pH in situations where renal regulation of acid base balance is impaired, e.g. by reduced plasma volume secondary to osmotic diuresis in DKA. Treatment includes rehydration, insulin replacement to allow energy derivation from glucose, rather than continued ketone production and electrolyte replacement, lost in the overwhelming diuresis.

Pathology in fatty acid oxidation

Generally, medium chain fatty acids such as those containing 8 or 10 carbon atoms are the easiest form to rapidly access. This access process requires a specific enzyme system including the action of medium chain acyl CoA dehydrogenase (MCAD). In a rare inborn error (incidence 1:10,000 in the UK), where this enzyme is defective, rapid access to energy in glucose deplete times is severely impaired, and hypoglycaemia cannot be counteracted by medium chain fatty acid metabolism, resulting in potentially fatal hypoglycaemia. This condition (known as MCADD—MCAD deficiency) is one of five currently screened for in newborn screening programmes in the UK on day 5 of life, as early recognition and parent education can prove potentially lifesaving if the baby becomes unwell and glucose requirement increases.

Fatty acid synthesis

Fat biosynthesis from sugars and amino acid carbon skeletons is initiated if liver glycogen stores are replete. The process occurs in the cytosol (in contrast to breakdown, which occurs within the mitochondrial matrix) and is catalysed by fatty acid synthase (FAS), a complex of enzymes comprising a dimer of two identical 260 kDa subunits. Each subunit possesses seven catalytic domains, with covalently bound intermediates handed from one domain to the next without leaving the complex.

The committed step for fat synthesis (Fig. 3.13) requires the ATP-dependent carboxylation of acetyl-CoA to malonyl-CoA; biotin is an essential co-factor for the carboxylase, which is allosterically activated by citrate. To initiate synthesis, an acetyl-CoA is linked to a component of one

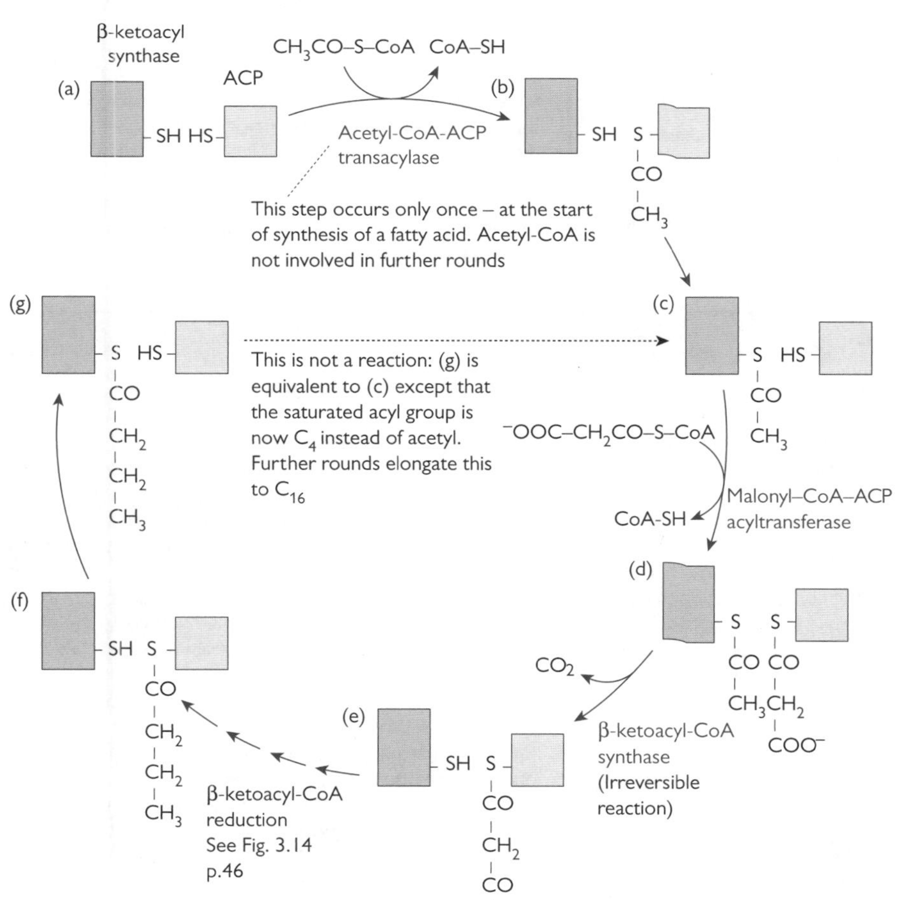

Fig. 3.13 The steps involved in the synthesis of fatty acids.

Reproduced from R Wilkins et al., *Oxford Handbook of Medical Sciences, Second Edition*, 2011, Figure 2.17, p. 122, by permission of Oxford University Press.

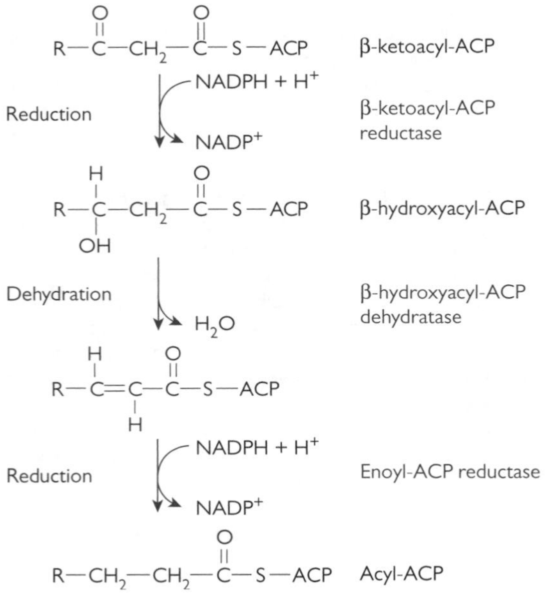

$R-C(=O)-CH_2-C(=O)-S-ACP$ β-ketoacyl-ACP

Reduction ($NADPH + H^+$ → $NADP^+$) β-ketoacyl-ACP reductase

$R-CH(OH)-CH_2-C(=O)-S-ACP$ β-hydroxyacyl-ACP

Dehydration (→ H_2O) β-hydroxyacyl-ACP dehydratase

$R-CH=CH-C(=O)-S-ACP$

Reduction ($NADPH + H^+$ → $NADP^+$) Enoyl-ACP reductase

$R-CH_2-CH_2-C(=O)-S-ACP$ Acyl-ACP

Fig. 3.14 Reductive steps in fatty acid synthesis, (e)–(f) in cycle shown in Fig. 3.13.

Reproduced from R Wilkins et al., *Oxford Handbook of Medical Sciences, Second Edition*, 2011, Figure 2.18, p. 123, by permission of Oxford University Press.

FAS monomer, the acyl carrier protein (ACP), via the linker molecule phosphopanthetheine and then passed to the condensing enzyme (CE) of the second monomer. Malonyl-CoA covalently binds to ACP of the first monomer and a sequence of condensation, reduction dehydration and reduction reactions ensues (Fig. 3.14). NADPH is used as the reductant. The chain transfers to CE of monomer 1 and a further malonyl-CoA covalently links to ACP of monomer 2, after which the sequence of four reactions repeats. This process of elongation continues until a C16 (palmitoyl) unit is formed, which is released as free palmitate by hydrolysis. Longer chain fatty acids and unsaturated fatty acids can subsequently be synthesized from palmitate in the smooth endoplasmic reticulum.

The balance between synthesis and degradation of fatty acids reflects the energy state of the cell. If ATP levels are high, inhibition of the TCA cycle leads to high levels of citrate in mitochondria, which exits in exchange for malate on a carrier protein. Once in the cytosol, the citrate is converted into acetyl-CoA (which undergoes carboxylation to yield malonyl-CoA for fatty acid synthesis) and oxaloacetate (which is converted back to pyruvate and returned to the mitochondrion). The process yields one of the two NADPH required for the FAS reaction (the second comes is derived from the pentose phosphate pathway). The carboxylase is regulated by AMP-sensitive kinase, which supresses activity when energy levels are low. The allosteric activation of the enzyme by citrate overcomes this supression, while high levels of palmitoyl-CoA antagonize the action of citrate (and inhibit the mitochondrial citrate carrier). The carboxylase is activated by insulin, and suppressed by glucagon and adrenaline. Finally, malonyl-CoA inhibits transferases, preventing uptake of substrates for β-oxidation into mitochondria.

Metabolic disorders

Major metabolic abnormalities that apply to the topics described in the previous section include those affecting food supply, in deficiency states and excess, and those affecting metabolic pathways, such as fatty acid oxidation defects, urea cycle defects, and glycogen storage disorders. Other disease states having an indirect metabolic effect on nutritional pathways include haemochromatosis (where liver function is affected, intrinsic to many important nutritional pathways), cystic fibrosis affecting the ability to absorb a wide range of dietary components due to GI pathology and various enzyme blocks/defects that prevent more specific deficiencies, including lactase deficiency preventing selective absorption of lactose sugars by lack of the absorptive enzyme.

Enzyme defects affecting nutritional status

Glycogen storage disorders

Glycogen is the first line energy reserve and principal storage carbohydrate used to spare glucose in fasting states. Hepatically, deposition averages around 50–120 g/kcal in optimal situations, with muscle glycogen available only for muscular activity (averaging 350–400 g in optimal circumstances) and not for release into the general circulation.

Glycogen metabolism is under the control of specific enzyme systems—*synthase* and *phosphorylase*—through allosteric control and hormonal effect. Allosteric interaction involves modulation of action by low molecular weight molecules that effect action through binding to the enzyme despite a lack of structural similarity to related coenzymes or substrate. This form of control is very commonly found in biosynthetic pathways, often at the most committed step within the reaction sequence. The main hormones involved include glucagon during fasting conditions to maintain glucose supply to obligate tissues, and insulin post-prandially to maximize energy substrate storage and anabolism after digestion.

Glycogen storage disorders describes a group of eight inherited metabolic disorders affecting type or storage of glycogen, resulting in multiple organ dysfunction due to abnormal glycogen deposition, and tendency to hypoglycaemia in some cases (Table 3.6).

Lactase deficiency

Lactose is the carbohydrate found in milk, consisting of a disaccharide of glucose and galactose. Its digestion requires

Table 3.6 Glycogen storage diseases and their pathophysiology

Glycogen storage disease	Alternative name	Enzyme defect	Clinical symptoms and signs
Type I	Von Gierke's disease 1:100,000 births	Glucose-6-phosphatase	Liver and renal tubular cells filled with abnormal glycogen deposits; tendency to hypoglycaemia, lactic acidosis, ketosis, and hyperlipidaemia; hepatic adenoma's, hypertension, and renal calculi
Type II: autosomal recessive	Pompe's disease: infantile, juvenile, and adult onset forms	Lysosomal α 1–4 and 1–6 glycosidase (acid maltase). Enzyme replacement treatment of α-glucosidase available	Glycogen accumulation in lysosomes results in early fatality in infantile onset
Type III: autosomal recessive	Cori's disease	Debranching enzyme	Branched insoluble polysaccharide accumulates to damages liver and/or muscle, and hypoglycaemia
Type IV	Amylopectinosis, Andersen	Branching enzyme	Accumulation of polysaccharide with limited branching in heart and liver, resulting in fatality in first 5 years of life
Type V	McArdle's syndrome	Muscle phosphorylase	Reduced exercise tolerance and lack of lactate build-up after exercise. High muscle glycogen content
Type VI	Hers' disease	Liver phosphorylase	High hepatic glycogen content but inability to access results in predisposition to hypoglycaemia
Type VII	Tarui's disease	Phosphofructokinase in muscle and rbc's	Reduced exercise tolerance and lack of lactate build-up after exercise. High muscle glycogen content, possible rhabdomyolysis with haemolytic anaemia features
Type IX		Liver phosphorylase kinase	High hepatic glycogen content but inability to access results in predisposition to hypoglycaemia

the enzyme lactase, which is most active in the first few months of life, reducing after weaning. Deficiency is much more common in those of African, Asian, and Inuit extraction than in northern European populations. Most situations of lactase deficiency are asymptomatic, but those presenting with nausea, bloating, and abdominal pain after milk ingestion should be further investigated by measurement of mucosal disaccharidase activity after intestinal biopsy for a definitive diagnosis. The treatment is avoidance of the offending substance, i.e. low lactose diet. In reality, this is often implemented without definitive diagnosis, if it solves the clinical symptoms.

Fructose intolerance

Found in 1:20,000 births and resulting from an autosomal recessive lack of fructose-1-phosphate aldolase (chromosome 9q22.3). This prevents breakdown of fructose in foods containing this substrate, resulting in nausea, vomiting, abdominal pain, hepatomegaly, lactic acidosis, and potentially progressing to liver failure, with proximal convoluted tubular Fanconi syndrome.

There is also a benign form resulting from a lack of fructokinase, which produces asymptomatic fructosuria after ingestion of fructose containing food substances.

Galactosaemia

Incidence 1:60,000 births, produced by lack of galactose-1-phosphate uridyl transferase (GALT) enzyme responsible for the conversion of galactose to glucose (chromosome 9p13). Symptoms begin at the start of milk feeding due to galactose build-up, resulting in failure to thrive, vomiting, diarrhoea and jaundice, with hepatomegaly and ascites, complicated by developmental delay in speech, language and general learning.

Wider metabolic disorders affecting nutritional status

Haemochromatosis

Incidence as high as 1:200 in northern Europeans (see Chapter 7).

Cystic fibrosis

Incidence 1:2500 in Caucasians mainly. An autosomally recessive inherited defect in chloride transporter function, resulting in respiratory and GI complications due to thickened mucous production and complicated by recurrent respiratory infections and pancreatic blockage by mucoviscid secretions (see Chapter 11). Lack of pancreatic enzyme action reduces fat absorption complicated by fat soluble vitamin deficiencies.

Further reading

Harpers Illustrated Biochemistry 29th Edition - Robert Murray, David Bender, Kathleen M. Botham, Peter J. Kennelly, Victor Rodwell, P. Anthony Weil. McGraw-Hill 2012. ISBN: 9780071765763 / 007176576X

Multiple choice questions

1. Which of the following statements is true?

A. Muscle lacks glucose-6-phosphatase (G6P) and therefore cannot generate glucose from glycogen.
B. The function of muscle glycogen is to provide glucose for the brain during starvation.
C. Skeletal muscle contains substantial glycogen stores, but cardiac muscle does not.
D. Glycogen synthesis in muscle is stimulated by myocyte contraction.
E. Muscle glycogen is stored in mitochondria.

2. Which of the following statements is true?

A. Liver synthesizes glycogen principally from fructose-6-phosphate.
B. Glycogenolysis in liver is regulated by covalent modification of glycogen phosphorylase.
C. Glycogenolysis in muscle is not regulated allosterically.
D. Liver glycogen is a highly hydrophobic molecule.
E. The adult human liver stores about 1 kg of glycogen.

3. Which of the following statements is true?

A. Glycogen is replenished during aerobic exercise.
B. Liver glycogen is broken down following high dietary fat intake.
C. Muscle glycogen can be replenished by conversion of triacylglycerols stored in adipose tissue.
D. Glycogen is stored in tissues other than muscle and liver.
E. Glycogen cannot be synthesized from amino acids.

4. Which of the following statements is true?

A. The pentose phosphate pathway produces NADH, which is used in fatty acid synthesis.
B. The pentose phosphate pathway produces NADPH, which is used in the β-oxidation of fatty acids.
C. The pentose phosphate pathway produces NADPH, which is used in fatty acid synthesis.
D. The pentose phosphate pathway produces NADH, which is used in the β-oxidation of fatty acids.
E. The pentose phosphate pathway produces both NADH and NADPH.

5. Which of the following statements is true?

A. One of the functions of the pentose phosphate pathway is to produce oxidizing power in order to oxidize glutathione
B. One of the functions of the pentose phosphate pathway is to produce reducing power in order to reduce glutathione
C. Oxidized glutathione is an important anti-oxidant
D. Reduced glutathione is an important anti-reductant
E. The pentose phosphate pathway is absent in erythrocytes glucose

6. Which of the following statements is true?

A. Glucose-6-phosphate dehydrogenase (G6PD) deficiency results in increased oxidative damage and haemolytic anaemia.
B. G6PD deficiency is Y-linked.
C. G6PD deficiency occurs mostly at high geographical latitudes.
D. Haemolysis associated with fava bean ingestion is observed in all affected individuals.
E. G6PD deficiency is treated with gene therapy.

7. Which of the following statements is true?

A. The electron transport chain creates an electron gradient across the inner mitochondrial membrane to energize phosphorylation.
B. The electron transport chain depends on the impermeability of the outer mitochondrial membrane to protons.
C. The electron transport chain creates a proton gradient across the inner mitochondrial membrane to energize phosphorylation.
D. The electron transport chain creates a NAD+ gradient across the inner mitochondrial membrane
E. The electron transport chain depends on impermeability of the outer mitochondrial membrane to electrons

8. Which of the following statements is true?

A. Oxidation of one NADH molecule results in phosphorylation of one ADP molecule.
B. Oxidation of one FADH2 molecule results in phosphorylation of one ADP molecule.

C. FADH2 may be oxidized by complex I of the electron transport chain.
D. All complexes of the electron transport chain are oxido-reductases.
E. All complexes of the electron transport chain can translocate protons.

9. Which of the following statements is true?

A. Protons are conducted back in to the mitochondrial matrix by uncoupling proteins.
B. Protons leak back through the inner mitochondrial membrane via a voltage-dependent leak current.
C. Proton transport across the inner mitochondrial membrane is an active (energy requiring) process.
D. The Fo ATP synthase component translocates 3 protons together.
E. ATP is generated in the intermembrane space.

10. Which of the following statements is true?

A. Electron carriers in the electron transport chain have manganese atoms in their active centres.
B. Cytochrome C is also known as ubiquinone.
C. Electron carriers in the electron transport chain contain iron-sulphur clusters.
D. Complex II has NAD-reductase activity.
E. Electron carriers in the electron transport chain are hydrophilic proteins.

For answers, please see Appendix: Answers to multiple choice questions, page 313.

CHAPTER 4

Immunology

Introduction and general principles

The immune system is fundamental to host defence against infection, and is important in protection against malignancy. Dysregulated immune responses are central to the pathophysiology of many autoimmune and inflammatory diseases.

The immune system comprises two overlapping components, the innate and adaptive systems (Table 4.1). The innate system includes physical barriers in addition to cells and soluble factors. The adaptive system consists of an extremely broad range of antigen-specific lymphocytes and antibodies.

Immune cells communicate by cell-cell contact and by secretion of soluble mediators including *cytokines*. Adaptive system components are displayed in bold in Table 4.2.

The innate and adaptive immune systems constantly interact:

- Antigen presenting cells of the innate immune system are needed to activate T cells.
- In turn, the adaptive immune system directs innate immune responses.

From an anatomical perspective, the immune system consists of the primary and secondary lymphoid organs, and the lymphatic system.

Primary lymphoid organs

- *Thymus:* maturation and selection of T cells.
- *Bone marrow:* maturation and selection of B cells and NK cells, and origin of all haematopoietic progenitor cells.

Secondary lymphoid organs

- *Spleen:* processes blood-borne antigens.
- *Lymph nodes:* process lymph-borne antigens.
- *Mucosal associated lymphoid tissue:* processes mucosal antigens.

Lymphatic system

Lymphatic vessels circulate interstitial fluid (lymph) from tissues and organs back to the circulation via the right thoracic duct. Groups of lymph nodes are found at intersections of these vessels in strategic sites (cervical, inguinal, axillary, hilar, para-aortic, etc.). T cells and B cells are present in lymph nodes, where they are primed by soluble lymph-borne antigens captured by lymph node-resident antigen presenting cells, and also by peripheral antigen presenting cells that have captured antigen and migrated to the lymph node from tissues.

Table 4.1 A comparison of the innate and adaptive immune system

Innate immune system	Adaptive immune system
Conserved	Recently evolved
Lymphocyte and antibody independent	Lymphocyte and antibody dependent
Non-specific	Antigen-specific (clonal)
Immediate onset	Slower onset (due to clonal proliferation
No self-tolerance	Self-tolerance
No memory	Memory (allowing faster responses on second encounter with antigen)

Table 4.2 The cellular and soluble components of the immune system

Cells	Main function (additional function)	Soluble	Main function
Granulocytes Neutrophils Eosinophils Basophils Mast cells	 Phagocytosis Cytotoxicity: extracellular pathogens Release of inflammatory mediators Release of inflammatory mediators	Complement pathway	Label pathogens for phagocytosis (opsonization) Cytotoxicity Cellular activation
Mononuclear phagocytes Monocyte/macrophages Dendritic cells	 Phagocytosis (antigen presentation) Antigen presentation (phagocytosis)	Cytokines	Intercellular signalling Cellular activation/suppression Cytotoxicity
Lymphocytes NK cells T cells B cells	 Cytotoxicity: intracellular pathogens **Co-ordinate immune response** **Produce antibody (antigen presentation)**	Chemokines	Direct cell movement Cellular activation
		Antibodies	**Label pathogens for phagocytosis (opsonization)** **Antibody-dependent cellular cytotoxicity** **Activate complement** **Cellular activation**
		Inflammatory mediators: Prostaglandins Leukotrienes Histamine	↑ Vascular permeability ↑ Blood flow Cellular activation

Barriers to infection

Intact physical and anatomical barriers are the initial lines of defence against microbial pathogens (Tables 4.3 and 4.4).

Disruption of normal barriers by medical intervention is central to the pathogenesis of the major healthcare-associated infections:

- *Intravenous cannulae:* bloodstream infection.
- *Endotracheal ventilation:* ventilator-associated pneumonia.
- *Urinary catheterization:* urinary tract infection.
- *Broad spectrum antimicrobials: C. difficile* infection.

Table 4.3 Anatomical versus biological barriers to infection

Anatomical barriers	Chemical and biological barriers
Skin	Lysozyme (mucosal secretions)
Upper airways cilia	Gastric acid (pH1)
Mucociliary escalator	Secretory IgA
Urinary stream and bladder emptying	Bacterial flora (skin, GI tract)

Table 4.4 Intrinsic barrier dysfunction is commonly associated with clinical infection

Barrier dysfunction	Causes	Consequence
Loss of skin integrity	Wounds (including burns) Chronic skin disease (psoriasis, eczema)	Skin and soft tissue infection Bacteraemia
Defective mucociliary escalator	Cigarette smoking Cystic fibrosis Kartagener's syndrome	Bronchitis and pneumonia
Achlorhydria	Atrophic gastritis Gastric acid-suppression	↑ Risk of gastroenteritis and *Clostridium difficile*-associated diarrhoea

Inflammation

Inflammation occurs in response to tissue damage or infection. Inflammatory responses are also triggered by cytokines produced by T cells, and by antibody-antigen binding (see 'Antibody-mediated immunity' and 'Cell-mediated immunity').

Inflammation involves:

- ↑ Vascular permeability (cytokines, inflammatory mediators).
- ↑ Blood flow (vasoactive mediators, e.g. histamine).
- Recruitment and activation of immune effector cells (cytokines, chemokines, adhesion molecules).

The purposes of inflammation

- Clearance of debris and pathogens by macrophages and neutrophils.
- Capture of antigens for adaptive immune priming by dendritic cells.
- Limitation of infection or damage.
- Wound healing, tissue remodelling and repair.

Innate triggering of inflammation involves release of fever-inducing pro-inflammatory cytokines such as tumour necrosis factor alpha (TNFα), interleukin 1 (IL-1) and IL-6 from sentinel macrophages or patrolling leucocytes. Specialized *pattern recognition receptors* (PRRs) expressed by these cells sense:

- *Damage-associated molecular patterns (DAMPs):* host intracellular components (DNA, ATP, intracellular proteins) signalling tissue damage or cellular stress.
- *Pathogen-associated molecular patterns (PAMPs): such as bacterial or fungal cell wall components or nucleic acid.*

PRR binding activates various intracellular signalling cascades → NFκB activation and cytokine production.

The toll-like receptors (TLRs) are a family of PRRs and are listed with their ligands:

- *TLR1:* lipopeptides (Gram –ve bacteria, mycobacteria).
- *TLR2:* lipoteichoic acid (Gram +ve bacteria), zymosan (fungi), lipoarabinomannan (mycobacteria).
- *TLR3:* dsRNA (viruses).
- *TLR4:* Lipopolysaccharide (LPS).
- *TLR5:* flagellin (bacteria).
- *TLR6:* di-acetyl lipopeptides (mycobacteria).
- *TLR7:* dsRNA (viruses).
- *TLR9:* CpG motifs (bacteria).

Innate soluble mediators active in acute inflammation include:

- Plasmin system → prothrombotic state.
- Kinin system.
- Contact system.
- Inflammatory mediators released by mast cell degranulation (e.g. histamine, 5-hydroxytrytamine, leukotrienes and prostaglandins) → ↑ vascular permeability and ↑ blood flow.
- Acute-phase proteins produced by the liver (e.g. mannose binding lectin, C-reactive protein, serum amyloid-P) → complement activation.
- Complement system.

The evolutionarily conserved complement system labels invading pathogens for phagocytosis (opsonization) and directly destroys pathogens by cytolysis.

Complement cascade activation (Table 4.5, Box 4.1) occurs in three pathways, all involving the amplification of the initial signal by positive feedback mechanisms. Complement inhibitors prevent excessive activation and protect host cells. The common final mechanism to these proteolytic cascades is the production of C3 convertase, which converts C3 to C3b, activating the terminal chain components C5–C9.

Complement activation results in:

- Opsonization by C3b and C4b.
- Membrane attack complex (MAC) formation, a complex of terminal chain complement proteins (C5b—C9), → cytolysis.
- Cellular activation, chemotaxis and activation of polymorphs (C5a), increased vascular permeability (C4, C2) and mast cell degranulation, mediated by C3a and C5a (also referred to as anaphylatoxins).

Table 4.5 The three pathways by which the complement cascade can be activated

	Trigger	Initial components	Pathway	Co-factors	C3 convertase	Inhibitory factors
Classical	Antibody in immune complexes	C1, C2, C4	Ca^{2+} dependent		C4b2a	C1 inhibitor C4bp Decay activating factor (DAF) Membrane cofactor protein (MCP)
Mannose-binding lectin	Mannose binding (and other lectins)	MBL, C2, C4	Ca^{2+} dependent	MASP 1 MASP 2	C4b2a	C1 inhibitor C4bp DAF MCP
Alternative	C3b binding to microbial cell surface	Factor B-C3b	Mg^{2+} dependent	Factor D	C3bBb	Factor H Factor I

BOX 4.1 PATHOLOGY ARISING FROM COMPLEMENT CASCADE DYSFUNCTION

Inherited deficiency of C1 inhibitor (C1inh) leads to recurrent severe swelling or angioedema (hereditary angioedema, HAE, autosomal dominant) through the uncontrolled generation of bradykinin following activation of the contact system by innocuous trauma, infection, or stress.

Clinical features

- Recurrent abdominal pain (GI oedema) and respiratory compromise (laryngeal oedema) as well as localized peripheral swelling.
- N C3, ↓ C4.
- Type I HAE = low or undetectable levels of C1inh, type II HAE (15%) = functional abnormality despite normal levels.
- Treatment is with recombinant C1inh during attacks.

Decay activating factor is a cell surface complement inhibitor attached to cells by a GPI-anchor protein. In paroxysmal nocturnal haemoglobinuria recurrent attacks of complement-mediated haemolysis occur due to deficiency of GPI-anchoring. The direct-antiglobulin test (Coomb's test) is negative. Humanized anti-C5 monoclonal antibody has been used for treatment. Deficiency in classical or alternative complement components or the membrane attack complex → recurrent infections with encapsulated bacteria such as *Neiserria meningitidis* (see 'Immunodeficiency').

Chemokines

These are cytokines that stimulate chemotaxis (cell movement) and cellular activation.

- Chemokine receptor expression by leucocytes is ↑ by pro-inflammatory cytokines within minutes to hours. Ligand-receptor interactions → cellular activation and trans-endothelial trafficking.
- The differential expression of chemokines by vascular endothelium results in the staged recruitment of leucocytes: first neutrophils, then mononuclear phagocytes, and then T and B cells.

Trans-endothelial migration of leucocytes depends on expression of adhesion molecules (selectins and integrins) on vascular endothelium.

- *Selectins* expressed on endothelium (e.g. E-selectin) slow the circulating leucocytes by transient interactions with leucocyte glycoproteins → chemokine receptor-ligand signalling and leucocyte activation.
- *Integrins* (e.g. leucocyte functional antigen 1, LFA-1) are ↑ on activated leucocytes and have ↑ binding affinity for intercellular adhesion molecules (ICAMs, part of the immunoglobulin superfamily e.g. ICAM-1) on the vascular endothelium. Stable interactions are formed by integrin-ICAM binding → leucocyte arrest → trans-endothelial migration.
- *Selectins and integrins* can be ↑ by cytokines at sites of inflammation, although are constitutively expressed at low levels (see Box 4.2).

Phagocytes

Monocytes, macrophages, and neutrophils phagocytose pathogens in opsonin dependent or independent pathways. Opsonization dependent pathways involve complement or antibody coating, and binding via complement receptors (CRs), or Fc receptors (FcRs). Opsonization independent pathways (mainly involving macrophages) involve PRRs such as:

- *Scavenger receptors* (SR) class A and B.
- *LPS receptor:* CD14.
- *C-type lectins:* including the mannose receptor (MR) and dectin-1.
- TLRs.

Phagocytosed pathogens are degraded by oxygen-dependent and -independent mechanisms.

- In *oxygen-dependent pathways*, reactive oxygen intermediates are produced by generation of the superoxide anion by NADPH oxidase → production of hydroxyl radicals and hydrogen peroxide (*respiratory burst*). This leads to a transient rise in pH in the phagosome, during which time cationic microbicidal proteins (defensins, cathelicidin) are most effective. Fusion with the lysosome leads to acidification of the phagolysosome → microbial damage. Many lysosomal proteases function optimally at low pH. Lysozyme and myeloperoxidase are pumped into the phagolysosome, the latter generating further toxic oxidants. In addition, nitric oxide synthesis from L-arginine, catalysed by inducible nitric oxide synthase, contributes to intracellular pathogen killing, extracellular inflammatory signalling and vasodilatation.
- *Oxygen-independent pathways* involve additional microbicidal peptides, lysozyme, and the lysosomal proteases (e.g. cathepsins, elastase).

Ultimately the phagolysosome disintegrates, and peptide fragments are processed for presentation by antigen-presenting cells (APCs), such as macrophages and dendritic cells (see 'Cell-mediated immunity'). However, some pathogens are capable of surviving within macrophages (e.g. mycobacteria), and this contributes to their pathogenesis (see 'Hypersensitivity'; see also Box 4.3).

BOX 4.2 LEUCOCYTE ADHESION DEFICIENCY

Deficiency of β2 integrin synthesis in Leucocyte Adhesion Deficiency → failure of neutrophil recruitment → recurrent bacterial and fungal infection (see 'Immunodeficiency').

BOX 4.3 PATHOLOGY ARISING FROM PHAGOCYTE DYSFUNCTION

Deficiency of NADPH oxidase → impaired catalase-positive bacteria (staphylococcus) killing in chronic granulomatous disease (see 'Immunodeficiency'). Impaired lysosomal trafficking/degranulation in Chédiak-Higashi syndrome→recurrent pyogenic infections (see 'Immunodeficiency').

Cytotoxic chemotherapy → neutropenia → ↑ susceptibility to bacterial and fungal infection.

Phagocytosis of pathogens and necrotic cells leads to activation of the phagocyte and pro-inflammatory cytokine production. The response to phagocytosis of apoptotic cells and debris is more variable, and may → anti-inflammatory cytokine production (IL-10, TGFß), which may contribute to the resolution of inflammation.

Wound healing and tissue remodelling

This is a contiguous process with acute inflammation and follows haemostasis and resolution of acute inflammation (including removal of particulates and debris by macrophages). A variety of growth factors such as epidermal growth factor 1 (EGF-1) and transforming growth factor beta (TGFß) are involved. Wound healing requires both proliferation and remodelling.

Proliferative phase

- Angiogenesis (endothelium).
- Collagen synthesis (fibroblasts).
- Granulation tissue formation (fibroblasts).
- Wound contraction (myofibroblasts).
- Epithelialization (epithelial cells).

Remodelling

- Replacement of type III collagen with type I to strengthen the extracellular matrix (ECM).
- Remodelling of collagen fibres along tissue lines.

Chronic inflammation

Persistence of the triggering antigen (autoimmune disease, chronic infection) → inflammatory responses without resolution or tissue remodelling → significant tissue damage. In chronic inflammatory responses, the main effector cells are macrophages and adaptive immune cells—T cells, B cells, and cytotoxic T lymphocytes.

Virus-specific innate soluble and cellular responses

TLR3 and TLR7 stimulation by dsRNA triggers macrophage activation. *Type I interferons* (IFNα/ß) are a group of antiviral proteins produced by virus-infected cells and specialized DCs that activate antiviral gene transcription to:

- Block viral protein synthesis and trigger apoptosis by bcl-2 and caspase-dependent mechanisms (dsRNA dependent protein kinase R).
- Degrade viral mRNA (2'5'-oligoadenylate synthetase).
- Block viral transcription (Mx protein).
- Up-regulate MHC I and II expression.

Type I interferons also activate *natural killer (NK) cells* and macrophages.

NK cells are innate immune effector cells of the lymphocyte lineage (derived from large granular lymphocytes) that do not express the T- or B-cell receptors. They contain cytotoxic granules containing granzymes and perforin, which can induce cell death in target cells. They express a variety of receptors including killer immunoglobulin-like receptors (KIRs) that recognize the absence of expression of the major histocompatibility complex I (MHC I). MHC I is constitutively expressed on all nucleated cells. NK cells kill virus infected cells (or tumour cells) in which MHC class I expression has been down-regulated to evade recognition by cytotoxic T lymphocytes. NK cells express Fc receptors. Antibody-labelled cells are killed by FcR bearing cells (NK cells, monocytes, neutrophils)—antibody-dependent cellular cytotoxicity (ADCC). NK cells produce IFNγ in response to virus infection.

Antibody-mediated immunity

Antibodies (Abs) produced by B cells are extremely effective in combatting extracellular pathogens by:

- Labelling pathogens for phagocytosis, complement mediated lysis, or antibody-dependent cellular cytotoxicity (see 'Inflammation').
- Neutralizing toxins.
- Binding to cell surface molecules on bacteria and viruses to prevent infection of host cells (neutralization).

Antibodies are soluble glycoproteins. The basic antibody unit consists of two light and two heavy chains. Each antibody has:

- Two clonal antigen-binding sites (FAb fragments) that match the conformation of the target epitope (an epitope is the portion of antigen recognized by specific antibodies or T cells of the adaptive immune system). The target epitope may be:
  - *Continuous*—a continuous sequence of linked amino acids.
  - *Conformational*—two disconnected amino acid sequences, which are recognized together by the Ab due to the conformation of the native antigen.
- A single heavy chain Fc segment (bound by FcRs on host immune effector cells). This segment (encoded by the constant gene region) determines antibody function, including:
  - Opsonization → phagocytosis (IgG).
  - Classical complement pathway activation (IgM, IgG).

Table 4.6 Properties of the five major classes of antibodies

Ab Class	Frequency in serum (%)	Subclasses	Structure	Function
IgA	10–15	IgA1–2	Secreted—dimer Serum—monomer	Mucosal immunity
IgD	1	–	Monomer	B-cell receptor
IgE	<0.01	–	Monomer	Parasite immunity
IgG	65–75	IgG1–4	Monomer	Secondary antibody response
IgM	15–20	–	Pentamer	Primary antibody response

- ADCC (IgG).
- Mast-cell degranulation (IgE).

Antibodies differ in structure (number of monomeric components), function, and frequency (Table 4.6).

Antibody binding is determined by:

- *Affinity:* the strength of epitope binding.
- *Avidity:* affinity multiplied by the number of epitopes the antibody recognizes.

The almost infinite variation of Ab epitope-binding site structures is achieved by random *somatic recombination* of the variable gene segments. Recombination is mediated by the recombination activating gene proteins RAG-1 and RAG-2. In contrast to T-cell receptors (TCR) rearrangement, the antibody antigen-binding region continues to recombine during mature B-cell proliferation (*somatic hypermutation*) to enhance the specificity and affinity of antigen binding. B cells producing antibodies with enhanced affinity avoid apoptosis. Those with reduced affinity undergo apoptosis (*clonal selection*). This process is *affinity maturation*, and occurs in the germinal centre of secondary lymphoid tissues.

B-cell maturation

B cells are derived from lymphoid progenitors. X-linked agammaglobulinaemia results in a deficiency of B cells and antibody production (see Box 4.4). During maturation in bone marrow, immature B cells undergo:

- *Positive selection:* only B cells with a functional rearrangement of *Ig* genes survive.
- *Negative selection:* self-reactive B cells undergo apoptosis.

The B-cell receptor (BCR) consists of surface IgM (IgD) together with a heterodimer of Igα and Igβ. B-cell activation is enhanced by the co-receptor complex involving CD21, CD19 and CD81.

BOX 4.4 X-LINKED AGAMMAGLOBULINAEMIA

X-linked agammaglobulinaemia leads to a congenital deficiency of B cells and all antibody classes→recurrent infections in infancy. Deficient antibodies are replaced by repeated infusions of pooled human immunoglobulin (IVIG).

The *primary antibody response* results in production of antigen-specific IgM. Helper T cells (Th cells) are required for *class switching* to allow antigen-specific IgG production in the *secondary antibody response*. Class switching occurs under the influence of cytokines produced by Th subsets. B cells can alter the class/isotype of antibody produced by rearranging different constant (*Fc*) gene segments, to produce different effector functions. In T-cell independent B-cell activation class switching does not occur, and the second exposure to antigen results in (mostly) IgM production.

B-cell activation

B-cell activation is either:

- *T-cell independent (TI):* mainly involving the B-1 ($CD5^+$) subset of B cells that predominate in the peritoneum:
  - TI-1 polyclonal stimulators (e.g. lipopolysaccharide (LPS) from Gram -ve bacteria).
  - TI-2 cross-link clonal BCRs (e.g. pneumococcal capsular polysaccharide).
- *T-cell dependent (TD):* antigen recognition by B cells and MHC II restricted Th cells with co-stimulation via CD40-CD40L (e.g the majority of antigens derived from extracellular bacteria and viruses). Failure of T cell signalling causes common variable immunoideficiency disorder (see Box 4.5).

Upon activation, B cells proliferate and develop into antibody-forming cells (AFCs) or memory B cells. Terminally differentiated AFCs (plasma cells) are antibody factories, no longer expressing Ig receptors. Memory B cells allow more rapid and amplified responses on second encounter with an antigen, producing antigen-specific IgG. TI activation is inefficient at generating memory B cells.

BOX 4.5 COMMON VARIABLE IMMUNODEFICIENCY DISORDERS

Common variable immunodeficiency disorders are caused by a failure of T cell signalling to B cells through an unknown mechanism → recurrent sinusitis, pneumonia and chronic diarrhoea. X-linked mutations in CD40L (a form of hyper IgM syndrome) → a combined immunodeficiency syndrome involving a broad range of pathogens including intracellular opportunistic infections (OI).

Cell-mediated immunity

Cell-mediated immunity is primarily concerned with defence against intracellular pathogens (e.g. TB and viruses, such as HIV). T cells are the key mediators of cellular immunity (see Box 4.6). Unique T cell receptors (TCRs) expressed by T cells determine their antigen specificity, and unlike B cells which can recognize epitopes in their native conformation, T cells only recognize processed peptides. The TCR is part of the immunoglobulin superfamily, and the process of diversifying the antigen-recognition repertoire of TCRs and antibodies is similar.

There are distinct T-cell populations

The T-cell receptor is a heterodimer of two chains, either α and β, or γ and δ, and forms a complex with CD3 (the TCR complex). The TCR complex can only recognize specific peptide antigens loaded onto specialized MHC molecules. TCR signalling is ↑ by association with a co-receptor expressed by the T cell (CD4 or CD8). The majority of T cells (> 95%) express the αβTCR and either CD4 or CD8. CD4 or CD8-MHC binding stabilizes peptide-MHC-TCR complex interactions.

- CD4 binds MHC class II expressed by antigen-presenting cells (APCs). Similarly, the TCR on $CD4^+$ T cells only recognizes antigens presented by MHC II expressing APCs.
- CD8 binds MHC I, expressed by all nucleated cells (erythrocytes do not have a nucleus and do not express MHC I). The TCR on CD8 T cells only recognizes antigen bound to MHC I.

$CD4^+$ T cells are a heterogeneous population, which co-ordinate the phenotype of cellular immune responses (known as helper T cells, or Th cells) and are involved in immune regulation (regulatory T cells, or T_{REGS}). Deficiency in CD4+ Th cells can be caused by HIV (see Box 4.7). $CD8^+$ T cells are important in defence against intracellular pathogens (particularly viruses) and tumour cells.

αβT-cell subsets

T helper cells (Th cells) have diverse functions that include activating cytotoxic T cells and macrophages, stimulating B-cell maturation, and influencing antibody class switching (see 'Antibody-mediated immunity'). Th cells are polarized into subsets by the cytokines they produce, and the functions they perform. Th1 cells produce IFNγ and TNFα to co-ordinate cell-mediated immune responses (effectors—macrophages, $CD8^+$ T cells, and NK cells) against intracellular pathogens, whilst Th2 cells co-ordinate antibody-mediated responses (effectors—B cells and eosinophils) to extracellular pathogens including parasites (e.g. schistosomiasis) through the production of IL-4 and IL-5. Th17 cells direct immune responses to pathogens at mucosal sites through production of IL-17 (and other cytokines). All activated Th cells produce IL-2, an important growth factor for T cells (see Table 4.7).

Regulatory T cells

Regulatory T cells (T_{REGS}) help prevent autoimmune disease by maintaining peripheral tolerance. They also have a role in regulation of inflammatory responses to prevent bystander damage (immunopathology). Pathogens may attempt to stimulate T_{REG} responses as an immune evasion strategy (e.g. HIV, malaria). T_{REGS} are antigen-specific, and produce

BOX 4.6 SEVERE COMBINED IMMUNODEFICIENCY

The virtual absence of T cells in severe combined immunodeficiency (SCID) is also associated with a functional B cell deficiency and is invariably fatal without bone-marrow transplantation.

BOX 4.7 CELL-MEDIATED IMMUNODEFICIENCY OF AIDS

HIV infects and kills $CD4^+$ Th cells, leading progressively to the cell-mediated immunodeficiency of AIDS. Antiretroviral drugs prevent viral replication allowing $CD4^+$ T cell immune reconstitution.

Table 4.7 T helper cell subtypes and their pathophysiology

Th subset	Principal cytokines	Function	Dysfunction	Cellular interactions
Th1	IFNγ, TNFα, IL-12	Cell-mediated immunity	Autoimmune disease	Macrophages, cytotoxic $CD8^+$ T lymphocytes (CTL)
Th2	IL-4, IL-5, IL-13	Antibody-mediated immunity, parasite defence	Atopy Autoimmune disease	B cells, eosinophils
Th17	IL-17, IL-21, IL-22	Mucosal antimicrobial immunity	Autoimmune disease	Multiple
T_{FH}	$CXCR5^+$	Humoral immunity		B cells
T_{REG}	IL-10, TGFβ	Immune regulation	Autoimmune disease	T cells, APC

the regulatory cytokines IL-10 and TGFß in response to antigen recognition. T_{REGS} may express either CD4 or CD8.

Naturally occurring $CD4^{+}CD25^{+}$ T_{REGS} display a breadth of TCR diversity comparable to effector T cells. T_{REGS} make up 5–10% of the total lymphocyte population. They exert their immunosuppressive effects through close contact with self-reactive or pathogen-specific effector cells and APCs in lymphoid or non-lymphoid tissues, and therefore they express a variety of tissue homing chemokines and adhesion molecules. They are differentiated from activated T cells (which can also express the IL-2R α chain CD25) by expression of the transcription factor forkhead box p3 (Foxp3).

Mutations in the *Foxp3* gene are associated with the rare and serious autoimmune inflammatory syndrome—immune dysregulation, polyendocrinopathy, enteropathy, X-linked syndrome (IPEX).

Peripherally-induced T_{REGS} are a subset of antigen-experienced T cells that display variable expression of CD25 and Foxp3, producing their inhibitory effects by secretion of anti-inflammatory cytokines (IL-10, TGFß). Induced T_{REGS} may be diverted down the regulatory path by exposure to IL-10 or TGFß in the cytokine microenvironment.

Cytotoxic T lymphocytes (CTLs)

Cytotoxic T lymphocytes respond to peptide-MHC I complexes on the surface of infected cells or tumours by killing the target cell, either by secretion of cytotoxic granule components (granzymes, perforin, see Box 4.8), cytokines that induce apoptosis (TNFα, IFNγ), or by expression of the death receptor ligand fasL. CTLs are usually $CD8^{+}$, although $CD4^{+}$ T cells may function as CTLs. They are thought to form a critical role in control of chronic virus infections such as HIV.

NKT cells

A subgroup of T cells express αβTCRs with limited antigen diversity and do not recognize peptide-MHC complexes, but are CD1d-restricted, and respond to lipid and glycolipid antigens. These T cells express the NK cell markers and produce granzyme, and are termed NKT cells. They produce a diverse array of cytokines such as IL-2, TNF-α, IFN-γ, IL-4, and GM-CSF. Their role is incompletely understood, but NKT cells are thought to play a role in peripheral tolerance.

γδT cells

5% of T cells express the γδTCR (and are termed γδT cells). γδT cells are enriched in the mucosa in comparison to lymphoid tissues, and recognize antigen by MHC-independent mechanisms. The role of γδT cells remains incompletely understood, but they span the innate and adaptive immune systems. They recognize PAMPs and DAMPs and may have phagocytic activity (innate immune functions). γδT cells have also been reported play a role in B-cell immunoglobulin class switching and αβT cell regulatory signalling (adaptive immune functions). γδ T cells are evolutionarily conserved, and play an important role in mucosal immunity.

T-cell development

T-cell progenitors originate from bone marrow lymphoid precursors and mature in the thymus, although extrathymic maturation has been observed. T-cell precursors are initially negative for CD4 and CD8 (double negative). They proliferate to become double positive ($CD4^{+}CD8^{+}$) thymocytes. During the proliferation stage, TCR variable region genes undergo *somatic recombination* to generate diverse antigen repertoires. Recombination is mediated by the recombination activating gene proteins RAG-1 and RAG-2 (see Box 4.9). The TCRs produced by such stochastic gene rearrangement must fulfil three criteria to prevent the thymocyte undergoing apoptosis:

- Functional TCR.
- Recognize self-MHC (either class II—CD4, or class I—CD8) with intermediate affinity (inadequate or excessive binding leads to apoptosis).
- Do not respond to self-peptides (self-tolerance).

Only ~5% of thymocytes become mature T cells (expressing only CD8 or CD4) and migrate to secondary lymphoid tissues. As not all self-reactive T cells are negatively selected during thymic maturation, other mechanisms of peripheral tolerance are required to prevent autoimmunity:

- *Anergy* induced by antigen recognition in the absence of co-stimulatory molecules provided by the target cell (see 'Antigen presentation and T-cell activation').
- Immune privileged tissue sites (e.g. brain, testes, cornea).
- Regulatory T cells (T_{REGS}).
- Immune ignorance (i.e. the self-reactive T cell does not encounter its specific antigen).

Antigen presentation and T-cell activation

T-cell activation is tightly regulated. Dendritic cells are specialized APCs that present antigens to naïve T cells. APCs acquire extracellular antigen by phagocytosis, pinocytosis, or receptor-mediated endocytosis in non-lymphoid tissues, and migrate to lymphoid tissues where they prime naïve T cells. Extracellular polypeptide antigens are processed and complexed with MHC II (or MHC I in a process known as

BOX 4.8 CHÉDIAK-HIGASHI SYNDROME

In Chédiak-Higashi syndrome CTL responses are also dysfunctional due to impaired exocytosis of cytotoxic granules containing granymes and perforin.

BOX 4.9 MUTATIONS IN RAG-1 OR RAG-2

Mutations in RAG-1 or RAG-2 result in potentially fatal severe combined immunodeficiency (SCID).

> **BOX 4.10 SUPERANTIGENS**
>
> Superantigens (such as the exotoxin staphylococcal toxic shock syndrome 1) are capable of broad activation of T cells without co-stimulatory signals by cross-linking the TCR-MHC, causing uncontrolled T cell activation → toxic shock syndrome MHC II deficiency→CD4+ T-cell immunodeficiency (see 'Immunodeficiency').

cross-presentation). Intracellular proteins are processed and presented with MHC I. Dendritic cells that have recognized danger signals through PRRs express the B7 co-stimulatory molecules (CD80 and CD86), which provide a co-stimulatory signal by binding CD28 on the T cell required for activation of the T cell. In the absence of co-stimulation, the T cell becomes resistant to further activation (*anergic*). Therefore, DCs can stimulate or suppress Ag-specific adaptive immune responses depending on the activation state of the APC, and the tissue micro-environment sampled. Macrophages and B cells can present antigen to activated T cells during infection, when co-stimulatory molecules and MHC II are ↑.

CD8+ T-cell activation is similar, but the second signal may be derived from pro-inflammatory cytokines produced by activated Th cells (see Box 4.10).

Upon activation, T cells proliferate and express IL-2, which is a growth factor for activated T cells. Proliferation usually requires maintained antigen exposure, although CD8+ T cells may continue to proliferate with brief exposure to antigen. Negative feedback mechanisms exist to trigger apoptosis of activated T cells to prevent uncontrolled activation:

- *Activation induced cell death (AICD):* FasL and TNFα.
- *Passive cell death (PCD):* withdrawal of growth factors after antigen clearance.

T_{REGS} and immunoregulatory cytokines, such as IL-10 and TGFß, can suppress T-cell activation. Progressive telomere shortening occurs during rounds of mitosis in activation-induced lymphocyte proliferation → mitosis arrest (prevents uncontrolled T-cell proliferation).

Immune senescence is a physiological ageing process → immunodeficiency of old age. Thymic involution and ↓ progenitor cells contribute to ↓ naïve T-cell population and ↓ antigen recognition repertoire against new pathogens. Excessive immune activation may → premature senescence (e.g. CMV, HIV).

T-cell memory

A key feature of the adaptive immune system is the ability to mount an amplified and more efficient response when encountering an antigen for the second time. This is mediated by memory T and B cells. About 5% of antigen-specific T cells do not undergo apoptosis after activation. These cells exhibit ↑ expression of the anti-apoptotic molecule bcl-2, and become long-lived memory cells.

- Central memory T cells (T_{CM}) predominate in LNs, mediated by the LN-homing chemokine receptor CCR7 and L-selectin CD62L.
- Effector memory cells (T_{EM}) are mainly resident in non-lymphoid tissues. T_{EM} rapidly differentiate into effector cells on contact with antigen.

HLA and susceptibility to disease

The human leucocyte antigen (HLA) genes encode for MHC I (A, B, and C) and MHC II (DP, DQ, and DR) molecules. The HLA region on chromosome 6 is the most polymorphic in the genome. This increases the range of potential pathogen epitopes that can be recognized by T cells. Protective HLA molecules are under continuous evolutionary selection. HLA B-53, over-represented among West African populations, is associated with reduced susceptibility to severe malaria.

Certain HLA haplotypes are associated with autoimmune disease:

- *HLA B-27:* seronegative arthritides.
- *HLA DR-3:* Sjogren's syndrome, autoimmune hepatitis, type 1 diabetes mellitus (T1DM), etc.
- *HLA DR-4:* rheumatoid arthritis, T1DM, etc.

Hypersensitivity

Hypersensitivity is defined as an excessive or inappropriate tissue-damaging immune response. This can occur in response to innocuous exogenous antigens (allergy) or self-antigens (autoimmunity) (see Table 4.8).

Allergy

Antibody-mediated

Antigen-specific IgE mediates host defence against parasites. However, when the IgE is directed against innocuous exogenous antigens/peptides the process is referred to as allergy, and the antigen is known as an allergen. Atopy is the (usually heritable) tendency to produce excess IgE in response to innocuous exogenous antigens. Hay fever and atopic dermatitis (eczema) are examples of IgE-mediated atopic disorders. Mast cells bind IgE via the high-affinity Fc receptor and following subsequent exposure, the allergen binds to the membrane bound IgE, cross-linking adjacent molecules triggering activation of the mast cell leading to degranulation (rapid release of histamine, cytokines and other preformed *inflammatory mediators*; see Box 4.11). Recruitment of Th2 cells and eosinophils follows (late response) and is responsive to corticosteroid therapy. IgE production by B cells is

Table 4.8 Mechanisms and diseases

Principal immune component	Classification (Gell—Coombs)	Effector mechanism	Example
Antibody	Type I (IgE, 'immediate')	Mast cell degranulation	IgE—atopic disorders
X-linked agammaglobulinaemia	Type II (IgG/IgM, 'antibody-mediated')	Phagocytosis	IgG—Autoimmune haemolysis, immune thrombocytopenia (ITP)
		ADCC/complement activation	IgG—Goodpastures syndrome
			IgM—Haemolytic transfusion reaction
		Neutrophil activation	IgG—Wegner's granulomatosis
		Receptor binding	IgG—Graves disease, myaesthenia gravis
Antigen-antibody (immune-complex)	Type III ('immune-complex mediated')	Complement activation and neutrophil recruitment/activation and tissue damage	SLE, extrinsic allergic alveolitis, cryoglobulinaemia
T cell	Type IV ('delayed')	Macrophage activation (granuloma)	Contact dermatitis, sarcoidosis, Crohn's

mediated by IL-4/IL-5 from Th2 cells. IFNγ and other Th1 cytokines suppress IgE production. Chronic airway inflammation in asthma (which can have an atopic component) is multifaceted and involves Th2 cells and eosinophils → smooth muscle hypertrophy, bronchial hyper-responsiveness and intermittent airflow obstruction.

Immune-complex mediated

The characteristic feature is immune-complex (IC) deposition in tissues. Immune complexes are formed by the combination of soluble antigen with antibody. These are coated with complement C3b and transported to the spleen bound to C3b receptors on erythrocytes for removal by splenic macrophages. If excessive IC formation (or inadequate removal) occurs these may be deposited in tissues (skin, kidney, joints) and small vessels, leading to damage. Deposition is influenced by the size and solubility of ICs. Circulating antigen may also deposit in tissues leading to subsequent formation of ICs within the tissue. Persistent or repeated antigen exposure drives IC formation and may result from:

- Microbial antigens – in chronic infection (e.g. hepatitis C)
- Auto-antigens – in autoimmune disease (e.g. dsDNA in SLE)
- Environmental antigens (inhaled) – (e.g. mould spores in extrinsic allergic *alveolitis*)

Complement activation by immune complexes → neutrophil recruitment/activation→ tissue damage. Where immune complexes are deposited within the wall of small blood vessels the consequence is immune-complex mediated vasculitis. The clinical phenotype of immune-complex disease depends on the organs and tissues affected, but may include arthritis, glomerulonephritis and skin rashes, in addition to systemic symptoms such as fever, malaise and myalgia.

Extrinsic allergic alveolitis is an IgG-mediated allergy where persistent/repeated exposure to the allergen (e.g. aspergillus precipitans in 'Farmer's lung' or avian precipitans in 'Pigeon fancier's lung') → immune-complex deposition → chronic inflammation and pulmonary interstitial fibrosis.

T Cell-mediated

This form of allergic response requires hapten-specific Th cells which activate macrophages → granulomatous inflammation. Haptens are exogenous molecules (such as

BOX 4.11 PATHOPHYSIOLOGY AND TREATMENT OF ANAPHYLAXIS

Anaphylaxis – vasodilatation with hypotension and cardiovascular shock, ↑ capillary permeability with tissue oedema, smooth muscle contraction (bronchoconstriction and or GI contraction). Immediate life-saving treatment with intramuscular epinephrine reverses the bronchoconstriction and vasodilatation. Allergen identification and avoidance, and self-administered epinephrine are recommended for individuals with a history of anaphylaxis. Corticosteroids inhibit the late response mediated by eosinophil recruitment and activation. Antihistamines, sodium cromoglycate (mast cell stabiliser) and leukotriene receptor antagonists are additional treatment options for this type of allergy.

Certain drugs (opiates, contrast media, vancomycin) cause IgE independent mast cell degranulation. This is known as the *anaphylactoid* reaction, but is clinically indistinguishable from anaphylaxis. Mast cell tryptase is elevated in both cases for up to 24 hours.

Allergen immunotherapy (desensitisation) for severe IgE-mediated allergy involves repeated s.c. injections of increasing doses of allergen → induce tolerance.

nickel) that are conjugated to self-proteins and presented to T cells by antigen-presenting cells (such as Langerhans cells). Examples of T cell-mediated allergies included contact dermatitis. Identification of the relevant allergen usually requires patch testing.

Autoimmunity

Antibody-mediated

Occurs due to antibodies directed against cell-surface or extracellular matrix antigens → complement activation and FcR mediated phagocytosis or ADCC (there is often considerable overlap). Frustrated phagocytosis results when phagocytes bind antibodies against large extracellular matrix compartments (e.g. basement membranes in *Goodpasture's syndrome*) resulting in exocytosis of lysosomal and granule contents → tissue damage.

ABO incompatibility (major transfusion reaction) occurs when IgM against the donor (allogenic) erythrocyte blood group antigen results in widespread complement activation, donor erythrocyte agglutination and intra-vascular haemolysis. Antibodies to blood groups A and B develop without previous exposure to allogens due to the presence of identical carbohydrate epitopes on microbial glycoproteins. Blood type O is considered the universal donor as there is universal tolerance to the O group antigen.

There are several other clinical examples of antibody-mediated autoimmunity, where autoantibodies to cellular or tissue autoantigens resulting in complement-mediated or FcR mediated cytotoxicity or phagocytosis:

- *Autoimmune haemolytic anaemia* (AIHA, IgG → FcR mediated phagocytosis or IgM → complement-mediated lysis)
- *Idiopathic/immune thrombocytopenia* (ITP, IgG → FcR-mediated phagocytosis)
- Lupus anticoagulant (anticardiolipin IgG/IgM – and other antiphospholipid antibodies – target phospholipids on platelet membranes leading to pro-coagulable state)
- *Wegner's granulomatosis* (antiproteinase-3 IgG, a neutrophil membrane protein → direct neutrophil activation and tissue damage)
- *Pemphigus vulgaris* (IgG against antiepithelial junction adhesion molecules (desmoglein-1 and desmoglein-3) → skin splitting - mechanism unclear)

Treatment of antibody-mediated autoimmune diseases may involve:

- Non-specific anti-inflammatory or immunosuppressive drugs (e.g. corticosteroids in ITP, AIHA)
- Splenectomy if FcR mediated splenic removal by macrophages is the major cause (e.g. AIHA, ITP)
- Plasmapheresis to temporarily remove the autoantibody (e.g. Wegner's, Goodpastures)
- High dose IV immunoglobulin (IVIG, e.g. ITP)
- Specific immunotherapy including humanised monoclonal antibodies (see 'Cytotoxics' and 'Immunosuppressive drugs')

(IgG) Autoantibodies may also target normal cell-surface receptors, acting as antagonists:

- Post-synaptic acetylcholine receptors in *myasthenia gravis* or pre-synaptic voltage gated Ca^{++} channels in *Lambert-Eaton syndrome* (reduced acetylcholine release)

or agonists:

- TSH receptor autoantibodies → thyrotoxicosis (*Grave's disease*)

Immune-complex mediated

A few examples of disorders mediated by dysregulated production and deposition of immune-complexes are:

- *Systemic lupus erythematosis* (SLE)
- *Cryoglobulinaemia* (e.g. hepatitis C, myeloma)
- Osler's nodes, Roth spots and immune-complex glomerulonephritis in subacute bacterial endocarditis

IC deposition leads to complement consumption (↓ C3 and C4). ICs can be visualised in tissue biopsies using immunofluorescence.

Complement deficiency syndromes are associated with impaired solubilisation of ICs, leading to IC deposition (see 'Immunodeficiency').

T Cell-mediated

Th1-mediated macrophage activation → granulomatous inflammation (e.g. *sarcoidosis* and *inflammatory bowel disease*), although the specific self-antigens responsible remain unknown. In chronic infection with pathogens that resist killing, such as mycobacteria, granulomatous inflammation occurs with persistent antigen exposure. Th1 cells produce IFNγ → macrophage activation. Activated macrophages differentiate into epitheleoid and multi nucleate giant cells and produce TNFα, driving granuloma formation. Treatment of T cell-mediated hypersensitivity involves non-specific anti-inflammatories (e.g corticosteroids) and immunosuppressives (e.g. azathioprine, cyclosporin), although specific monoclonal antibody therapy plays an increasingly important role in severe cases (e.g. anti-TNFα monoclonal antibodies in Crohn's disease). See Box 4.12.

BOX 4.12 TUBERCULIN AND HYPERSENSITIVITY

The tuberculin skin test (TST) detects a dermal T cell-mediated delayed hypersensitivity response to injected mycobacterial antigens. IFNγ-release assays (IGRAs) detect IFNγ produced by TB-specific $CD4^+$ T cells *ex vivo*, indicating latent TB infection. It is important to screen individuals for latent TB with TST or IGRA before commencing anti-TNF monoclonal antibody therapy (see 'Immunological drugs').

Immunodeficiency

- Primary (inherited).
- Acquired (HIV infection, immunosuppressive drugs, malnutrition).

Primary immunodeficiency

Deficiency of any component of the innate or adaptive immune system may produce clinical consequences. Immunodeficiency should be considered in severe, persistent, unusual, or recurrent infections (mnemonic SPUR).

T Cell Immunodeficiency

Leads to recurrent infection with intracellular opportunistic pathogens (VZV, CMV, pneumocystis, mycobacteria, GI parasites—opportunistic infections, OI).

Antibody immunodeficiency

Leads to recurrent infection with extracellular encapsulated bacteria (e.g. *S. pneumoniae, S. aureus, H. influenza*). Syndromes linked to humoral immunodeficiency are described in Table 4.9 whilst syndromes linked to cellular immunodefiiciency are summarised in Table 4.10.

Innate immunodeficiency

Leads to spectrum of pathogens similar to humoral immunodeficiency (see Table 4.11).

Secondary immunodeficiency

- HIV infection (see Chapter 5 'Human immundeficiency virus', in 'Viruses').
- Immunosuppressive drugs (see 'Immunological drugs').

Table 4.9 Syndromes linked to humoral immunodeficiency

Syndrome	Deficiency	Cause	Consequence	Association
Secretory IgA deficiency	IgA	Unclear	Respiratory/GI tract infection	Autoimmunity
X-linked agammaglobulinaemia	B cells, all Igs	*XL:* deletion of *btk* gene	Recurrent sinusitis, pneumonia, otitis media after 6 months Bronchiectasis Presents in infancy, IVIG necessary	–
Hyper IgM	*XL:* B cell and T cell *AR:* B cell, IgG, IgA	*XL:* CD40L mutations *AR:* activation induced cytidine deaminase gene (B cell deficiency)	*XL:* combined immunodeficiency, may require BMT *AR:* recurrent sinusitis, pneumonia, otitis media after 6 months. Bronchiectasis. Presents in infancy, IVIG necessary	–
IgG subclass deficiency	IgG1-3 IgG4 deficiency tends not to be clinically relevant	Unclear	Recurrent sinusitis, pneumonia, chronic diarrhoea.*Treatment and diagnosis controversial:* only use IVIG if functional responses impaired	–
Thymoma with hypogammaglobulinaemia (may be regarded as secondary antibody deficiency)	All Igs	Benign or malignant tumour of thymus	Recurrent sinusitis, pneumonia, chronic diarrhoea Onset aged 40-60 Mediastinal mass	Pure red cell aplasia Myaesthenia gravis
Common variable immunodeficiency disorders (CVID)	Acquired defect in T-cell signalling to B cells	Unclear Associated with HLA-B8 and HLA-DR3	Recurrent sinusitis, pneumonia, chronic diarrhoea Bronchiectasis Intestinal parasites (e.g. *Giardia*) Onset in adulthood, treated with IVIG	Autoimmunity

- Malignancy (particularly haematological malignancies, myeloma).
- Metabolic disease (diabetes).
- Autoimmune diseases (rheumatoid arthritis, SLE).
- Drugs (phenytoin, colchicine).
- Nephrotic syndrome (Ig loss).
- Malnutrition.

Malnutrition

Has broad immunosuppressive effects, but predominantly affects cell-mediated immunity. In protein-energy malnutrition, a reduction in $CD4^+$ T cells and reduced $CD4^+/CD8^+$ ratio also → impaired antibody responses. Phagocytosis is also impaired. Opportunistic pathogens dominate, as in cell-mediated immunodeficiency. Many micronutrients (including vitamin A, zinc, selenium) are required for effective immune function.

Table 4.10 Syndromes linked to cellular immunodeficiency

Syndrome	Deficiency	Cause	Consequence	Association
Severe combined immunodeficiency (SCID)	Virtual absence of T-cells, thymic aplasia. Functional B-cell deficiency	XL defect in IL-2 receptor gene. *AR:* RAG-1 or RAG-2 deletion	Severe OI from birth, including PCP and mucosal candidiasis, overwhelming BCG if vaccinated, death within 2 years without BMT	–
Adenosine deaminase deficiency (subtype of SCID)	Virtual absence of T-cells, thymic aplasia. Functional B-cell deficiency	AR: accumulation of toxic purine metabolites in lymphoid stem cells	Severe OI from birth, including PCP and mucosal candidiasis, overwhelming BCG if vaccinated, death within 2 years without BMT	–
Purine nucleoside phosphorylase deficiency (subtype of SCID)	Virtual absence of T-cells, thymic aplasia Functional B-cell deficiency	AR: Accumulation of toxic purine metabolites in lymphoid stem cells	Severe OI from birth including PCP and mucosal candidiasis, overwhelming BCG if vaccinated, death within 2 years without BMT	-
MHC II deficiency	Deficiency of CD4+ T-cells	*AR:* deficiency of MHC II promoter proteins	Recurrent GI infections from infancy	–
Hereditary ataxia telangiectasia	T-cell number and function reduced, Variable IgA, IgG2 and IgG4 deficiency	AR: chromosomal defects on 7 and 14 (TCR and heavy chain Ig regions)	Severe respiratory tract infections	Susceptibility to ionizing radiation Ataxia Telangiectasia
Wiskott–Aldrich syndrome	Defective cytoskeletal T-cell function. Thrombocytopenia ↑ IgA, IgE, reduced IgM	XL	Recurrent pyogenic and OI	Severe eczema
DiGeorge syndrome	Thymic aplasia. Reduction in T-cell numbers	Deletion of chromosome 22q11.2	Variable susceptibility to infection	Cardiac malformations, cleft palate, hypocalcaemia

Table 4.11 Syndromes linked to innate immunodeficiency

Syndrome	Deficiency	Cause	Consequence	Associations
Classical pathway deficiency	C1q, C1s, C2, C4	*AR:* mutation in *C1q, C1s, C2,* or *C4* genes	Immune complex disease	SLE
Complement C3	C3	*AR:* mutation in *C3* gene	Recurrent pyogenic infection in childhood	–
C5–8 (terminal chain complement)	C5–8	*AR:* mutation in C5–8 genes	Recurrent *Neisseria* infection, requires vaccination	–
Mannose-binding lectin	MBL levels <0.1 μg/mL	Several distinct SNPs in MBL gene	Minimal in adulthood (10% of population affected)	↑ Risk of bacterial infections if HIV infected
Alternative pathway deficiency	*AP properdin or fD:* impaired amplification via AP activation	*AR:* mutation in *fD* gene*XL:* mutation in properdin gene	Recurrent *Neisseria* infection, requires vaccination	–
Leucocyte adhesion deficiency (LAD)	*Type 1:* LFA-1, CR3 and p150,95 deficiency.*Type 2:* failure of selectin synthesis. Impaired trans- endothelial migration. High peripheral blood neutrophil count	*Type 1:* ß-2 integrin gene mutation.*Type 2:* AR deficiency of fucosylated carbohydrate ligands	Delayed separation of the cord Recurrent pyogenic infection in childhood Spectrum of severity (BMT for most severe phenotype)	–
Chédiak–Higashi syndrome	Impaired phagolysosome formation due to intracellular defects of lysosome trafficking and degranulation, impaired degranulation of CTL	*AR:* deletion in *CHS1* gene encoding lysosome trafficking regulator protein LYST	Recurrent pyogenic infection in childhood. Accelerated phase (lymphoproliferative disorder) in adulthood associated with viral infection	Albinism, peripheral neuropathy, neutropenia
Chronic granulomatous disease (CGD)	*Defective NADPH oxidase:* impaired respiratory burst, results in type IV hypersensitivity and granuloma formation	*XL:* defect in cytochrome b_{558}.*AR:* defect in cytochrome b_{558}, $p47^{phox}$ or $p67^{phox}$	Staphylococcal pneumonia, abscesses, aspergillus infection. Treated with IFNγ	–
IFNγ deficiency	IL-12. IL-12R. IFNγR deficiency	*AR:* mutation in IL-12, IL-12R or IFNγR genes	Unable to form granulomas, susceptible to mycobacterial and salmonella infection. Treated with IFNγ	–

Transplantation

An expanding treatment modality for end-stage organ failure:

- Kidney.
- Bone marrow.
- Liver.
- Heart.
- Lung.
- Heart–lung.
- Skin (autograft).
- Pancreas.
- Small bowel.
- Complex tissue (e.g. hand, face).

Rejection of transplanted foreign tissue (allograft) is mediated by the adaptive immune system recognizing the tissue as foreign and destroying it with inflammatory responses. Immune-privileged tissue transplants (e.g. corneal) do not usually undergo rejection. Skin grafts are usually autografts. However, without immunosuppressive therapy, rejection is inevitable in all but identically HLA-matched allografts. With better HLA matching, less intense immunosuppression is required to prevent rejection.

Rejection has three phases:

- *Hyperacute:* hours, antibody mediated (ABO incompatibility)—treated by surgical removal.
- *Acute:* days to weeks, mediated by donor DCs presenting foreign antigen-MHC to host T cells. Predominantly cellular infiltrates, or complement deposition (C4d), may be seen on tissue biopsy.
- *Chronic—months to years:* predominantly arteriosclerosis (chronic allograft vasculopathy) with limited immunological component. Responds poorly to immunosuppression. Bronchiolitis obliterans is a form of chronic lung transplant rejection → progressive airflow obstruction.

Immunosuppressive therapies used to prevent rejection are summarized in 'Immunological drugs'. The combination of an antiproliferative agent (e.g. azathioprine), a calcineurin inhibitor (e.g. cyclosporin), and an anti-inflammatory agent (e.g. prednisolone) is typically used.

Graft versus host disease

Most rejection is host versus graft, mediated by host T lymphocytes recognizing donor MHC molecules. However, graft versus host disease (GvHD) arises following bone marrow transplantation, when donor T cells react to host MHC molecules → severe skin and gut tissue damage. GvHD requires enhanced immunosuppression. The risk of GvHD is reduced by adequate HLA matching and T-cell depletion of the graft.

Immunological tests

In general, immunological tests (see Table 4.12) are measures of:

- Quantity (e.g. Ig levels, lymphocyte subsets).
- Function (e.g. Ig response to immunization, complement function).

Table 4.12 Tests for different components of the immune system

	Test	Description	Abnormal In
Inflammation	ESR	Rate of sedimentation of erythrocytes in tube (mm/hr)	Inflammatory conditions: non-specific
	CRP (pneumococcal complement-reactive protein)	ELISA and other immunoassays. Increase within 6-12 hours, peaking at 48 hours	Inflammatory conditions: non-specific. CRP not usually elevated in SLE unless infection present (or polyserositis) CRP ↑↑ in pneumococcal infection.
	Procalcitonin	Precursor peptide of calcitonin. Normally undetectable in health, measured by commercial immunoassays Released within 2-3 hours, peaking at 6-12 hours of bacterial infection	Sensitive and specific for bacterial infection Used in research studies to differentiate septic from cardiogenic shock, and to limit antibiotic prescribing in respiratory infection
Complement	Individual Levels (C3, C4, etc.)	Measured by nephelometry, ELISA	C3, C4 ↓ by complement consumption in Type III hypersensitivity (immune-complex deposition) Individual components ↓ by deficiency
	AP50 total haemolytic component	Functional activity of alternative pathway: Mg^{2+} dependent lysis of rabbit RBCs by test serum	Alternative pathway component deficiency
	CH50 total haemolytic component	Functional activity of classical pathway: Ca^{2+} dependent lysis of IgM-sensitized sheep RBCs by test serum	Classical pathway component deficiency

(*continued*)

Table 4.12 Tests for different components of the immune system (*continued*)

	Test	Description	Abnormal In
	C3 nephritic factor	Indicated for unexplained ↓ C3 Identifies autoantibody to C3 convertase	Mesangial capillary nephritis in renal failure Present in some individuals with lipoatrophy
	C1 inhibitor: immunochemical	ELISA	Type I hereditary angioedema
	C1 inhibitor: functional	Chromogenic assay of C1 functional activity	Type I and II hereditary angioedema
Antibodies	Antibody levels	Nephelometry, ELISA	↓ Hypogammaglobulinaemia (all causes) ↑ IgA: alcoholic liver disease ↑ IgM: acute infection, primary biliary cirrhosis ↑ IgG: chronic infection, chronic inflammation, autoimmune hepatitis etc Polyclonal ↑: HIV
	IgG subsets	Immunoassay (various)	IgG subclass deficiency
	Serum (urine) electrophoresis	Electrophoresis for Ig light chains (Bence–Jones proteins)	MGUS Multiple myeloma, Waldenstrom's macroglobulinaemia
	Functional Abs	Specific antibody response to protein or polysaccharide vaccines	Humoral immunodeficiency
Cell-mediated	Lymphocyte subsets	Flow cytometry. Surface staining for CD3, CD4, CD8, CD19, CD56	HIV monitoring CVID diagnosis SCID diagnosis Malnutrition
	Beta-2 microglobulin	MHC I component	Elevated in lymphoma, myeloma etc i.e. increased turnover of lymphocytes
Phagocytosis	Phagocytosis	DHR tests	Negative in chronic granulomatous disease
Allergy	Total IgE	Immunoassay (ELISA)	Atopy, parasitic infection
	Allergen-specific IgE	Identifies allergen-specific IgE	Atopic conditions
	Tryptase	Immunoassay	Anaphylaxis Anaphylactoid reactions Mastocytosis
	Skin prick test	Intra-epidermal injection of allergen panel with histamine positive control and negative control	Atopic conditions
Autoantibodies	Coombs' test (direct antiglobulin test)	RBC autoantibodies RBC washed and incubated with antiglobulin (Coomb's reagent)	Autoimmune haemolytic anaemia
	Rheumatoid Factor	Autoantibodies directed against Fc component of IgG	Rheumatoid arthritis (80%)
	c-ANCA	Immunofluorescence/ELISA	Wegener's granulomatosis
	Anti Proteinase-3 (PR3)	ELISA	Wegener's granulomatosis (more specific than c-ANCA)

Table 4.12 Tests for different components of the immune system (*continued*)

	Test	Description	Abnormal In
	p-ANCA	Immunofluorescence/ELISA	Churg-Strauss Syndrome Microscopic polyarteritis, Polyarteritis nodosa, Primary sclerosing cholangitis, Glomerulonephritis
	Anti Myeloperoxidase (MPO)	ELISA	Churg-Strauss Syndrome Microscopic polyarteritis etc. (more specific than p-ANCA)
	Anti-TTG (tissue transglutaminase)	ELISA for anti-TTG IgA (use IgG if IgA deficiency)	Coeliac disease
	Anti-nuclear antibody	Immunofluorescence, ELISA	Various – SLE, scleroderma, mixed connective tissue disease etc.
	Anti-dsDNA	Immunoblot, ELISA, (immunodiffusion)	SLE
	Anti-RNP (ribonucleoprotein)	Immunoblot, ELISA (immunodiffusion)	Mixed connective tissue disease
	Anti-Smith (Sm)	Immunoblot, ELISA (immunodiffusion)	SLE (only 25%)
	Anti-Ro	Immunoblot, ELISA (immunodiffusion)	Sjogren's syndrome
	Anti-La	Immunoblot, ELISA (immunodiffusion)	Sjogren's syndrome
	Anti-Scl-70	Immunoblot, ELISA (immunodiffusion)	Scleroderma
	Anti-histone	Immunoblot, ELISA	SLE (H1 and H2B) and drug-induced lupus (H2A-H2B and H3-H4)
	Anti-smooth muscle	Immunoblot, ELISA	Autoimmune hepatitis, sclerosing cholangitis
	Anti-mitochondrial	Immunoblot, ELISA	Primary biliary sclerosis
	Anti-liver kidney microsomal-1	Immunoblot, ELISA	Autoimmune hepatitis
Immune complexes	Immunofluorescence on tissue biopsies	Immunofluorescence for autoantibody (e.g. pemphigus or immune complexes (e.g. lupus nephritis) in tissues	Antibody or immune complex mediated disorders
	Cryoglobulins	Spectrophotometry of cryoglobulins – cryocrit Subsequent immunofixation/ELISA	Type I-III cryoglobulinaemia Associated with low C4 Hepatitis B, C and type III hypersensitivity
	Precipitans (avian, fungal)	Immunoassay for specific IgG	ABPA (type I + III hypersensitivity) EAA Invasive aspergillosis (not sensitive)

Immunological drugs

For a table of immunological drugs and their properties (see Table 4.13).

Table 4.13 Immunological drugs

	Therapy	Mechanism(s) of action	Effects	Toxicity	Indications	Interactions
Anti-inflammatories	Paracetamol	Prostaglandin inhibitor	Antipyretic. Analgesic	Hepatotoxicity		–
	Aspirin	Prostaglandin inhibitor (COX-1)	Antipyretic. Analgesic. Antiplatelet	GI haemorrhage		Caution with anticoagulants
	NSAIDs	Prostaglandin inhibitor (COX-1)	Antipyretic. Analgesic	GI haemorrhage Interstitial nephritis Hyperkalaemia		Caution with anticoagulants
	Corticosteroid	Mediated via intracellular glucocorticoid receptor (involved in regulation of 1% of total genes)	Antipyretic. Inhibits T-cell activation, induces lymphocyte and eosinophil apoptosis, reduce pro-inflammatory cytokine secretion, reduce adhesion molecule expression	Mood disturbance. GI haemorrhage. Hypertension. Osteoporosis. Avascular necrosis. Skin thinning. NIDDM	Allograft rejection type I–IV hypersensitivity. Reduce CNS inflammation (meningitis, SOL) GvHD	*Metabolized via CYP450:* ↑ levels with inhibitors of CYP450 (erythromycin, carbamazepine, ritonavir), ↓ levels with inducers of CYP450 (rifampicin, phenytoin, efavirenz)
Antiproliferative agents	Azathioprine	Purine antagonist (competes with inosine monophosphate)	Active on dividing cells. Preferentially inhibits T-cell proliferation, also reduces B-cell numbers and NK cell function	Hepatotoxicity. Bone marrow toxicity. Hypersensitivity reactions	Allograft rejection Type I–IV hypersensitivity. Steroid-sparing agent	Allopurinol increases toxicity. Check TPMT levels pre-treatment
	Methotrexate	Folate antagonist	Inhibits immunoglobulin synthesis. Inhibits neutrophil activation (anti-inflammatory)	Hepatotoxicity. Lung fibrosis. Bone marrow toxicity	Allograft rejection. Treatment of hypersensitivity. Type I–IV. Steroid-sparing agent	Aspirin and NSAIDs may increase levels
	Lefluonamide	Inhibits pyrimidine nucleotide synthesis	Inhibits T and B-cell proliferation. Inhibits antibody production	Hypertension. Bone marrow toxicity	Treatment of hypersensitivity type I–IV	Toxicity ↑ with methotrexate
	Mycophenolate mofetil	Reversible inhibitor of inosine monophosphate	Inhibits T and B-cell proliferation. Inhibits adhesion factor expression	GI disturbance GI haemorrhage	Allograft rejection. Treatment of hypersensitivity type II–III	Levels ↓ by rifampicin
Alkylating agent	Cyclophosphamide	DNA cross-linking agent	Reduces B and T-cell numbers and function	Bone marrow toxicity. Haemorrhagic cystitis	Type III hypersensitivity. Multiple sclerosis. Allograft rejection	↑ Risk of cytotoxicity with pentostatin and clofazimine (agranulocytosis)
Calcineurin inhibitors	Cyclosporin	Bind to cyclophilins inhibiting calcineurin	Inhibits T-cell proliferation, B-cell function and antigen presentation	Hypertension. Renal dysfunction. Hyperkalaemia ↑ risk of skin cancer	Allograft rejection. Treatment of hypersensitivity type I–IV. Steroid-sparing agent GvHD	Drugs causing renal dysfunction and hyperkalaemia (e.g. ACE inhibitors, NSAIDs). Metabolized by CYP450

Table 4.13 Cytotoxics and immunosuppressive drugs (*continued*)

	Therapy	Mechanism(s) of action	Effects	Toxicity	Indications	Interactions
	Tacrolimus	Bind to FK inhibiting calcineurin	Inhibits T-cell proliferation, B-cell function and antigen presentation	GI disturbance. Renal dysfunction. Cardiomyopathy	Allograft rejection. Treatment of hypersensitivity type I–IV	Drugs causing renal dysfunction. Metabolized by CYP450 (see above)
mTOR inhibitors	Rapamycin (sirolimus)	Inhibition of IL-2 dependent signal transduction pathways	Varied effects, may decrease IL-2 response, but may increase memory responses. Inhibits vascular smooth muscle proliferation	Lipid abnormalities. Bone marrow toxicity. Thromboembolism	Allograft rejection	Metabolized by CYP450 (see above)
Monoclonal antibodies and/or fusion proteins	Rituximab	Anti-CD20 mAb	Depletes B cells	Cytokine release syndrome. Hypotension, dysrhythmia, bone marrow toxicity PML	Type II–III hypersensitivity	Caution with other immunosuppressive therapy
	Alemtuzumab	Anti-CD52 mAb	Depletes B cells, T cells, NK cells, granulocytes, monocytes	Cytokine release syndrome. Hypotension, dysrhythmia, bone marrow toxicity	Allograft rejection GvHD. Hypersensitivity	Caution with other immunosuppressive therapy
	Infliximab, Adalimumab	Anti-TNFα mAb	Inhibits TNFα	As above + TB reactivation (screen for latent TB)	Treatment of hypersensitivity type III–IV	Caution with other immunosuppressive therapy
	Certolizumab pegol	Anti-TNFα pegylated FAb fragment	Inhibits TNFα	As above	Treatment of hypersensitivity type III–IV	Caution with other immunosuppressive therapy
	Etanercept	Fusion protein of TNFR2 with IgG1 Fc	Inhibits TNFα (soluble TNF receptor)	As above	Treatment of hypersensitivity type III–IV	Caution with other immunosuppressive therapy
	Abatacept	*Fusion protein of CTLA-4 and IgG:* inhibits B7 co-stimulation	Prevents co-stimulation by APC via B7 binding	As above	Type III–IV hypersensitivity	Caution with other immunosuppressive therapy
	Tocilizumab	Anti Il-6R mAb	Binds IL-6R	As above	Rheumatoid arthritis	Caution with other immunosuppressive therapy
	Natalizumab	Anti-α4 integrin	Inhibits leucocyte migration	PML. Systemic symptoms	Relapsing: remitting MS Crohn's disease	Caution with other immunosuppressive therapy
Cytokines	Pegylated Interferon α	Recombinant IFNα	Type I IFN	Bone marrow toxicity, fatigue, skin rashes, depression, lowers seizure threshold	Chronic HCV and HBV infection	Myelosuppressive drugs
	Interferon ß	Recombinant IFNß	Type I IFN	Bone marrow toxicity, fatigue, skin rashes, depression, lowers seizure threshold	Relapsing: remitting MS	Myelosuppressive drugs

Multiple choice questions

1. Which of the following are *not* recognized barriers to infection?

A. Secretory IgA.
B. Defensins.
C. Lysozyme.
D. Airway cilia.
E. Bladder emptying.

2. Which of the following is true of trans-endothelial migration?

A. Cellular activation is mediated by adhesins.
B. Selectins are secreted proteins responsible for regulating cellular migration within tissues.
C. Arrest of leucocytes is mediated by ICAM-LFA-1 interaction.
D. Chemotaxins are not involved in cellular activation.
E. Up-regulation of chemotaxin receptors mediates leucocyte arrest.

3. In T-cell development (select one):

A. $CD4^+$ T cells are selected for high binding affinity to MHC II.
B. $CD8^+$ T cells are selected for binding to self-peptides loaded on MHC I.
C. Immature thymocytes are $CD4^-CD8^-$ or $CD4^+CD8^+$.
D. Antigen specificity is determined by CD3.
E. T-cell development is independent of IL-7.

4. Which one of the following statements regarding antibodies is false:

A. IgG is the major serum cytokine.
B. IgM predominates in the primary response.
C. IgA is secreted as a monomer.
D. IgE is present at low levels in the serum.
E. IgD forms the B-cell receptor.

5. Regarding hypersensitivity reactions (select one):

A. Anaphylaxis is a type II hypersensitivity reaction.
B. The tuberculin skin test is an example of delayed-type hypersensitivity.
C. Type III hypersensitivity is characterized by elevated serum complement C3.
D. Extrinsic allergic alveolitis is an example of type I hypersensitivity.
E. Mast cell degranulation is a key effector response in type II hypersensitivity.

6. Which of the following is likely to be most effective in the treatment of hyperacute allograft rejection?

A. Surgical graft removal.
B. Corticosteroid.
C. Rituximab (anti-CD20 mAb).
D. Calcineurin inhibitor.
E. Azathioprine.

7. A 2-year-old is investigated for recurrent pneumonia and otitis media, following a recent admission with *S. pneumoniae* bacteraemia. The following tests of complement are reported:

- C3: 4 mg/dL (N 65–190 mg/dL).
- C4: 43 mg/dL (N 15–50 mg/dL).

Total haemolytic component CH50: 52 U/L (N 150–250 U/L). Which of the following is the most likely diagnosis?

A. C1 inhibitor deficiency.
B. Terminal chain component deficiency.
C. Immune complex deposition disorder.
D. C3 deficiency.
E. C1r deficiency.

8. A 34-year-old female zookeeper is investigated for episodic haemoptysis and nasal stuffiness.

Hb 10.1	Urea 12.2	CXR—diffuse interstitial changes	c-ANCA (awaited)
MCV 89	Creat 298	Urinalysis: Protein: +++	p-ANCA (awaited)
Neut 7.2	Albumin 32	Blood: +++	Anti-PR-3 +ve
Lymp 1.4	CRP 140	*Urine protein:* 1.2 g/24 hr	Anti-MPO –ve
Eos 0.6	ESR 98	*Microscopy:* RBC casts	Anti-GBM –ve

What is the most likely diagnosis:

A. Churg–Strauss syndrome.
B. Hanta virus infection.
C. Goodpasture's syndrome.
D. Extrinsic allergic alveolitis.
E. Wegner's granulomatosis.

9. Which of the following is considered a function of NKT cells?

A. Mucosal immunity.
B. Immune regulation.
C. Antibody-dependent cellular cytotoxicity.
D. Killing virus-infected cells.
E. IL-17 production.

10. Calcineurin inhibitors:

A. Include sirolimus.
B. Induce DNA cross-links.
C. Inhibit IL-2 dependent signal transduction.
D. Bind cyclophilin/FK.
E. Include mycophenolate mofetil.

For answers, please see Appendix: Answers to multiple choice questions, page 313.

CHAPTER 5

Infectious diseases

Bacteria

Bacteria are single celled prokaryotic micro organisms (i.e. they lack a membrane-bound nucleus). They are cocci, bacilli, or spiral in shape. Almost all bacteria have a cell wall made of peptidoglycan. Bacteria may be divided into two groups: Gram positive (+ve) or Gram negative (-ve) on their ability of this cell wall to retain a complex of crystal violet and iodine—the Gram stain. Some bacteria have very waxy envelopes that make them acid-fast, meaning that once stained with strong carbol fuchsin dye, they resist decolourization with acid (Ziehl–Neelsen stain). Some bacteria are enclosed within a capsule which helps them resist phagocytosis (Table 5.1).

Bacteria vary in their oxygen requirements. *Anaerobic* bacteria have a lack of catalase and superoxide dimutase enzyme, and so have decreased ability to eliminate toxic products of aerobic metabolism. *Obligate anaerobes* have an absolute requirement for oxygen and are killed by traces of oxygen (e.g. bacteroides fragilis). *Facultative anaerobes* can survive in the absence, as well as the presence of oxygen (e.g. *E. coli*). *Aerotolerant* organisms can survive in air, but grow better anaerobically (e.g. *Clostridium*) and *micro-aerophyllic* organisms require lower concentrations of oxygen to grow (e.g. *Campylobacter*).

Virulence mechanisms

The capacity of an organism to cause disease is determined by its intrinsic virulence factors. These mechanisms include:

- *Adhesion:*
  - Creation of biofilm.
  - Attachment to host cell receptors.
- *Cell damage:*
  - Toxin mediated.
  - Enzyme mediated.
  - Direct invasion.
- *Evasion from host defences:*
  - *Structure*—e.g. bacterial capsule inhibits phagocytosis.
  - *Inhibition of host immune responses*—e.g. producing proteins that bind host antibodies.

Endotoxins and exotoxins

Toxins are key mediators of bacterial virulence. *Exotoxins* are polypeptides secreted by certain gram +ve and gram –ve organisms (Table 5.2). *Endotoxins* are an integral part of gram negative organisms' cell wall, typically released on cell death, usually composed of lipopolysaccharide and important for mediated Gram –ve associated septic shock (see Figs 5.1–5.6 for classification of Gram +ve and Gram –ve cocci, rods and organisms).

Resistance to anti-microbial agents

Resistance to antimicrobial agents increases the virulence of bacteria. Potential mechanisms of antibiotic resistance in bacterium include;

- Production of enzymes that inactivate the antibiotic, e.g. β lactamases.
- Modification of the antibiotic target, e.g. penicillin-binding proteins in cell wall.

Table 5.1 Key encapsulated and intracellular bacterium

Encapsulated bacterium	Bacterium lacking a cell wall	Intracellular bacterium
Haemophilus influenza *Strep. pneumoniae* *Neisseria meningitides* *Klebsiella pneumonia* *Salmonella typhi*	*Mycoplasma* spp.*	*Obligate: Chlamydia* spp. and *Rickettsia* *Optional: Mycobacterium* spp. and *Brucella* spp.

*Mycoplasma are therefore not seen on gram stain and are resistant to antibiotics targeting the cell wall synthesis

Table 5.2 Key exotoxins producing organisms

Organism	Type of exotoxin	Action	Disease
Staphylococcus aureus †Laboratory tests to aid identification of organism	Enterotoxins	Superantigen	Food poisoning
	Toxic shock syndrome toxin	Superantigen	Toxic shock syndrome
	Exfoliative toxins		Scalded skin syndrome
	Coagulase†	Clots plasma	
	DNAse†	Hydrolyses DNA	
	Catalase†	Hydrolyses hydrogen peroxide	
Streptococcus pyogenes	Haemolytic		
Vibrio cholerae	Enterotoxin	Increased cAMP production	Cholera
Clostridium botulinum	Neurotoxin	Blocks acetylcholine release at neuromuscular junction	Botulism and diarrhoea
Clostridium difficile	*Toxin A:* enterotoxin *Toxin B:* cytotoxin		
Clostridium perfringens			Gas gangrene and food poisoning
Clostridium tetani	Tetanospasm	Block GABA and glycine release	Tetanus
Bacillus cerus	Enterotoxins	Superantigen and increased cAMP production	Food poisoning
Bacillus anthracis	Cytotoxin	Increased cAMP production	Cutaneous and pulmonary anthrax
Corynebacterium		Inhibits protein synthesis	Diphtheria
Shigella		Inhibits protein synthesis	Dysentery
E. coli	Enterotoxins	Increased cAMP production	
E. coli 0157	*Shigella*-like toxin		
Salmonella typhi and *S. paratyphi*	Enterotoxins		
Legionella pneumophilia	Numerous	Cell lysis	
Pseudomonas aeruginosa		Inhibits protein synthesis	
Bordetella pertussis	Pertussis toxin	Increased cAMP production	Whooping cough
*Aspergillus flavus**	Aflatoxin B1	Carcinogenic	Hepatocellular carcinoma
*Entamoeba histolytica**	Enterotoxin	Cell lysis	Amoebic dysentery

*Not bacterium.

- Decreased permeability of the bacterial cell wall to the antibiotic.
- Active export of the antibiotic from bacteria by 'efflux pump'.

Bacterium can develop antibiotic resistance through a chromosomal mutation during replication or by acquiring new genetic material in a number of potential ways:

- *Transformation:* certain bacteria (e.g. *Strep. pneumoniae*, *H. influenza*) are able to 'take up' free DNA fragments from related species across their cell wall.
- *Conjugation:* bacterial 'mating'. Direct transfer of genetic material (e.g. plasmids) between bacterium involving cell-to-cell contact. The most important mechanism for transfer drug resistance genes, e.g. spread of extended beta lactam (ESBL) resistance.
- *Transduction:* transfer of genetic material by infection with a bacteriophage, e.g. penicillin resistance in *Staphylococcus*.

Spirochaetes

These are spiral-shaped bacteria that are extremely difficult to culture. Diagnosis is usually by serological testing. The main pathogenic genera are *Treponema pallidum* subspecies, *Borrelia* and *Leptospira* (see Table 5.3).

They remain highly sensitive to penicillins and tetracyclines. *Jarisch–Herxheimer* reactions can rarely occur mediated by pro-inflammatory cytokine release (TNF-alpha) in response to killing of organisms by antibiotic.

All endemic treponema infections (yaws, pinta, bejel) give false positive syphilis serology.

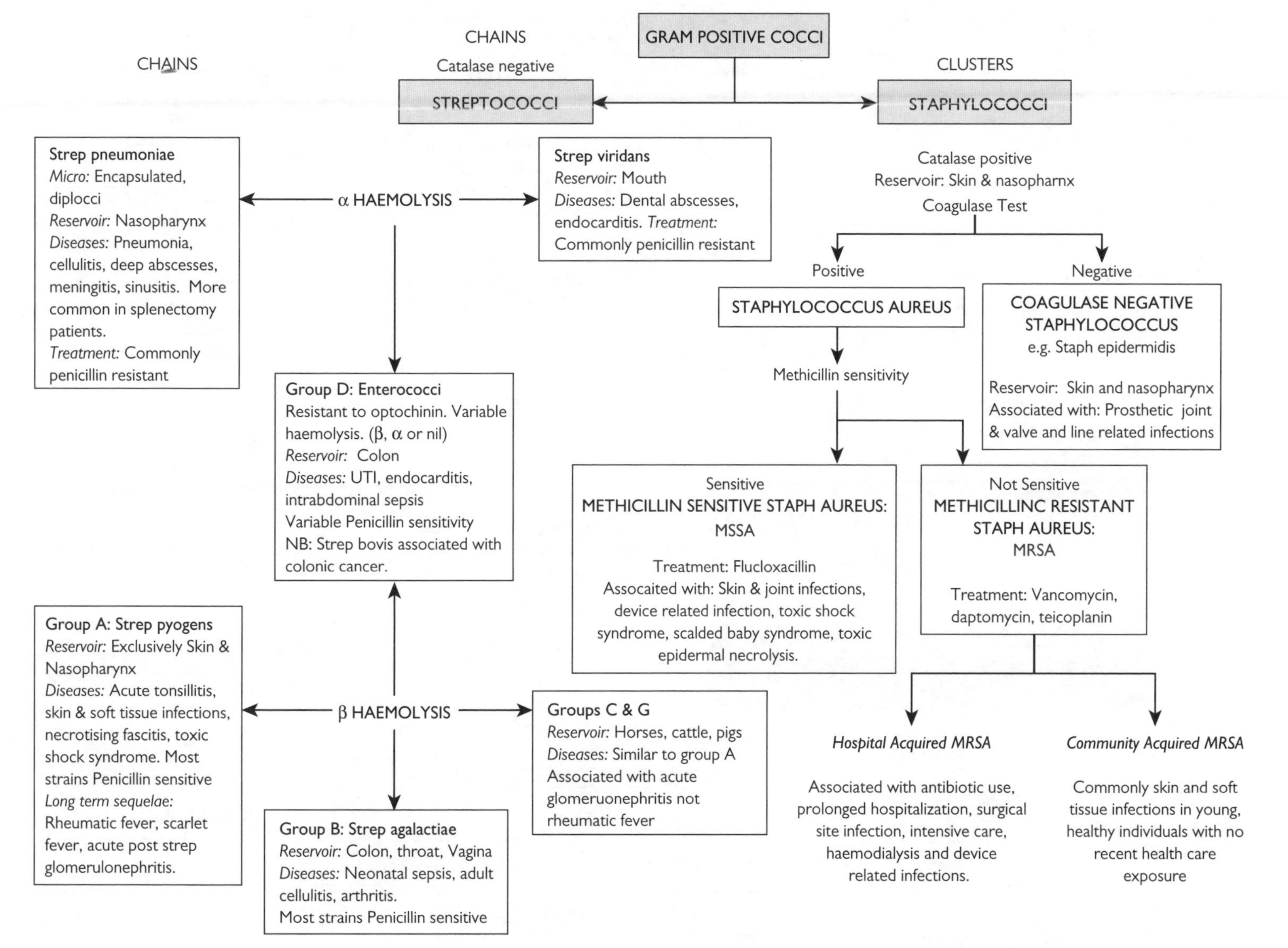

Fig. 5.1 Classification of gram positive cocci.

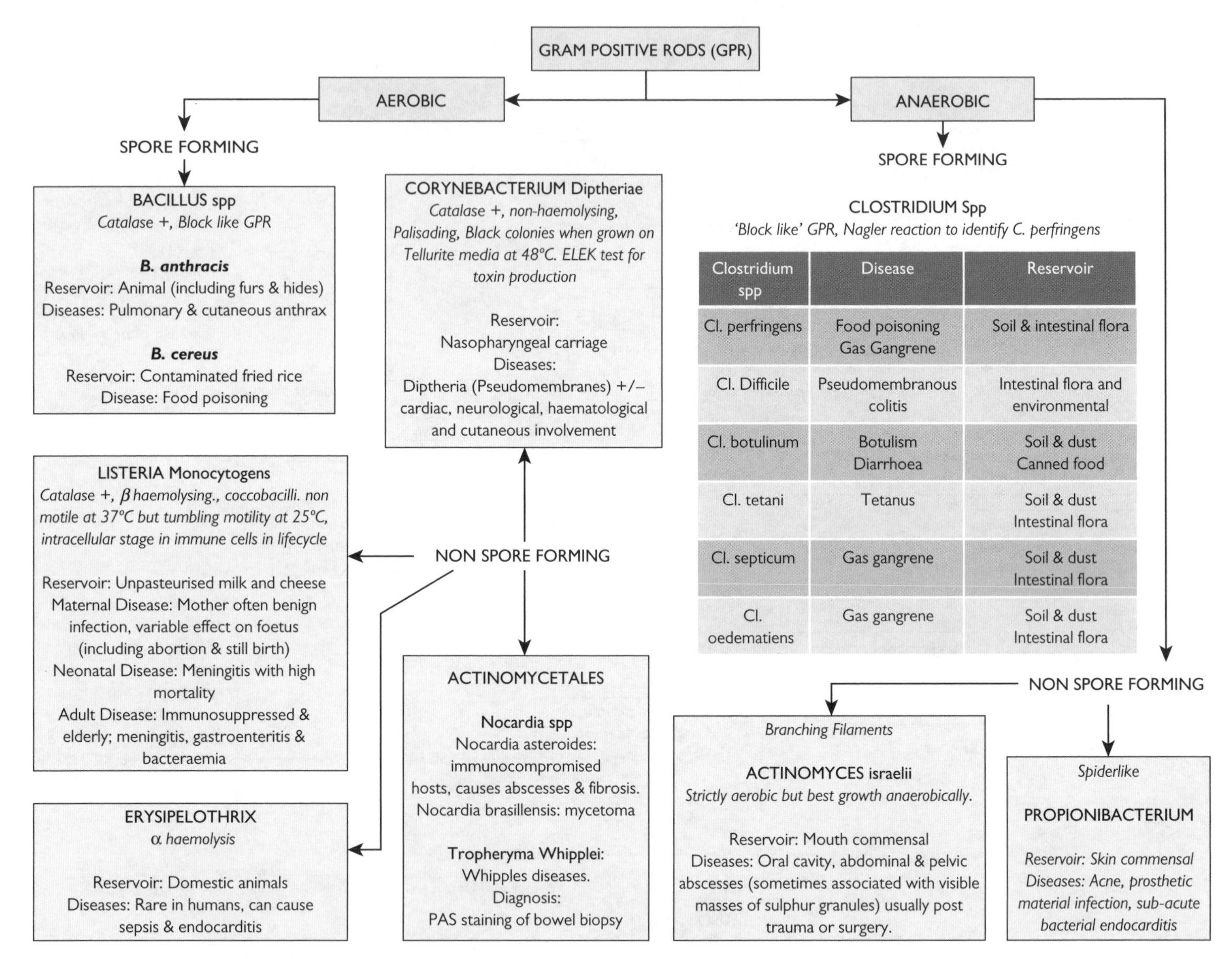

Clostridium spp	Disease	Reservoir
Cl. perfringens	Food poisoning Gas Gangrene	Soil & intestinal flora
Cl. Difficile	Pseudomembranous colitis	Intestinal flora and environmental
Cl. botulinum	Botulism Diarrhoea	Soil & dust Canned food
Cl. tetani	Tetanus	Soil & dust Intestinal flora
Cl. septicum	Gas gangrene	Soil & dust Intestinal flora
Cl. oedematiens	Gas gangrene	Soil & dust Intestinal flora

Fig. 5.2 Classification of gram positive rods.

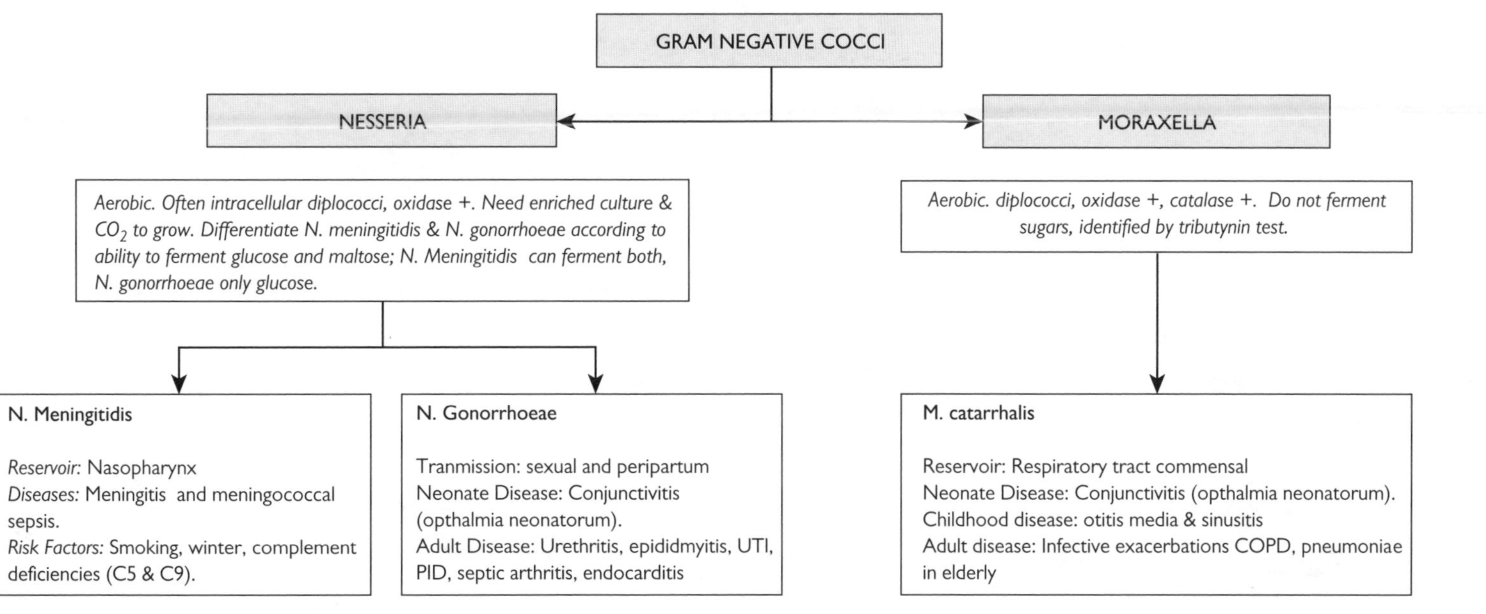

Fig. 5.3 Classification of gram negative cocci.

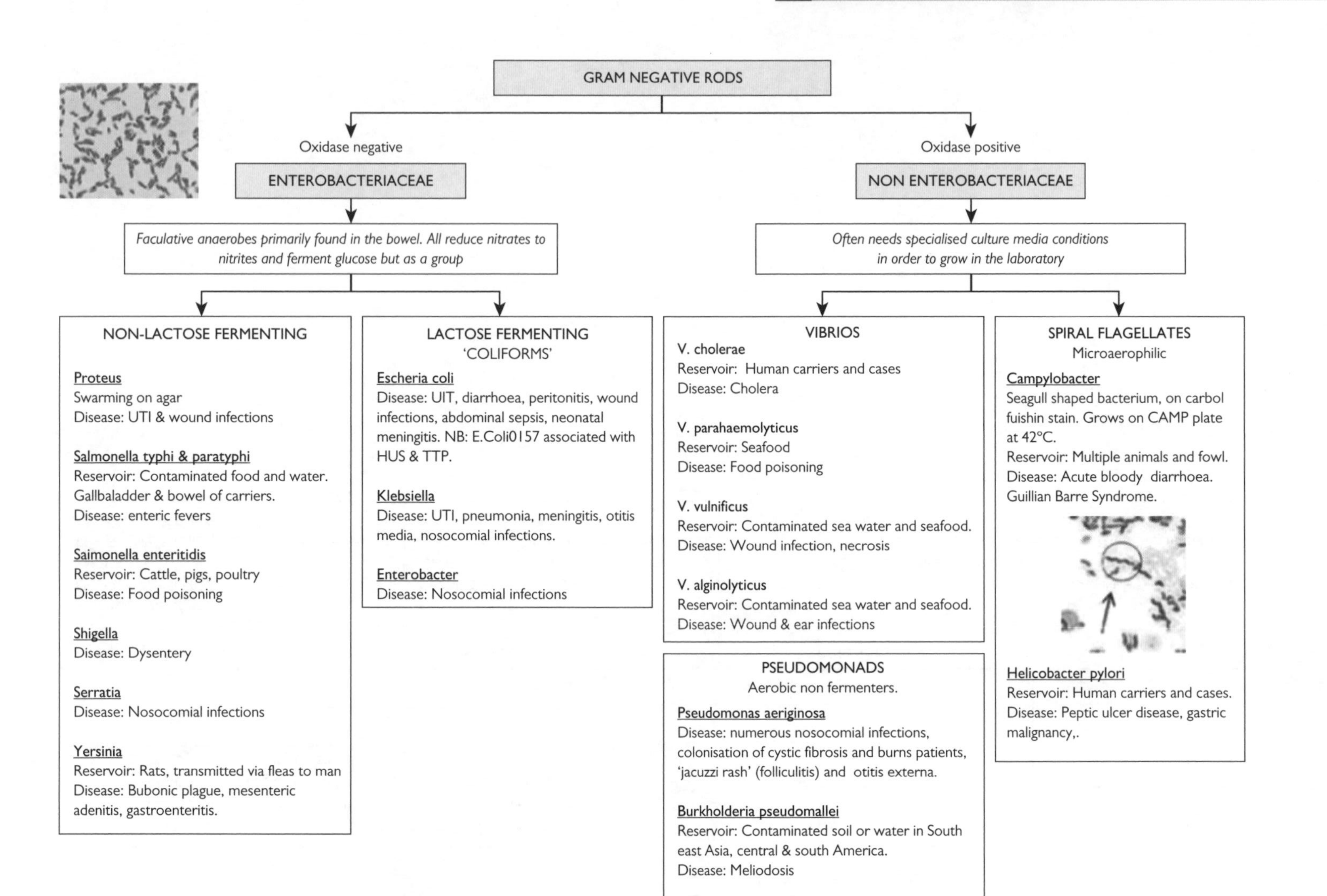

Fig. 5.4 Classification of gram positive rods.

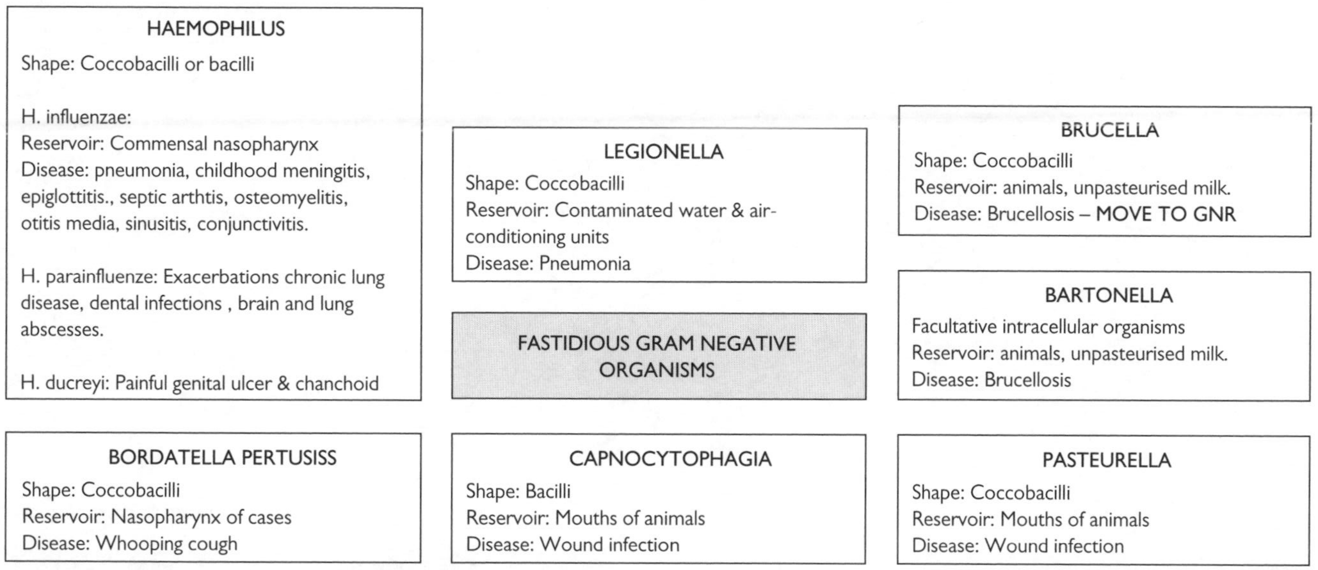

HAEMOPHILUS

Shape: Coccobacilli or bacilli

H. influenzae:
Reservoir: Commensal nasopharynx
Disease: pneumonia, childhood meningitis, epiglottitis., septic arthtis, osteomyelitis, otitis media, sinusitis, conjunctivitis.

H. parainfluenze: Exacerbations chronic lung disease, dental infections , brain and lung abscesses.

H. ducreyi: Painful genital ulcer & chanchoid

LEGIONELLA

Shape: Coccobacilli
Reservoir: Contaminated water & air-conditioning units
Disease: Pneumonia

BRUCELLA

Shape: Coccobacilli
Reservoir: animals, unpasteurised milk.
Disease: Brucellosis – **MOVE TO GNR**

FASTIDIOUS GRAM NEGATIVE ORGANISMS

BARTONELLA

Facultative intracellular organisms
Reservoir: animals, unpasteurised milk.
Disease: Brucellosis

BORDATELLA PERTUSISS

Shape: Coccobacilli
Reservoir: Nasopharynx of cases
Disease: Whooping cough

CAPNOCYTOPHAGIA

Shape: Bacilli
Reservoir: Mouths of animals
Disease: Wound infection

PASTEURELLA

Shape: Coccobacilli
Reservoir: Mouths of animals
Disease: Wound infection

Fig. 5.5 Classification of fastidious gram negative organisms.

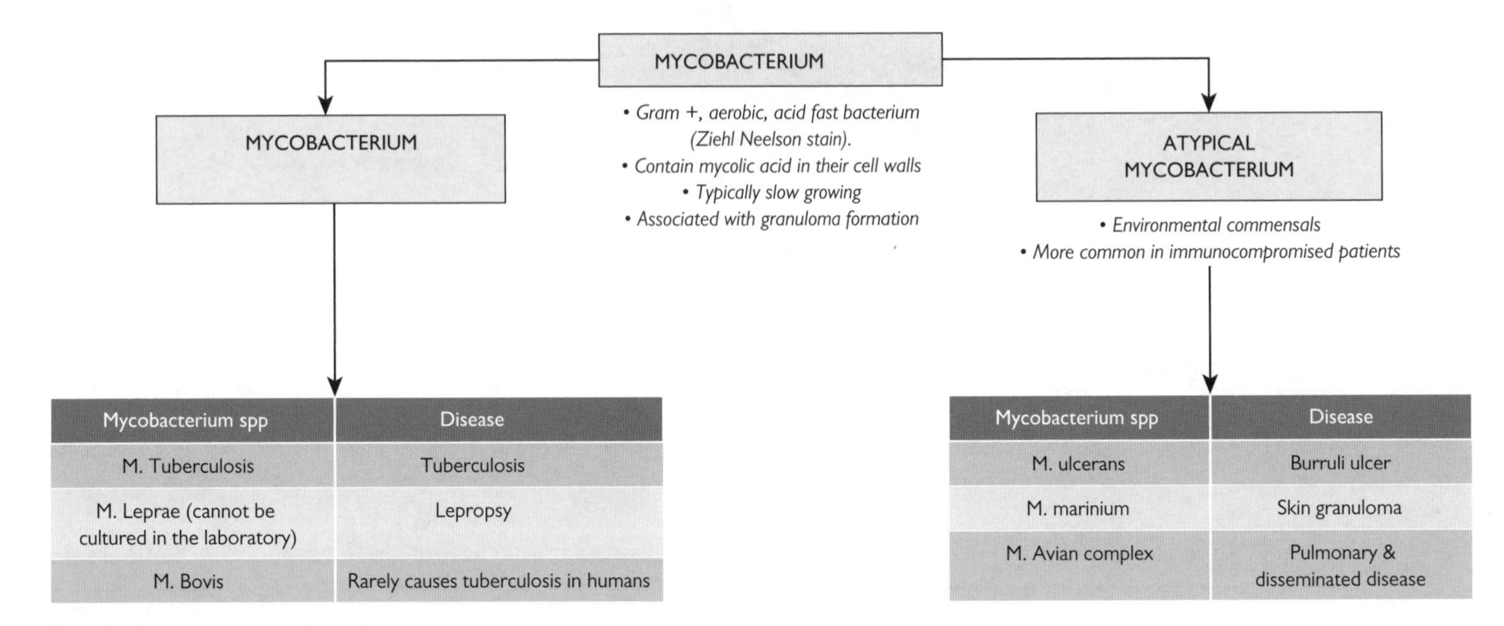

Mycobacterium spp	Disease
M. Tuberculosis	Tuberculosis
M. Leprae (cannot be cultured in the laboratory)	Lepropsy
M. Bovis	Rarely causes tuberculosis in humans

Mycobacterium spp	Disease
M. ulcerans	Burruli ulcer
M. marinium	Skin granuloma
M. Avian complex	Pulmonary & disseminated disease

Fig. 5.6 Classification of mycobacterium.

Table 5.3 Selected Spirochaetes

Genus/species	Disease	Transmission	Clinical features	Diagnosis	Treatment
Treponema pallidum ssp.					
T. pallidum	Syphilis	Mucosal contact (sexual)	*Early:* *Primary:* painless ulcer ± adenopathy *Secondary:* Palmo-plantar skin rash, systemic upset *Late:* Neurosyphilis-meningoencephalitis; chorioretinitis; tabes dorsalis Cardiac involvement; Gummata	Dark-field microscopy (swab): Spirochaetes *Serology:* VDRL/RPR + EIA + TPPA	IV/IM penicillin *Early:* IM benzathene penicillin × 1 *Late:* IM procaine (daily)/benzathene penicillin (×3) IV benzylpenicillin + probenicid Monitor VDRL over time for treatment response (should become negative)
T. pertunae	Yaws	Mucosal (non-sexual)	Skin and bone involvement Tropics	Serology (see above)	IV penicillin (or doxycycline)
T. endemicum	Endemic syphilis 'Bejel'	Mucosal (non-sexual)	Skin and bone involvement Sub-tropics (India, Africa, etc.)	Serology (see above)	IV penicillin (or doxycycline)
T. carateum	Pinta	Skin/mucosal contact	Skin changes only Latin America	Serology (see above)	IV penicillin (or doxycycline)
Borrelia					
B. burgdorferi	Lyme disease	Tick (Ixodes)	*Early:* Erythema chronicum migrans (central-clearing rash) Cardiac and neurological involvement possible (cranial, peripheral nerve lesions, transient carditis) *Late:* Arthritis (chronic synovitis) Neuroboreliosis (painful radiculopathy) Carditis (complete heart block)	*ECM:* clinical *Others:* blood ± CSF ELISA plus Western Blot (false negative serology extremely unusual) CSF PCR rarely helpful	Oral doxycycline IV ceftriaxone for CVS/CNS or late-stage infections Treat complications
B. recurrentis (epidemic)	Relapsing fever (louse-borne)	Louse	Recurrent fever, systemic upset, hepato-splenic and CNS involvement	Microscopy (blood film) Serology	Doxycycline (single dose) or penicillin
B. hermsii (endemic)	Relapsing fever (tick-borne)	Tick (Ortnithodorus)	Recurrent fever, systemic upset, followed by severe shock (can be fatal)	Microscopy (blood film) Serology	Tetracycline or doxycycline
Leptospira					
L. interrogans (including serovar ictohaemorrhagicae)	Leptospirosis	Mucosal (exposure to rat urine in freshwater)	Febrile illness with hepatosplenomegaly, conjunctival injection, myalgia; Aseptic meningitis; Hepato-renal dysfunction; Weil's disease: hepatorenal failure with jaundice in severe disease (5% of cases, mortality 40%)	Serology Urine antigen detection	*Mild:* Doxycycline Severe (Weil's disease): IV penicillin

Viruses

Introduction

The term virus (Latin, *poison*) describes small (20–300 nm) particles containing genetic material, which depend on living host cells for replication. They consist of nucleic acid (DNA or RNA) contained within a protein structure (Capsid) ± surrounded by a host-derived lipid membrane (Envelope). Some virus particles (virions) also contain additional enzymes (non-structural proteins) involved in replication. Viruses spread within hosts by *cell-free* diffusion or direct *cell-to-cell* contact. Dissemination routes between hosts include:

- Mucosal contact.
- Respiratory droplet.
- Faecal-oral.
- Insect vector (mosquito, tick—arbovirus).
- Blood-borne.
- Vertical.

Some are also transmitted to humans from animals (zoonotic).

Replication

Retroviruses must reverse transcribe RNA to DNA prior to integration.

Virus replication is error prone and occurs rapidly. Mutation rates are consequently very high. Host-immune responses ± antiviral drugs exert selection pressure on rapidly mutating viruses. This confers a fitness advantage on immune-escape or drug-resistant mutants, leading to failure of immune control or therapy.

HIV rapidly develops resistance to single antiretroviral drugs. Combination antiretroviral drug therapy (cART, typically 3 active drugs) suppresses replication and protects individual drugs from drug resistance mutations. In addition, influenza A undergoes constant mutation of its surface proteins (haemaglutinin (H), neuraminidase (N)) to evade host antibody responses (*antigenic drift*) → seasonal *epidemics*. *Reassortment* with another strain (which may infect another species, e.g. avian influenza) causes dramatic change in HN proteins (*antigenic shift*) → *pandemics*.

Pathogenesis

Viral pathology is mediated by:

- Cellular cytotoxicity.
- Host immune response.
- Viral manipulation/destruction of host immunity → secondary infection.

Host defence

Both *innate* and *adaptive* responses (see Chapter 4, 'Immunology') are important in host defence against viruses.

Type I interferons (IFN-alpha and beta)

Activate transcription of host anti-viral genes (*interferon-stimulated genes*) conferring an antiviral phenotype to host cells.

- *Natural killer (NK) cells:* lymphocyte lineage cells that recognize and kill virus-infected cells in which constitutive MHC Class I molecule expression is down-regulated by the virus.
- *Antigen-presenting cells (APC)* are immune sentinels that detect viruses and produce pro-inflammatory cytokines and type I IFNs. They link the innate and adaptive immune system by processing and presenting viral antigens to CD4+ and CD8+ T lymphocytes.

Adaptive responses include:

- *Cytotoxic T lymphocytes (CTL):* kill virus infected cells through recognition of specific viral peptide antigen bound to MHC Class I.
- *Neutralizing antibodies* produced by B lymphocytes bind to viral receptors preventing entry into cells, opsonize for complement-mediated phagocytosis, mediate antibody-dependent cellular cytotoxicity ± direct complement cytolysis.

Virus classification

By structural characteristics

- *Genome:*
  - DNA/RNA.
  - Double/single strand.
  - Positive or negative sense (positive sense RNA can be directly translated, negative sense requires complimentary mRNA transcription).
  - Linear/circular.
  - Requirement for reverse transcription (RT creates DNA from RNA, which is integrated into the host genome).
- *Capsid geometry*
  - Icosahedral.
  - Helical.
  - Complex (for example pox viruses have either an ovoid or brick-shaped nucleocapsid containing a biconcave core and two lateral bodies).
- Presence/absence of envelope (enveloped viruses survive less well outside hosts).

By taxonomy

- Order (-virales).
- Family (-viridae).
- Subfamily (-virinae).
- Genus (-virus) and species.

Specific infections

Examples of important viruses and their clinical features are summarized in Tables 5.4 and 5.5.

Table 5.4 DNA viruses

Family	Structure	Transmission	Clinical features	Diagnosis	Treatment	Vaccine
Adenoviridae (e.g. *Adenovirus*)	ds linear DNA. Icosahedral non-enveloped	Respiratory	Conjunctivitis; common cold; pharyngitis; pneumonia; hepatitis; and gastroenteritis Severe in immunocompromise	Serology Virus isolation IF	Supportive	–
Hepnadnaviridae (e.g. *Hepatitis B*)	dsDNA Enveloped	Blood-borne Vertical	Acute and chronic hepatitis; cirrhosis; hepatocellular carcinoma; extra-hepatic (renal disease, arthropathy)	Antigen detection. Serology. PCR	*Antivirals:* tenofovir; entecavir; lamivudine; adefovir. IFN-alpha. Immunize contacts	Yes (HBsAg subunit)
Herpesviridae (e.g. *Herpes simplex virus (HSV)-1/2; Epstein–Barr Virus; CMV; VZV; human Herpes virus-8*)	ds linear DNA. Icosahedral enveloped All establish latent infections, which can reactivate during immunocompromise, e.g. steroid therapy, malignancy, old age, etc.	*Orogenital:* HSV *Respiratory secretions:* EBV, CMV, VZV. *Congenital:* CMV, VZV	*Recurrent orogenital ulceration: HSV-1/2:* Chickenpox (varicella). *VZV* initial infection, pneumonitis risk ↑ in adult smokers, pregnancy *Shingles (herpes zoster):* VZV reactivation. *Ramsay–Hunt syndrome:* VZV reactivation (CN VII). *Meningitis:* HSV-2, VZV. *Encephalitis:* HSV-1 commonest cause, VZV. *Mononucleosis ('glandular fever'—pharyngitis, lymphadenopathy, fatigue):* EBV, CMV. *Hepatitis:* EBV, CMV. *Autoimmune haemolytic anaemia:* EBV. *Congenital infection:* CMV, VZV. *Kaposi sarcoma:* HHV-8. *Castleman's disease:* HHV-8.	*Heterophile antibodies (Paul–Bunnell, monospot):* EBV (negative in 10–15%). PCR (CSF, respiratory secretions). Serology (IgM)	*HSV:* acyclovir, Foscarnet (acyclovir resistance). *VZV:* supportive, acyclovir, anticonvulsants for post-herpetic neuralgia. *EBV:* supportive ± steroids for severe complications. *CMV:* ganciclovir, Foscarnet. *HHV-8:* treat complications (KS, Castleman's) with chemoradiotherapy (KS), and rituximab (Castleman's)	Yes (VZV, live-attenuated vaccine, VZIG – passive immunization)

Table 5.4 DNA viruses (*continued*)

Family	Structure	Transmission	Clinical features	Diagnosis	Treatment	Vaccine
Parvoviridae (e.g. *Parvovirus B19*)	ss linear DNA. Icosahedral non-enveloped. Highly resistant to degradation	Respiratory secretions Blood-borne Vertical	*'Slapped cheek'*: infants. *Fever, rash, arthralgia:* adults. Severe anaemia in haemoglobinopathy (transient aplastic crisis, TAC), and immunocompromise (pure red cell aplasia, PRCA). *Congenital infection:* hydrops foetalis	PCR Serology (IgM)	Supportive. Blood transfusion in severe anaemia. Isolation (TAC, PRCA)	–
Papoviridae (e.g. *Papillomavirus* and Polyomavirus: *BK* and *JC virus*)	ds DNA. Icosahedral non-enveloped	Inoculation (skin and anogenital mucosa)	*Papilloma:* 'warts'. *Cervical carcinoma: HPV*-16 and -18. *Progressive multifocal leucoencephalopathy (PML): JC virus* reactivation. *Haemorrhagic cystitis: BK virus* reactivation	Clinical Histology. PCR urine (BK) and CSF (JC)	*Topical therapy:* cryoptherapy, podophyllin toxin. Correct immunocompromisec ART for HIV+ with PML	Yes (quadravalent—6, 11, 16, 18) and bivalent (16 and 18
Poxviridae (e.g. *Variola* and *Molluscum contagiosum*)	Large dsDNA viruses. Capable of replication in cytoplasm	*Respiratory:* Variola. *Close contact:* Molluscum	*Papular, umbilicated lesions:* Molluscum *Smallpox* (*Variola major*) has been eradicated	*Clinical histology:* PCR (skin lesions in smallpox)	*Topical therapy:* cryoptherapy	Yes (Vaccinia, live virus derived from cowpox)

Table 5.5 RNA viruses

Family	Structure	Transmission	Clinical Features	Diagnosis	Treatment	Vaccine
Arenaviridae: e.g. *Lassa, Junin, Mapucho*	ssRNA enveloped	Zoonotic (rat urine—Lassa)	*VHF:* fever, haemorrhage, shock. *Lassa:* pharyngitis, back pain. Onset within 21 days of travel to (rural) endemic area	Serology PCR	Supportive Ribavirin Strict isolation (negative pressure unit) Important to inform lab, CCDC, and do malaria film in CL3 lab	–
Bunyaviridae: e.g. *Hantavirus, Rift-Valley fever*	ssRNA helical enveloped	Zoonotic	*Hantavirus haemorrhagic pulmonary-renal syndrome:* ARF, pulmonary infiltrates, ↓TLCO), incubation period 5–40 days. *Hantaan:* ARF + shock)	Serology PCR	Supportive Ribavirin Dialysis	–
Calciviridae: e.g. *Norovirus*	ss linear RNA. Icosahedral non-enveloped	Faecal-oral. Resistant to heat, acid, and ether	*Gastroenteritis:* profuse vomiting with short incubation period. *Outbreaks:* cruise-ships, hospitals	PCR (stool)	Supportive Isolation	–
Coronaviridae: e.g. SARS-coronavirus	ssRNA Helical Enveloped	Respiratory	Usually mild URTI Occasionally severe viral pneumonia ± MOF (SARS-coronavirus, onset 2-10 days following visit to endemic region)	Serology PCR	Supportive Ribavirin Strict isolation (negative pressure unit) for SARS	–
Flaviviridae: e.g. *Hepatitis C, Yellow fever, Dengue, Japanese encephalitis*	ssRNA spherical enveloped	Blood-borne (Hepatitis C). Mosquito vector	*Acute and chronic hepatitis:* Hepatitis C. *Cryoglobulinaemia:* Hepatitis C. *Fever, rash, arthralgia (biphasic):* Dengue fever. *VHF (with jaundice):* Yellow fever. *Encephalitis:* Japanese encephalitis, severe, mortality 30%	Serology PCR (blood, CSF)	Supportive Pegylated IFN-alpha and ribavirin (Hepatitis C)	Yes (Yellow fever – live attenuated - and Japanese encephalitis)

Table 5.5 RNA viruses (*continued*)

Family	Structure	Transmission	Clinical Features	Diagnosis	Treatment	Vaccine
Filoviridae: e.g. *Marburg, Ebola*	ss linear RNA. Filamentous enveloped	Close contact with blood or blood-contaminated secretions. Animal reservoir unknown	VHF within 21 days of return from endemic country Usually exposure history, e.g. healthcare worker	PCR, IF (CL4 lab)	Supportive Strict isolation (negative pressure until transfer to Trexler Unit). Important to inform laboratory, CCDC, and do malaria film in CL3 laboratory. High mortality	–
Orthomyxoviridae: e.g. *Influenza A, B*	ssRNA enveloped	Respiratory. Also zoonotic (pigs, birds)	Influenza (fever, headache, myalgia). Viral pneumonia ± secondary bacterial pneumonia. Rarely myocarditis, encephalitis, Reye's syndrome	PCR on respiratory secretions (throat/nasal swab)	Supportive (may require critical care for H1N1 ± ECMO). Neuraminidase inhibitors (oseltamavir, inhaled zanamivir in pregnancy)	Yes (killed)
Paromyxoviridae: e.g. *measles, mumps, RSV, para-influenza*	ssRNA helical enveloped	Respiratory	*Measles:* viral exanthema, pharyngitis, Koplick's spots (buccal mucosa), immunocompromise, encephalitis, very rarely SSPE. *Mumps:* parotitis (minor ↑ amylase); orchitis; pancreatitis (major ↑ amylase), meningitis	PCR (respiratory secretions, CSF). Serology (IgM)	Supportive. Ribavirin for RSV	Yes (measles, mumps – live attenuated)
Picorniviridae: e.g. *Rhinoviruses, Enteroviruses* (incl. poliovirus, echovirus, Coxsackie A/B), *Hepatitis A*	ss linear RNA Icosahedral non-enveloped	Respiratory. Faecal-oral. Resistant to detergents	*Meningitis:* Entroviruses *Encephalitis:* Enteroviruses *Common cold:* Rhinoviruses. *Hand-foot-and-mouth disease (vesicular rash palms, soles):* Coxsackie. *Polio:* meningitis, anterior horn cell (motor) infection – regional flaccid paralysis (LMN). *Acute hepatitis:* Hepatitis A. *Pericarditis:* Coxsackie	PCR (CSF, respiratory secretions) virus isolation, serology	Supportive Novel antivirals for enterovirus infection in development	Yes: IPV, OPV

(*continued*)

Table 5.5 RNA viruses (*continued*)

Family	Structure	Transmission	Clinical Features	Diagnosis	Treatment	Vaccine
Reoviridae: e.g. *Rotavirus*	ssRNA virus Icosahedral non-enveloped double capsid	Faecal-oral	Most common cause of gastroenteritis (particularly infants) Nursing home outbreaks	ELISA for antigen, PCR	Supportive	In development
Retroviridae: e.g. HIV-1/2, HTLV-1/2	ssRNA (two copies) enveloped retroviruses	Mucosal (sexual) Blood-borne Vertical	*HIV—primary infection:* mononucleosis-like presentation ('seroconversion illness'). *HIV—chronic infection:* asymptomatic immunocompromise → AIDS, indicator illnesses raise suspicion (see 'Human immunodeficiency virus'). *HTLV:* adult T cell leukaemia (Dx histology), tropical spastic paraparesis (Dx MRI)	ELISA and WB for anti-HIV/HTLV Ab p24 Antigen PCR for HIV vRNA	Combination antiretroviral therapy (cART, HIV only) Treatment of specific complications	–
Rhabdoviridae: e.g. *Rabies*	ssRNA enveloped bullet-shaped	*Zoonotic:* animal bite, saliva (mammals e.g. bats, dogs)	Encephalitis. Long incubation period (days to years). *Furious (80%):* delirium, autonomic features, hydrophobia → coma. *Paralytic (20%):* ascending symmetrical paralysis → coma	IF of skin biopsy (nape of neck), PCR Negri bodies at autopsy	Post-exposure prophylaxis (hyperimmune globulin, and vaccine at 0, 3, 7, 14, and 28 days). Milwaukee protocol (induced coma, ribavirin, amantadine); single case report of success	Yes (diploid cell)
Togaviridae: e.g. Rubella, Alphaviruses, Chikungunya, various equine encephalitis viruses	ssRNA viruses Icosahedral enveloped	Respiratory (Rubella) Mosquito vector (Alphaviruses)	*Rubella:* viral exanthema; congenital infection. *Alphaviruses:* 'New World': encephalitis with exposure history. *'Old World'. Chikungunya, Ross River virus:* fever, rash, arthralgia	IgM Serology, PCR, *in vitro* inoculation	Supportive Supportive	Yes (live attenuated) –

Human immunodeficiency virus

HIV infects CD4+ T cells and macrophages. Depletion of CD4+ cells (particularly in the *gut-associated lymphoid tissue*, See Chapter 4, 'Immunology') and *chronic immune activation* result in a profound *cell-mediated immunodeficiency* syndrome, characterized by multiple *opportunistic infections* and malignancies (see Table 5.6; AIDS-defining illnesses).

However, the introduction of potent combination antiretroviral therapy (cART) has transformed HIV into a chronic disease with near-normal life expectancy. Such improvements are compromised by late diagnosis of HIV, meaning all physicians must be aware of the potential for HIV and offer testing widely for indicator conditions (see Table 5.7). The epidemiology of HIV is changing in the UK, and HIV is increasingly diagnosed in older, heterosexual populations.

Combination antiretroviral therapy (cART, usually two nucleotide reverse transcriptase inhibitor (NRTI) plus one non-nucleotide reverse transcriptase inhibitor (NNRTI) or protease inhibitor (PI) is associated with:

- Numerous challenging *drug–drug interactions* with other therapies (see www.hiv-druginteractions.org and Table 5.8)
- Must be taken life-long without interruption, and
- Causes significant side effects and **toxicity**.

The aim of cART is to suppress viral replication (plasma *viral load*, measured by PCR, of below 40 HIV RNA copies per mL blood,) to allow recovery of the CD4+ T cell compartment (immune reconstitution). Not infrequently, when patients commence cART with a profoundly depleted immune system (e.g. *CD4 count* <50 cells/uL), immune reconstitution can lead to paradoxical inflammatory responses to opportunistic pathogens previously 'ignored' by the immune system (this is termed the *immune reconstitution inflammatory syndrome* (IRIS), and occasionally requires steroid therapy if severe).

Resistance mutations compromise the efficacy of cART, and poor cART *adherence* increases the risk of drug-resistance, therefore, *tailoring therapy* (particularly regarding side-effect and toxicity profiles to the individual is crucial. Resistance and/or poor adherence are reflected in loss of control of viral replication, leading to *virological failure* (*rebound* of the plasma viral load). Attention to patient adherence and testing for *resistance mutations* are mandatory in virological failure. A new cART regimen is then designed to regain viral control.

Viral hepatitis

Acute viral hepatitis is caused by many viral pathogens:

- Hepatitis A, B, C, and E. Hepatitis D (delta) is a subvirion only able to replicate in someone already infected with Hepatitis B.
- CMV, Epstein–Barr virus (EBV).
- HSV, measles, rubella, Coxsackie, adenovirus, yellow fever, Arboviruses, etc.

Appropriate screening tests for the most common causes are:

- Hepatitis A IgM (positive in acute Hepatitis A).
- Hepatitis B surface antigen, HBsAg. If positive the anti-HBC IgM will distinguish between acute (positive anti-HBC IgM) and chronic (negative anti-HBC IgM).

Table 5.6 WHO/CDC classification of AIDS-defining illnesses in HIV

Infections	Malignancies	Other
Viral		
CMV: retinitis/pneumonitis/oesophagitis/colitis. *HSV*: visceral any duration or chronic ulcer >1/12	Lymphoproliferative. Lymphoma (NHL, diffuse B cell, Burkitt's, primary CNS)	HIV encephalopathy. Progressive multifocal leucoencephalopathy (PML). HIV wasting syndrome
Bacterial		
Recurrent pneumonia Non-typhoidal salmonella (invasive)	Other Kaposi's sarcoma Invasive cervical carcinoma	
Mycobacterial		
Mycobacterium tuberculosis (any site), *Mycobacterium avium* complex, or *kansasii* (disseminated or extrapulmonary)		
Parasitic		
Coccidioidomycosis (disseminated or extrapulmonary). Cryptococcosis (extrapulmonary). Cryptosporidiosis (> 1/12). Isosporosis (> 1/12). Toxoplasmosis (CNS)		
Fungal		
Candidiasis (pulmonary, oesophageal). *Pneumocystis jiroveci* pneumonia (PCP). Histoplasmosis (disseminated or extrapulmonary)		

Data from '1993 Revised Classification System for HIV Infection and Expanded Surveillance Case Definition for AIDS Among Adolescents and Adults', *Morbidity and Mortality Weekly Report*, December 18, 1992, 41(RR-17).

Table 5.7 Indicator conditions for HIV testing in adults (adapted from BHIVA testing guidelines, 2008)

Specialty	Indicator condition(s)
Respiratory	Bacterial pneumonia; aspergillosis
Neurology	Aseptic meningitis/encephalitis; cerebral abscess; SOL unknown cause; Guillain–Barré syndrome; transverse myelitis; peripheral neuropathy; dementia (early onset); leucoencephalopathy
Dermatology	Severe or recalcitrant seborrhoeic dermatitis/psoriasis; multidermatomal *Herpes zoster*
Gastroenterology	Oral candidiasis; oral hairy leucoplakia; chronic diarrhoea of unknown cause; hepatitis B or C infection; anal carcinoma or intraepithelial dysplasia
Oncology	Lung cancer; head and neck cancer; seminoma; Hodgkin's disease; Castleman's disease
Gynaecology	Cervical intraepithelial neoplasia ≥grade 2; vaginal intraepithelial neoplasia
Haematology	Unexplained thrombocytopenia, neutropenia, lymphopenia
Ophthalmology	Infective retinal diseases; unexplained retinopathy
Ear, nose, and throat	Lymphadenopathy of unknown cause; chronic parotitis; lympho-epithelial parotid cysts
Other	Pyrexia of unknown origin (PUO); any STI; mononucleosis-like illness (primary HIV)

Table 5.8 Indications for HIV therapy (adapted from British HIV Association (BHIVA) treatment guidelines, 2013)

Condition	Indication to start antiretroviral treatment
Chronic HIV infection:	treat if CD4 cell count is < 350 cells/mL
AIDS diagnosis	treat irrespective of CD4 cell count
HIV-related co-morbidity eg. HIV-associated nephropathy, idiopathic thrombocytopenic purpura, symptomatic HIV-associated neurocognitive disorders	treat irrespective of CD4 cell count
Coinfection with hepatitis B or C virus	treat if CD4 cell count is <500 cells/mL
Non-AIDS-defining malignancies requiring immunosuppressive radiotherapy or chemotherapy	treat when coinfection with hepatitis B if CD4 cell count is >500 cells/mL and treatment of hepatitis B is indicated
AIDS-defining infection, or with a serious bacterial infection	treat within 2 weeks of initiation of specific antimicrobial chemotherapy. if CD4 cell count <200 cells/mL
Primary HIV infection	treat if neurological involvement, any AIDS-defining illness, or confirmed CD4 cell count <350 cells/mL

Data from The British HIV Association (BHICA), the British Association for Sexual Health and HIV (BASHH), and the British Infection Society (BIS). Treatment of HIV-1 positive adults with antiretroviral therapy 2012 (updated November 2013). http://www.bhiva.org/TreatmentofHIV1_2012.aspx

- Hepatitis C antibody, HCV Ab.

If these screening tests are negative, proceed to test for other causes as clinically indicated.

Fungi

Mycoses (fungal infections) are common eukaryotic pathogens (see Table 5.9). They contain chitin and ergosterol in their cell walls (rather than cholesterol) and most antifungal agents target these fungal-specific components. Morphologically, they appear as *yeasts* (single-cells) or *moulds* (branched multicellular organisms). Some have the potential to adopt both morphological characteristics (*dimorphic*). Fungi cause skin, soft-tissue, and *disseminated infections* (invasive and affecting any organ), and are mainly a problem in individuals with compromised *cell-mediated immunity* (see Chapter 4, cell–mediated immunity; See also Table 5.10).

Table 5.9 Classification of medically important mycoses

Moulds	Yeasts	Dimorphic fungi
Aspergillus	*Candida*	*Coccidiodes*
Dermatophytes	*Cryptococcus*	*Histoplasma*
Zygomycota	*Malassezia*	*Penicillium*
	Pneumocystis	*Sporothryx*

Table 5.10 Selected important mycoses

Genus/species	Pathogen	Risk factors	Clinical features	Diagnosis	Treatment	Prophylaxis
Yeasts						
Candida	*C. albicans* *C. parapsilosis* *C. kruseii*	Steroids. Antibiotics. Diabetes. Neutropenia. IV catheter	Mucocutaneous. Candidaemia. Endocarditis. Endophthalmitis. Abscesses	Culture. Oesophago-gastro duodenoscopy (OGD) Beta-glucan test Imaging	*Mucocutaneous:* Topical or azole. *Invasive:* fluconazole, or caspofungin, or amphotericin B. Surgery	Fluconazole
Cryptococcus	*C. neoformans*	HIV. Transplant. Lymphoma	Skin Pulmonary. Meningitis (↑ICP). Cerebral abscess (cryptococoma). Bone	*Microscopy (CSF):* India ink stain. Antigen test (serum + CSF). Culture	Amphotericin B plus flucytosine. Repeat lumbar puncture (LP). CSF shunt may be required	Fluconazole
Malassezia	*M. furfur*	–	Pityriasis versicolor. Seborrhoeic dermatitis	*Skin scraping:* UV fluorescence; clinical	Clotrimazole topical	–
Pneumocystis	*P. jiroveci*	HIV. Transplant. Chemotherapy	Skin. Pneumonia. Pneumothorax (immune-compromised) Extrapulmonary	CXR. Induced sputum or BAL – IF ± PCR. Histology (silver stain)	Co-trimoxazole (high dose). Steroids if PaO_2 <9.3 kPa Alternatively, give clindamycin plus primaquine, dapsone, or pentamidine (IV)	Co-trimoxazole, or pentamidine (neb), or dapsone
Moulds						
Aspergillus	*A. fumigatus.* *A. flavus.* *A. niger*	Diabetes. Asthma (ABPA). Burns. HIV. Leukaemia. Neutropenia. TB cavity	Cutaneous ABPA. Aspergilloma. Invasive. Aspergillosis (pulmonary or extra-pulmonary)	*Invasive:* culture; CT scan (pulmonary IA); bronchoscopy; galactomannan/beta-glucan test. *ABPA: Aspergillus precipitans*	*Invasive:* amphotericin B, or voriconazole, or caspofungin. *Aspergilloma:* surgery. *ABPA:* steroids + itraconazole	*Invasive:* posiconazole, or voriconazole, or itraconazole
Dermatophyte	Various (ringworm)	Sporting activities	Tinea pedis, etc. Onychomycosis (nail)	*Skin scraping:* treat with KOH, observe hyphae	*Tinea:* topical. *Onychomycosis:* itraconazole or terbinafine	–
Zygomycota	Mucor Rhizopus Rhizomucor	DKA. Neutropenia	*Mucormycosis:* Invasive rhinocerebral infection (rapidly fatal)	*Culture:* tissue biopsy to identify organism	Amphotericin B (resistant to voriconazole). Surgical debridement	

(continued)

Table 5.10 Selected important mycoses (*continued*)

Genus/species	Pathogen	Risk factors	Clinical features	Diagnosis	Treatment	Prophylaxis
Dimorphic fungi						
Coccidiodes	*C. immitis* (Americas only)	HIV. Transplant. Lymphoma	*Pulmonary*: similar to histoplasmosis. *Disseminated*: any organ, particularly skin, bone, meninges	Serology. Culture.	Amphotericin B or fluconazole	Itraconazole or fluconazole
Histoplasma	*H. capsulatum* (mainly USA, but worldwide) *H. capsulatum* var. *dubiosii* (Africa)	Exposure to bat/bird guano (e.g. exploring caves) HIV	*Cutaneous ± bone: H. dubiosii.* *Pulmonary*: mimicks TB (BHL ± cavitation). *Disseminated*: any organ	Culture. Urine antigen. Serology	Itraconazole or amphotericin B (1st line in disseminated disease)	Itraconazole (HIV)
Penicillium	*P. marnefii* (SE Asia)	HIV Other immunocompromise	Cutaneous. Pulmonary (cavitation). Disseminated	Microscopy. Culture histology	*Cutaneous:* itraconazole *Other:* amphotericin B	*Disseminated:* itraconazole
Sporothryx	*S. schenckii*	Occupational (cutaneous). Alcoholism (pulmonary). HIV (disseminated)	*Cutaneous:* ulcerating lesions spread along lymphatics. Pulmonary. Disseminated	Culture. Histology	*Cutaneous:* itraconazole *Other:* amphotericin B	*Disseminated:* itraconazole

Protozoa and helminths

- Eukaryotic organisms, usually with complex life cycles.
- Responsible for a host of important tropical and cosmopolitan diseases.
- Most are diagnosed by microscopy (for ova/cysts and parasites) ± antigen tests, and/or serology.
- Cutaneous larva migrans, a serpinginous intensely itchy skin rash, is caused by human infection with dog hookworm larvae (treat with Ivermectin® or albendazole).

Classification

Protozoa

- *Flagellates (with a flagellum):* e.g. leishmaniasis, trypanosomiasis, giardiasis (see Table 5.11).
- *Sporozoan (no flagellum):* e.g. malaria, toxoplasmosis (Table 5.12).

Helminths (worms)

- *Nematodes (round worms):*
  - *Intestinal*—e.g. hookworm, strongyloidiasis.
  - *Tissue*—e.g. filariasis and oncocerchiasis.
- *Flat worms:*
  - *Cestodes (tapeworms)*—e.g. cystercercosis, hydatid disease.
  - *Trematodes (flukes)*—e.g. liver flukes, schistosomiasis.

(See Table 5.13)

Host response to infection

The normal host response to infection is a complex process that serves to localize and control pathogen invasion, and initiate repair of injured tissue. This consists of the innate and adaptive immune responses.

Innate immune response

An evolutionally conserved host defence mechanism, present from birth and activated by molecular components found only in micro-organisms. These mechanisms are not learned, adapted, or permanently heightened as a result of exposure to micro-organisms and provide the first line of defence to infection. Cells of the innate immune system (including phagocytes, mast cells and natural killer cells) attracted by chemotactic signals use pattern recognition receptors (PRRs) to recognize pathogen associated molecular patterns (PAMPs) on micro-organisms. Using cytokines, enzymes and proteins these cells then initiate and regulate the inflammatory immune response, clear away dying and damaged cells, and present antigen to and activate the adaptive immune response. Swelling, redness, heat, and pain, the cardinal signs of inflammation, are products of the innate immune response.

Adaptive immune response

A lymphocyte-mediated response specific for a particular foreign antigen that demonstrates tolerance of self-antigens. Antibody and cell-mediated immune responses demonstrate immunological memory, i.e. the immune response become more rapid, durable, and potent with each infection (see Chapter 4 'Introduction and general principles' see also Table 5.14).

The immune response to infection is usually localized and tightly regulated by pro- and anti-inflammatory cytokines released by macrophages. In some circumstances, this inflammatory response becomes generalized, exaggerated, and uncontrolled, resulting in a systemic pro-inflammatory reaction leading to generalized tissue damage—a syndrome termed sepsis (Fig. 5.7, Table 5.15). Sepsis can occur as a result of both Gram –ve and Gram +ve bacterial infections; components of the bacterial cell wall bind to toll-like receptors on innate immune cells, leading to the production of a large number of pro-inflammatory molecules. Nitric oxide is a key mediator of the hypotension associated with septic shock and with TNFα, IL-1, IL-6, and IL-8 is important for mediating the capillary and alveolar endothelial damage that leads to the enhanced microvascular permeability and pathological interstitial oedema seen in acute respiratory distress syndrome.

Principals of vaccination

Vaccination of a significant portion of a population prevents transmission of disease and can provide a measure of protection for individuals who do not have immunity. This is known as "*herd immunity*" and generally requires at least 75-85% of the population to be immunized depending on the disease. Table 5.16 summarizes the routine childhood immunization schedule used in the UK.

Active immunity via vaccination can be obtained by using a live attenuated variation of the organism against which vaccination is required, an inactivated version or by using a

Table 5.11 Selected Flagellate Protozoa

Genus/species	Infective stages	Specific infections	Geographical distribution	Transmission	Clinical features	Diagnostic tests	Treatment	Prevention
Trichomonas spp.	Flagellated organisms	*T. vaginalis*	Worldwide	Sexual	Dysuria, discharge	Microscopy (wet-mount)	Metronidazole. Partner notification	Safe sex practices. Condoms
Entamoeba spp. Amoebiasis	Trophozoite. Cyst	*E. histolytica*	Tropics > temperate	Faecal-oral (sexual)	Bloody diarrhoea (dysentery). Amoebic liver abscess. Metastatic abscesses (e.g. brain, lung)	*Microscopy (wet-mount):* trophozoites or cysts. Serology (invasive). Imaging. Colonoscopy	Metronidazole plus diloxanide furoate, for luminal carriage	Safe water. Hand hygiene
Giardia spp. Giardiasis	Cyst. Trophozoite	*G. lamblia*	Worldwide	Faecal-oral	Watery diarrhoea, abdominal pain, flatulence, malabsorption	*Microscopy (wet-mount):* trophozoites or cysts. Faecal antigen tests. String test. OGD	Metronidazole, tinidazole, or nitazoxanide	Safe water. Hand hygiene
Leishmania spp. Leishmanisis	Promastigotes (sandfly). Amastigotes (macrophages)	*Cutaneous:* *L. major* *L. tropica* *L. aethiopica* *L. braziliensis* *L. Mexicana* Mucocutaneous: *L. braziliensis* Visceral *(kala-azar):* *L. donovani* *L. infantum*	Middle-East, India, Asia, Africa Mediterranean Latin America Latin America As cutaneous	Sandfly vector. Animal reservoir (dogs)	*Cutaneous:* chronic skin ulceration. *Mucocutaneous:* destruction of nasopharyngeal mucosa *Visceral:* massive hepato-splenomagaly, fever, adenopathy (East African), pancytopenia	*Biopsy:* skin (cutaneous), spleen, bone-marrow (visceral). Microscopy for amastigotes and PCR to identify organism	*Cutaneous:* supportive (old world), topical or cryotherapy *L. Braziliensis:* sodium stibogluconate (toxic) *Visceral:* sodium stibogluconate or liposomal amphotericin B	Avoidance of bites. Vector control
Trypanosoma spp. *Sleeping sickness:* African trypanosomiasis *Chagas' disease:* American trypanosomiasis	Trypomastigotes	*T. bruceii* var. *gambiense* *T. bruceii* var. *rhodesiense* *T. cruzii*	W Africa E Africa Latin America	Tsetse fly, *Glossinia palpalis* *G. moristans* Reduviid bug Blood transfusion	*African stage 1:* fever, chancre, regional adenopathy. *African stage 2:* meningo-encephalitis *American:* cardiomyopathy and dilatation of hollow organs	*Microscopy:* blood, lymph, buffy coat for trypanosomes. CSF examination (↑protein, IgM, WCC). Serology (American)	*African stage 1:* pentamidine; or eflornithine—*gambiense*; Suramin—*rhodesiense* *African stage 2:* melarsoprol (mortalilty 5%) or eflornithine—*gambiense* *American:* nifurtimox or benznidazole; treat complications	Avoidance of bites Vector control Screening blood products

Table 5.12 Selected Sporozoan Protozoa

Genus/species	Infective stages	Specific- infections	Geographical distribution	Transmission	Clinical features	Diagnostic tests	Treatment	Prevention
Plasmodium spp. Malaria	*Asexual:* sporozoite (mosquito) → liver. Schizont ± hypnozoite → merozoite → trophozoite → merozoite (all RBCs) *Sexual:* male and female gametocytes (RBCs) → sporozoite (mosquito)	*P. falciparum* (mortality) *P. vivax* (relapse) *P. ovale* (relapse) *P. malariae* (relapse) *P. knowalesi* (mainly macaques)	Africa, Asia, W Pacific Latin America, Asia, W Pacific W Africa, Asia Africa, SE Asia, W Pacific SE Asia	Anopheles mosquitoes	*All:* Fever, chills, myalgia, headache, nausea and vomiting, hepato-splenomegaly *P. falciparum:* jaundice, coma, haemolytic anaemia ('blackwater fever') History of travel	Thick/thin blood film microscopy × 3 min. Ring forms (all). Erythrocytic schizonts, Shuffners dots (vivax or ovale). Rapid antigen tests PCR	*P. falciparum:* uncomplicated—po quinine + doxycycline, or atovaquone and/or proguanil, or artemether and/or lumefantrin *Complicated:* iv quinine ± artemesinin (depending on availability) *Non-falciparum:* chloroquine + primaquine to prevent relapse (vivax and ovale) Supportive therapy	*Avoiding mosquito bites:* bed nets, DEET. Antimalarial chemoprophylaxis. *P. falciparum:* doxycycline, mefloquine, or atovaquone and/or proguanil. *Non-falciparum:* chloroquine. Vector control
Babesia spp. Babesiosis		*B. microtti*	Europe, USA	Tick bite (Ixodes)	Fever, hepato-splenomegaly; severe in splenectomy	*Microscopy:* ring forms, Maltese cross in erythrocytes	Quinine and clindamycin	Avoidance of tick bites
Cryptosporidium spp.	Oocysts → sporozoites → merozoites	*C. parvum*	Worldwide	Faecal-oral	Watery diarrhoea, prolonged if IC	*Stool microscopy:* oocysts	Supportive. Nitazoxanide for IC, plus correct underlying cause	Safe water. Hand hygiene
Toxoplasma gondii Toxoplasmosis	Sporulated oocysts. Tissue cysts (bradyzoites). Tachyzoites	—	Worldwide	Ingestion of raw or poorly cooked meat. Contact with cat faeces. Transplacental	Asymptomatic. Mononucleosis. Choroidoretinitis. Fulminant disease in immune-compromised	Toxoplasma IgM or rising IgG titre	*Pregnancy:* spiramycin. *Immunocompromised:* sulphadiazine plus pyrimethamine or clindamycin plus pyrimethamine	Thorough cooking of meat. Safe disposal of cat litter

Table 5.13 Selected Helminths (worms)

Genus/species	Infective stage	Specific infections	Geographical distribution	Transmission	Clinical features	Diagnostic tests	Treatment	Prevention
Nematodes (roundworm)								
Ascaris spp. Ascariasis	Ova → worms	*A. lumbricoides*	Worldwide	Faecal-oral	*Asymptomatic lung migration:* Loeffler's syndrome (CXR infiltrates, eosinophilia). GI obstruction with large infections	*Stool microscopy:* ova	Mebendazole or albendazole	Sanitation. Hand hygiene
Hookworm	Larvae → adult worms → ova (soil) → larvae	*Ancyclostoma duodenale. Necator americanus*	Worldwide	Invasion of larvae through skin. Vertical	Loeffler's syndrome. Iron-deficiency anaemia	*Stool microscopy:* ova	Mebendazole or albendazole	Avoid walking barefoot
Strongyloides spp. Strongyloidiasis	Larvae → adult worms → ova (soil) → larvae	*Strongyloides stercoralis*	Tropics > temperate	Invasion of larvae through skin. Faecal-oral	Skin rash (larva currens). Loeffler's syndrome. *Hyperinfection syndrome (in IC):* shock, ARDS, Gm –ve bacteraemia	*Microscopy:* stool, duodenal aspirate. Serology (false negative in hyperinfection)	Albendazole	Avoid walking barefoot
Toxocara spp.	Ova (soil) ingested → larvae (infiltrate tissue)	*Toxocara canus. Toxocara cati*	Worldwide	Ingestion of ova	Endophthalmitis. Visceral larva migrans (fever, eosinophilia, urticaria)	Histology. Serology (sero-positivity common)	Thiabendazole ± steroids	Deworming dogs and cats
Filariae: *Wuchereria* and *Brugia* spp. Lymphatic filariasis	Microfilaria (mosquito) → filariae → ova → microfilaria	*W. bancrofti* *B. malayi* *B. timori*	Tropics. S and SE Asia. E Indonesia	Mosquito vector (multiple species)	Lymphatic filariasis (adenophathy and lymphoedema—'elephantiasis')	*Microscopy (blood film):* microfilariae. Serology. Histology	Diethylcarbamazine (DEC) or Ivermectin® (doxycycline treats symbiotic *Wolbachia* bacterium)	Avoidance of bites Vector control
Onchocerca volvulus Onchocerciasis	Microfilaria (mosquito) → filariae → ova	*O. volvulus*	Africa. S America	Black fly *Simulium* sp.	Skin lesions (rash, depigmentation, nodules). Keratitis, corneal fibrosis	*Microscopy (wet mount) of skin snips:* microfilariae	Ivermectin® (DEC causes Mazzotti reaction)	Avoidance of bites Vector control
Loa loa Loiasis	Microfilaria (mosquito) → filariae → ova → microfilaria	*L. loa*	W Africa	*Chyrysops* fly	Subcutaneous swellings (calabar swellings); occasionally migration across sclera	*Microscopy (blood film):* microfilariae	Ivermectin (DEC causes encephalopathy if high infection burden)	Avoidance of bites Vector control

Table 5.13 Selected Helminths (worms) (*continued*)

Genus/species	Infective stage	Specific infections	Geographical distribution	Transmission	Clinical features	Diagnostic tests	Treatment	Prevention
Cestodes (tapeworm)								
Taenia spp. Neuro-cystercercosis	Encysted larvae → adult worm → ova	*T. solium* (pork) *T. saginatum* (beef)	Tropics > temperate	Ingestion of undercooked meat (encysted larvae) or eggs	Asymptomatic. Mild GI symptoms. Seizures (CNS encysted larvae—*T. solium*)	*Microscopy (stool)*: ova, serology. Imaging for tissue cysts	Albendazole or praziquantel ± steroids. Antiepileptics	Thorough cooking of meat
Echinococcus spp. Hydatid disease	Encysted larvae → adult worm → ova	*E. granulosis* *E. vogeli*	Worldwide	Ingestion of ova from infected dog, sheep etc.	Asymptomatic unless cyst rupture (severe allergic reaction); liver > lung	Microscopy. Serology. Imaging	Praziquantel ± albendazole. Surgery. PAIR (puncture, aspiration, injection, re-aspiration)	–
Trematodes (flukes)								
Schistosoma spp. Schistosomiasis (Bilharzia)	Cercariae → adult worm → ova	*S. mansoni* *S. japonicum* *S. haematobium* *S. mekongi* *S. intercalcatum*	Africa Asia Africa Asia Africa	Invasion of cercariae through skin (in freshwater)	*Katayama fever (acute)*: fever, eosinophilia, rash, hepato-splenomegaly. *Chronic*: haematuria, bladder carcinoma, or hepatic fibrosis/portal hypertension. Rarely CNS infection	*Microscopy*: urine, stool, rectal snips for ova. Serology. Histology	Praziquantel (± steroids for Katayama fever)	Avoidance of fresh water in endemic regions. Treatment of human hosts
Fasciola spp. Liver fluke	Encysted metacercariae → larvae → adult fluke	*F. hepaticum*: liver fluke of sheep and cattle	Worldwide	Ingestion of encysted metacercariae	*Acute*: fever, eosinophilia, hepatomegaly, RUQ pain. *Chronic*: asymptomatic or biliary obstruction	*Microscopy (stool or bile)*: Ova. Serology	Triclabendazole or nitazoxanide	

Table 5.14 Comparison of innate and adaptive immune responses

	Innate immune response	Adaptive immune response
Components	Physical barriers. Phagocytes. Complement system. Inflammatory mediators (including TNFα, nitric oxide, prostaglandins, and IL-1)	*Humoral response:* B cells. *Cell-mediated response:* T cells
Immunological memory	No	Yes
Speed of response	Rapid—within minutes	Slower—days to weeks
Specificity for antigen	Non-specific	Antigen stpecific
Self-tolerance	N/A	Yes

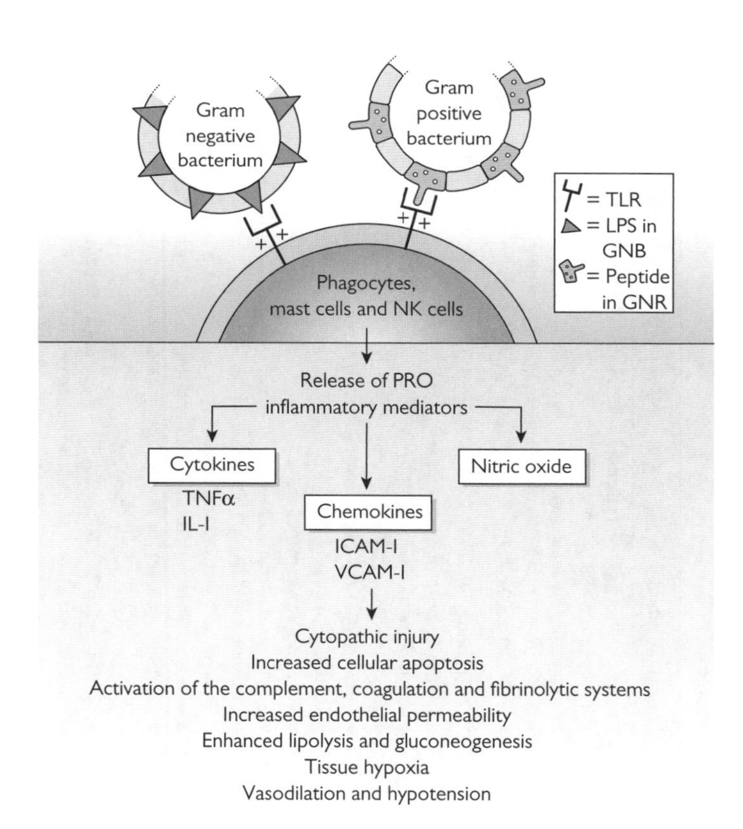

Fig. 5.7 Immunological mechanisms of sepsis.

sub-unit or single antigen from the organism. This compares to passive immunizations via immunoglobulin and is used when there is a high risk of infection and insufficient time for the body to develop its own immune response, or to reduce the symptoms of ongoing or immunosuppressive diseases.

Currently available active and passive vaccinations are summarized in Table 5.17 and a comparison of the features of live and inactivated vaccines is included in Table 5.18.

There are very few contraindications to vaccination, and these are listed in Table 5.19.

Table 5.15 Definitions of septic syndromes

Syndrome	Clinical definition
Systemic inflammatory response syndrome (SIRS)	*≥2 of the following clinical features:* • Temperature >38.5°C or <35°C. • Heart rate >90 beats/min. • Respiratory rate >20 breaths/min or $PaCO_2$ <32 mmHg. • WBC >12,000 cells/mm^3, <4000 cells/mm^3, or >10% immature (band) forms.
Sepsis	SIRS in response to culture positive infection or focus of infection identified by visual inspection, e.g. wound with purulent discharge
Severe sepsis	*Sepsis and ≥1 of the following features:* • Areas of mottled skin. • Capillary refilling ≥3 sec. • Urine output <0.5 mL/kg for at least 1 hr, or renal replacement therapy. • Lactate >2 mmol/L. • Abrupt change in mental status. • Abnormal electroencephalographic (EEG) findings. • Platelet count <100,000 platelets/mL. • Disseminated intravascular coagulation. • Acute lung injury or acute respiratory distress syndrome (ARDS). • Cardiac dysfunction, as defined by echocardiography or direct measurement of the cardiac index.
Septic shock	*Severe sepsis and ≥1 of the following:* • Systemic mean BP <60 mmHg (or <80 mmHg if the patient has baseline hypertension) despite adequate fluid resuscitation. • Maintaining the systemic mean BP >60 mmHg (or >80 mmHg if the patient has baseline hypertension) requires dopamine >5 micrograms/kg per min, norepinephrine <0.25 micrograms/kg/min, or epinephrine <0.25 micrograms/kg/min despite adequate fluid resuscitation.
Refractory shock	Septic shock and requires inotropes (dopamine >15 micrograms/kg/min, norepinephrine >0.25 micrograms/kg/min or epinephrine >0.25 micrograms/kg/min) to maintain the systemic mean BP >60 mmHg (or >80 mmHg if the patient has baseline hypertension) despite adequate fluid resuscitation

Table 5.16 UK immunization schedule

Age	Vaccines recommended
Routine UK childhood immunization schedule	
2 months	DTP, polio, Hib, pneumococcus, rotavirus
3 months	DTP, polio, Hib, Men C, rotavirus
4 months	DTP, polio, Hib, pneumococcus, Men C
12–13 months	MMR, Hib, pneumococcus, Men C
2, 3, and 4 years	flu vaccination
3 years, 4 months	MMR, DTP, polio
12–13 years girls	HPV
13–15 years	Men C
13–18 years	Tetanus, diphtheria, polio
18–25 (students)	Men C
65 years and over	Flu (annually), pneumococcal
70 years	Herpes Zoster
Non-routine UK childhood immunization schedule	
At birth, and 1, 2, and 12 months	Hepatitis B
At birth	TB

Meningitis B vaccine to be introduced as routine vaccination for infants in 2015.

Source: UK EPI, Department of Health, 2015.

Abbreviations: DTP, diphtheria, tetanus, pertussis. Hib, *Haemophilus influenzae* type b. Men C, meningococcus C. MMR, measles, mumps, rubella. HPV, human papilloma virus. BCG, Bacillus Calmette–Guérin.

Table 5.17 Currently available active and passive vaccinations

Live attenuated	Inactivated	Subunit
Active vaccination—antigen		
BCG Measles Mumps Rubella Varicella zoster Polio (oral) Typhoid Rotavirus Yellow Fever Smallpox Influenza	Hepatitis A Japanese Encephalitis Influenza Polio	*Virus-like particles:* Human papilloma virus *Surface antigen:* Hepatitis B *Toxoid:* Tetanus Cholera Diphtheria *Capsular polysaccharide:* Men A&C Pneumococcus *H. influenzae* b Typhoid
Passive vaccination—immunoglobulin		
Targeting pathogen		Targeting toxin
Rabies Tetanus Varicella zoster Measles Rubella Hepatitis B Mumps		Diphtheria Botulism

Table 5.18 Comparison of the features of live and inactivated vaccines

	Live vaccines	Inactivated vaccines
Cell-mediated immunity	Yes	Weak or none
Humoral immunity	IgA and IgG	IgG
Duration of response	Boosting often unnecessary	Boosting often required
Immunogenicity	Potent	Poor—often requires adjuvant
Safety of vaccine	• Possible reversion to virulence. • Possible spread to non-immune individuals. • Unsafe in immunocompromised.	Safe if completely inactivated
Stability at room temperature	Low	High

Table 5.19 Contraindications to vaccination

All vaccines	Live vaccines
Allergy to vaccine component Reaction to previous dose of vaccine	Pregnancy Immunocompromise including: • HIV. • Haematological and solid tumours. • Long-term immunosuppressive treatment. • Congenital immunodeficiency. • Pregnancy.

Laboratory assays

HIV-1 tests

- *Enzyme-linked immunosorbent assay (ELISA)* followed by a confirmatory western blot assay. This has a high sensitivity (>99.5%) and specificity (99.9%). In acute infection, seroconversion occurs after around 4 weeks, but can take up to 6 months. This is known as the 'window period'.
- *Antigen tests:* testing for Gag protein (p24) can detect HIV before seroconversion.
- *RNA:* highly sensitive quantitative PCR assays allow accurate measurement of HIV copies in peripheral blood (copies/mL).
- *CD4 count:* measured by flow cytometry. The total number (cells/μL) and percentage of CD4+ T cells in the peripheral blood is a surrogate marker of immune status.

Hepatitis B tests

For the interpretation of Hepatitis B tests, see Table 5.20.

Syphilis serology

There are several components to syphilis testing. The enzyme immunoassay (IgG and IgM) is used as a screening test. This is combined with non-specific cardiolipin tests (the venereal disease research laboratory or VDRL test, and the rapid plasma reagin or RPR test) and treponema-specific agglutination tests (*Treponema pallidum* particle agglutination or TPPA assay,, and *Treponema pallidum* hemaglutination or THPA assay). The prozone phenomena refers to false negative VDRL/RPR with extremely high titres of antibody in early infection (Table 5.21).

Interpretation of cerebral spinal fluid

For the interpretation of cerebral spinal fluid, see Table 5.22.

Polymerase chain reaction

PCR is a highly sensitive method of detecting target nucleic acid in a clinical sample. It is mostly used in the detection of slow growing bacterium (e.g. anaerobes or mycobacterium) or organisms difficult to culture in the laboratory (e.g. viruses, chlamydia).

Table 5.20 Interpretation of hepatitis B tests

	HBsAg	HBeAg	Anti-HBS	Anti-HBC IgM	Anti-HBC IgG	HBV DNA
Acute hepatitis B	+	+	–	+	–/+	+
Chronic hepatitis B	+	+/–	–	–	+	+
Prior hepatitis B	–	–	+	–	+	–
Inactive carrier state	+	–	–	–	+	–/+
Hepatitis B vaccinated	–	–	+	–	–	–

Table 5.21 Interpretation of hepatitis B tests

Test	Early		Late	Treated
	Primary	Secondary		
VDRL/RPR	+/–	+	+/–	–
EIA IgM	+	+	–	–
EIA IgG	+	+	+	+
TPHA/TPPA	+	+	+	+

Table 5.22 Interpretation of cerebrospinal fluid samples

Agent	Appearance	WBC	Glucose*	Protein (mg/dL)	Additional tests
Bacterial meningitis	Turbid	Raised (>80% PMNs)	Reduced	Elevated	Specific pathogen demonstrated in 60% of Gram stains and 80% of cultures
Viral meningitis	Clear	Raised (lymphocytes)	Normal	May be slightly elevated	PCR assays
Tuberculous meningitis	Clear or turbid	Raised (lymphocytes)	Reduced	Elevated	Ziehl–Neelsen stain, culture for mycobacterium, PCR
Cryptococcal meningitis	Clear or turbid	Raised (lymphocytes)	Reduced	Elevated	India ink stain, cryptococcal antigen, culture
Aseptic meningitis	Clear	Raised (lymphocytes)	Normal	May be slightly elevated	

*CSF glucose is reduced if ≤60% of serum glucose taken simultaneously.

Infection control and public health: notifications

For diseases notifiable (to Local Authority Proper Officers) under the Health Protection (Notification) Regulations 2010 (see Table 5.23).

Antimicrobial pharmacology

A summary of antimicrobial agents can be found in Tables 5.24–5.30

Table 5.23 Notifiable diseases in the UK (2010)

Clinical syndromes	Pathogens
Acute encephalitis Acute meningitis Acute infectious hepatitis Food poisoning Haemolytic uraemic syndrome Infectious bloody diarrhoea Viral haemorrhagic fever	Acute poliomyelitis Anthrax Bordetella pertussis Botulism Brucellosis Cholera Diphtheria Invasive group A strep and scarlet fever Legionnaire's disease Leprosy Malaria Measles Meningococcal septicaemia Plague Rabies SARS Smallpox Tetanus Typhoid or paratyphoid Tuberculosis Typhus Yellow fever

As of April 2010, it is no longer a requirement to notify the following diseases: dysentery, ophthalmia neonatorum, leptospirosis, and relapsing fever.

Data from Health Protection Legislation (England) Guidance 2010, Department of Health, Crown Copyright.

Table 5.24 Antimicrobial agents: antibiotics—β-lactam agents

Drug	Route	Action	Spectrum of activity	Mechanism of action	Side effects	Empirical use	Notes
'Ordinary' penicillins: e.g. Benzylpenicillin (Pen G) & Phenoxymethyl penicillin (Pen-V)	*Pen G:* parenteral only. *Pen-V:* oral. Variable absorption in adults	Bacteriocidal	*Sensitive:* Strep, *Clostridium* spp., *Neisseria* (resistance increasing), treponemes, leptospira, *Listeria monocytogens*, many anaerobes (excluding bacteroides fragilis). *Resistant: Pseudomonas, H. influenzae*, MRSA	Bind to penicillin-binding proteins (PBPs) and inhibit cell wall synthesis	Hypersensitivity rash, interstitial nephritis, fever, anaphylaxsis, cerebral toxicity with high dose	Tonsillitis	Reduce dose in ESRF
Broader spectrum penicillins: e.g. ampicillin, amoxicillin, co-amoxiclav (amoxicillin + clavulanic acid*)	*Ampicillin:* best IV. *Amoxicillin:* best oral, better absorbed than Pen-V *Co-amoxiclav:* iv and po	Bacteriocidal	As 'ordinary' penicillins, but better action against *Enterococcus* spp. and action against some Gram –ves (including *E. coli*, *H. influenzae*, *Brucella*, and *Salmonella* spp.)	Bind to penicillin binding proteins (PBPs) and inhibit cell wall synthesis	'Ampicillin rash' in acute EBV. Anaphylaxsis. Nausea. Diarrhoea. *Clostridium difficile*. Cholestatic jaundice with Co-amoxiclav	Community Acquired Pneumonia	Reduce dose in renal impairement. Caution use of co-amoxiclav in hepatic failure
Flucloxacillin	Oral or iv	Bacteriocidal	Use for staphylococci and mixed infections with Strep. Inactive against *Enterococcus* and MRSA	As penicillin. Resistant to β-lactamases	Rare neutropenia. Reversible renal and hepatic (cholestatic) dysfunction	Soft tissue infections	No reduction in renal impairment
Gram negative β lactamase-resistance penicillins: e.g. piperacillin, tazocin (piperacillin + tazobactam*)	Parenteral only	Bacteriocidal	Active against many *Pseudomonas* spp. in addition to spectrum of co-amoxiclav. Less active against Gram +ve cocci, anaerobes and 'hard coliforms'	As penicillin. Resistant to β-lactamases	Sodium load. Occasional reversible platelet dysfunction and liver abnormalities. Rare convulsions (commoner in renal failure, previous CNS disease and old age)	Severe sepsis	Reduce dose in renal impairment
Carbapenems: e.g. meropenem	Parenteral only	Bacteriocidal	Meropenem good activity against virtually all bacteria groups excluding MRSA, *Enterococcus faecium*	As penicillin. Resistant to β-lactamases	Low risk of cross-reaction with penicillin allergy. Occasional reversible liver dysfunction, nausea	Severe sepsis	Reduce dose in renal impairment
Monobactam: e.g. Aztreonam	Parenteral only	Bacteriocidal	Aztreonam good activity against Gram –ve organisms, poor activity against Gram +ve organisms and anaerobes	As penicillin. Resistant to β-lactamases	No cross-reaction with penicillin allergy. Nausea, vomiting, diarrhoea. Occasional reversible neutropenia, thrombocytopenia, liver dysfunction		Reduce dose in renal impairment

(*continued*)

Table 5.24 Antimicrobial agents: antibiotics—β-lactam agents (*continued*)

Drug	Route	Action	Spectrum of activity	Mechanism of action	Side effects	Empirical use	Notes
1st generation cephalosporins: e.g. cefalexin, cefradrin	Oral	Bacteriocidal	Active against *Strep. pneumonia*, *Moraxella catarrhalis*, and most *E. coli*. Not active against enterococci, poor activity against *H. influenzae*	As penicillin. Resistant to β-lactamases	10% risk cross-reactivity with penicillin. Diarrhoea, *C. difficile*, fever, rashes, erythema multiforme, arthralgia, reversible hepatitis, or cholestasis	Uncomplicated URTI, UTI, and soft tissue infections	Reduce dose in renal impairment
2nd generation cephalosporins: e.g. cefoxitin, cepfuroxime	Oral and parenteral	Bacteriocidal	More resistant to β-lactamases than 1st generation drugs. Good activity against, *Staph. aureus*, *Strep. pneumonia*, *Neisseria* spp., *H. influenza*. Not active against enterococci	As penicillin. Resistant to β-lactamases	As 1st generation cephalosporins		Reduce dose in renal impairment
3rd Generation cephalosporins: e.g. cefotaxime, ceftriaxone, ceftazidime	Parenteral only	Bacteriocidal	As 2nd generation with increased activity against Gram –ve organisms. Ceftazidime is active against *P. aeruginosa*	As penicillin. Resistant to β-lactamases	As 1st generation cephalosporins		Reduce dose in renal impairment
4th generation cephalosporins: e.g. cefixime, cefpodoxime	Oral	Bacteriocidal	Similar range to 3rd generation cephalosporins	As penicillin. Resistant to β-lactamases	As 1st generation cephalosporins	Use restricted due to cost and frequency of adverse events	Reduce dose in renal impairment

Table 5.25 Antimicrobial agents: antibiotics—other

Drug	Route	Action	Spectrum of activity	Mechanism of action	Side effects	Empirical use	Notes
Glycopeptides: e.g. vancomycin, teicoplanin	Oral and parenteral	Bacteriocidal	Good action against virtually all Gram +ve organisms. No action against Gram –ve organisms (cannot cross cell wall)	Inhibit cell wall synthesis by binding to end of pentapeptide chains and preventing incorporation of new subunits in growing cell wall	Renal and oto-toxicity, occasional neutropenia. Rapid infusion of vancomycin associated with 'red man' syndrome	MRSA, *Staph. epidermidis, C. difficile*, severe infection in pencillin allergic patients	Therapeutic monitoring of drug levels necessary. Reduce dose in renal impairment.
Oxazolidinones: e.g. Linezolid	Oral	Bacteriostatic	Gram +ve organisms including MRSA and glycopeptide-resistant strains. No action against Gram –ve organisms	Inhibit protein synthesis by binding to 50S ribosomal unit	Diarrhoea, nausea, taste disturbance, headache, anaemia, leucopenia, and thrombocytopenia	Serious Gram +ve infections, including MRSA	Do not give concomitantly with MAO inhibitor drugs. Patients should avoid tyramine rich foods. Check full blood count (FBC) weekly during therapy. Avoid in uncontrolled hypertension, serious psychiatric disease, thyrotoxicosis, carcinoid, or phaeochromocytoma
Daptomycin	Parenteral	Bacteriocidal	Gram +ve organisms, including MRSA and glycopeptide resistant strains. No action against Gram –ve organisms	Disrupt bacterial cell membrane function	Anaemia, diarrhoea, nausea, vomiting, myopathy, Eosinophilic pneumonia, hypersensitivity	Severe MRSA or Vancomycin-resistant enterococci (VRE) infections (not pneumonia—inactivated by pulmonary surfactant)	Reduce dose in renal impairment. Monitor CK. Use with caution in patients receiving other myopathy-inducing drugs, e.g. HMG-CoA reductase inhibitors
Aminoglycosides: e.g. gentamicin, amicakin, tobramycin, netilmicin, streptomycin	Parenteral	Bacteriocidal	Gram –ve organisms and many *Pseudomonas* spp. Lower activity against *Staphylococcus* and *Streptococcus*. Poor anaerobic action	Inhibit protein synthesis by binding to 30S ribosomal unit	Nephrotoxicity (synergy with other nephrotoxic drugs, ototoxicity (8th nerve)	Gram –ve infection. Synergy with penicillin for endocarditis	Monitor levels. Reduce dose in renal impairment. Avoid in myasthenia gravis
Quinolones: e.g. ciprofloxacin, ofloxacin, levofloxacin	Oral and parenteral (excellent bioavailability)	Bacteriostatic	Broad spectrum, including *Pseudomonas* spp. Poor anaerobic action	Inhibition of DNA synthesis	Convulsions, diarrhoea, *C. difficile*, photosensitivity, confusion, hallucinations, tendonitis	Oral agent for *Pseudomonas* spp. infections.	Reduce dose in renal impairment.

(*continued*)

Table 5.25 Antimicrobial agents: antibiotics—other (*continued*)

Drug	Route	Action	Spectrum of activity	Mechanism of action	Side effects	Empirical use	Notes
Macrolides: e.g. erythromycin, clarithromycin, azithromycin	Oral and parenteral	Depends on drug	Similar spectrum to penicillins. Also *Mycoplasma* sp., *Legionalla pneumophilia, Chlamydia*	Inhibit protein synthesis by binding to 50S ribosomal unit	Phlebitis, gastric upset, diarrhoea, C. *difficile,* rash, fever, eosinophilia, ototoxicity (at high doses)	Penicillin allergy	
Lincosamides: e.g. clindamycin	Oral and parenteral	Bacteriostatic	Many Gram +ve organisms and obligate anaerobes	Inhibit protein synthesis by binding to 50S ribosomal unit	Diarrhoea, *C. difficile,* rash, fever, eosinophilia	Necrotizing fasciitis and penicillin allergy	
Tetracyclines: e.g. doxycyline, minocycline, lymecycline, tetracycline	Oral	Bacteriostatic	Broad action, but increasing resistance. Drugs of choice for *Chlamydia* spp., *Coxiella burnetti, Mycoplasma* spp., *Crucella* spp., rickettsial infection	Inhibit protein synthesis by binding to 30S ribosomal unit	GI disturbance	COPD exacerbations, MRSA	Avoid in renal impairment (except doxycyline)
Antifolate: e.g. trimethoprim, co-trimoxazole	Oral	Bacteriostatic	Gram –ve organisms, variable Staph. cover, poor streptococcal cover	Inhibition of folic acid and, therefore, nucleic acid synthesis	Nausea, vomiting, fever, rash, leucopenia, eosinophilia.	*Pneumocystis carinii*	Reduce dose in renal impairment.
Nitroimidazoles: e.g. metronidazole	Oral and parenteral	Bacteriocidal	Obligate anaerobes and protozoan	Disrupt DNA structure	Antabuse effect, nausea, metallic taste, peripheral neuropathy	*C. difficile,* anaerobic infections	Reduce dose in renal impairment

*Has no intrinsic antimicrobial action, but irreversibly inhibits many β-lactamases that degrade penicillins.

Table 5.26 Antimicrobial agents: anti-tuberculous drugs

Drug	Route	Action	Mechanism of action	Side effects	Notes
Isoniazid	Oral	Bacteriocidal	Kills rapid and intermediate growing mycobacterial populations	Hepatitis. Peripheral neuropathy. Agranulocytosis. SLE syndrome	Administer with pyridoxine in individuals with risk of peripheral neuropathy. Interacts with multiple other drugs. Avoid in acute liver disease
Rifampicin	Oral	Bacteriocidal	Kills all mycobacterium, including dormant populations.	Hepatitis. Rash. Nephritis. Rash. Flu-like syndrome	Multiple drug interactions (including oral contraceptive, digoxin, β-blockers, warfarin, protease inhibitors)
Pyrazinamide	Oral	Bacteriocidal	Kills slow growing mycobacterial populations	Hepatitis. Nausea and vomiting. Myalgia and arthralgia	Dose reduce in renal failure. Avoid in acute gout and severe hepatic impairment
Ethambutol	Oral	Bacteriostatic	Kills all mycobacterial populations	Optic neuropathy (red-green colour blindness or change in visual acuity)	Dose reduce in renal failure
Streptomycin	im	Bacteriocidal	Kills slow growing mycobacterial populations	Renal impairment. Ototoxicity	

Table 5.27 Antiretroviral drugs

Drug	Route	Mechanism	Activity	Side effects	Notes (interactions)
Nucleoside reverse transcriptase inhibitors (NRTI) Two NRTIs combined with either NNRTI or PI as first line therapy. Cause mitochondrial toxicity—lipoatrophy, neuropathy, pancreatitis, lactic acidosis, hepatic steatosis					
Abacavir (ABC)	po	Inhibition of viral reverse transcription by incorporation into elongating vDNA causing chain termination	HIV Hep B (3TC and FTC)	*Fatal hypersensitivity (HS):* avoid if HLA B5701; possible ↑ CVD risk	*Caution:* pregnancy; never re-challenge if HS reaction
Didanosine (ddI)	po			Mitchondrial toxicity. Possible ↑ CVD risk	Ribavirin: pancreatitis; allopurinol; *Caution:* pregnancy
Emtricitabine (FTC)	po			Minimal	
Lamivudine(3TC)	po			Minimal	(Zalcitabine – interference) YMDD mutation – Hep B
Stavudine (d4T)	po			Mitchondrial toxicity	*Zidovudine:* interference
Zidovudine (AZT)	po/iv			Anaemia ↑MCV; Headache	*Stavidine:* interference
Nucleotide reverse transcriptase inhibitors (NRTI)					
Tenofovir (TDF)	po	As NRTI	HIV Hep B	Renal tubular dysfunction. Osteopenia	Avoid with ddI

(*continued*)

Table 5.27 Antiretroviral drugs (*continued*)

Drug	Route	Mechanism	Activity	Side effects	Notes (interactions)
Non-nucleoside reverse transcriptase inhibitors (NNRTI) Low genetic barrier to drug resistance. Extremely potent P450 CYP3A inducers.					
Nevirapine (NVP)	po	As NRTI	HIV	Rash; fatal hepatotoxicity *Avoid if:* CD4>350 (female) CD4>250 (male)	*Potent P450 CYP3A inducer:* ↑ metabolism of antimicrobials; warfarin; anticonvulsants; cyclosporin; anti-arryhthmics, etc.
Efavirenz (EFV)	po			Neuropsychiatric SE. Dyslipidaemia. Diabetogenic. Lipohypertrophy	As nevirapine. Co-formulated with TDF/FTC in single tablet once daily (Atripla).
Protease inhibitors (PI) *High genetic barrier to resistance. Class side effects—lipohypertrophy; diabetogenic. Trials of monotherapy ongoing.* Most co-formulated with low dose ritonavir given its potent P450 CYP3A inhibition (boosted PI).					
Atazanavir (ATV)	po	Inhibition of protease enzyme (responsible for cleaving nascent capsid proteins for viral assembly), preventing packaging and release of new virions	HIV (also activity against Leishmania)	↑ Bilirubin	As Ritonavir if co-formulated
Fosamprenavir (FOS-APV)	po			Rash (avoid if sulpha allergy)	As Ritonavir if co-formulated
Darunavir (DRV)	po			Hepatitis; ↑ CK	As Ritonavir if co-formulated
Indinavir (IDV)	po			Renal stones	Rarely used
Lopinivir (LPV)	po			GI; dyslipidaemia	As Ritonavir if co-formulated
Ritonavir (RTV)	po			GI; dyslipidaemia	*Potent P450 CYP3A inhibitor:* ↑↑ levels of antimicrobials; warfarin; anticonvulsants; cyclosporin; anti-arryhthmics, etc. Can be fatal (midazolam)
Saquinavir (SQV)	po			GI; dyslipidaemia	As Ritonavir if co-formulated
Tipranavir (TPV)	po			Hepatotoxicity; SAH	As Ritonavir if co-formulated
Integrase inhibitor					
Raltegravir (RAL)	po	Inhibit integrase enzyme, preventing integration of vDNA into host DNA	HIV	Hepatitis; ↑ CK	Metabolized by glucoronidation via UGT1A1
Entry inhibitor					
Maravaroc (MVC)	po	Small molecule inhibitor of human chemokine receptor (CCR5) binding	R5-tropic strains of HIV	Hepatotoxicity	Metabolized by CYP3A
Fusion inhibitor					
Enfurvitide (T-20)	sc	Inhibits gp41-membrane fusion	HIV	Injection site reactions. GI toxicity. Bacterial pneumonia	

Table 5.28 Antiviral drugs

Drug	Route	Mechanism	Activity	Side effects	Notes (interactions)
Neuranimidase inhibitors					
Oseltamavir	po	Block budding from cell	Influenza A/B	GI upset; CNS (delirium)	Avoid in pregnancy
Zanamavir	Inhalation			Minimal; cough, sinusitis	Avoid if underlying respiratory disease Use in pregnancy
Adamantines					
Amantadine	po	Poorly understood—prevents uncoating	Influenza A	CNS (agitation/delirium/seizures)	High level resistance
Rimantadine	po				High level resistance
Nucleoside analogues All can cause mitochondrial toxicity and flares of Hepatitis B on discontinuation					
Adefovir	po	Incorporation into elongating vDNA (RNA – ribavirin) causing chain termination	Hepatitis B	Minimal; rarely nephrotoxicity	–
Cidofivir	po		CMV/JCV (BKV)	Nephrotoxicity	Avoid concomitant nephrotoxic drugs
Entecavir	po		Hepatitis B	Minimal	Some HIV activity—do not use as Hepatitis B monotherapy in HIV co-infection
Ribavirin	po/inhalation		Hepatitis C RSV Lassa	Haemolytic anaemia	Teratogenic ddI—causes pancreatitis *Caution:* cardiac disease
Telbivudine	PO		Hepatitis B	Minimal	
Guanosine analogues					
Acyclovir	iv/po	Incorporation into elongating vDNA causing chain termination, activated by viral thymidine kinase (TK)	HSV VZV	Minimal; rarely: crystallises in urine, seizures	Resistance-mediated by TK mutations. Dose adjust in renal failure
Famciclovir	po		HSV/VZV	As acyclovir	As acyclovir
Valaciclovir	po		HSV/VZV	As ganciclovir	As acyclovir
Ganciclovir	iv/intra-ocular/po		CMV	Pancytopenia	Resistance-mediated by TK mutations. Teratogenic. Dose reduce in renal failure
Valganciclovir	po		CMV	As ganciclovir	As acyclovir
Interferons					
Interferon alpha/pegylated IFN-alpha	sc	*Stimulate* transcription of ISGs	Hep B/C (HIV)	Depression; flu-like symptoms; exacerbation of psoriasis, diabetic retinopathy; seizures; hypothyroidism; cytopenias	Avoid in poorly-controlled epilepsy or diabetic retinopathy
Miscellaneous					
Foscarnet	iv	Inhibits pyrophosphate binding to viral DNA polymerase	HSV CMV	Nephrotoxicity, hypokalaemia	Reduce dose in renal impairment and avoid concomitant nephrotoxic drugs. Use for resistant HSV/CMV infections

Table 5.29 Antimalarial drugs

Drug	Route	Mechanism	Activity	Side effects	Notes (interactions)
Quinine	po/iv	Inhibits breakdown of haem	Blood stage	Cinchonism (tinnitus, vertigo, vomiting, rash). Hypoglycaemia	Omit loading dose if previously taking mefloquine. Reduce dose in renal impairment
Mefloquine	po	As quinine	Blood stage	Neuropsychiatric; arrhythmia	*Avoid*: history of psychiatric illness; prophylaxis only
Aminoquinolones					
Amodiaquine	po	Unclear	Blood stage	As chloroquine	Rarely used
Chloroquine	po	Unclear	Blood stage	Itching, exacerbation of psoriasis	High level resistance *P. falciparum 1st line*: non-falciparum
Primaquine	po	Blocks oxidative metabolism	Hypnozoites (non-falciparum)	Haemolytic anaemia in G6PD deficiency	Use to prevent relapse (non-falciparum). *Avoid*: G6PD deficiency. Test for G6PD prior to use
Artemesinin derivatives					
Artemether-lumefantrine	po	Unclear, mediated by peroxide bridge	Blood stage	GI upset, headache, dizziness	Prolongs QTc *Avoid*: family history of sudden cardiac death *Metabolized*: P450 CYP3A4
Artesunate	iv/im	As artemether	Blood stage	As artemether	As artemether. Severe *P. falciparum* (given with quinine due to production reliability issues)
Antibiotics					
Clindamycin	po	Inhibits protein synthesis	Blood stage	Antibiotic-associated diarrhoea. Skin rash	Use with quinine for treatment of *P. falciparum*
Doxycycline	po	Inhibits protein synthesis	Blood stage	GI upset, photosensitivity	Treatment (+ quinine) or prophylaxis.*Avoid*: children, pregnancy
Others					
Atovaquone-proguanil	po	Dihydrofolate reductase inhibitor	Liver and blood stage	*Minimal*: GI upset	Treatment or prophylaxis

Table 5.30 Antimicrobial agents: anti-fungal drugs

Drug	Route	Spectrum of activity	Mechanism of action	Side effects	Notes
Echinocardins: e.g. caspofungin, micafungin	iv only	*Candida* and *Aspergillus*. Not *active* against *Cryptococcus* and dermatophytes	Inhibits synthesis of cell wall component, decreasing cell wall integrity	Hepatotoxicity, infusion reactions, headache, drugs interactions, histamine type reactions	Resistance described for some Candida spp.
Polyenes: e.g. amphotericin B, liposomal amphotericin B, nystatin	Ampotericin iv. Nystatin topical only.	Broad including invasive aspergillosis, *Candida*, cryptococcal, histoplasma, blastomyces, coccidioides, zygommycosis	Bind to ergosterol in cell membrane to form a pore, increasing permeability	Acute infusion related chills, rigor and hypotension. Dose-dependent renal toxicity. Phlebitis at injection site. Hypokalaemia	Lipid formulations are associated with improved side effect profile, but increased cost.
Azoles: triazoles, e.g.. fluconazole, itraconazole, voriconazole, posaconazole	iv and oral	Broad, excluding non-*Candida albicans* spp. Fluconazole is not active against Aspergillus fumagatus	Inhibit synthesis of ergosterol	Hepatotoxic. Nephrotoxic. Drug interactions. Nausea and vomiting. Torsades de pointes. Rashes	Excellent oral bioavailability. Multiple drug interactions (including warfarin, rifampicin, and immunosuppressive agents)
Azoles: imidazoles, e.g. ketoconzole, clotrimazole, miconazole		Broad, excluding non-*Candida albicans* spp. and *Aspergillus fumagatus*	Inhibit synthesis of ergosterol	As for triazoles. Gynaecomastia (ketoconazole)	Excellent oral bioavailability. Multiple drug interactions
Pyrimadine: e.g. flucytosine		Candida Crytococcus Aspergillus	Nucleoside analogue inhibiting DNA synthesis	Bone marrow suppression. Nephrotoxicity. Hepatotoxicity	Only used in combination therapies in order to minimize generation of resistance
Griseofulvin		Onychomycoses	Binds to fungal polymerized microtubules to inhibit mitosis	Headache. Hepatitis. Photosensitivity	Drug interactions (including warfarin)
Pentamidine		*Pneumocystis jiroveci*	Inhibits DNA syntheses; mechanism unknown	Fatigue, dizziness, decreased appetite, dyspnoea	
Allylamines: e.g. terbinafine		Onychomycoses	Inhibit synthesis of ergosterol	Gastrointestinal	

Multiple choice questions

1. A 25-year-old man who admits to having unprotected sexual intercourse with a number of partners is diagnosed with syphilis. He is treated with a 14-day course of doxycycline. Serology results are as follows:
   - *Pre-treatment:* VDRL positive; TPHA titre 1:256.
   - *Post-treatment:* VDRL negative; TPHA titre 1:16.

   What would you recommend?

   A. Repeat doxycycline.
   B. Give azithromycin.
   C. Do nothing.
   D. Give ceftriaxone (im).
   E. Give ciprofloxacin.

2. A 30-year-old man is due to start treatment for hepatitis C with pegylated interferon alpha and ribavirin. Which of the following is a recognized adverse effects/concerns regarding treatment of this patient?

   A. Erythema multiforme.
   B. Teratogenicity.
   C. Hypertrophic cardiomyopathy.
   D. Visual field defects.
   E. Early dementia.

3. Which of the following is *not* a notifiable disease in the UK under the Health Protection (Notification) Regulations 2010?

   A. Legionaire's disease.
   B. Tuberculosis.
   C. Smallpox.
   D. Malaria.
   E. *Staphylococcus aureus* infective endocarditis.

4. A 16-year-old woman presents with headache and neck stiffness of 3 days duration. Lumbar puncture results are as follows:
   - WCC 400 × 106/L (80% lymphocytes).
   - RCC 25 × 106/L.
   - Protein 0.63 g/L.
   - Glu 4.8 mmol/L (serum 5.4 mmol/L).

   Gram stain reveals no organisms. What is the most likely diagnosis?

   A. *Mycobacterium tuberculosis.*
   B. *Haemophilus influenza.*
   C. *Streptococcus pneumoniae.*
   D. Enterovirus.
   E. *Neisseria meningitides.*

5. Against which of the following diseases is a live attenuated vaccine routinely used

   A. Japanese encephalitis.
   B. TB.
   C. HPV.
   D. Hepatitis B.
   E. Botulism.

6. Which of the following diseases is caused by a helminth?

   A. Schistosomiasis
   B. Malaria
   C. Toxoplasmosis
   D. Chagas disease
   E. Leishmaniasis

7. Which of the following bacteria are correctly classified?

   A. *Strep. Pneumoniae*: Gram positive cocci, catalase positive
   B. *Listeria Monocytogenes*: Gram positive rod, anaerobic
   C. *E. coli*: Gram negative cocci
   D. *N. meningitidis*: Gram –ve rod, lactose fermenter
   E. *Enterococci*: Gram positive cocci, catalase negative

8. Which of the following is a Non-nucleotide reverse transcriptase inhibitor (NNRTI)?

   A. Nevirapine.
   B. Didanosine.
   C. Ritonavir.
   D. Lamivudine.
   E. Indinavir.

9. Which of the following drugs can cause optic neuropathy?

A. Isoniazid.
B. Rifampacin.
C. Pyrazinamide.
D. Ethambutol.
E. Streptomycin.

10. Which of the following antibiotics inhibit bacterial protein synthesis?

A. Vancomycin.
B. Ceftazadine.
C. Gentamicin.
D. Meropenem.
E. Coamoxiclav.

For answers, please see Appendix: Answers to multiple choice questions, page 313.

CHAPTER 6

Statistics and epidemiology

Descriptive population statistics

Descriptive statistics is the process of using numbers to summarize or better understand a set of data. In clinical science, almost all data sets can be described as either categorical or continuous. When an attribute is either present or absent in a population, e.g. rash or no rash, this is known as *categorical*, or discrete, data. Categorical variables sometimes have more than two categories, for example macular rash, papular rash, no rash. However, when an attribute is measured on an interval scale, e.g. peak expiratory flow rate, the data is known as *continuous* data. This distinction is important as it determines the likely distribution of the data and, therefore, which statistical methods are used for analysis. In medicine, continuous data are often dichotomized into categorical data by assigning values either side of a defined cut-off value (e.g. 'healthy' if peak expiratory flow rate is above 75%, 'disease' if below).

Normal (or Gaussian) distribution

Many continuous variables, such as height, IQ, and plasma sodium concentration, have a Normal distribution in the population. Plotting the probability distribution of the variable yields the familiar bell-shaped curve (Fig. 6.1). Continuous variables are evaluated using *parametric* methods. If a distribution appears to be positively or negatively *skewed* it can often be transformed to a Normal distribution by taking the logarithm, reciprocal, or square root, of each observation.

Non-normal distribution

Continuous variables that are not Normally distributed or for which no assumptions about distribution can be made are evaluated using *non-parametric* methods. Examples might be patients' pain scores after surgery (probably positively skewed) or duration of pregnancy of live births (probably negatively skewed).

Binomial distribution

Categorical data have a binomial (or if more than two categories, multinomial) distribution. The probability of the number of successes in a sequence of individual observations (such as rash versus no rash in a sequence of *n* patients, or heads versus tails in a series of coin tosses) is plotted against *n*. It is quite different from the Normal distribution, yet if the sample size is large enough the shapes of the graphs will look similar. The binomial distribution in Fig. 6.2 shows the probability of observing a given number of heads (or tails) in 40 successive coin tosses. In other words, the binomial probability distribution for $p=0.5$, $n=40$.

Poisson distribution

Categorical data about the number of some discrete event occurring over a specified time, e.g. number of epileptic seizures per year, follow the Poisson distribution. This

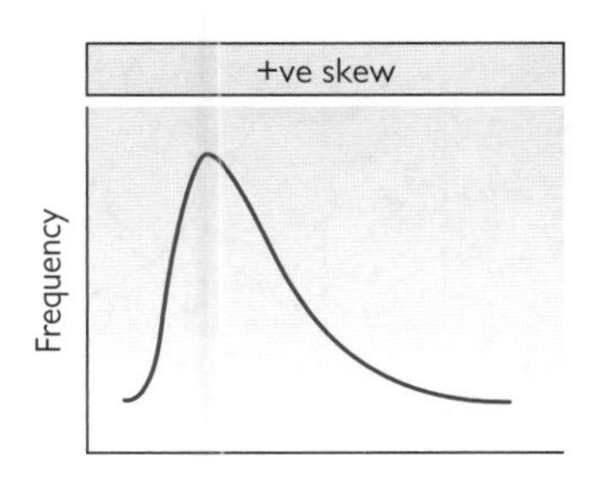

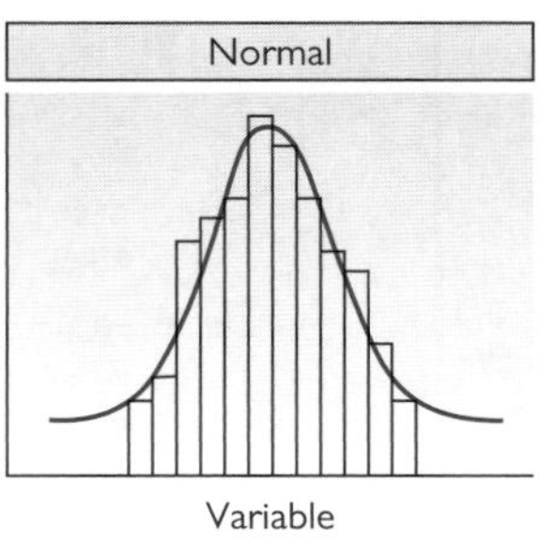

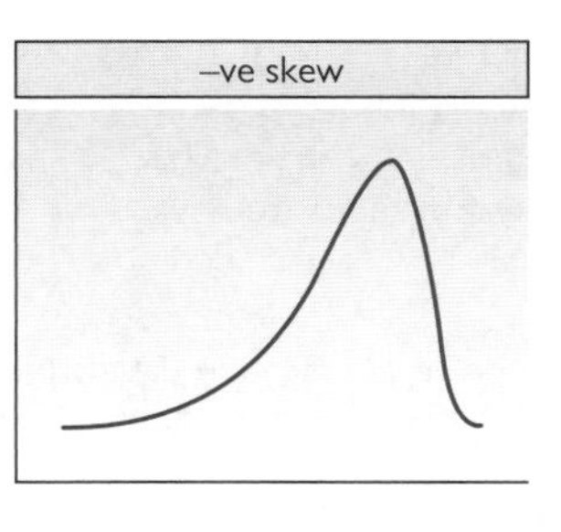

Fig. 6.1 The shape of frequency distributions of continuous variables can be positively, normal and negatively skewed.

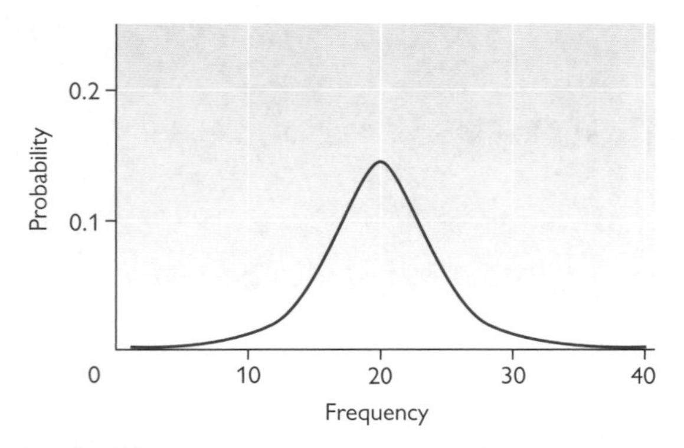

Fig. 6.2 A binomial distribution with n=40, p=0.5.

distribution usually arises in the context of an event with a low probability in a very large population, and in which there is no theoretical limit to the number of events that could occur.

Summarizing continuous data

Continuous data are summarized in terms of both central tendency and variation.

Central tendency

There are three measures of *central tendency*: mean, median, and mode.

- The *mean* (μ) is the arithmetic average, obtaining by summing all the values and dividing by the number of observations, $\mu = \Sigma\chi/n$.
- The *median* is the middle point of all the values, in other words 50% of the data lie below and 50% above the median.
- The *mode* is the most commonly observed value. Some distributions can be multimodal (several peak values).

Suppose we have the following results from an experiment repeated eight times: 32, 11, 12, 18, 22, 22, 24, 19. Then:

- Mean = sum of values/8 = 20.
- Median = midpoint of values = 19 + 22/2 = 20.5.
- Mode = 22.

When a distribution is *skewed*, the mean is a poor measure of central tendency because it is susceptible to strong influence from outliers, therefore, the median should be used.

- *Normal:* mean = median = mode.
- + *Skew:* mean > median >= mode (usually).
- – *Skew:* mean < median <= mode (usually).

Variation

Measures of *variation* differ whether the data is Normally or non-Normally distributed. The *range* states the lowest and highest data points (the 0th and 100th percentile), without giving any information about the spread of the data. A better indication of this might be the *interquartile range*, which states the 25th and 75th percentiles, thus giving an indication of the spread of the middle 50% of values. The *n*th percentile is the point below which *n*% of the data lie. When stated together with the median, the interquartile range provides a good assessment of variation for a non-Normally distributed data set.

In a Normally distributed data set, the data are symmetrically spread around the median (which equals the mean) and, therefore, we can use variance and standard deviation (SD) to succinctly describe variation (Fig. 6.3). The *standard deviation* (σ) provides a measure of the spread of values (χ_1, χ_2, χ_3 ...) around the mean, calculated by taking the square root of the average squared difference between each value and the mean, or $\sigma = \sqrt{[\Sigma(\chi-\mu)^2/n]}$. It is approximately equivalent to the average difference between the sample value and the mean. The more tightly grouped the values, the smaller the σ will be. The *variance* is σ^2.

For all Normally distributed data, approximately 68% of data lie within +/− 1 σ of the mean, 95.5% within 2 σ, and 99.7% within 3 σ. The 95% confidence interval (CI) for a single observation in a Normally distributed sample is the mean +/− 1.96 σ. This is the range within which we can be 95% confident that any given value from our sample will fall. Changing the multiplier from 1.96 to 2.58 includes exactly 99% of the distribution.

When a population is repeatedly sampled, the data sets obtained will differ. For example, if we measure the blood pressures of 100 people, and then replicate the experiment on another 100 people, we would expect the two means to vary. How much the mean varies on repeated sampling gives us a measure of how reliably the sample mean estimates the true population mean. The *standard error of the mean* (SEM) is a measure of the expected spread of these sample means—in other words how reproducible the mean is. SEM = $\sigma/\sqrt{n}$, where *n* is the number of observations. The following distinction is important: SD is a measure of variation between individual observations, whereas standard error is a measure of variation of the mean, or other statistic, derived from a sample of observations.

Just as described previously we calculated the 95% CI for a single observation in a sample, we can also calculate a 95%

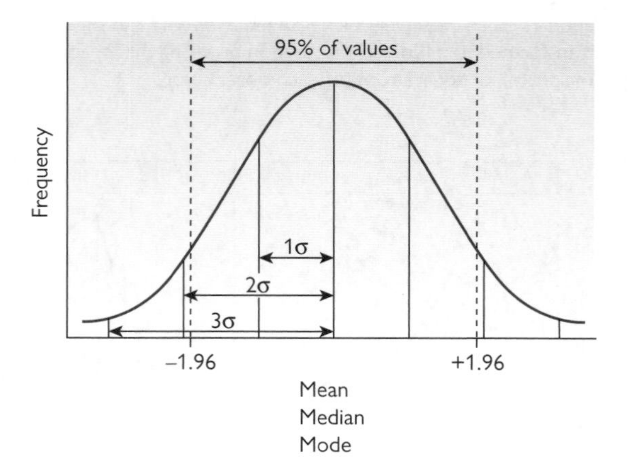

Fig. 6.3 The mean and standard deviation of a normally distributed variable illustrated on a frequency distribution.

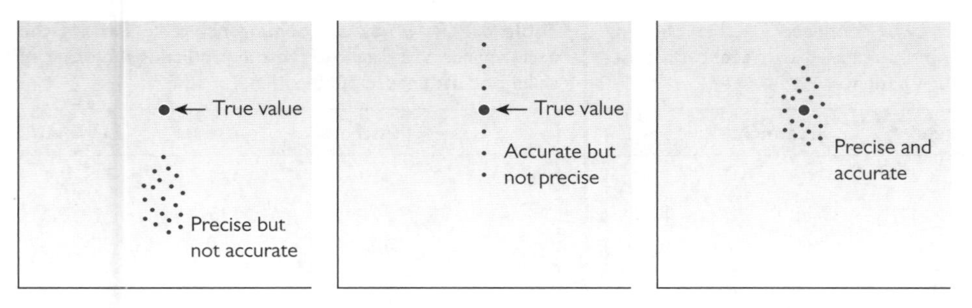

Fig. 6.4 The difference between precision and accuracy of assay measurements in relation to the true value.

CI for the mean, within which it is 95% probable that a new sample mean will lie, by calculating the mean +/− 1.96 SEM. It should be noted that as sample size, *n*, falls below about 100, this approximation becomes less exact because the distribution of means is less likely to approximate the Normal distribution, and so the Students *t* distribution should be used. This will calculate a multiplier based on sample size, which approaches to 1.96 as *n* increases.

Clinical measurements and assays

Statistics that describe variability and uncertainty are particularly relevant when evaluating clinical measurements and laboratory assays. The reliability of an assay can be summarized by two terms. *Precision* is the term used to describe repeatability or reproducibility of a measurement or assay. *Accuracy* refers to the closeness of an observation to its true value. For example, a new troponin assay could be precise, giving very similar values on repeat sampling from the same patient, yet inaccurate, because the values do not reflect the patient's true troponin level (Fig. 6.4).

Summarizing categorical data

For a binomial distribution, where the probability of the attribute being present is p (and therefore the probability of it being absent is $1-p$), the mean is np and the variance is $np(1-p)$. As n increases, the binomial distribution approaches a Normal distribution with mean np and variance $np(1-p)$. For a Poisson distribution, the mean and variance are equal and, for very large samples, it approaches a Normal distribution with mean equal to variance.

When summarizing categorical data, the frequency distributions of each attribute are typically displayed in a *contingency table* from which effect size statistics can be calculated.

Effect size statistics

Effect size statistics deal with concepts of probability, odds and risk. For example, Table 6.1 is a two-by-two contingency table showing the data on 2000 adults with or without atrial fibrillation (AF), recruited in equal numbers, who were observed for 1 year to see if they suffered a cerebrovascular accident (CVA).

Based on these data, the *probability* of an adult having a CVA if they have AF is 31/1000=0.031, whereas without AF it is 0.009. Put differently, the estimated annual *risk* of CVA for adults in AF is 3.1%.

Table 6.1 A two-by-two contingency table showing the relationship between AF and CVA in 2000 patients

	CVA yes	CVA no	Totals
AF yes	31	969	1000
AF no	9	991	1000
Totals	40	1960	2000

The *odds* of an event is the probability of it occurring compared to the probability of it not occurring, or for an event with probability p, the odds are $p/1-p$.

Therefore, the odds of an adult having a CVA if they have AF is 31/969=0.032, and the odds of an adult having a CVA if they don't have AF is 9/991=0.009. The *odds ratio*, another way to express risk, is the ratio of the odds in the exposed group to the odds in the unexposed group=0.032/0.009=3.56. A patient in AF is 3.56 times more likely to have a CVA per year than one without AF.

Evaluating randomized controlled trial data

Effect size statistics are also needed to evaluate data from trials of therapeutic interventions. Suppose a randomized controlled trial of a new medication for post-operative nausea yields the data given in Table 6.2.

On first glance, it can be seen that there were a total of 48 nauseated patients of which 36 occurred in the placebo group and 12 in the treatment group, so the

Table 6.2 A two-by-two contingency table showing the effect of a treatment compared to placebo on post-operative nausea in 1094 patients

	Placebo	Treatment	Totals
Nausea	36	12	48
No nausea	512	534	1046
Totals	548	546	1094

medication appears to work. The following statistics are usually calculated.

- Event rate: the *control event rate* (CER), or the probability of the event in the control group, is 36/548=0.066. In other words the risk of nausea in the control group is 6.6%. The *experimental event rate* (EER) is 12/546=0.022.
- *Relative risk: RR*=EER/CER=0.022/0.066=0.33. In other words, the risk of nausea with the medication is 33% of the risk without medication. Compare this with the odds ratio (described earlier), which is 12/534÷36/512=0.32. You may have noticed that the odds ratio gives a good estimate of relative risk. This is providing that the number of trial subjects is large and the event is quite rare. The mathematical difference is to do with ratios—the relative risk uses event rates in the intervention group compared to the whole study population, whereas the odds ratio uses event rates in the intervention group compared with controls.
- *Relative risk reduction: RRR* is 1 – RR, or can also be calculated from CER – EER/CER=0.066 – 0.022/0.066=0.66. The medication reduces the risk of nausea by 66%, which sounds very efficacious. The problem with RRR is that it does not take into account the baseline risk of nausea, which is actually quite low at 6.6%.
- *Absolute risk reduction: ARR* is calculated as CER – EER=0.044, in other words, the absolute occurrence of nausea is 4.4% less with medication.
- *Number needed to treat:* This is calculated from the ARR and therefore gives us information about absolute benefit, rather than relative benefit, which can be particularly misleading if the CER of a condition is low. *NNT*= 1/ARR=23 so 23 post-operative patients would need to be treated to prevent one incidence of nausea. When analysing data about harm, rather than benefit, such as the occurrence of a side effect, the calculation yields a number needed to harm (NNH).
- *Patient expected event rate:* this is useful if you believe that the event rate for your particular patient is different than the CER. For example, you might estimate a pregnant patient to be twice as prone to post-operative nausea as normal. Hence, the estimated *PEER* is 0.132, and the patients at risk of readmission (PARR) is therefore PEER×RRR=0.087. The NNT for your particular patient type is lower at 11.

Table 6.3 A two-by-two contingency table showing the performance of a diagnostic test in predicting the onset of childhood asthmas in 1000 patients

	Asthma yes	Asthma no	Totals
Test+ve	90	169	259
Test–ve	6	735	741
Totals	96	904	1000

Evaluating diagnostic tests

The contingency table is also used when summarizing categorical data about diagnostic tests and screening programmes. For example, suppose there is a new blood test to predict subsequent onset of childhood asthma, which yields the results shown in Table 6.3 in 1000 randomly selected babies.

Of 1000 babies, 96 subsequently developed asthma, so the *pre-test probability* is 9.6%. How useful was the blood test at detecting these? It successfully identified 90 out of 96 cases and there were 6 *false negatives*. In other words the proportion of *true positives* that were correctly detected by the test, the *sensitivity*, was good at 93.7%. How useful was the blood test at ruling out future asthma cases? It successfully ruled out asthma in 735 of 904 babies, and there were 169 *false positives*. In other words, the proportion of *true negatives* that were correctly identified, the *specificity*, was moderate, 81.3%.

- *SnNout:* for a test with high sensitivity, if the test is negative, it rules the diagnosis out.
- *SpPin:* for a test with a high specificity, if the test is positive, it rules the diagnosis in.

For a test that produces a continuous measurement (such as the D dimer test), how is the cut-off value chosen? The area under the *receiver operating characteristic* (ROC) curve reflects the relationship between sensitivity and specificity for a given test (Fig. 6.5). Sensitivity (true positive rate) on the *y*-axis is plotted against 1 – specificity (false positive rate) on the *x*-axis. High-quality tests will have an area under the ROC approaching 1, and high-quality publications about clinical tests will provide information about the area under the ROC. The perfect test, with no false positive or false negative results, would be represented by a line from the origin up the *y*-axis and across the top of the plot, whilst a test that produces false positives and true positives at an equal rate would produce a diagonal $y=x$ line.

Sensitivity and specificity are characteristics of the diagnostic test, not the population being studied. To interpret sensitivity and specificity in individual patient terms, it is useful to ask: 'Does this positive test mean my child will get asthma?' to which the answer is: 'Not necessarily' because, of 259 positive tests, only 90 babies, or 34.7% get asthma. This is the *positive predictive value* (PPV). What about asking 'Does this negative test mean my child won't get asthma?' The *negative predictive value* (NPV), 735 out

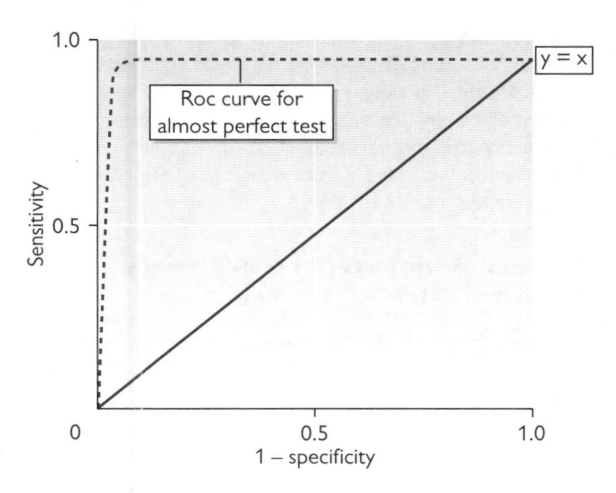

Fig. 6.5 A receiver operating characteristic (ROC) curve for a test plotting sensitivity against false positive rate (1-specificity).

Table 6.4 A two-by-two contingency table showing the performance of a diagnostic test in identifying a disease

	Disease yes	Disease no	Totals
Test+ve	a	b	a+b
Test−ve	c	d	c+d
Totals	a+c	b+d	a+b+c+d

a = True positives; b = false positives; c = false negatives; d = true negatives.
Sensitivity = a/a + c.
Specificity = d/b + d.
Positive predictive value = a/a + b.
Negative predictive value = d/c + d.
Likelihood ratio$^{(+)}$ *for ruling in a diagnosis* = sensitivity/1 − specificity = a/(a + c) ÷ b/(b + d).
Likelihood ratio$^{(-)}$ *for ruling out a diagnosis* = 1 − sensitivity/specificity = c/(a + c) ÷ d/(b + d).
Post-test odds = pre-test odds × LR.
Pre-test odds = pre-test probability/(1 − pre-test probability).
Post-test probability = post-test odds/(post-test odds + 1).

of 741, is 99.2% so the answer is 'this negative test makes it highly unlikely. For every 100 babies like yours, 99 do not develop asthma'.

The prevalence of the condition in the population being studied is crucially important when interpreting PPV and NPV. If, instead of testing all newborn babies, we tested all 2-year-olds who had already suffered three or more episodes of wheeze in their lives, we would get very different values (although the sensitivity and specificity of our test would stay the same) because this population is already much more likely to develop asthma. In other words their *pre-test probability* is higher. How do we work out the *post-test probability*?

For a given condition and a given diagnostic test, the pre-test probability and post-test probability are related to the *pre-test odds* and *post-test odds*, respectively, as follows: if the probability of an event is p, the odds are $p/1 - p$.

The pre- and post-test odds are related to each other by a useful term called the *likelihood ratio*, which is a measure of the diagnostic value of a test. A test with a high LR$^{(+)}$ (>5) is good at increasing certainty about the presence of a disorder, and a low LR$^{(-)}$ (<0.2) is good at increasing certainty about the absence of a disorder, but LRs around 1 are unhelpful.

Odds of disease after test = odds of disease before test × likelihood ratio

The *likelihood ratio* (LR) can also be estimated from sensitivity and specificity:

$$\text{For ruling in a diagnosis, } LR^{(+)} = \text{sensitivity} / (1 - \text{specificity})$$

$$\text{For ruling out a diagnosis, } LR^{(-)} = (1 - \text{sensitivity}) / \text{specificity}$$

In this example about asthma, LR = 5.01.

The statistical terms and formulae relating to diagnostic tests are summarized in Table 6.4.

Inferential statistics

Hypothesis testing involves making estimations or predictions about something unknown using some prior knowledge, thus moving from descriptive statistics to inferential statistics. It necessitates making assumptions and therefore dealing with error and significance.

Null hypotheses

The basis for this is the *null hypothesis*, which is the hypothesis that there is no difference between two groups of data. In clinical science, the two groups usually differ in respect of a medical intervention. The *alternative hypothesis* is that the two groups are not equal, in other words that there is a true difference between the two groups.

To test a null hypothesis, a *p value* is calculated using a statistical 'significance test' (these are described later in 'Significance tests'). The p value is the probability of getting a data set at least as extreme as that observed if the null hypothesis is true. The larger the p value, the more likely it is that the data have arisen by chance alone (that the null hypothesis is true) and do not represent a real difference between the groups. If the p value is small, it is more likely that the alternative hypothesis is favoured. Tests can either be one- or two-tailed, depending on the null hypothesis being tested. A one-tailed hypothesis specifies the direction of a difference or correlation (treatment A is *not superior* to treatment B) and can be tested with a smaller sample than a two-tailed hypothesis (treatment A *equivalent* to treatment B).

A p value < 0.05 means that, if the null hypothesis is true, there is a less than 1 in 20 chance of the observed data arising by chance. In other words, it is over 95% probable that the two groups of data genuinely differ and, therefore, the null hypothesis should be rejected in favour of the alternative hypothesis. The two groups are said to be significantly different. For medical interventions, it is conventional to set the significance level at 0.05. However, for some types of research (for example, genome-wide association studies) the significance level is set much lower. The principle is that the null hypothesis should only be rejected when a chance error is very unlikely as we do not want to conclude that a treatment is effective (or a gene polymorphism associated with a disease) when it is not.

Type I error

When the null hypothesis is wrongly rejected when it is actually true, it is known as a *type I error*. This is a false positive result, where the two interventions are wrongly deemed to be different when they are actually not. The probability of a type I error is α, and in the example given earlier, it would be 0.05. This means that if you repeated a trial of an effective intervention trial 20 times, a negative result would be expected once on average.

Type II error

A *type II error* is a false negative result, where the two interventions are genuinely different, but they have been wrongly deemed to be equivalent (the null hypothesis is wrongly accepted). The probability of a type II error is β. In medicine, a type II error may be preferable than a type I error because it is less harmful to reject an effective intervention than to adopt an ineffective one.

The *power* of a study is $1 - \beta$. This is the probability that the difference between the interventions, if one exists, will be shown to be statistically significant (that the null hypothesis is rejected when it is, indeed, false). Having a larger sample size will increase the power.

Significance tests

Significance tests are mathematical functions which compute an observed value of a test statistic from experimental data. The p value required to determine significance is derived from this test statistic. The type (categorical, continuous) and distribution (Normal, non-Normal, binomial) of the data determines which significance test should be used. In practice, computer programs are used to do these calculations.

Parametric tests (for Normally-distributed data)

- *Unpaired student* t*-test:* this test is used to compare the means of two independent groups of values. For example, we could compare the mean weights of two groups of patients having received different weight reduction treatments to see if they are significantly different.
- *Analysis of variance (ANOVA) test:* ANOVA enables the means of more than two groups to be compared instead of using multiple t-tests, which would increase the chance of committing a type I error.
- *Paired Student* t*-test:* this test is used to compare the means of values obtained from a single group at two different points in time. For example, we could compare the mean weight of a group of patients before and after a specific treatment to see if it is significantly reduced (or increased). It is 'paired' because each patient contributes one data point to each group.

Non-parametric tests (for non-Normally-distributed data)

- *Mann Whitney U-test:* this non-parametric test is used to compare the medians of two independent groups, equivalent to the unpaired Student *t*-test.
- *Wilcoxon matched pairs test:* this non-parametric test is used to compare the medians obtained from a single group at two different points in time.
- *Kruskal–Wallis test:* this is the non-parametric equivalent of ANOVA.

Tests for categorical data

- *Chi-square test:* this test is used to compare the proportions of two or more groups with a particular attribute. For example, we could compare the proportion of people suffering a cerebrovascular accident in two groups receiving statin or no statin to see if they are significantly different. An odds ratio of 1, or whose 95% CI includes the value 1, implies that there is no difference between the two groups.
- It is important to appreciate that statistical significance does not imply clinical significance. In a very large trial of a new weight loss therapy we might say with great confidence that the intervention group lost more weight (say $p < 0.0001$), but that the mean weight loss was only 200 g. Effect-size statistics (described previously) allow quantification of risk and benefit on an individual patient basis.

Tests of correlation

Correlation tests are used to evaluate the strength of a linear relationship between two variables measured in a single group (without making any implication about cause and effect). For example, we might want to investigate whether serum glucose is related to core body temperature. We would use Pearson's correlation coefficient because we expect the variables to be Normally distributed. The Spearman's rank correlation coefficient is the non-parametric equivalent test of correlation.

A correlation coefficient (r) can be between –1.0 and +1.0, where zero indicates no relationship. A large positive r (+0.5 to +1.0) indicates a strong positive relationship (blood glucose rises and falls with body temperature), whereas a large negative r (–0.5 to –1.0) indicates a strong inverse relationship (blood glucose rises as body temperature falls). If it is believed that the relationship between a dependent and an independent variable is non-linear, it might be necessary to transform the data using logarithms or square roots. Alternatively, there may be multiple confounding factors involved for which multiple regression is needed.

Multiple regression analysis

This is necessary to determine relationships between continuous variables if there are multiple confounding variables. The analysis derives a model to describe the relationship between x and y and allow prediction of y for any given x, but taking into account any non-linearity and the confounding effect of variable z. Several correlation coefficients are computed, to express the independent risk attributable to each variable. For example, regression analysis would be required to analyse the complex relationship between multiple cardiovascular risk factors and incidence of heart disease, and develop a risk prediction model.

Degrees of freedom

Significance testing requires estimates of various parameters to be made, however, each estimate reduces the certainty of the resulting statistic. The degrees of freedom is the number of independent values in the final calculation of a statistic that are free to vary. The more degrees of freedom (DF), the more likely the result is to achieve significance. For an unpaired *t*-test, DF=total number of observations − 2. For a paired *t*-test, DF=no of pairs of observations − 1. For a correlation coefficient, DF=no of pairs of observations − 2. For a chi-square test, DF=(number of rows − 1) × no of columns − 1).

Study design

When designing a clinical study or trial, many factors need to be taken into account, the overall objective being to maximize the chances of testing the hypothesis, whilst minimizing bias. Broadly, they fall into two categories—observational studies and interventional trials.

Observational studies

Cross-sectional study

Like a census, this aims to provide data about population health, normal ranges of biological parameters, and disease prevalence or severity by observing the entire population, or a representative subset, at a single point in time. The disadvantage of retrospective data collection is that it is susceptible to recall bias.

In this kind of study we can determine *prevalence*, which is the total number of cases of a condition existing within a population, often quoted as cases per 1000 or per 100,000 people. When the study is performed over a specified time interval, or repeated, we can also estimate *incidence*, which is the number of new cases occurring in a given period of time, often quoted as cases per 1000 per year. Rates such as birth rate, mortality rate, and age-specific mortality rate are determined in this way.

Case-control study

This is a specific type of cross–sectional study, usually retrospective, in which cases of a specific disease (for example, new variant Creutzfeld–Jacob disease) are identified and matched to controls who do not have the disease. Data are then collected to identify any differences between the two groups (for example, prior surgical procedures or prior beef consumption). Case control studies are ideal for studying associations between an exposure and an outcome when the outcome is uncommon or if the outcome occurs decades after exposure. They allow calculation of the odds ratio for exposure and outcome. However, unlike in a whole population study absolute risk cannot be quantified.

A cohort study

This is typically prospective and longitudinal (although can be conducted retrospectively from records) and involves following a defined group of people (for example, exposed to a particular toxin) for a set time to determine association with a future outcome (for example, developing mental illness). The comparator group may be otherwise similar unexposed people or members of the general population. Cohort studies are ideal for studying associations between an exposure and an outcome when the exposure is uncommon and, additionally, they allow calculation of absolute and relative risk (but not odds ratio). However, they can take many years if the outcome is delayed.

Interventional trials

Clinical trials

These are used to test a hypothesis that a particular healthcare intervention is different from another or from no intervention. They occur in multiple phases. The initial objective is to evaluate the safety of the healthcare intervention or find out the optimal dose, but the ultimate aim is to test its efficacy or effectiveness.

- *Phase I:* the first stage of human testing in which a small group of healthy volunteers is given the intervention under close monitoring to evaluate safety, tolerability, and in the case of drugs, pharmacodynamics.
- *Phase II:* larger trials in both healthy volunteers and patients in which safety and tolerability continue to be assessed, but efficacy is also evaluated.
- *Phase III:* even larger multicentre randomized controlled trials (RCT) to definitively assess efficacy against the gold standard.
- *Phase IV:* post-marketing surveillance trials in which safety data continue to be collected and specific issues, such as drug interactions and pregnancy may be evaluated, even after the intervention is licensed.

Sample size

The *sample size* in a *phase II* or *III clinical trial* is critical, and must be determined knowing the incidence of the disease in question, the potential effect of the intervention (estimated from earlier studies), the significance level deemed acceptable, and the variance of the outcome measure. The ideal clinical trial would have large numbers of a relevant sample population, appropriate follow-up, and would be randomized, double-blinded, and have a placebo-controlled comparator group. Due to economical, logistical, and intervention-specific issues this is not always possible.

Randomization

Randomization to study groups removes any allocation bias to which the researchers might be prone. It also improves the chances of having comparably matched groups. Block randomization is usually done to keep group sizes approximately equal as the trial proceeds, in case the trial is terminated early or interim analysis is planned. Variable block sizes ensure researchers cannot predict the final allocation in a given block. Stratified random allocation is used to increase the matching between groups in smaller trials. In cluster randomization, the allocation is done by centre, rather than by subject. After randomization the subjects in each group are cared for and followed-up identically except for the intervention in question. The process of randomization can be complex involving computer generated sequences and anonymous telephone centres, or more simple with sequentially numbered opaque sealed envelopes.

- In an *open trial* everybody knows which intervention is being given.
- In a *single blind trial* either the subject or the researcher is not blinded. This is usually either because the placebo does not perfectly mimic the intervention (for example, the drug has a detectable side effect) or because the researcher has to know the full facts (for example, to do real versus sham electroconvulsive therapy).
- A *double blind trial* usually achieves the highest standard of scientific rigor because it eliminates both conscious and unconscious bias on the part of the researcher and the subject.
- A *cross-over study* involves each patient receiving both (or all) of the interventions being compared and, therefore, acts as their own control. The order in which they receive the interventions must be randomized and there is usually a 'washout period' between different drugs.

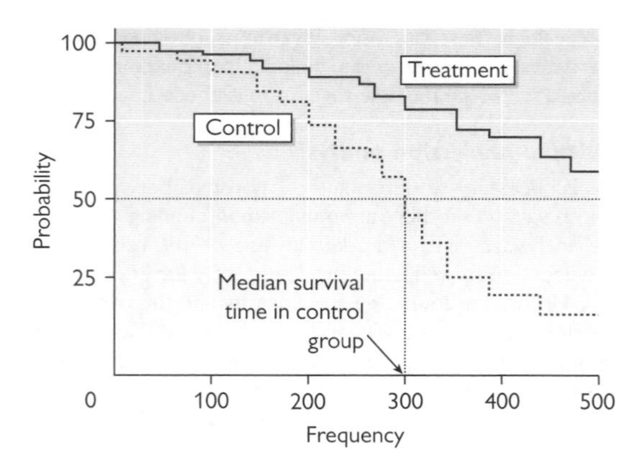

Fig. 6.6 A Kaplan-Meier graph plotting survival over time.

- *A placebo-controlled* design accounts for bias caused by the *placebo effect*, whereby patients do better when they think they are receiving a treatment than when they are not, even if the treatment is an inactive substance.

Follow-up

The *follow-up* period must be long enough to allow the outcomes of the trial to occur, which requires prior knowledge about the natural history of the condition being studied. Drop-out rates must be sufficiently low so as not to bring into doubt the results of the trial, and equivalent in both the control and intervention groups. Additionally, it is essential all subjects are analysed in the groups to which they were initially assigned, even if they end up crossing-over or dropping out of the trial. This is known as *intention-to-treat* analysis. Failure to do this usually biases the results in favour of the poorer intervention.

Survival curves

The time from treatment to disease recurrence or from treatment to death is often a primary outcome measure in interventional studies. These data are best displayed on Kaplan–Meier survival curves, where probability of survival (or recurrence) is plotted against time elapsed (Fig. 6.6). The cumulative survival probability at a selected time point can be estimated from the graph. Alternatively, the median survival time can be estimated as the time interval indicated by a survival probability of 50%. A plot of control and intervention groups on the same graph allows direct comparison.

Evidence-based medicine

This is defined as the explicit use of current best evidence gained from the scientific method to guide clinical decisions. The inferential statistics described earlier, especially post-test odds and number needed to treat, will help to decide if a patient would benefit from a particular diagnostic test or intervention. This is assuming that the methodology of the trial was sound, that the trial was designed to answer the relevant clinical question (internal validity), and that the patient in question is similar enough to the trial subjects for the results to be applicable (external validity). Finally, the patient will have their own values and preferences that must be considered.

Different types of medical evidence are graded according to their rigor and freedom from bias. The highest level of evidence is that obtained from randomized controlled trials, whilst the lowest level is that obtained from case reports or expert opinion. Various grading schemes and categories of recommendations exist, and the following is adapted from widely accepted guidance published by the Oxford Centre for Evidence Based Medicine:

- *Grade A:* consistent level 1 studies, namely randomized controlled trials.
- *Grade B:* consistent level 2 (cohort) or level 3 (case control) studies *or* extrapolations from level 1 studies.
- *Grade C:* level 4 studies, namely case series, *or* extrapolations from level 2 or 3 studies.
- *Grade D:* expert opinion without explicit critical appraisal, or based on physiology, bench research or first principles, *or* inconclusive studies at any level.

Systematic review and meta-analysis

A *systematic review* is a paper that collects and summarizes all of the evidence surrounding a particular clinical question. The term 'systematic' refers to a clearly defined methodology for searching and identifying all potentially relevant literature, critically evaluating it, and selecting it for inclusion based on predefined quality criteria. This distinguishes a systematic review from the more commentary style expert reviews found in many journals.

A systematic review may include a *meta-analysis* of results, whereby statistical methods are used to integrate multiple studies by analysing all the data from the included literature to reach a more powerful estimate of effect size. In meta-analyses of randomized controlled trials of interventions, the outcome data from each trial are usually illustrated as a series of odds ratios with their confidence intervals on a graph known as a forest plot.

Further reading

Howick J, Chalmers I, Glasziou P, *et al.* *The Oxford 2011 Table of Evidence*. Oxford Centre for Evidence-Based Medicine. http://www.cebm.net/index.aspx?o=5653

Multiple choice questions

1. Which of the following statistical tests is appropriate for comparing means between two independent parametric variables?

A. Repeated measures ANOVA with Tukey's *post-hoc* analysis.
B. Mann–Whitney *U*-test.
C. Unpaired *t*-test assuming unequal variances.
D. Wilcoxon matched pairs test.
E. Kruskal–Wallis test.

2. If the null hypothesis is wrongly rejected when it is actually true, this an example of:

A. A test with a high power.
B. A test with a type II error.
C. A test with a high negative predictive value.
D. A test with a type I error.
E. A test with data, which must be non-parametric.

3. The performance of a new predictive test for a disease is evaluated with the following results:

	Those with disease	Those without disease
Test positive	98	902
Test negative	2	98

Which of the following statements is correct?

A. The test has a high sensitivity.
B. The test has a high positive predictive value.
C. The test has a high specificity.
D. The test has a low negative predictive value.
E. The test is not useful clinically.

4. An intervention reduces the risk of death from 10 in 1000 to 5 in 1000. The number needed to treat to prevent one death is:

A. 1000.
B. 200.
C. 5.
D. 990.
E. 15.

5. The following measurements are made of systolic blood pressure in a sample of patients on a hospital ward: 80, 90, 90, 90, 95, 100, 130, 140, 150, 160, 160, 160, 170.

A. The median value is 100.
B. The data is normally distributed.
C. The data is bimodal.
D. The mean is higher than the median.
E. The range is smaller than the standard error.

6. Drug A reduces the risk of contracting a disease from 10 in 10,000 to 5 in 10,000 in trial A, whilst in a separate trial drug B reduces the risk of contracting the same disease from 3 in 1000 in 2 in 1000. Which of the following statements are true?

A. The absolute risk reduction of drug A is greater than drug B.
B. The relative risk reduction of drug A is less than drug B.
C. Assuming that both drugs have an additive effect and the actual risk of contracting the disease is 6 in 1000, taking both drugs together will reduce the risk to 5 in 10,000.
D. Assuming that both drugs have an additive effect and the actual risk of contracting the disease is 6 in 1000, taking both drugs will reduce the risk to 2 in 1000.
E. The incidence of the disease in the control arm of trial A is 10 in 10,000.

7. Which of the following data sets are categorical?

A. Height.
B. Plasma brain type natriuretic peptide (BNP).
C. Weight.
D. Age.
E. Sex.

8. A receiver operating characteristic curve:

A. Plots the probability of survival against time from intervention or start of treatment.
B. Reflects the relationship between sensitivity and specificity for a given test.
C. Describes the distribution and skew of data.
D. Can only be used for categorical data.
E. Demonstrates the degree of correlation between two variables.

9. Calculating an appropriate sample size for a randomized placebo controlled trial is based upon all the following variables except:

A. The required power of the trial.
B. The incidence of the disease being studied.
C. The estimated impact of the intervention.
D. The variance of the outcome measure.
E. Whether it is a phase II or phase III trial.

10. All of the following are a measure of spread of data except:

A. Correlation coefficient.
B. Standard deviation.
C. Interquartile range.
D. Variance.
E. Range.

For answers, please see Appendix: Answers to multiple choice questions, page 313.

CHAPTER 7

Haematology

Introduction

Blood is a suspension of several cell types in a proteinaceous aqueous medium known as plasma. It transports oxygen in red cells and essential ions, amino acids and proteins in plasma for cellular respiration, while removing the waste products of this process. As a transport medium it also carries hormones and other signalling molecules from where they are produced to their target organs, while white blood cells and platelets help protect against infection and repair damaged tissue.

Plasma is an iso-osmotic aqueous medium, the basic constituents of which are sodium and potassium salts, glucose, and plasma proteins. Plasma is isolated from the cellular fractions of blood by centrifugation in the presence of an anticoagulant to prevent the blood from clotting. Serum is similar to plasma, but is isolated by allowing the blood to clot; as a result, serum does not include clotting factors.

Red blood cells

Erythrocytes are the most abundant cell type in the blood (Table 7.1). They are anucleate and account for ~40% of total blood volume in healthy adults (the haematocrit). They develop in the bone marrow from large, nucleated normoblastic cells that differentiate into mature red cells in response to renally produced erythropoietin. Healthy red blood cells are a biconcave discoid shape (~8 μm in diameter) that is sufficiently flexible to allow them to pass through capillaries, which can be as narrow as 3 μm. They have a life span of 18–120 days in the circulation before being broken down by macrophages in the spleen and, to a smaller extent, in the liver and bone marrow. An increased red cell mass is known as polycythaemia and can be secondary to chronic hypoxia and high levels of erythropoietin (e.g. from high altitude or chronic pulmonary disease) or from a myeloproliferative condition of the bone marrow itself (e.g. polycythaemia rubra vera).

Haemoglobin

Red blood cells contain haemoglobin, a complex protein comprising four polypeptide chains each of which contains a haem- group and form a subunit. In the fetus the main type of haemoglobin is HbF (2α and 2γ chains), while in the first year of life adult haemaglobin A (2α and 2β in adults) gradually replaces this. About 4% of haemoglobin in the adult is HbA2 (2α and 2δ chains). Diseases associated with abnormal production of haemoglobin polypeptide chains are summarized in Box 7.1).

The haem- group of haemoglobin consists of a Fe^{2+} in a protoprorphyrin ring. In order to bind O_2 efficiently, haem iron is kept in its reduced (Fe^{2+}) form as opposed to the met (Fe^{3+}) form by NADPH-fuelled methaemoglobin reductase and the abundant endogenous antioxidant, glutathione (gsh). The haem- groups are synthesized in the mitochondria of maturing red blood cells and in the liver in a process requiring circulating iron bound to transferrin. Protoporphyrin is synthesized via a metabolic pathway, which starts with the combination of glycine and succinyl CoA to form d-amino laevulinic acid (ALA); the rate-limiting step. Two ALAs are then combined to form porphobilinogen (PBG). Inherited disorders in the synthesis of haem from porphobilinogen are known as the 'Porphyrias' and the enzyme defects are highlighted in the summary diagram of haem synthesis in Fig. 7.1.

The hepatic porphyrias (acute intermittent porphyria, porphyria variegate, and hereditary coproporphyria lead to increased ALA and PBG in the urine as well as increased urine and faecal porphyrins, whereas erythropoietic porphyrias lead to increased urine and faecal porphyrins only.

Failure to incorporate Fe^{2+} into haemoglobin can lead to iron deposition into mitochondria around the nuclei. Red cells then appear as 'ring sideroblasts' in a condition known as sideroblastic anaemia, which can either be inherited or acquired (such as in lead poisoning).

Iron, found in meat, liver, and cereals, is taken up in the upper small intestine and transported in the plasma in the

Table 7.1 The cellular elements of whole blood

Cell type	Site of production	Typical cell count (l−1)	Comments and function
Erythrocytes (red cells)	Bone marrow	5×10^{12} (men) 4.5×10^{12} (women)	Transport of O_2 and CO_2
Leukocytes (differential count)		7×10^{9}	
Granulocytes			
Neutrophils	Bone marrow	5.0×10^{9} (40–75%)	Phagocytes—engulf bacteria and other foreign particles
Eosinophils	Bone marrow	100×10^{6} (1–6%)	Congregate around sites of inflammation—have antihistamine properties Very short lived in blood
Basophils	Bone marrow	40×10^{6} (<1%)	Circulating mast cells—produce histamine and heparin
Agranulocytes			
Monocytes	Bone marrow	0.4×10^{9} (2–10%)	Phagocytes—become macrophages when they migrate to the tissues
Lymphocytes	Bone marrow, lymphoid tissue, thymus, spleen	1.5×10^{9} (20–45%)	Production of antibodies
Platelets	Bone marrow	250×10^{9}	Aggregate at sites of injury and initiate hemostatis

Note that, while mean values are given, these are subject to considerable individual variation. The approximate percentage of individual types of leukocyte are given after the number per liter—this is called the differential white cell count.

BOX 7.1 HAEMOGLOBINOPATHIES: ABNORMAL PRODUCTION OF POLYPEPTIDE CHAINS

- *Sickle cell disease:* abnormal β chain production (valine to glutamate substitution at position 6) leads to HbS production. Heterozygotes produce up to 40% HbS with the rest HbA while homozygotes produce HbS with HbF and HbA2.
- *Thalassaemias:* are characterized by small amounts of otherwise normal polypeptide chains causing anaemia. α-Thalassaemia (*HBA*$_1$ and *HBA*$_2$ genes on chromosome 16) is lethal for homozygotes, but insignificant in heterozygotes and is prevalent in peoples of Western African and South Asian descent. β-thalassaemia (*HBB* gene on chromosome 11) is prevalent among Mediterranean peoples. Homozygotes (major) can have pronounced anaemia, while heterozygotes (minor) have a more subtle phenotype that, like sickle cell heterozygotes, may confer a degree of protection against malaria, thus perpetuating the mutation

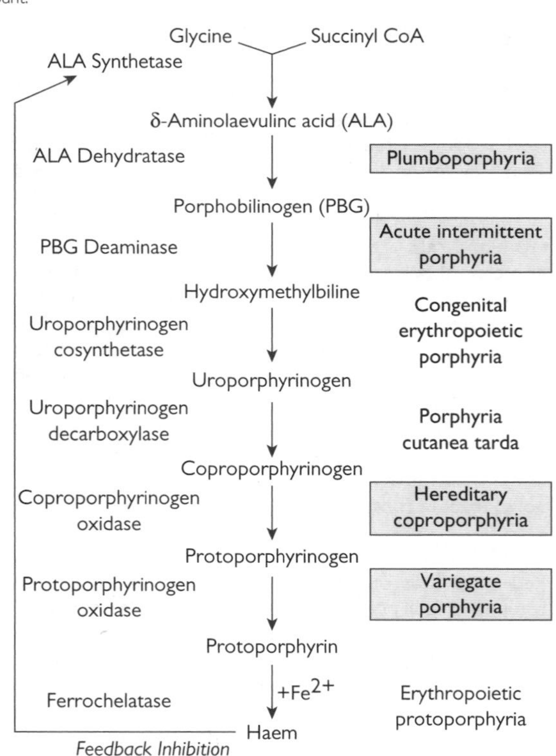

Fig. 7.1 Metabolic pathways of haem synthesis.

Reproduced from MFM James and RJ Hift, 'Porphyrias', *British Journal of Anaesthesia*, 2000, 85, pp. 143–153, by permission of Oxford University Press

Fe^{3+} form bound to transferrin (which is usually about a third saturated). Transferrin-bound iron can be stored as ferritin in the plasma, liver, spleen, and bone marrow. Iron deficiency either due to insufficient dietary source or on-going bleeding, is therefore diagnosed by a reduced plasma iron in the context of a low plasma ferritin level, and high plasma transferrin or high total iron binding capacity. Conversely, mutations in transferrin, its receptor or proteins that regulate the interaction of transferrin with its receptor (e.g. *HFE* gene) can cause excess iron deposition in organs such as the liver, pancreas, and heart in a condition known as hereditary haemochromatosis.

Anaemias and abnormal red cell shape (poikilocytosis)

Haemoglobin concentration is usually 13–17 g/dL in males and 12–15 g/dL in females (due to the loss of blood from menstruation). A low haemoglobin concentration or anaemia is usually viewed in the context of the red cell size.

Macrocytosis

A mean cell volume >100 fl can be associated with a megaloblastic bone marrow in conditions where there are problems with DNA synthesis such as Vitamin B12, folate deficiency and secondary to cytotoxic drugs. In these conditions, red cell number and haemoglobin concentration are usually low and basophilic nuclear remnants of DNA can be found in circulating erythrocytes, which have not been expelled during bone marrow erythropoiesis. These are known as Howell–Jolly bodies, which can also be seen in association with myelodysplasia, hereditary spherocytosis, and asplenia. A macrocytosis with a normoblastic bone marrow is seen in liver disease, alcohol excess (although this can be via folate deficiency) and myxodema.

Microcytosis

A mean cell volume <76 fl is usually associated with hypochromia, in that the mean corpuscular haemoglobin concentration is also low. The most common cause of this is iron deficiency, but it can also be seen in thalassaemia heterozygotes (trait) and in sideroblastic anaemias (see under haem- metabolism)

Normocytic anaemias

Normocytic anaemias can occur as a result of an increase in plasma volume (e.g. pregnancy, iv fluid administration), during acute blood loss, and also during chronic disease. In response to inflammatory mediators in the latter, the liver produces increased amounts of hepcidin. Hepcidin, in turn, stops ferroportin from releasing iron stores. In addition, inflammatory mediators may also inhibit erythropoiesis to produce anaemia. Complete bone marrow failure can lead to aplastic anaemia and can be a result of chemotherapy, bone marrow irradiation, or in response to hepatitis causing viruses that are also toxic to bone marrow stem cells.

Haemolysis

Haemolysis is another cause of a normocytic anaemia. This is characterized by pre-hepatic jaundice with raised plasma bilirubin and lactate dehydrogenase (LDH) together with haemosiderin and urobilinogen present in the urine. Fragmented 'schistocytes' and an increased number of immature reticulocytes are often seen on blood film. The condition is classified as to whether haemolysis occurs intravascularly or mainly extravascularly in the reticuloendothelial system (see Box 7.2). A direct antiglobin (Coombs' test) can help distinguish between an autoimmune haemolytic anaemia and other causes. The patient's red cells are washed and incubated with antihuman globulin (or Coombs' reagent). If immunoglobulin or complement factors are fixed to the red cells the antihuman globulin will agglutinate the cells, which can be directly visualized, producing a positive result.

BOX 7.2 THE PRINCIPLE CAUSES OF RED CELL HAEMOLYSIS

Intravascular haemolyisis

- Infections (e.g. malaria).
- Mirco-angiopathic haemolytic anaemias.
- Early haemolytic transfusion reaction (see 'Blood groups').
- G6PD deficiency.
- Paroxysmal nocturnal haemoglobinuria.

Extravascular haemolysis

- Hereditary spherocytosis.
- Haemoglobinopathies.
- Autoimmune haemolytic anaemia.

Blood groups

Red blood cells, along with many other cells in the body, express antigens on their cell membranes. These antigens are glycoproteins (proteins linked to carbohydrate chains), the precise structures of which are determined at a genetic level. In humans, there are two types of antigen that can be expressed, each with a different sugar residue at a specific locus in its carbohydrate chain—type A has an acetylgalactosamine, whereas type B has galactose. Blood groups are assigned according to which of these antigens is expressed in an individual, hence, the blood groups A, B, AB (where both are expressed), and O (where neither are expressed). In terms of Mendelian inheritance, A and B are co-dominant, while O is recessive. The blood group of an individual determines the antibodies that they will produce against red blood cell antigens and the compatibility of blood used for transfusion.

There are a large number of other antigens on red blood cells many of which have not yet been fully characterized. Rhesus antigens constitute a group of glycoproteins that are expressed in most people (85% Caucasians and 99% Orientals are Rhesus positive, Rh+). The Rhesus system only becomes an issue in the case where a Rhesus negative (Rh–) mother gives birth to a Rh+ child that is of the same ABO blood group as the mother. In the event of some red blood cells from the fetus crossing into the mother's circulation during childbirth, the cells will not be destroyed by the mother's immune system because they are of the same ABO group. However, the surviving cells will induce the mother to produce antibodies against Rh antigens and while the first child is unaffected, should the mother have a second Rh+ child, her immune system will destroy the red blood cells of the child, leading to haemolytic disease. The issue is overcome in modern medicine by screening pregnant women for Rh and injecting them with Rh+ antibodies within 36 hr of childbirth to destroy any fetal red blood cells before her immune system has time to generate antibodies of her own.

White blood cells

The primary function of leucocytes is to fight infection. They can be divided into two classes:

- Lymphocytes that act in concert with immunoglobulins and the complement system to instigate immunity.
- Phagocytes that contribute to inflammatory processes and actively ingest invading pathogens, diseased host cells, and cellular debris.

The origins of WBCs, as well as erythrocytes and platelets, are outlined in Fig. 7.2.

Lymphocytes and natural killer cells

Lymphocytes are derived from stem cells, which differentiate into lymphoid stem cells in response to specific cytokines (e.g. interleukin 3, il-3) and growth factors (e.g. granulocyte-macrophage colony stimulating factor, GM-CStF), release of which is stimulated by infection. In this way, the body responds rapidly by generating more WBCs to help deal with the crisis. All of the main causes of a lymphocytosis are summarized in Box 7.3. Lymphoid stem cells differentiate into B lymphocytes (in the bone marrow) and T lymphocytes (in the thymus). B lymphocytes are responsible for generating antibodies for immunity and are characterized by expression of specific surface markers (CD19, 20, and 22). T lymphocytes express CD4 or CD8 surface markers (amongst others), and have the ability to distinguish between healthy cells that belong to the host individual ('self'), and foreign or diseased cells ('non-self'). CD4-Expressing lymphocytes help to produce antibodies ('helper cells'), while CD8 expressing lymphocytes initiate cell-mediated immunity against intracellular organisms. Mature B and T cells circulate in the bloodstream, but are able to migrate into tissues to fight infection, and also gravitate towards the lymph nodes and spleen via the lymphatic system, resulting in localized swelling of the nodes during infection. Lymphocytes flow back into the bloodstream via the thoracic duct into the superior vena cava. NK cells are also derived from lymphoid stem cells in the bone marrow. NK cells are designed to search and destroy cells that are infected by viruses or are cancerous.

The phagocytes: granulocytes and monocytes

Phagocytes are derived from haemopoeitic stem cells, which differentiate into myeloid stem cells in the bone marrow. The fate of myeloid stem cells is determined by the relative abundance of specific monocyte, granulocyte, or eosinophil-derived growth factors and interleukins.

Neutrophils

These granulocytes have a very distinctive nuclear arrangement consisting of densely packed chromosomal material in 2–5 distinct lobes. The cytoplasm of neutrophils is packed with primary granules containing a range of enzymes that generate highly toxic oxygen-related species, including superoxide and hydrogen peroxide (e.g. myeloperoxidase) and secondary granules contain enzymes that act to lyse cells and digest their contents, (e.g. lysozyme, collagenase) or deprive them of essential iron (lactoferrin). The primary function of neutrophils is the identification, phagocytosis, and killing of invading pathogens. Mature neutrophils only circulate for about 10 hr, before they undergo apopotosis and are cleared by macrophages. The main causes of neutrophilia and neutropenia are summarized in Boxes 7.4 and 7.5 respectively.

Eosinophils

Eosinophils are very similar in structure, function, and origin to neutrophils. Their distinguishing feature is their 2–3-lobed dense nucleus and they are often associated with allergic reactions and defence against parasites. See Box 7.6 for causes of eosinophila.

Monocytes and macrophages

Both neutrophils and monocytes, originate from myeloid progenitor cells, which differentiate into granulocyte stem cells. Monocytes circulate in a quiescent form for up to 2 days before they migrate into tissues and differentiate into macrophages. Macrophages are the scavengers of the immune system and are particularly prevalent in the liver (where they are sometimes called Kupffer cells) and the lungs. However, they accumulate in specific sites of infection to help kill invading pathogens and to clear cellular debris from the site. See Box 7.7 for causes of monocytosis.

Basophils

Basophils are rarely found in peripheral blood and when they enter tissues, they become mast cells that are involved in the recruitment of other inflammatory cells to sites of infection or damage. These cells are packed with histamine and heparin-containing granules that can obscure the nucleus.

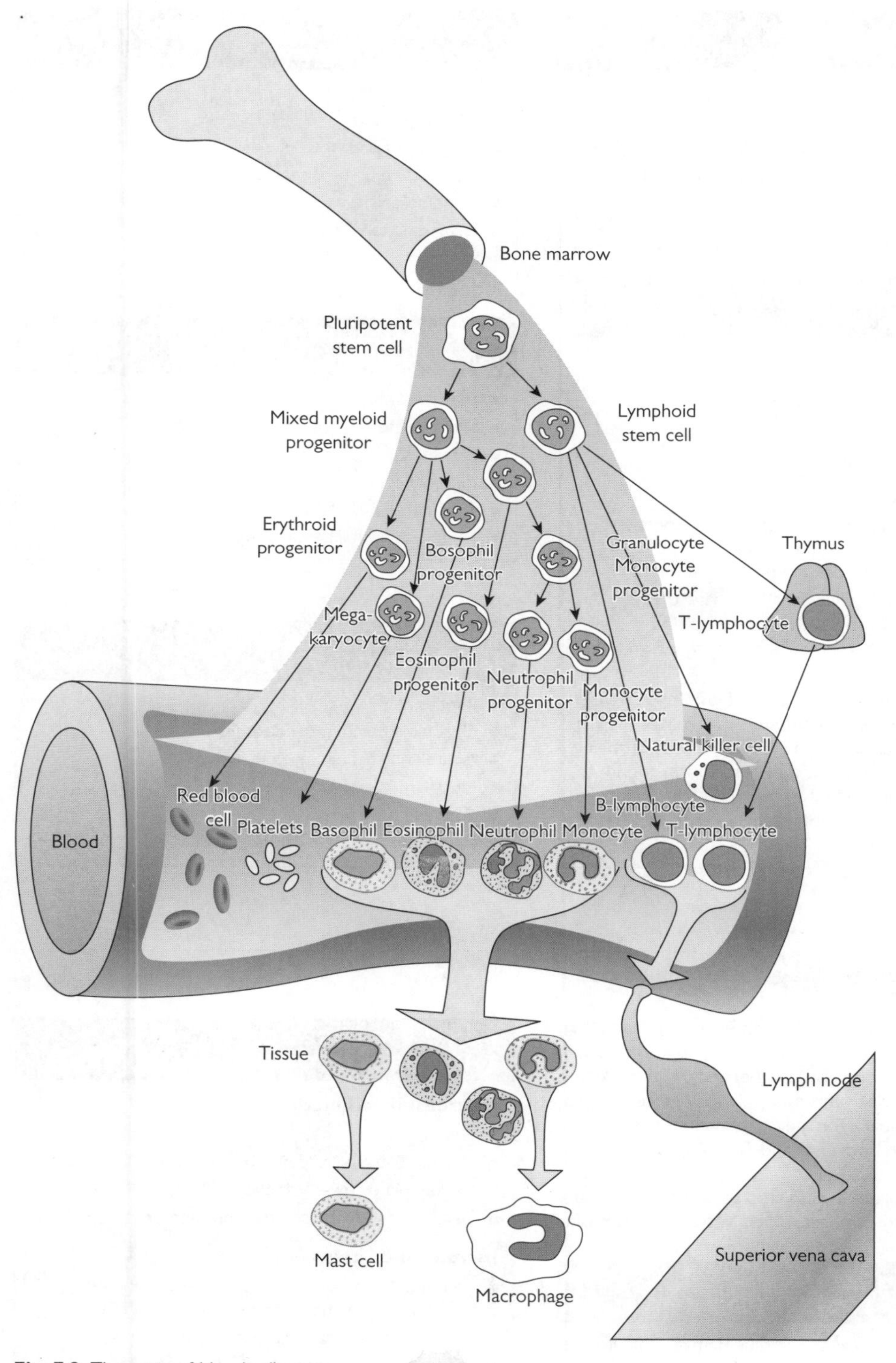

Fig. 7.2 The origin of blood cells.

Reproduced from R Wilkins et al., *Oxford Handbook of Medical Sciences, Second Edition*, 2011, Figure 6.23, p. 413, by permission of Oxford University Press.

BOX 7.3 CAUSES OF LYMPHOCYTOSIS (>3.5 × 10^9/L)

- Viral infections.
- Thyrotoxicosis.
- Chronic lymphocytic leukaemia (95% are B cell).
- Acute lymphoblastic leukaemia (predominantly in children, cytogenetic chromosomal abnormalities, especially translocations, in 75% of cases).

BOX 7.4 CAUSES OF NEUTROPHILIA (>7.5 × 10^9/L)

- Bacterial infections.
- Any cause of inflammation or necrosis.
- Malignancy.
- Metabolic disorders.
- Corticosteroid.
- *Myeloproliferative disorders:*
  - *Acute myeloproliferative leukaemia*—cytogenetic abnormalities in 60–70% of cases, presence of Auer rods in blast cells common.
  - *Chronic myeloid leukaemia*—90% have the Philadelphia chromosome a translocation between the *Abl* gene on chromosome 9 and the *Bcr* gene on chromosome 22.
  - *Polycythaemia rubra vera, myelofibrosis, and essential thrombocythaemia*—associated with mutations in Janus Kinase 2 (JAK2) in 80, 50, and 20% of their cases, respectively. It is also occasionally found in cases of CML. JAK2 signalling is essential for several cytokine receptor families, including the GM-CSF family.

BOX 7.5 CAUSES OF NEUTROPENIA (<2 × 10^9/L)

- Viral infections.
- Chemotherapy.
- Marrow infiltration.
- Connective tissue disease.
- Hypersplenism.
- Drug reactions (e.g. carbimazole).

BOX 7.6 CAUSES OF EOSINOPHILIA (>0.5 × 10^9/L)

- Allergies.
- Skin disease.
- Parasites.
- Malignancy.
- Tropical eosinophilia.
- Hypereosinophilic syndrome.

BOX 7.7 CAUSES OF MONOCYTOSIS (>0.8 × 10^9/L)

- Infections.
- Chronic inflammatory disease.
- Acute and chronic myeloid leukemia.
- Hodgkins disease.
- Post-chemotherapy.
- Drug reactions (e.g. carbimazole).

Platelets and the coagulation cascade

Platelets are anucleate small sub-cellular fragments that are derived from megakaryocytes in the bone marrow in response to thrombopoietin synthesized in the kidneys and liver. Platelets clear thrombopoietin themselves providing negative feedback for their production. See Box 7.8 for causes of thrombocytosis and Box 7.9 for causes of thrombocytopenia.

The function of platelets is to stop blood loss after injury by forming a plug in damaged blood vessels and releasing

BOX 7.8 CAUSES OF THROMBOCYTOSIS (>500 × 10^9/L)

- In response to any cause of tissue damage, inflammation, or thrombosis.
- Essential thrombocythaemia.

BOX 7.9 CAUSES OF THROMBOCYTOPENIA (<150 × 10^9/L)

Decreased production

- Sepsis.
- Vitamin B12/folate deficiency.
- Leukaemia or myelodysplasia.
- Liver failure (decreased thrombopoietin production).

Increased destruction

- Immune thrombocytopenic purpura (ITP) and thrombotic thrombocytopenic purpura (TTP).
- Disseminated intravascular coagulation (DIC).
- Heparin-induced thrombocytopenia (HIT).
- SLE/antiphospholipid syndrome.

agents, e.g. thrombin, that contribute to rapid clot formation. They also release signals to recruit and activate further platelets, e.g. ADP, thromboxane A2, 5-hydroxytryptamine (5-HT) and to attract inflammatory cells, e.g. platelet-derived growth factor (PDGF) to the site of injury in order to ward off any potential infection.

There are three components of haemostasis:

- Platelet activation to form a loose plug as a stop-gap measure.
- Local vasoconstriction to reduce blood flow to the affected area.
- Activation of the coagulation cascade to convert soluble fibrinogen to fibrin strands that form a mesh around the platelet plug and trap other blood cells to generate a more permanent repair to the damaged vessel.

These processes are closely interlinked—platelet activation in response to exposed collagen at the wound results in their synthesizing the vasoconstrictor and platelet activator, thromboxane A2 (TXA2), and their release of granules containing the vasoconstrictors (adrenaline and 5-hydroxyryptamine (5-HT), as well as inflammatory mediators, e.g. platelet-activating factor (PAF), PDGF. Meanwhile, collagen and platelets stimulate the intrinsic pathway for blood coagulation, while the tissue damage stimulates the extrinsic pathway. These pathways converge to convert prothrombin (so-called factor II) to thrombin (Factor II activated (IIa)), which acts to convert fibrinogen to fibrin and to further recruit platelets.

Platelet activation

There are a range of different glycoprotein (gp) receptors on platelet membranes, which recognize and bind to a variety of ligands, including collagen and von Willebrand factor (vWF)—a factor secreted by the endothelium in response to injury. Mutations in von Willebrand factor can cause von Willebrand's disease as summarized in Box 7.10. Stimulation of these receptors triggers the platelet activation pathway (Fig. 7.3), resulting in an

BOX 7.10 VON WILLEBRAND'S DISEASE

A mutation in von Willebrand factor (vWF) gene on chromosome 12 predisposes to bleeding. vWF is made in endothelial cells and acts as a protective carrier for factor VIII to prevent its breakdown. It also binds to collagen and other platelet receptor when they are activated and releases factor viii in the presence of thrombin to target platelets and activated clotting at the site of exposed vascular subendothelium.

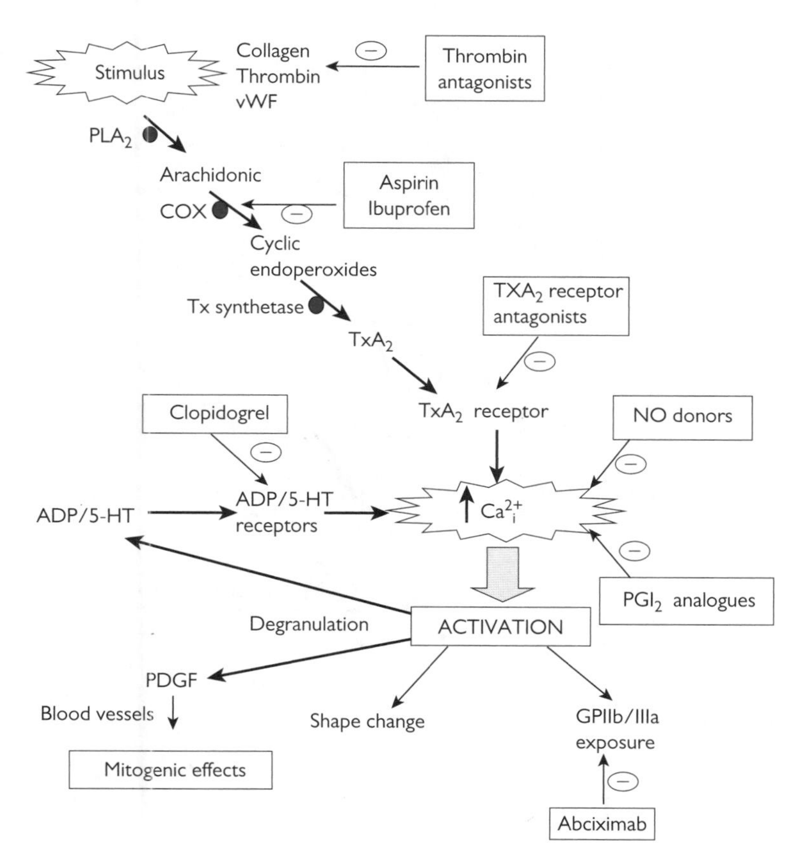

Fig. 7.3 Platelet activation pathways and therapeutic interventions.

Reproduced from R Wilkins et al., *Oxford Handbook of Medical Sciences, Second Edition*, 2011, Figure 6.44, p. 465, by permission of Oxford University Press.

increase in intracellular Ca^{2+}, the trigger responsible for the following cellular effects:

- *Shape change:* pseudopodia emerge from the normal smooth discoid platelet surface, vastly increasing the surface area, and consequently, the adhesiveness of the platelets.
- *Degranulation:* release of vasoconstrictor and platelet activating factors to cause vasoconstriction and platelet recruitment, respectively.
- *gpIIb/IIIa exposure:* a conformational change in the membrane leads to the exposure of the otherwise hidden glycoprotein, gpIIb/IIIa, which binds to fibrinogen to help stabilize the platelet plug.

Coagulation

Coagulation consists of two cascade pathways (see Fig. 7.4) that converge to generate the activated serine protease, thrombin (factor IIa), which is responsible for the polymerization of soluble fibrinogen into fibrin strands. The purpose of the cascade systems is to amplify the signal—activation of a small amount of one factor in the cascade generates large amounts of the next factor downstream, and so on. The result is rapid formation of large amounts of fibrin in response to what may have been a fairly weak initial signal. Each step in the cascade involves the activation of normally inactive circulating enzymes (known as 'factors'), most of which are serine proteases. As each factor becomes activated, it catalyses a specific proteolytic event in the subsequent factor in the cascade to activate it. Fibrin formed from soluble fibrinogen is finally stabilized by the action of factor XIIIa. The most common inherited disease of clotting factors is haemophilia as described in Box 7.11.

Thrombosis and endogenous anti-thrombotic mechanisms

Haemostasis is clearly a crucial process to very rapidly form a temporary patch in damaged blood vessels, in advance of the healing process affecting a permanent repair. However, it is essential that the haemostatic process is only stimulated in damaged vessels and that inappropriate clotting (known

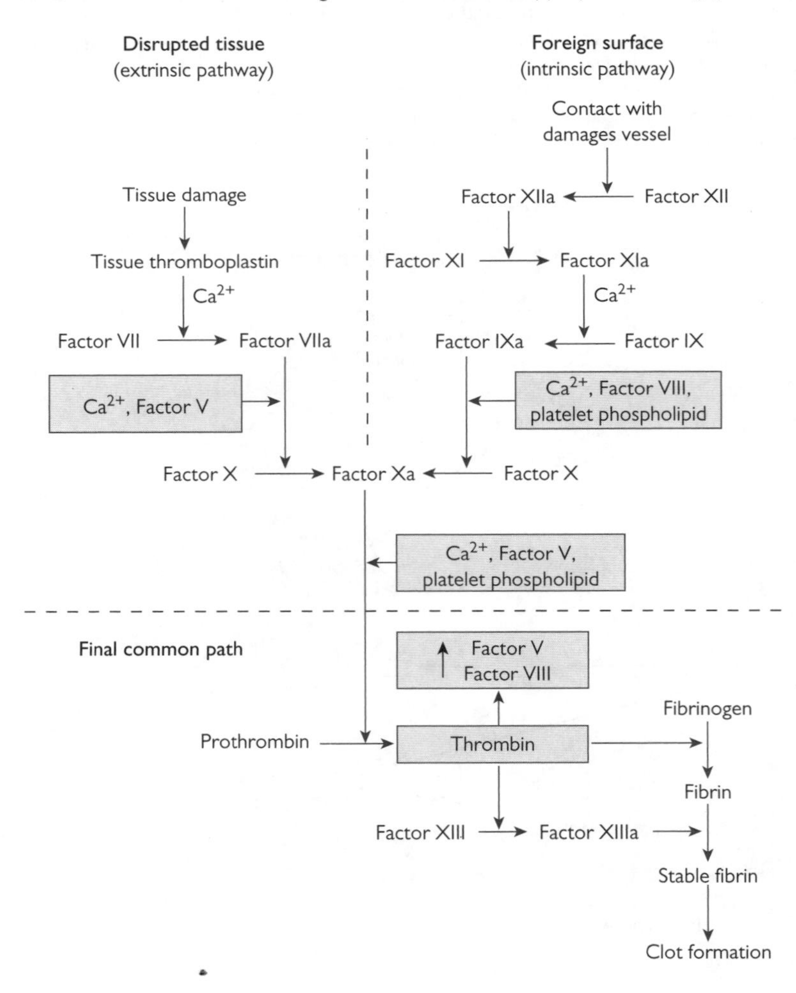

Fig. 7.4 The extrinsic and intrinsic pathways leading to the formation of a blood clot. Note the central roles played by Factor Xa and thrombin in the process of blood coagulation.

Reproduced from G Pocock and CD Richards, *Human Physiology: The Basis of Medicine, Third Edition*, 2006, Figure 13.11, p. 240, by permission of Oxford University Press

BOX 7.11 HAEMOPHILIA

Haemophilia is a sex-linked genetic disorder that affects men only and constitutes an inability to synthesize factor VIII (classical haemophilia) or more rarely, factor IX (haemophilia B or Christmas disease). Treatment is with recombinant factor VIII and IX, although with acute bleeds viral inactivated coagulation factor concentrate, tranexamic acid (a fibrinolytic inhibitor) and DDAVP (a synthetic analogue of ADH that can release factor VIII from storage within endothelial cells) can be used.

as thrombosis), which would prevent blood flowing to tissues and organs, is avoided.

Antithrombin III (ATIII) is central to preventing thrombosis by binding to the active site of all of the factors involved in the coagulation cascade and inhibiting their action.

The endothelial lining of blood vessels is now recognized to be central to preventing thrombosis in undamaged vessels by a number of mechanisms (Fig. 7.5):

- Presenting a physical barrier that separates platelets and coagulation factors in the blood from stimulatory collagen in the sub-endothelial layers of the blood vessel.
- Secretion of heparan sulphate on the luminal surface to activate ATIII and prevent activation of the clotting factors.
- Synthesis of powerful inhibitors of platelet activation. Prostacyclin (PGI2) and nitric oxide (NO) act synergistically to prevent the increase in intra-platelet Ca^{2+} essential for activation.
- Expression of the enzyme CD39 on the luminal surface to convert the platelet activator, ADP, to inactive adenosine monophosphate (AMP).
- Release of tissue plasminogen activator (t-PA) to convert plasminogen to plasmin, which cleaves fibrin strands, earning t-PA the title 'clot-buster'.

Damage to, or dysfunction of, the endothelium compromises some or all of these protective effects and also leads to the release of the platelet activator, vWF, and the t-PA inhibitor, plasminogen activator inhibitor-1 (PAI-1). This is believed to be a vital step in a number of pathological conditions that cause thrombosis, with potentially fatal consequences. The site (arterial or venous) of thrombus generation is important in determining the morphology and cardiovascular impact of thrombosis:

- *Arterial thrombi* are predominantly composed of activated platelets (so-called 'white thrombus') with some fibrin.

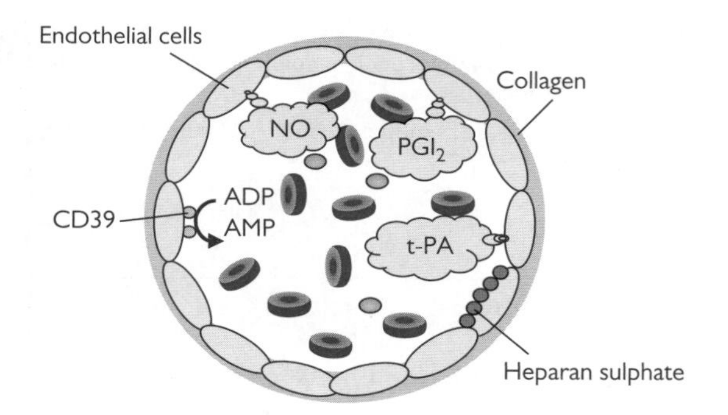

Fig. 7.5 Anti-platelet and anti-coagulation properties of the endothelium.

Reproduced from R Wilkins et al., *Oxford Handbook of Medical Sciences, Second Edition*, 2011, Figure 6.46, p. 467, by permission of Oxford University Press.

They can be caused by atherosclerotic plaque rupture, left atrial appendage blood stasis in atrial fibrillation, stasis surrounding a large akinetic prothrombotic myocardial infarction scar, or release of debris during vascular surgery or interventional cardiology procedures. They may remain at the initial site of thrombosis or be carried downstream as an embolus.

- *Venous thrombi* are mainly fibrin with few platelets and a large proportion of red blood cells that become trapped in the mesh (red thrombus). Venous thrombi tend to form in conditions where venous flow has stopped (deep vein thrombosis caused by extended physical inactivity, such as long flights). Venous thrombi are susceptible to distal embolization to the lungs as a pulmonary embolism, or if a right to left intracardiac shunt exists, such as a patent foramen ovale, as a paradoxical embolism into the systemic circulation. See Box 7.12 for causes of thrombophilia.

Anti-platelet and anticoagulant drugs are covered in Chapter 10, Cardiovascular pharmacology.

BOX 7.12 CAUSES OF THROMBOPHILIA

- *Congenital:* Factor V Leiden (most common in the UK), antithrombin III, protein C and protein S deficiency.
- *Acquired:* antiphospholipid syndrome, lupus anticoagulant, essential thrombocythaemia, polycythaemia.
- *Pre-disposition:* immobility, obesity, smoking, contraceptive pill, pregnancy, malignancy.

Drug-induced haematological reactions

- *Aplastic anaemia/neutropenia:* cytotoxic chemotherapy, carbimazole, propylthiouracil, phenytoin, carbamazepine, chloramphenicol, quinine, non-steroidal anti-inflammatory drugs (NSAIDS).
- *Thrombocytopenia:* heparin, sodium valproate, penicillin, sulphonamides, quinine, NSAIDS, ranitidine, gold salts.

- *Haemolytic anaemia (especially if g6pd deficiency):* primaquine, hydroxychloroquine, sulphonamides, sulfasalazine, penicillin, aspirin.
- *Folate deficiency:* methotrexate, 6-mercaptopurine, phenytoin.
- *B12 deficiency:* colchicine, cholestramine, H2 antagonists, PPIs, phenytoin, metformin.
- *Methaemoglobinaemia:* antibiotics (trimethoprim, sulphonamides), local anaesthetics (e.g. benzocaine), metoclopramide, dapsone.

Multiple choice questions

1. A mother is blood type A and a father blood type B. Which blood type is their offspring most likely to be?

A. A.
B. B.
C. O.
D. AB.
E. Any of the above.

2. A 35-year-old man presents with a Hb of 8 g/dL and a mean cell volume (MCV) of 85 fl. This is associated with a raised urinary urobilinogen and a positive direct coombs test. The most likely diagnosis is:

A. Microangiopathic haemolytic anaemia.
B. Glucose-6-phosphate dehydrogenase deficiency.
C. Autoimmune haemolytic anaemia.
D. Paroxysmal nocturnal haemoglobinuria.
E. Hereditary spherocytosis.

3. Which of the following statements regarding HbA is true:

A. Failure to incorporate iron into HbA produces 'ring sideroblasts'
B. HbA consists of 2α and 2δ chains.
C. HbA is the main type of Hb in the fetus
D. HbA has a Hill co-efficient for binding of oxygen of 4.
E. De-oxygenated HbA contains iron mainly kept in its Fe^{3+}, rather than Fe^{2+} form.

4. Vitamin K-dependent clotting factors include all of the following except:

A. II.
B. III.
C. VII.
D. IX.
E. X.

5. The most common congenital cause of thrombophilia in the UK is:

A. Antithrombin III deficiency.
B. Protein S deficiency.
C. Antiphospholipid syndrome.
D. Factor V Leiden.
E. Protein C deficiency.

6. The following clotting factors are only involved in the intrinsic pathway of the clotting cascade:

A. IX.
B. X.
C. II.
D. VII.
E. V.

7. Which of following disorders are *not* associated with mutations in janus kinase 2 (JAK2)?

A. Polycythaemia rubra vera.
B. Myelofibrosis.
C. Essential thrombocythaemia.
D. CML.
E. Christmas disease.

8. The Philadelphia chromosome:

A. Is sufficiently specific for the diagnosis of CML.
B. Is a reciprocal translocation between chromosome 9 and 21.
C. Creates a fusion oncogene by combining *Abl1* and *Bcr*.
D. Is linked to the presence of Auer rods in blast cells.
E. Gene product is a JAK2 kinase coupled receptor.

9. A 40-year-old woman with asthma and a chronic widespread blistering rash on her elbows and knees presented with worsening asthma following a 1-month history of a flu-like illness. On examination she was centrally cyanosed, and on auscultation of the chest there was good air entry, but widespread expiratory wheeze. Pulse oximetry on room air shows 88% saturation, while an arterial blood gas, also on room air, demonstrates a PO_2 of 14.5 kPa. The most likely diagnosis is:

 A. Pneumocystitis pneumonia.
 B. Methaemaglobinaemia induced by dapsone.
 C. Congestive cardiac failure.
 D. Iron deficiency anaemia.
 E. AML.

10. A 60-year-old man was day 5 post-aortic valve replacement, but was proving difficult to wean from ventilator support due to high oxygen requirements. A CTPA demonstrates a pulmonary embolism despite adequate anti-coagulation with low molecular weight heparin. Blood tests demonstrate Hb = 11 g/dL, WCC = 13×10^9/L, platelets = 10×10^9/L. What is the most likely cause of the PE?

 A. Immobility.
 B. Malignancy.
 C. Disseminated intravascular coagulation.
 D. Heparin-induced thrombocytopenia.
 E. Thrombotic thrombocytopenic purpura (TTP).

For answers, please see Appendix: Answers to multiple choice questions, page 313.

CHAPTER 8

Clinical pharmacology

Principles of drug action

Receptors

Sixty per cent of current drugs act upon cell surface receptors. These are proteins that recognize and respond to specific signalling molecules (or ligands) to change cellular function. Such receptors are either G protein coupled receptors, ligand gated ion channels, or have endogenous enzyme activity themselves (e.g. tyrosine kinase coupled receptors, such as the insulin receptor). However, receptors can also be enzymes in the cytoplasm of the cell whereby ligand binding changes their activity, or nuclear receptors where binding can modulate gene expression. Even extracellular enzymes, e.g. those involved in the breakdown or metabolism of hormones, can be considered as receptors and are modified by the action of drugs.

Endogenous ligands range from simple inorganic molecules (e.g. nitric oxide), to complex organic molecules, including amino acids (e.g. glutamate), peptides (e.g. atrial natriuretic peptide), and cholesterol derivatives (e.g. cortisol). Drugs are exogenous ligands that either mimic (agonists) or block (antagonists) the effects of their natural counterparts. The concept of a drug as a chemical substance has also been recently widened with the clinical use of monoclonal antibodies, which may target individual endogenous ligands (such as TNF-alpha), either by mimicking their receptor (etanercept) or by acting directly against the ligand itself (infliximab).

Ligand binding and responses

Binding of a ligand (A) to a specific receptor (R) is often a reversible interaction that results in the formation of a ligand-receptor complex (AR), represented by the following equation:

$$A + R \underset{k_{-1}}{\overset{k_{+1}}{\rightleftharpoons}} AR \qquad 8.1$$

The interaction can be considered in equilibrium such that k_{-1}/k_{+1} is the association constant (K_A) and is characteristic for a particular drug for a given receptor. K_A equals the amount of drug required to occupy 50% of the receptor population. How well a ligand binds to a given receptor, or its affinity for the receptor, is inversely proportional to the K_A (see Fig. 8.1A).

The proportion of receptors occupied at equilibrium (P_A) is therefore dependent on both the equilibrium constant and the concentration of ligand present, and is described by the Hill–Langmuir equation:

$$P_A = \frac{[A]}{[A]+K_A} \qquad 8.2$$

If more than one ligand molecule (n) binds to any given receptor, then this equation can be modified as follows

$$P_A = \frac{[A]^n}{[A]^n + K_A^n} \qquad 8.3$$

n is known as the Hill co-efficient and if it is greater than one per binding site, this implies negative co-operativity, whereas a Hill co-efficient less than the number of binding sites suggests positive co-operativity in that binding of one ligand increases the affinity of binding for the next. A good example of this is oxygen molecules binding to haemoglobin where n is 2.8 rather than 4 (see Chapter 11, 'Respiratory medicine').

The response of the cell or organ is generally a function of the number of receptors bound (N_A). Different drugs may bind equally as well to a receptor (i.e. have the same affinity), but have different efficacy or ability to bring about a cellular response. For example, an antagonist may bind equally as well as an agonist, but on its own bring about no cellular response (i.e. it has zero efficacy). Other agonists may have different degrees of efficacy. An example of this would be morphine as a full agonist at the μ opioid receptor compared with buprenorphine, which has lower efficacy and is, therefore, considered a partial agonist. A partial agonist will have different effects depending on the presence of the endogenous ligand. For example, tamoxifen is a partial agonist at oestrogen receptors. In premenopausal women who have high circulating levels of oestrogen, tamoxifen binds to oestrogen receptors but because it is only a partial agonist, by displacing the full agonist, oestrogen, the net

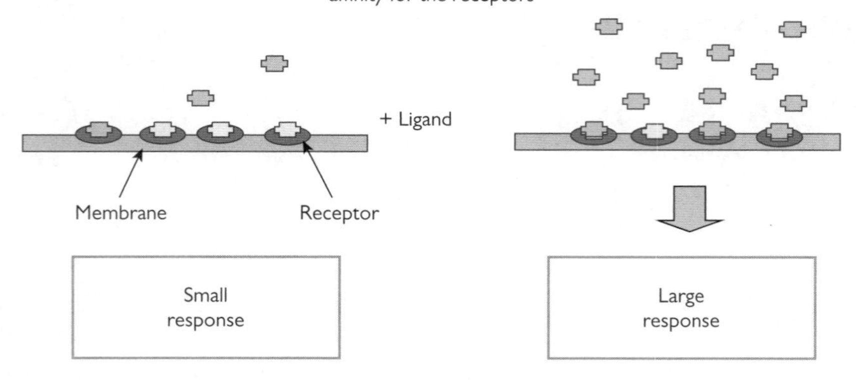

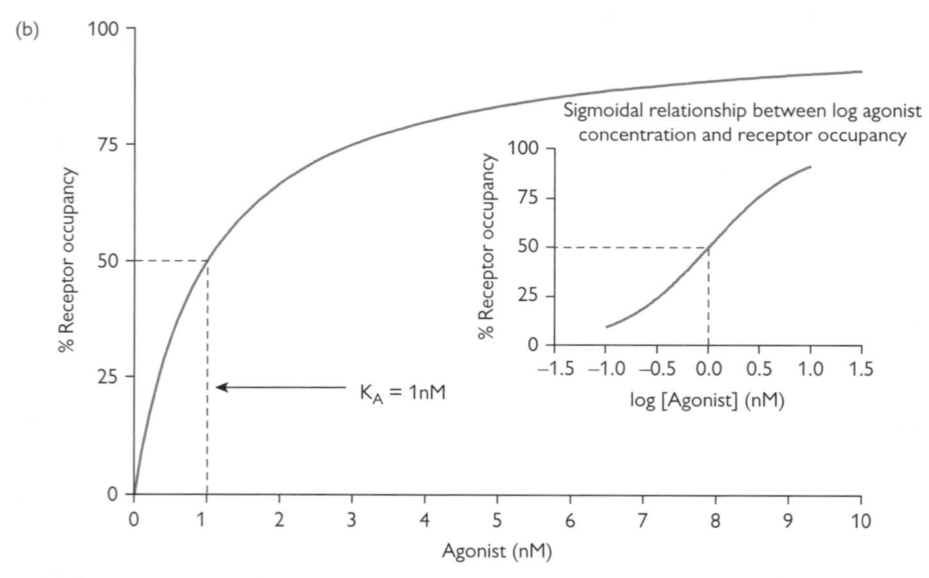

Fig. 8.1A Ligand binding. (a) Law of mass action. (b) The relationship between agonist concentration and receptor occupancy for an idealized agonist. This relationship is specific for a given drug and receptors in a particular tissue.

effect is apparent antagonism. In post-menopausal women in whom oestrogen levels are low, tamoxifen allows sufficient residual agonist effect to provide a degree of bone protection not seen with aromatase inhibitors. Efficacy (ε) can be considered as the proportionality constant between the number of receptors bound and the response.

$$\text{Response} = f(\varepsilon \cdot N_A) \quad 8.4$$

As P_A, the proportion of the total number of receptors occupied is N_A/N_{TOTAL}, then

$$\text{Response} = f\left[\frac{\varepsilon \cdot N_{TOTAL} \cdot [A]}{[A] + K_A}\right] \quad 8.5$$

Response is often plotted against dose of the agonist [A] in a dose–response curve, often on a logarithmic scale.

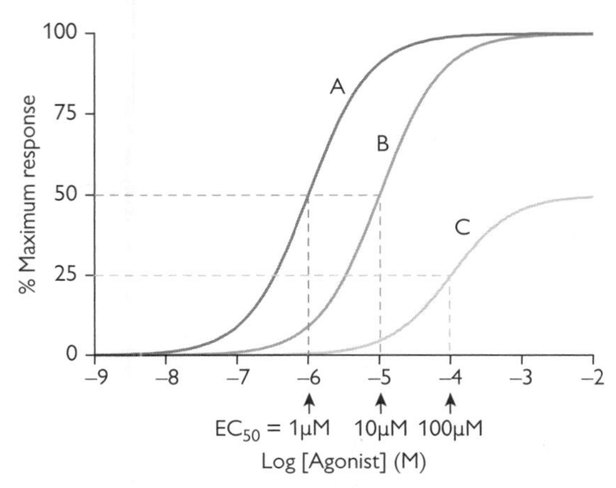

Fig. 8.1B Log concentration response curves for idealized examples of full (A and B) and partial (C) agonists.

Reproduced from R Wilkins et al., *Oxford Handbook of Medical Sciences, Second Edition*, 2011, Figure 1.40, p. 81, by permission of Oxford University Press.

The concentration required to produce 50% of the maximal response for that drug (the EC_{50}) is therefore related to both the affinity and efficacy of a given agonist (see Fig. 8.1B). If a drug produces an inhibitory response (i.e. it is an inverse agonist), the term IC_{50} is used to describe the concentration of an inhibitor required to cause 50% inhibition of the response. Before molecular genetics, classification of receptors was based on 'potency' series of known agonists, rather than on the amino acid sequence homology of the receptor. Potency is a relative term, which incorporates affinity and efficacy, and is inversely proportional to the EC_{50}. For example, bumetanide and furosemide have equal efficacy, but bumetanide is more potent (i.e. you need less of it to achieve the same diuretic effect, but the ceiling is the same for the two drugs).

Continual stimulation of receptors can lead to receptor desensitization and eventually internalization of the receptors. An example of this is with the β_1-adrenergic receptor, which after continued stimulation, becomes phosphorylated by a β-adrenergic receptor (or G protein receptor) kinase (βARK1 otherwise known as GRK2). Binding of β-arrestin-1 then leads to desensitization of the receptor and its internalization via endocytosis. The activity of β-arrestin and βARK-1 are influenced by levels of cAMP, the second messenger of the β1 receptor itself.

Antagonists

Antagonists bind to receptors (and, therefore, have affinity), but bring about no response in their own right (have zero efficacy). If they are competitive and reversible, they compete with the endogenous agonist for the same binding site. This results in a right ward shift in the dose response curve for the agonist (Fig. 8.2A). The dissociation constant (K_D) of a competitive antagonist can be established from experiments using

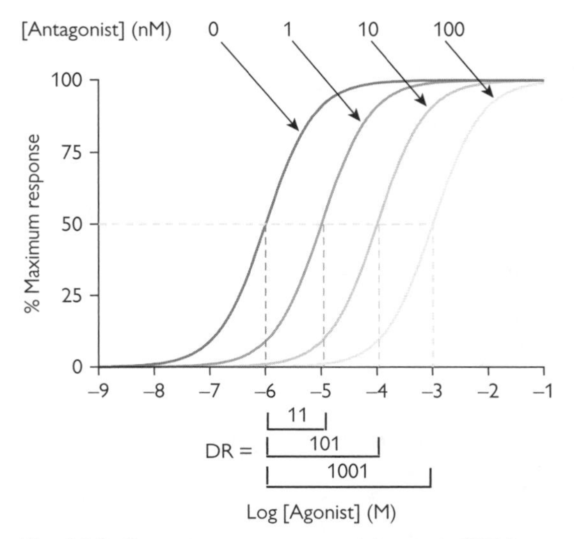

Fig. 8.2A Competitive antagonism and dose ratio (DR) for several concentrations (1–100nM) of an idealized competitive antagonist.

Reproduced from R Wilkins et al., *Oxford Handbook of Medical Sciences, Second Edition*, 2011, Figure 1.42, p. 83, by permission of Oxford University Press.

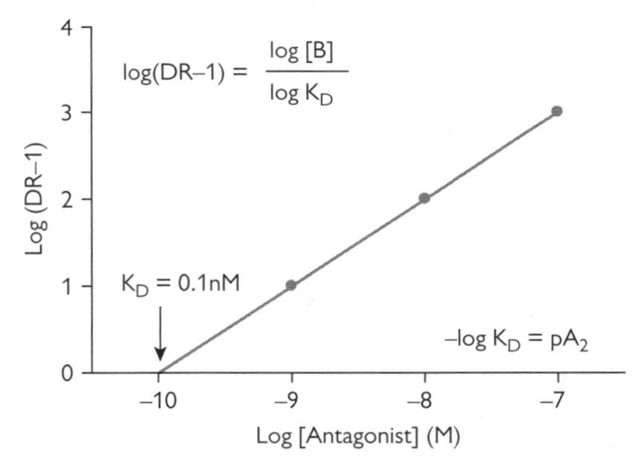

Fig. 8.2B Schild equation and plot to establish the dissociation constant (KD) for the competitive antagonist (B) shown in Figure 8.2A.

Reproduced from R Wilkins et al., *Oxford Handbook of Medical Sciences, Second Edition*, 2011, Figure 1.43, p. 83, by permission of Oxford University Press.

an established agonist in the presence of different antagonist concentrations to determine the dose ratio (DR; the ratio of agonist required to generate a given response in the presence of a known antagonist concentration compared to that in the absence of antagonist. Using the Schild equation or the Arunlakshana & Schild plot (Fig. 8.2B), the K_D (sometimes also referred to as the K_B) can be determined. The K_D for a true competitive antagonist should be independent of antagonist

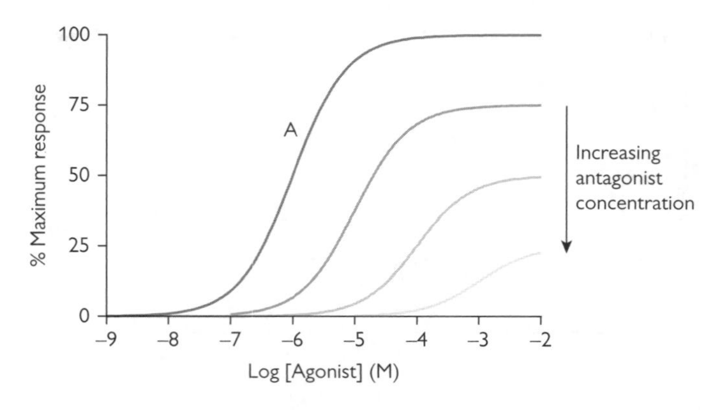

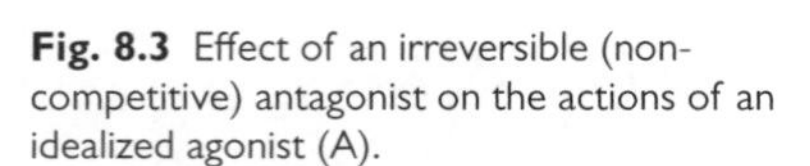
Fig. 8.3 Effect of an irreversible (non-competitive) antagonist on the actions of an idealized agonist (A).

Reproduced from R Wilkins et al., *Oxford Handbook of Medical Sciences, Second Edition*, 2011, Figure 1.44, p. 83, by permission of Oxford University Press.

concentration and, therefore, the gradient of the plotted line should equal 1.0.

If competitive and irreversible then at low doses the antagonist will shift the dose–response curve of the agonist to the right and at higher doses will start to reduce the maximal response. This is because occupancy of only 30% of the total number of receptors is generally required for a maximal response to the agonist.

Non-competitive antagonists bind to a region of the receptor other than the agonist-binding site. These antagonists prevent activation of the transduction mechanism required to evoke a response, and, therefore reduce the maximum response of the agonist (see Fig. 8.3). Physiological antagonists act via a different receptor and 2nd messenger system entirely to reverse the effect of an agonist.

Pharmacokinetics and monitoring drug therapy

In order for a drug to have a physiological effect *in vivo*, a sufficient concentration must be delivered to the relevant receptors at its site of action. The chemical characteristics of the drug will determine how well it is absorbed into the bloodstream, how it distributes in the body, and how quickly it will be metabolized and excreted. Knowledge of these processes will therefore determine the route and frequency of administration, as well as the best formulation of the drug.

Administration and absorption

A drug can either be administered systemically for ultimate transport in the blood stream to its site of action, or targeted to a localized area where the drug is to act, such as using inhaled and nebulized bronchodilators in asthma. Other examples of local administration include intrathecal injections, dermatological creams, eye drops, and eardrops. Table 8.1 illustrates the main systemic routes of administration and their pros and cons.

Distribution

Once in the blood many drugs are bound to plasma proteins. Drugs may complete for binding to albumin and displace each other leading to adverse effects. An example of this is warfarin that can be displaced by drugs such as tolbutamide and lead to an increased risk of haemorrhage.

Drugs may also distribute into other compartments depending on their relative solubility in aqueous and lipid environments (the partition coefficient). Lipid soluble drugs, for example, may also distribute into adipose tissue, which can give the drug a particularly long half-life due to the poor blood supply to fat. Chronic use of such drugs may build up an additional reservoir in adipose tissue, which can then be displaced by administration of another lipid-soluble drug (such as with cannabis use and some general anaesthetics).

Another example of where lipophilicity can influence the distribution of a drug is ion trapping of drugs that are weak acids or bases. In this way, the pH of the compartment will determine whether the drug is in an ionized or lipid soluble non-ionized form. For this reason, orally administered acidic drugs are absorbed primarily in the stomach (pH 3), whilst oral basic drugs are absorbed in the small intestine (pH 9). For example, a weakly acidic drug like aspirin (pKa = 3.5) is absorbed in the stomach (pH ~3), where it passes first into the epithelial barrier layer and then into the blood (both of which pH ~7.4). The pKa for aspirin determines that it is mainly in the non-ionized form at this low pH, and can therefore readily diffuse across the epithelial cell membrane. Once inside the cell, however, the higher pH will cause a large proportion of the drug to ionize, rendering it unable to diffuse back through the membrane into the stomach compartment. As a result, when the non-ionized form of the drug reaches equilibrium between the two compartments (stomach and intracellular), a large amount of drug is effectively 'trapped' within the cell in the ionic form. A similar principle is exploited by using sodium bicarbonate

Table 8.1 Advantages and disadvantages of different routes of administration of pharmacological agents

Route	Advantages	Disadvantages
Oral	No special equipment or patient supervision	Breakdown of drug by enzymes or pH changes. Absorption dependent on GI transit time (problems with diarrhoea or vomiting). Interactions with food. Not useful peri-operatively when nil by mouth. 1st pass metabolism once entering portal circulation
Rectal	Rapid absorption into the blood stream. Can be given to unconscious patients	Unpleasant administration. Only suitable for some drugs
Sublingual	Rapid absorption into the blood stream, avoids first pass metabolism	Only suitable for some drugs
Intravenous	Rapid, reliable absorption. Infusion rate can be controlled to control pharmacodynamics. Can be given to unconscious patients	Requires iv cannula. Risk of infection at cannula site
Sub-cutaneous/ intramuscular	Patient can be trained to administer. Can be given to unconscious patients	Less predictable absorption and less rapid onset than iv administration. Potential irritation to skin or muscle

administration to alkalinize the urine in aspirin over dose to promote urinary clearance.

Whilst the plasma concentration of a drug that is confined to the bloodstream will accurately reflect the amount of drug in the body for a drug heavily absorbed in body fat, this will vastly under-estimate the amount of drug in the body. The apparent 'volume of distribution' of a drug is calculated using the amount of drug administered and the concentration of the drug measured in the blood. By this method a volume of distribution equal to blood volume implies a highly hydrophilic drug that is likely to be protein bound (e.g. Warfarin), whilst a value close to total body water implies distribution throughout body tissues (e.g. ethanol). An extremely high value beyond that of total body water implies the drug is highly lipophilic and dissolved in body fat (e.g. chloroquine).

Metabolism and excretion

The amount of drug that reaches the tissue is dependent on absorption kinetics (described previously), its distribution within the body, and blood flow to and from the target tissue, as well as the rate of metabolism and subsequent excretion (or elimination of the drug).

The main site of drug metabolism is the liver, but it can also occur in other sites (for example, the gut). The aim of drug metabolism is first to reduce its biological activity (phase 1 enzymes) by oxidation, reduction, or hydrolysis. Then phase 2 reactions increase water solubility by conjugation via acetylation, methylation, sulphation, or glucuronidation, to aid excretion in the urine or bile. Phase 1 reactions are carried out by the mixed function oxidase system particularly in hepatic microsomes, which is made up of NADPH oxidase, cytochrome P450, and cytochrome P450 reductase. Knowledge of these metabolic pathways is important when dealing with pro-drugs (e.g. clopidogrel) that are then metabolized to their active form, rather than being inactivated following oral administration before reaching the systemic circulation by 'first pass' metabolism.

Genetic variation in the rate at which drug metabolism exists amongst the population and the most well-known example of this is with deficiency in N-acetyltransferase, which is associated with HLA DR4 ('slow acetylators'). Although this is common (up to 50% of the population in the UK), it is associated with adverse drug effects, such as drug-induced lupus and isoniazid-induced peripheral neuropathy. Conversely, rapid acetylators are prone to adverse effects from drug metabolites, such as isoniazid-induced hepatitis. Another example is genetic polymorphism in alcohol dehydrogenase (ADH) and aldehyde dehydrogenase (ALDH), which may explain the racial variation in the rate of metabolism and tolerance to alcohol (e.g. in the hepatic mitochondrial form ALDH2 in oriental populations).

Some drugs inhibit cytochrome P450 and this forms the basis of potential drug interactions with other hepatically-metabolized drugs (especially carbamazepine, cyclosporin, phenytoin, theophylines, and warfarin). Others are capable of inducing liver enzymes, which can result in the more rapid inactivation of drugs such as warfarin, phenytoin, the oral contraceptive pill, and hydrocortisone. Examples are illustrated in Table 8.2.

Plasma kinetics

The aim of a dosing strategy is to rapidly increase the plasma concentration into the therapeutic range and maintain it within the range with subsequent doses. Knowledge of the kinetics of elimination of a drug is therefore extremely important. Elimination of the vast majority of drugs follows first order kinetics in that the rate at which the plasma concentration falls over time is dependent on its concentration, and the time it takes for half of the drug to be eliminated (the half-life) remains constant. It is a feature of drugs with

Table 8.2 Inhibitors and inducers of different cytochrome P450 sub-types

Family	Important isoforms	Inhibitor	Inducer
CYP1	CYP1A2	Ciprofloxacin Disulfiram Cimetidine	Phenytoin Carbamazepine
CYP2	CYP2B6	Clopidogrel Fluoxetine	Phenytoin Barbiturates
	CYP2C9	Fluconazole Amiodarone	Rifampacin
	CYP2C19	Omeprazole Fluvoxamine	Phenytoin Carbamazepine
	CYP2D6	Quinine Cimetidine Paroxetine	No really important inducers of 2D6
CYP3	CYP3A4,5,7	Allopurinol Amiodarone Disulfiram Erythromycin Valporate Cimetidine Clarithromycin Grapefruit juice	St Johns Wort Phenytoin Carbamazepine Barbiturates Rifampacin Sulphonylureas

first order elimination kinetics (e.g. digoxin or heparin) that a larger loading dose followed by repeated doses at consistent intervals will ultimately result in generation of 'steady-state conditions', where the inter-dosing plasma concentration fluctuates between consistent maximum and minimum levels (Fig. 8.4). If the enzymes required to metabolize a drug become saturated at very low levels, then the drug will show zero order kinetics in that the rate of clearance is independent of its concentration (e.g. phenytoin). A plot of plasma alcohol or salicylate concentration, e.g. against time gives a straight line without a constant half-life, making predicting plasma levels with repeated dosing difficult to achieve.

Mechanisms of drug interactions

Drug interactions can therefore take several forms:

- *Receptor:* a drug can antagonize the effect of another drug by acting as a partial agonist, inverse agonist, or antagonist at the same receptor as another drug.
- *Pharmacodynamic:* a drug can have additive, synergistic or inhibitory effect on another drug by acting via different receptors in the same organ or system to alter physiology.
- *Pharmacokinetic:* one drug may alter the absorption, distribution, metabolism, or excretion of another drug as described in the previous section.

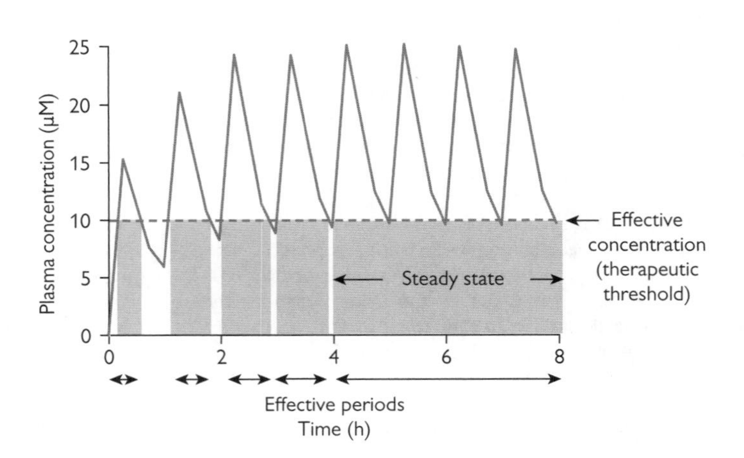

Fig. 8.4 An example of the plasma concentration profile for repeated oral drug dosing (1-h intervals) of a drug with a half-life of ~30min. Note how repeated doses progressively increase the duration of the effective periods until steady state is reached.

Reproduced from R Wilkins et al., *Oxford Handbook of Medical Sciences, Second Edition,* 2011, Figure 1.48, p. 89, by permission of Oxford University Press.

Therapeutics in particular conditions

The elderly

With ageing, both the pharmacodynamics and pharmacokinetics of how our bodies can handle drugs change in several important ways:

- *Reduced renal clearance:* drugs such as digoxin can easily accumulate and become toxic and care must also be taken given the reduction in baseline glomerular filtration rate with age with nephrotoxic drugs (such as NSAIDS and ACE inhibitors).
- *Reduced liver function:* can lead to increased bioavailability of drugs due to loss of first pass metabolism, e.g. with propranolol or verapamil. Diseases in the elderly that reduce plasma protein levels can complicate this further, particularly for drugs such as warfarin, sulphonylureas, and phenytoin.
- *Altered volume of distribution:* a lower body fat content can impact on how lipophilic drugs (such as diazepam) and hydrophilic drugs (such as digoxin) distribute.

The physiology of ageing may also mean that that potency of the drug and its therapeutic window may alter such that side effects become more likely. This is particularly the case for drugs acting on the central nervous system, such as benzodiazepines, opioids, and antipsychotics that may have more profound effects on alertness, mental function, and balance, but also antihypertensive drugs that are more likely to cause postural hypotension.

Ageing also means that patients are more likely to suffer from multiple, often chronic, illnesses and may, therefore, be prescribed multiple medications (polypharmacy), and may also be taking over-the-counter medications or herbal/dietary supplements. Altered pharmacodynamics and pharmacokinetics as described previously make it more likely that there will be adverse drug interactions. Medications should therefore be prescribed only when necessary, started at the lowest possible dose and titrated upwards, and be regularly reviewed in the context of all the medications (prescription or otherwise) the patient is taking. Unfortunately, those over 80 years of age are rarely included in randomized controlled trials and, therefore, evidence regarding efficacy is also often lacking. This should not always be seen as a reason not to prescribe, rather a reminder that potential risks and benefits should be balanced in particular circumstances.

Ageing may also be confounded by deterioration in sight, hearing, and dexterity, which may impact on the patient's ability to correctly administer multiple medications. This can be confounded by poor communication with the patient on the part of the health-care professional. The increased prevalence of dementia with age also needs also to be considered as this, too, can greatly hinder safe self-administration of the correct dose of drug at the appropriate frequency. Long-acting formulations of a medication may therefore be preferred, and 'pill organizers' or 'dosette boxes', prepared by the pharmacy, or with the help of carers or relatives, may prove useful in these circumstances. If, in some circumstances, administration may need to be supervised in order to be safe.

Pregnancy and breastfeeding

Administration of drugs in the first trimester of pregnancy can carry the risk of teratogenic effects to the foetus (e.g. alcohol, warfarin, angiotensin converting enzyme inhibitors, phenytoin, valproate, carbamazapine, lithium). Conversely, drugs administration later in pregnancy may affect the foetus if they are able to cross the placenta (e.g. carbimazole leading to hypothyroidism, aminoglycosides causing ototoxicity, opiates causing respiratory depression). The UK teratology information service provides useful guidance, which can be found at www.uktis.org.

The physiological changes that occur in the mother during pregnancy can also alter the pharmacokinetics of drugs. Gastric motility is slowed, which can increase the absorption of drugs such as digoxin, plasma volume increases with a net decrease in albumin concentration (increasing plasma protein binding of drugs such as phenytoin, but decreasing concentrations of drugs such as propranolol), and liver metabolism can be increased by the induction of enzymes by progesterone.

Drugs can also be excreted in breastmilk and may affect young infants who have under-developed metabolic pathways and capacity for drug excretion. Examples of these include amiodarone (thyroid abnormalities), cytotoxics (haematological abnormalities), lithium (movement disorders), and oestrogens (feminization of male infants). However, drugs such as warfarin, β-blockers, tricyclic antidepressants, penicillins, and cephalosporins are not excreted in breastmilk. Note that dopamine agonists, such as bromocriptine and apomorphine, can suppress lactation itself.

Renal failure

In acute renal failure, drugs with nephrotoxic side effects may exacerbate renal dysfunction, and such drugs may also cause an acute deterioration in patients with a degree of chronic renal failure. Examples of such drugs include:

- ACE inhibitors, aldosterone antagonists, and other antihypertensive drugs that reduce renal perfusion.
- Drugs causing direct tubular toxicity, such as aminoglycosides, NSAIDs, ACE inhibitors, cyclosporin, lithium salts, radio-opaque contrast.
- Drugs causing interstitial nephritis, such as sulphonamides, cephalosporins, NSAIDs, rifampicin, omeprazole, penicillin.
- Drugs causing diabetes insipidus, such as lithium salts, amphotericin B.

Drugs that are renally excreted may accumulate and cause toxicity especially in advanced renal impairment. Examples of these include penicillins and cephalosporins, erythromycin, lithium, and digoxin. Appropriate dose adjustment is therefore essential. Other drugs rely on renal tubular function to exert an effect and are, therefore, less useful in renal failure (nitrofurantoin, loop diuretics).

Hepatic failure

Hepatic failure has several consequences that can impact on drug toxicity:

- *Impaired hepatic metabolism can affect many drugs:* this can make patients very sensitive to the sedative properties of drugs such as opioids and benzodiazepines.
- *Impaired biliary excretion of drugs:* such as rifampicin can lead to their plasma accumulation.
- *Hypoalbuminaemia reduces the plasma binding of drugs such as phenytoin:* this affects the interpretation of plasma concentrations, rather than the maintenance dosage.
- *Reduced clotting factor synthesis:* increases the risk of bleeding in patients taking anti-coagulants.
- *Secondary hyperaldosteronism* and its associated fluid overload in advanced liver disease can be exacerbated by steroids and nephrotoxic drugs

Common overdoses

See www.toxbase.org

Paracetamol

Initially, patients may be asymptomatic, or suffer nausea and vomiting, but after 48–72 hr liver and renal failure can occur. Toxicity arises as the pathways of conjugation by glucuronidation and sulphonation become saturated. The drug is then metabolized by cytochrome P450 to form a toxic intermediate metabolite, which initially is conjugated with sulph-hydryl groups from glutathione, but in over-dosage these stores become depleted. At this point, the toxic intermediaries can cause liver necrosis. Raised international normalized ratio (INR) and hypoglycaemia can result from liver damage and an INR >3.0, plasma pH <7.3, lactate >3.5 mmol/L, and raised creatinine within 24 hr after ingestion are poor prognostic markers. N-acetyl cysteine replenishes liver stores of glutathione and protects against toxicity. The *British National Formulary* (see www.bnf.org) gives guidance on administration of N-acetyl cysteine depending on plasma paracetamol levels in relation to time from ingestion. Note that concurrent use of other hepatically metabolized drugs increases the risk of liver failure.

Tricyclic antidepressants

These drugs have sympathomimetic and anti-cholinergic actions (causing a dry mouth, pupillary dilation, and confusion). They also produce tachycardia with prolongation of the QTc on the ECG, which predisposes to *torsades-de-pointes*. This should be managed with correction of fluid and electrolytes, and with severely prolonged QTc, iv bicarbonate may be useful. Tricyclic antidepressants also lower seizure threshold and cause abnormalities of thermoregulation.

Salicylate

Due to its acidotic nature salicylates initially stimulate the medullary respiratory centre, and cause a respiratory alkalosis with sweating and tinnitus. Eventually, a metabolic acidosis and acute renal failure can ensue as oxidative phosphorylation is uncoupled by high levels of intra-cellular salicylate. Treatment is to give activated charcoal, iv fluids, and correction of electrolytes and, if severe, haemodialysis.

Ethylene glycol

Poisoning produces a metabolic acidosis with a raised anion gap as the ethylene glycol is broken down to oxalate. As well as producing cerebellar type symptoms similar to alcohol intoxication, calcium oxalate crystal can produce acute tubular necrosis and renal failure. Ethanol or fomepizole can inhibit the metabolism of ethylene glycol, and sodium bicarbonate may help reduce acidosis. *In extremis*, haemodialysis may be required to remove the ethylene glycol, correct the metabolic acidosis and the acute renal failure.

Ecstasy (MDMA)

Overdose is characterized by hyperthermia, hypertension, tachycardia, and agitation. The drug acts to stimulate adrenergic and 5-HT_{2A} receptors, as well as stimulate the release of ADH. In extreme overdose cases this leads to rhabdomyolysis, hyponatraemia, and convulsions arising from cerebral oedema, which may be treated with benzodiazepines, and correction of electrolytes and water overload.

Digoxin

Although acute toxicity does occur, often over-dosage is chronic accompanied by interaction with other drugs, hypokalaemia, or renal failure. Symptoms range from nausea and vomiting, diarrhoea, headache, alteration in colour perception (xanthopsia) to hallucinations and delirium. In acute toxicity, activated charcoal may be useful within the first hour, but measuring plasma digoxin levels at presentation and 6 hr after ingestion is still essential. Overdose can be characterized by profound AV block and in extreme cases ventricular tachycardia. This should be treated with correction of electrolytes, iv magnesium, and in the case of heart block, atropine and temporary pacing if compromised. Hyperkalaemia and renal failure may also ensue. Because of its large volume of distribution, haemodialysis is of no use in managing digoxin overdose, although associated severe renal failure may require it. Where there is hyperkalaemia, arrhythmias, or high plasma digoxin levels, digoxin specific antibodies (e.g. Digibind or DigiFab) are indicated. Never give calcium to correct hyperkalaemia in the presence of digoxin toxicity. Note that plasma levels of digoxin will be unreliable for up to week after administration of digoxin specific antibodies.

Carbon monoxide

As carbon monoxide binds more than 200 times more tightly to haemoglobin than oxygen, it essentially causes tissue hypoxia. Normal plasma carboxyhaemoglobin levels are less than 6% even in smokers. However, levels of 10–30% are associated with headaches and exertional dyspnoea, whilst levels above 30% can result in hypotension, tachycardia, confusion, hyperpyrexia, and eventually focal neurology, seizures, and coma. Even after treatment, long-term neurological sequelae can develop, such as amnesia, dementia, and Parkinsonism. Treatment is with 100% oxygen and, in severe cases, hyperbaric oxygen (at 2.5 atmospheres) to reduce the half-life of carbon monoxide (from 4 hr to 22 min).

Multiple choice questions

1. The ability of a drug once bound to bring about an effect is known as:

A. Affinity.
B. K50.
C. Efficacy.
D. Potency.
E. Co-operativity.

2. The apparent volume of distribution of which of the following drugs would be 15001?

A. Warfarin.
B. Ethanol.
C. Gentamicin.
D. Chloroquine.
E. Ibuprofen.

3. Which of the following is *not* a prodrug?

A. Lithium.
B. Enalapril.
C. Levodopa.
D. Clopidogrel.
E. Heroin.

4. Which of the following is an inhibitor of cytochrome P450?

A. Phenytoin.
B. Carbamazepine.
C. Rifampacin.
D. St Johns Wort.
E. Erythromycin.

5. Which of the following drugs are *not* known to be teratogenic?

A. Warfarin.
B. Paracetamol.
C. Phenytoin.
D. Sodium valproate.
E. Lithium.

6. Which of the following drugs have first order elimination kinetics?

A. Ethanol.
B. Digoxin.
C. Aspirin.
D. Theophylline.
E. Tolbutamide.

7. Which of the following are poor prognostic markers early in paracetamol overdose?

A. INR>2.
B. Plasma pH >7.3.
C. Plasma bilirubin >200.
D. Lactate >3.5mmol/L.
E. Creatinine <120 μmol/L.

8. Which of the following are common recognized manifestations of digoxin toxicity?

A. Visual disturbance.
B. Peripheral neuropathy.
C. Myopathy.
D. Splenomegaly.
E. Megaloblastic anaemia.

9. **Which of the following drugs do not need dose adjustment with renal failure?**

A. Gentamicin.
B. Furosemide.
C. Ceftriaxone.
D. Lithium.
E. Vancomycin.

10. **Which of the following do *not* have known interactions with warfarin?**

A. St John's wort.
B. Grapefruit juice.
C. Garlic.
D. Metronidazole.
E. Bisoprolol.

For answers, please see Appendix: Answers to multiple choice questions, page 313.

CHAPTER 9

Rheumatology

Introduction

The rheumatic disorders are a diverse group of conditions that can affect organ systems outside the joint. Broadly, they can be divided into degenerative osteoarthritis, autoimmune diseases, such as rheumatoid arthritis (RA) and systemic lupus erythematosus (SLE), and inflammatory conditions, such as gout. The past 20 years have seen dramatic advances in the understanding and treatment of the autoimmune rheumatic diseases with a significant impact on outcomes for patients.

Anatomy

The articular joint is a complex structure with tightly regulated homeostasis. It consists of several key structures that work together (see Fig. 9.1). Damage to one of its components can lead to disruption of others, especially if the mechanical integrity is affected.

- *Articular cartilage* is a matrix of collagen and proteoglycans, which acts both as a shock absorber for the joint and allows the articulation of the adjacent bones by forming a smooth surface. Chondrocytes are the only cell type found in this structure, and they are capable of both laying down and breaking up articular cartilage depending on signals from their environment, such as sheer stress, acid-base balance, and oxygen concentration. Destruction of this structure in rheumatoid and osteoarthritis results in loss of function and pain.

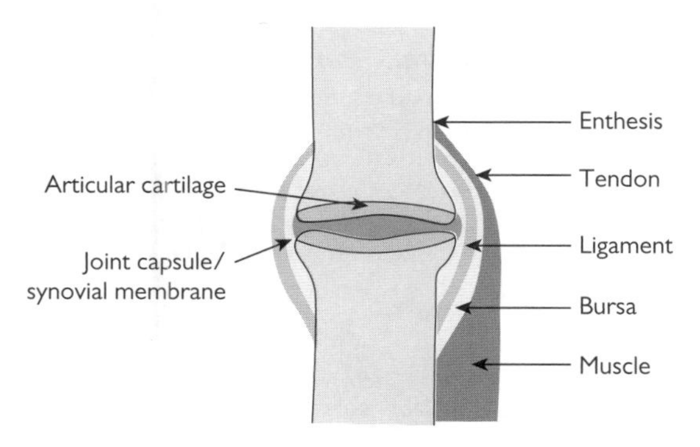

Fig. 9.1 Anatomy of the articular joint.

- *The synovial membrane* is a thin layer of tissue, which lines the joint capsule and tendon sheaths. It acts as a physical barrier in the joint, controlling the environment. The intimal layer of the membrane contains fibroblasts and macrophages. Fibroblasts produce synovial fluid, which consists of a long chain hydrophilic polymer called hyaluronan and a lubricating substance (lubricin). Macrophages clear the debris in the joint and initiate tissue repair if homeostasis is disturbed.

  Inflammation in RA starts at the synovium. Macrophages that normally direct tissue repair are also able to secrete a range of inflammatory cytokines, which recruit other immune cells to the area. This results in a pro-inflammatory positive feedback loop, and the production of matrix metalloproteinases by synovial fibroblasts and chondrocytes, which drive tissue destruction.

- *Ligaments* are structures that connect one bone to another to form a joint. They are comprised of dense fibrous connective tissue and their main role is to provide mechanical stability. They can form part of the articular capsule (capsular ligaments), or be inside the capsule (intracapsular ligaments such as the cruciate ligaments of the knee).
- *Tendons* are the structures that connect muscle to bone. They have a very similar structure to ligaments, but in addition have elastic properties that allow them to facilitate the smooth transmission of force from muscle to joint. Injuries of tendons are very common and termed tendonopathies. They can be caused by over-use or abnormal loading, resulting in weakening of the structures and, in some cases, rupture. In RA, the proteases

released by the inflammatory environment can also cause damage to the tendons. This occurs particularly in the small joints of the hands, leading to laxity and rupture, and the eventual subluxation and characteristic deformities seen in rheumatoid hands.

- *The Enthesis* is the point where a tendon, muscle, or ligament attaches to bone. This can be a simple fibrous enthesis where the tendon attaches directly to bone or a more complex fibrocartilaginous enthesis, where the tendon changes its structure through four intermediate structures during the transition from fibrous connective tissue to bone. The enthesis is often a site of inflammation in the seronegative spondyloarthritidies, such as psoriatic arthritis and ankylosing spondylitis.
- *Bursae* are small fluid filled sacs lined by synovial membrane. They reduce friction between the various structures in joints, such as bones and tendons, to allow free movement. Inflammation of these structures is termed bursitis and can be visualized on imaging (e.g. ultrasound or MRI) because the production of synovial fluid increases.

Pathology

Osteoarthritis

Osteoarthritis is the commonest cause of human joint disease worldwide, causing significant morbidity. It affects approximately 15% of the population over the age of 55. The pathological process is thought to be a chronic loss of cartilage with peri-articular bone reaction driven by chondrocyte dysfunction. A characteristic feature of the disease is new bone formation in the form of osteophytes, which can be seen clinically in the hands, particularly at the distal interphalangeal joints where they are known as 'Heberden's nodes'. The disease can follow a relapsing and remitting course, particularly in the hands, where patients can experience flares of pain associated with redness and swelling. Treatment at present is symptomatic.

Risk factors

- Inflammatory and crystal arthritis leading to secondary osteoarthritis (OA).
- *Metabolic disorders:* haemochromatosis, acromegaly, hyperparathyroidism, alkaptonuria.
- Smoking (especially in knee OA).
- Previous injury (especially in hips).
- Occupation, limited evidence, but often seen in manual workers, e.g. builders and dock workers.
- Female preponderance over the age of 50.
- Hip OA is more common in European populations.
- Obesity is a risk factor for knee OA.

Common joints affected

- *Hands:*
  - Distal interphalangeal joints.
  - Thumb carpometocarpal joints.
- Shoulders, often associated with degeneration of the rotator cuff.
- Knees, especially patello-femoral and medial tibio-femoral compartments.
- Hips.
- Spine, although wide discordance between radiological appearances and symptoms.

Radiological changes

- Joint space narrowing.
- Sclerosis.
- Osteophyte formation.
- Subchondral cysts.

Crystal arthropathies

The commonest crystal arthropathies are gout and calcium pyrophosphate deposition disease (pseudogout).

Gout

Gout is a disease caused by hyperuricaemia, leading to deposition of uric acid crystals in the joints and other tissues. These can be seen on polarized light microscopy of synovial fluid and are negatively birefringent. Direct visualization of the needle-shaped crystals in the synovial fluid is the gold standard test for confirming the diagnosis of gout, as raised serum uric acid levels are common and often asymptomatic. Gout is a fairly common condition affecting 10–15% of men over the age of 40 in western populations. It is thought to be caused by a genetic predisposition towards higher serum uric acid levels and western lifestyles.

Uric acid metabolism

Urate is derived from purines that are ingested in food and the endogenous products of purine nucleotides, which are the building blocks of RNA and DNA. Large increases in serum urate can also occur at times of high cell turnover or massive cell lysis, e.g. during chemotherapy for haematological malignancies. Urate is eliminated via the kidneys and gut (see Fig. 9.2).

Pathology

Above a concentration on 0.42 mmol/L, plasma is saturated with urate. This is a stable solution, which does not crystallize due to the presence of other plasma constituents.

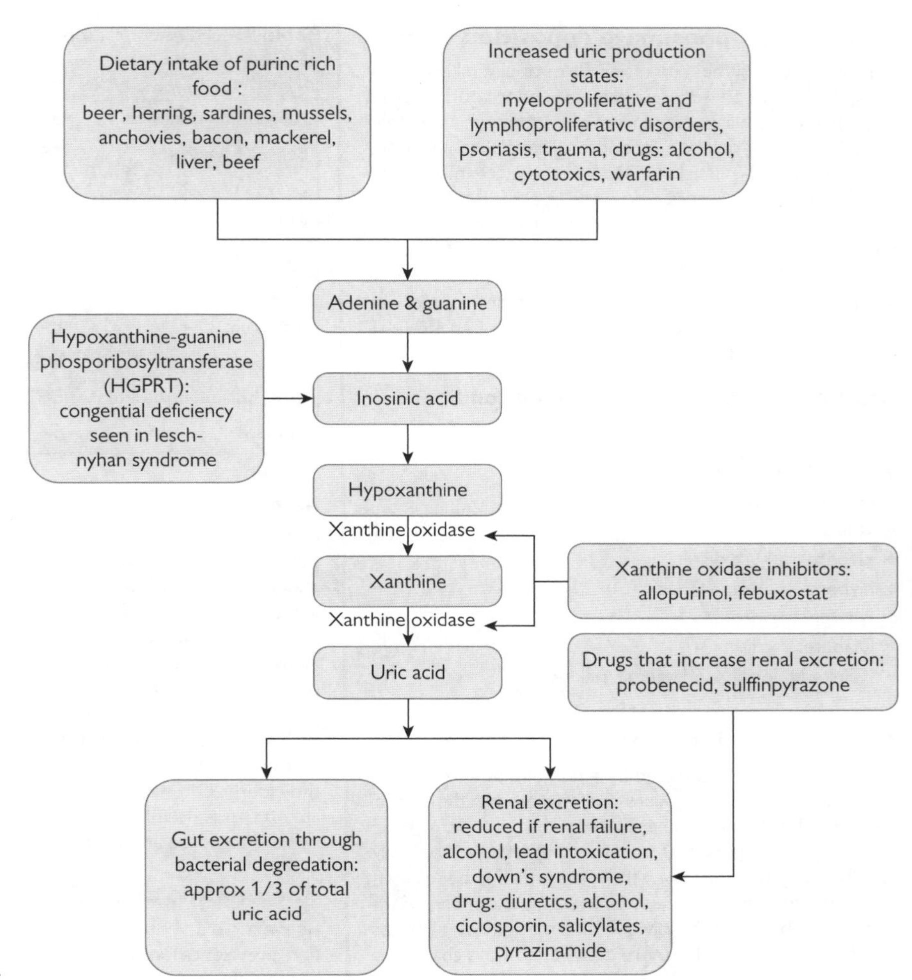

Fig. 9.2 Uric acid metabolism and excretion.

However, the solubility of urate decreases with lower temperatures and with acidic pH. It is postulated that in the synovial fluid, especially at the peripheral joints of the feet, the conditions are more favourable for monosodium urate crystal formation if the synovial fluid is saturated with urate. The triggers for attacks of gout remain poorly understood.

The crystals are potent immune system activators and trigger an inflammatory response characterized by the release of interleukin-1β. With repeated attacks tissue destruction occurs and over many years, a typical pattern of juxta-articular erosions is seen.

Manifestations of gout outside the joint

- *Tophi:* these are depositions of monosodium urate crystals in the soft tissues often around the joints. Typical site are the hands, elbows and ears.
- *Renal:* gout affects the kidneys in three ways:
  - *Urate nephropathy*—this is damage caused directly by the deposition of crystals and the inflammation triggered as a result.
  - *Uric acid nephropathy*—occurring acutely in patients who are dehydrated and acutely unwell with sepsis.
  - *Uric acid stones*—these are radiolucent and are common even in the absence of hyperuricaemia.

Management

- Acute attacks are treated with non-steroidal anti-inflammatory drugs (NSAIDs).
- Colchicine and glucocorticoids may be used if NSAIDs have to be avoided. The commonest example is renal impairment, which often co-exists with gout.
- Prophylaxis is usually in the form of a xanthine oxidase inhibitor, such as allopurinol or febuxostat, but these can trigger acute attacks of gout when first initiated.

Calcium pyrophosphate deposition disease

This is the second most common form of crystal arthropathy and the pathophysiology is not well understood. There is a spectrum of clinical disease from asymptomatic radiological calcification of cartilage (chondrocalcinosis) to inflammatory polyarthritis mimicking RA. It is most common in the elderly and rarely occurs below the age of 60. There are many associations which are listed in 'Calcium pyrophosphate associated conditions'. Polarized light microscopy reveals positively birefringent rhomboid crystals. There is no specific management apart from symptom control and intra-articular glucocorticoid injections are often useful if the flare is limited to one or two joints.

Calcium pyrophosphate-associated conditions

- Hypomagnesaemia.
- Hypophosphataemia.
- Haemochromatosis.
- Wilson's disease.
- Hyperparathyroidism.
- Hypercalcaemia.
- Bartter's syndrome.
- Diabetes mellitus.
- X-linked hypophosphataemic rickets.

Autoimmune inflammatory disorders

Joints are commonly affected by a number of autoimmune systemic diseases. The causes and triggers for the loss of immune self-tolerance in these conditions is a topic of much research, but remains largely elusive. In particular, there are very few clues to explain why the joints are affected so often.

Broadly-speaking, the rheumatological autoimmune inflammatory disorders can be divided into the following groups. These will be discussed in more detail later in this chapter.

- Rheumatoid arthritis.
- Spondyloarthropathies.
- Connective tissue diseases.
- Vasculitis.

Genetics

Recent advances from the human genome project and other genome wide association studies have implicated a number of genotypes associated with developing these autoimmune diseases. In general, the genetic polymorphisms associated with the diseases are centred around the human leukocyte antigen genes, which code for major histocompatibility complex (MHC) proteins. The normal function of MHC proteins is to process and present antigen for immune cells activation. However, these genetic polymorphisms only account for a small proportion of the risk of developing autoimmune rheumatic diseases with the remainder of the risk being attributable to environmental factors most of which remain unknown. Table 9.1 summarizes some of these gene associations with the relevant disease.

Table 9.1 HLA association with rheumatological diseases

Disease	HLA	Relative risk
Ankylosing spondylitis	B27	>150
Behçet's syndrome	B5	8
Grave's disease	DR3	4
Rheumatoid arthritis	DR4	9
Juvenile idiopathic arthritis	DR8	8
Coeliac disease	DQ2	30
Narcolepsy	DR2	40
Multiple sclerosis	DQ6	12
Type 1 diabetes mellitus	DR3	14
Psoriasis	C6	7

Autoantibodies

Many autoimmune diseases are associated with the production of auto-antibodies (Table 9.2). In some cases, these antibodies are known to be pathogenic, but in others they are a by-product of an active immune system and, therefore, can be found in other chronic inflammatory states. Auto-antibodies serve as useful biomarkers for the diagnosis of certain diseases. Rheumatoid factor was one of the first auto-antibodies to be identified; it is an IgM molecule against the Fc portion of human IgG. It is present in 5–25% of the normal population and more commonly found in the elderly. Often the amount of rheumatoid factor detectable (titre) is useful as high titre rheumatoid factor is much more likely to be associated with autoimmune disease.

Rheumatoid arthritis

Rheumatoid arthritis is a relatively common (1–3% population prevalence) inflammatory arthritis, which can present in a number of ways. Like other autoimmune diseases, it is more likely to affect women than men (3:1). The peak onset is during the 5th decade of life. Classically, it leads to a deforming symmetrical polyarthritis involving the small joints of the hands and feet. The classical deformed rheumatoid hand appearance is fortunately on the decline due to advances in therapy over the last 20 years.

RA can also involve extra-articular organs such as the eyes, skin, and lungs. In the clinic, the disease is often subdivided into sero-negative (meaning rheumatoid factor negative) and sero-positive disease. However, the presence of rheumatoid factor is not essential for making the diagnosis, but the prognosis is worse if rheumatoid factor is positive. More recently, anti-citrullinated protein antibodies (ACPA), like anti-CCP have become widely available and they offer a much better specificity for RA compared with rheumatoid factor. The presence of ACPAs also seems to correlate with the *HLA-DR4* susceptibility gene inheritance (the so-called shared epitope). ACPA antibodies may be present in the blood of susceptible individuals up to 9 years before the onset of the clinical disease.

Table 9.2 Autoantibodies associated with rheumatological diseases

Antibody	Main disease association	Other association
Rheumatoid factor	Rheumatoid arthritis (70%)	Normal population (5–25%). Chronic infection, e.g. syphilis, leprosy, endocarditis, TB. Cryoglobulinaemia. Sarcoidosis. Autoimmune liver disease. Sjögren's (80%). SLE (20–40%)
Anti-cyclic citrullinated peptide (ACPA)	Rheumatoid arthritis (70–80%)	Psoriatic arthritis (10–15%)
Anti-double-stranded DNA (dsDNA)	SLE (80%); predictor of renal involvement	Titre fluctuates with disease activity
Anti-cardiolipin	Anti-phospholipid syndrome	SLE (40%). Low titres found in sepsis
Anti-nuclear antibody (ANA)	SLE (>99%). Rheumatoid arthritis (50%)	Normal population (10–15%). Silicone breast implants (30%). Drug induced lupus. Connective tissue disorders where an ENA is present: • Systemic sclerosis • Sjogren's • Dermatomyositis
Extractable nuclear antigens (ENA): test if ANA positive		
Anti-Smith (anti-sm)	SLE (20%)	Specific to SLE only
Anti-Ro	Sjögren's	Cutaneous lupus. Associated with neonatal heart block during pregnancy in SLE
Anti-La	Sjögren's	Cutaneous lupus
Anti-ribonuclear protein (anti-RNP)	Mixed connective tissue disease	SLE
Anti-scl-70 also known as anti-topoisomerase	Systemic sclerosis	Associated with worse prognosis
Anti centromere	Systemic sclerosis	Associated with limited cutaneous phenotype (better prognosis)
Anti Jo1	Dermatomyositis (anti-synthetase syndromes)	Often associated interstitial lung disease
ANCA associated vasculitis		
ANCA	Now only used as a screening test. If positive test for PR3/MPO (see 'Small/medium vessel vasculitis' section)	• If cANCA (cytoplasmic) more likely to be granulomatosis with polyangiitis (formerly Wegner's). • If pANCA (peri-nuclear) more likely to be eosinophillic granulomatosis with polyangiitis (formerly Churg–Strauss) or microscopic polyangiitis. • ANCA without PR3/MPO can be associated with chronic infection or inflammation
Proteinase-3 (PR3)	Specific for granulomatosis with polyangiitis (formerly Wegner's)	
Myeloperoxidase (MPO)	Eosinophillic granulomatosis with polyangiitis (formerly Churg–Strauss)	• Crescentic glomerulonephritis. • Microscopic polyangiitis

Apart from genetic susceptibility, the only other well established risk factor for the development of RA is smoking, especially in genetically susceptible individuals. Moreover, patients who continue to smoke have a worse prognosis and are less likely to respond to therapy. In addition, RA is now an established risk factor (independent of smoking) for atherosclerotic cardiovascular disease due to the chronic inflammatory state. Cardiovascular disease is the main cause of early mortality in RA. See Table 9.3 for a summary of risk factors and prognosis in RA

Pathophysiology

At the cellular level, the inflamed RA joint is a complex mix of immune cells and cytokines. The majority of the tissue damage is mediated by proteases released from the chondrocytes and synovial fibroblasts, which are activated by the cytokine milieu. Innate immune cells, such as neutrophils and macrophages are recruited to the site and release prostaglandins, causing pain and further tissue damage from reactive oxygen species. The two key cytokines released by the macrophages in particular are TNF-α, which drives the inflammatory process and IL-6, which also activates the acute phase response and leads to systemic effects, such as weight loss and fever. The targeting of the innate immune system cytokines with monoclonal antibodies against IL-6 (tocilizumab) and TNF-α (infliximab, adalimumab, and etanercept) has proved to be very successful in the treatment of RA.

Adaptive immune cells are also recruited and begin to establish tertiary lymphoid organs. B cells act as antigen presenting cells for T cell activation and release immune complexes that may be contributing to the disease process. Therapies targeting B cells (rituximab) and T helper cell co-stimulation (abatacept) have also proved very effective.

Rheumatoid arthritis presentation and classification

The onset of RA can be variable making it a difficult condition to diagnose without specialist input. The following are well recognized patters of presentation

Table 9.3 Risk factors and marker of prognosis in RA

	Risk factors	
Markers of poor prognosis in RA	Established risk factors for developing RA	Possible risk factors
Smoking	Smoking	Poor dentition
Seropositvity (ACPA or RF). Extra-articular features	*HLA DR4* inheritance (especially the inheritance of 2 alleles)	Obesity
Female sex		Alterations in the gut microbiota
HLA-DR4 inheritance		
Insidious onset		
Early erosions		

- *Insidious (weeks/months):* often associated with worse prognosis probably due to delay in diagnosis.
- *Acute.*
- *Systemic:* accompanied by very raised inflammatory markers, fevers and weight loss.
- *Palindromic:* episodes occurring over several hours with complete resolution between attacks. This presentation is associated with the best long-term prognosis.
- *Polymyalgic:* upper limb proximal pain and stiffness similar to polymyalgia rheumatic.

In 2010 the American College of Rheumatology revised their classification criteria for RA to improve early disease detection (Table 9.4). This was in recognition of an increasing volume of evidence that suggests early effective therapy prevents longer term disability.

Table 9.4 The 2010 American College of Rheumatology-European League Against Rheumatism classification criteria for RA

Target population (who should be tested) • Patients who have at least one joint with definite clinical synovitis (swelling) • Patients with synovitis not explained by another disease *Classification criteria for RA (score-based algorithm: add score of categories A–D)* Score of 6 or greater is needed for classification of definite RA	
	Score
Joint involvement	
1 large joint	0
2–10 large joints	1
1–3 small joints (with or without large joint involvement)	2
4–10 small joints (with or without large joint involvement)	3
>10 joints (at least one small joint)	5
Serology	
Negative RF and negative ACPA	0
Low positive RF or low positive ACPA	2
High positive RF or high positive ACPA	3
Acute phase reactants	
Normal CRP and normal ESR	0
High CRP or high ESR	1
Duration of symptoms	
<6 weeks duration	0
>6 weeks duration	1

BOX 9.1 EXTRA-ARTICULAR MANIFESTATIONS OF RHEUMATOID ARTHRITIS

Tendons

- Rheumatoid nodules occur in 20% of sero-positive patients and are found mainly in the extensor surfaces of the forearms. They can worsen with methotrexate therapy.
- Tendon rupture in the hands is common and indication for surgical referral.

Skin

- Commonest presentation is palmar erythema.
- Leucocytoclastic vasculitis occurs especially in smokers.
- Erythema nodosum and pyoderma gangrenosum can occur rarely.

Ocular involvement

- Episcleritis.
- A painful form of scleritis can occur in rheumatoid vasculitis leading to scleromalacia.
- Dry eyes secondary to overlap Sjögren's syndrome occur in 10%.

Pulmonary disease

- Pleural effusions.
- Rheumatoid nodules can occur in the lung and are difficult to distinguish radiographically from malignancy.
- Interstitial fibrosis can occur rarely.
- Bronchiolitis obliterans is often fatal, but very rare.

Cardiovascular disease

- RA is an independent risk factor for atherosclerotic disease.
- Cardiovascular complications are the leading cause of early mortality.
- Pericardial disease is rare and often asymptomatic.

Haematological complications

- Anaemia of chronic disease is common, but other causes such as myelosuppression from drugs and occult GI bleeds from NSAIDs should be taken into account.
- Felty's syndrome (splenomegaly, neutropenia, and RA) is very rare <1% and associated with a positive ANA.
- Lymphadenopathy is common but often asymptomatic. It can cause anxiety as it is often picked up incidentally on CT.

Neurological involvement

- Mononeuritis multiplex is associated with rheumatoid vasculitis and is very rare.
- Nerve entrapment from joint deformity at the wrist and elbow is common.
- Cervical subluxation due to atlanto-axial disease is very rare, but should not be missed.

Bone

- RA is an independent risk factor for osteoporosis.
- Chronic glucocorticoid use can also contribute to fracture risk.

Systemic complications of chronic inflammation

- Weight loss is common.
- Secondary amyloidosis is now rare with better systemic therapy. The most commonly associated organ is the kidney.
- Patients with active RA have an increased risk of infection especially after surgery.

Rheumatoid arthritis outside the joint

RA is associated with a range of extra-articular manifestations which are summarized in Box 9.1.

Management of rheumatoid arthritis

The specific therapies are covered later in this chapter in 'Drugs used in the treatment of rheumatological conditions'. The accepted general principal is early aggressive management with combination disease modifying anti-rheumatic therapies and escalation to biologics to induce disease remission. Evidence suggests early aggressive management leads to better outcomes in terms of long-term joint damage and disability.

Autoimmune inflammatory disorders: spondyloarthropathies

This group of inflammatory disorders has a very strong association with HLA-B27 inheritance. HLA-B27 prevalence in western Caucasian populations is estimated to be 8–10%, but not all people with HLA-B27 go on to develop spondyloarthrits (Table 9.5). It seems a second event is needed for loss of tolerance. Unpicking the molecular events that lead to disease developments is the subject of much research.

Table 9.5 HLA-B27 association with the spondyloarthritidies

Old classification of spondyloarthritidies	HLA-B27 prevalence
Ankylosing spondylitis	90%
Reactive arthritis (formerly Reiter's syndrome)	70%
Enteropathic arthritis	50%
Psoriatic arthritis	20%

BOX 9.2 CLINICAL FEATURES SPONDYLOARTHRITIS

Spine

- *Sacroilitis:*
  - Main symptom is inflammatory back pain, which is worse in the second half of the night and improves with exercise.
  - Alternating buttock pain and early morning stiffness also help differentiate inflammatory back pain from mechanical back pain.
  - X-ray changes of sclerosis, erosions, and fusion are difficult to interpret and take years to develop, MRI STIR sequences are now the gold standard investigation for early detection.
  - MRI also detects inflammatory Romanus lesions at the corners of vertebrae, which progress to new bone formation (bridging syndesmophytes) and the late classic features of bamboo spine.

Joints

- A large joint oligo-arthritis is most common.
- Enthesitis is also seen frequently and can be difficult to manage.
- Dactylitis (sausage-like inflamed fingers or toes).

Skin

- Psoriasis with all of its potential presentations.
- Psoriatic nail changes of pitting, ridging, and onycholysis.
- Erythema nodosum and pyoderma gangrenosum are rare.

Eyes

- Anterior uveitis, which is painful and can be sight-threatening if untreated.
- In reactive arthritis conjunctivitis is seen.

Gut

- The association with Crohn's disease and ulcerative colitis is well established.
- Up to 65% of patients with ankylosing spondylitis can have subclinical colitis.

Cardiovascular

- Aortitis and aortic valve incompetence are rare features of ankylosing spondylitis.
- AV node block is very rare.

Respiratory

- Apical lung fibrosis is very rarely seen.

Systemic

- Fatigue is a common symptom.
- Systemic amyloid is rare.

Classically, this group of disorders was classified into four distinct diseases, but more recently, this classification has been changed by international consensus and patients are diagnosed as having spondyloarthritis with axial (spine) or peripheral involvement typically involving enthesitis and dactylitis (Fig. 9.3). As the disease progresses the phenotype can often change in the same individual and other organ systems can be involved (Box 9.2).

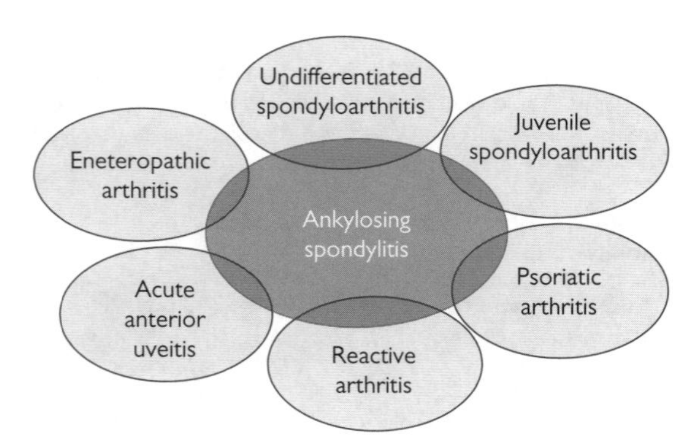

Fig. 9.3 ASAS consensus classification of spondyloarthritis.

Data from J Sieper et al., 'The Assessment of SpondyloArthritis international Society (ASAS) handbook: a guide to assess spondyloarthritis', *Annals of the Rheumatic Diseases: The Eular Journal*, 2009, 68, Suppl 2, pp. ii1–ii44

Management of spondyloarthritis

The management largely depends on the phenotype and axial disease can be dissociated from peripheral joint disease.

Axial disease

- Physiotherapy is very important for improving function and reducing the progression of spinal fusion.
- Long-term NSAIDs also slow the rate of disease progression. In ankylosing spondylitis their long-term benefit is deemed greater than their potential adverse effects on the cardiovascular system.
- Anti-TNF agents are currently the only licenced biological therapies and their use has transformed the management of axial disease with dramatic benefits for patients. However, 1/3 of patients do not respond and currently anti-TNF therapy is reserved for the most severe cases due to cost implications.

Peripheral disease

- Intra-articular glucocorticoids are useful for oligo-arthritis.
- Systemic glucocorticoids are also useful for short-term control of flares, but must be used with caution if there is skin psoriasis, as they can cause a flare in the skin disease.
- Disease-modifying anti-rheumatic drugs are used for long-term control of peripheral symptoms. Sulfasalazine, methotrexate, and leflunomide are the three main drugs used in the clinical setting, and they will be covered later in this chapter.

Autoimmune inflammatory disorders: psoriatic arthritis

Skin psoriasis affects 1–2% of the population and 10% of these develop psoriatic arthritis. The joint disease can precede the skin disease by up to 2 years. Nail changes may be the only psoriatic feature present. The development of a progressive erosive arthropathy only occurs in 20–30% of cases. 10–15% of patients have a positive rheumatoid factor or ACPA.

There are 5 clinical patterns but the phenotype changes over time in the majority of cases and the clinical pattern does not predict the prognosis.

- Distal interphalangeal joint arthritis
- Symmetric polyarthritis similar to RA
- Asymmetric oligoarthritis
- Sacroiliac joint involvement
- Arthritis mutilans

Treatment follows the same principles as peripheral spondyloarthritis (SpA). Methotrexate is good for controlling the skin disease but recent studies suggest it may not be effective at slowing down joint erosions.

Autoimmune inflammatory disorders: reactive arthritis

This condition is distinct from spondyloarthritis. It is an immune-mediated inflammatory arthritis with a very clear trigger from infections outside the joint. Treatment of the underlying infection does not necessarily result in resolution of the arthritis.

- Common organisms that trigger reactive arthritis are *Chlamydia*, *Yersinia*, *Salmonella*, *Shigella*, and *Campylobacter*.
- The arthritis normally involves a few large joints and typically presents within 4 weeks of the infection.
- The age of onset is 15–40 years and is more common in men.
- The classical triad of arthritis, conjunctivitis, and urethritis only occurs in one-third of cases.
- Other features include circinate balanitis, keratoderma blenorrhagica, iritis, enthesitis (particularly Achilles), and systemic features of fever and raised inflammatory markers.

Prognosis

- Eighty per cent of cases resolve within 6 months and require symptomatic NSAID therapy/intra-articular glucocorticoids.
- Fifteen per cent have recurrent episodes after 6 months, often triggered by infection. This is termed recurrent reactive arthritis and occurs in HLA-B27 positive individuals.
- Five per cent of individuals go on to develop a spondyloarthritis and require long-term treatment as detailed in 'Autoimmune inflammatory disorders: spondyloarthropathies'.

Autoimmune inflammatory disorders: systemic lupus erythematosus

SLE is the archetypal multi-system autoimmune disease. It predominantly affects women in the 3rd and 4th decade of life. In the majority of cases, symptoms are mild and chronic, but in approximately 10% of cases the disease can be severe and life-threatening. The disease is characterized by the development of auto-antibodies as listed in the previous section of this chapter. ANA is the key antibody for making a diagnosis and the existence of ANA negative lupus is only reserved for discussion in academic circles. Antibodies against dsDNA, Ro, La, and the Smith antigen (anti-Sm) are also commonly seen. These intracellular antigens are typically expressed on the cell surface during apoptosis and the reason for auto-antibody production by B cells is not yet understood. However, the depletion of B cells using monoclonal antibodies has proved to be quite successful in the management of severe SLE.

SLE can affect any major organ system in the body as summarized in Box 9.3. The features numbered 1 to 11 are included in the ACR classification criteria. At least four features out of the 11 need to be present for a diagnosis of SLE.

Management of SLE

- Hydroxychloroquine is the mainstay of therapy for mild cases. It is useful for managing skin disease, arthralgia, and fatigue. Additionally, it improves the prognosis and protects against developing life-threatening complications.
- Anticoagulation in the context of thrombotic events. Aspirin may be useful in patients with positive anti-phospholipid antibodies who have not had thrombotic events.
- Women of child-bearing age considering pregnancy should have pre-pregnancy counselling by a specialist obstetric team and a closely-monitored pregnancy.
- Glucocorticoids are useful in small oral doses for the management of small flares and intravenously in large doses for the treatment of severe flares.
- Azathioprine and mycophenolate mofetil are used as steroid sparing agents. Methotrexate is also often used especially in musculoskeletal manifestations.
- Intravenous cyclophosphamide is used to treat life- or organ-threatening complications.
- Anti-B cell therapies rituximab (anti CD-20 monoclonal antibody) and belimumab (anti-B cell activating factor (BAFF)) are emerging new therapies, but their use remains limited due to cost implications.
- Plasma exchange is reserved for life-threatening cases.

Autoimmune inflammatory disorders: Sjögren's syndrome

This is a chronic autoimmune disease characterized by lymphocyte infiltration of exocrine glands. The condition can be primary or occur secondary to other autoimmune diseases especially RA and SLE with overlapping features. Sjögren's

BOX 9.3 MANIFESTATIONS OF SLE BY ORGAN SYSTEM

1-11 indicate that these categories are included in the ACR classification criteria. At least four features out of the 11 need to be present for a diagnosis of SLE'

Skin (80% of cases)

- Malar rash[1] (up to 35% of cases).
- Chronic discoid rash[2].
- Photosensitive rash[3].
- Oral ulcers[4].
- Non-scarring alopecia.
- Vasculitis of digits.

Musculoskeletal (90% of cases)

- Arthralgia[5] (swelling and synovitis is rare).
- *Tendonitis:* can lead to non-erosive deformity (Jaccoud's arthropathy).
- Myalgia common, but true myositis <5%.

Cardiorespiratory (30–60% of cases)

- Serositis[6] (pleuritis or pericarditis).
- Libman–Sachs endocarditis rarely presents with symptoms.
- Increased risk of atherosclerotic disease.
- Interstitial fibrosis.
- Pulmonary vasculitis.
- Pulmonary hypertension in the presence of anti-phospholipid Abs.

Renal[7] (30–60% of cases)

- *WHO classification:*
  - *Class I (5%)*—minimal mesangial glomerulonephritis.
  - *Class II (20%)*—mesangial proliferative.
  - *Class III (25%)*—focal proliferative.
  - *Class IV (40%)*—diffuse proliferative.
  - *Class V (10%)*—membranous nephritis.

Neurological

The true prevalence of features depends on the definition.

- Seizures or psychosis[8] (~5%).
- Peripheral neuropathy (10%).
- Depression and anxiety very common, but difficult to differentiate from depression secondary to chronic illness.

Haematological[9]

Up to 70% of cases. Raised ESR, anaemia of chronic disease and lymphadenopathy occur, but do not count in classification criteria.

- Haemolytic anaemia.
- Leucopenia $<4.0\times10^9$/L on two or more occasions.
- Lymphopenia $<1.5\times10^9$/L on two or more occasions.
- Thrombocytopenia $<100\times10^9$/L.

Immunological[10,11]

ANA positivity scores one for the classification criteria plus maximum of one more point for any of the other following findings:

- *Raised dsDNA:* also predicts renal involvement and can fluctuate with disease activity.
- *Anti-Sm:* only in 20%, but highly specific.
- Antiphospholipid antibodies.
- Anti-cardiolipin antibodies.
- Lupus anticoagulants.
- Anti-β2 microglobulin antibodies.

Vascular

- Raynaud's phenomenon is common.
- Venous and arterial thrombosis in anti-phospholipid syndrome. Also recurrent miscarriages.
- Cutaneous vasculitis is rare and associated with low complement levels.

Gastrointestinal

- Hepatomegaly (25%).
- Splenomegaly (10%).
- Pancreatitis (rare).

Biochemical: hypergammaglobulinaemia (60%)

- Hypoalbuminaemia (50%).

Systemic: fatigue is very common

- Weight loss.

can also co-exist with other autoimmune diseases, in particular, primary biliary cirrhosis and autoimmune thyroid disease. Anti-Ro and anti-La antibodies are typical. In addition, many patients will also have a positive ANA and rheumatoid factor.

Most patients have the typical sicca syndrome features of dry eyes, dry mouth, and dyspareunia, secondary to vaginal dryness. This may be associated with parotid gland swelling and arthralgia is a common extraglandular manifestation of primary Sjögren's. The prognosis in these cases is good and the treatment is symptomatic with artificial tears and moistening sprays and gels. Hydroxychloroquine can be useful for the joint symptoms.

Approximately one-third of cases can be associated with more severe manifestations requiring the use of immunosuppressive drugs:

- Polyclonal hypergammaglobulinaemia, with systemic features of raised CRP, fevers, and weight loss.
- Asymptomatic lung involvement occurs in 25%, most commonly in the guise of organizing pneumonia. Lymphocytic interstitial pneumonitis (LIP) is a very rare, but serious complication.
- 30% of patients develop distal renal tubular acidosis with associated renal stones.

- There is a 40-fold increase in the rate of B-cell lymphomas. The salivary glands are the main site of lymphomatous change and persistent lymphadenopathy or gland enlargement should be investigated with biopsy.

Autoimmune inflammatory disorders: systemic sclerosis

Systemic sclerosis is a rare autoimmune disease characterized by skin thickening (scleroderma), severe Raynaud's often with digital ischaemia, and internal organ involvement. The disease is classified according to the extent of skin involvement. The disease starts at the finger tips and progresses up the arms. Skin changes beyond the elbow classify the disease as diffuse with a worse prognosis, while involvement only distal to the elbow is limited disease. Both limited and diffuse disease can involve the internal organs.

The pathophysiology of the disease is complex with features of inflammation, fibrosis, and vascular dysfunction. The autoantibody profile is important in predicting prognosis and the pattern of internal organ involvement (Box 9.4). Only two (anti Scl-70 and anti centromere) out of six associated autoantibodies are routinely available for testing in UK laboratory ENA panels, but a nucleolar staining pattern on ANA immunofluorescence is highly suggestive.

Autoimmune inflammatory disorders: inflammatory myositis

This is a group of inflammatory muscle disorders mediated by auto-antibodies. The presence of characteristic skin lesions is the key difference between the traditional labels of dermatomyositis and polymyositis. More recently, this group of disorders has been reclassified according to autoantibody profile (Box 9.5). The newly-described anti-synthetase syndrome is characterized by the presence of anti-Jo-1 antibodies and presents with a prodromal systemic illness followed by the classic triad of muscle, skin, and lung involvement. Other anti-synthetase antibodies are also described, but are very rare and not available for routine testing. Anti-SRP antibodies are associated with only muscle involvement and present abruptly.

Inflammatory myopathies and malignancy

Studies show the presence of malignancy in up to 15% of patients with inflammatory myopathy. The increased risk is only in those over the age of 45. More recently, this has been shown to be linked to a paraneoplastic autoantibody anti TIF-1-gamma antibody.

BOX 9.4 CLINICAL FEATURES AND AUTOANTIBODY ASSOCIATIONS OF SYSTEMIC SCLEROSIS

Skin

Changes occur with both **anti-centromere** and **anti-scl-70**, and are more likely to develop a diffuse phenotype if anti-scl-70 positive.

- The skin changes of scleroderma are difficult to treat and can cause flexion deformities.
- Raynaud's can precede disease by many years.
- Digital ulcers secondary to vascular dysfunction. Treated with:
  - Intravenous iloprost.
  - Sildenafil is also used.
  - Bosentan is a newly-licensed endothelin receptor antagonist.
- Nail bed capillary dilatation.
- Calcinosis (more likely in *anti-centromere*).
- Hair loss common in affected areas of skin.
- Mechanic's hands with *anti-PM-scl* antibody (not available for routine testing).

Gastrointestinal

This is a feature of all types of systemic sclerosis.

- Oesophageal reflux is most common and may contribute to lung disease through micro-aspiration. Aggressive anti-reflux treatment is required, often using combination proton pump inhibitors (PPI) and ranitidine.
- *Oesophageal dysmotility:* prokinetics such as metoclopramide can be useful.
- Bacterial overgrowth can be treated with antibiotics.

Musculoskeletal

- Overlap myositis occurs with *anti-PM-scl* antibody, although not often severe.
- An erosive arthritis is also a feature of this antibody.

Pulmonary

- Interstitial lung disease seen with *anti-scl-70* and *anti-PM-scl*, and is treated using systemic immunosupression with cyclophosphamide and mycophenolate mofetil.
- Pulmonary arterial hypertension can be a feature of all types of systemic sclerosis and occur insidiously. Regular screening with echocardiography is essential.

Renal

- Scleroderma renal crisis presents with accelerated hypertension.
- Mostly occurs with *anti-scl-70* and *anti-RNA-polymerase-III* (not available for routine testing).
- Early treatment with ACE inhibitors is essential.

BOX 9.5 KEY CLINICAL FEATURES OF INFLAMMATORY MYOPATHIES

Skin
- *Mechanic's hands:* patho-pneumonic feature of anti-synthetase syndrome (symmetric fissuring of the skin on the dorso-lateral aspects of the index and middle fingers).
- Raynaud's phenomenon.
- Nail bed capillary dilatation.
- Nail bed hypertrophy.
- *Gottron's papules:* erythematous or violacious plaques on the dorsum of the hands over the MCP joints.
- *Heliotrope rash:* purple/lilac-coloured suffusion around the eyes.
- Macular eruption on chest wall (V sign) and back of neck/shoulders (shawl sign).

Lungs
- Patients may present with shortness of breath due to respiratory muscle weakness or interstitial lung disease.
- Respiratory muscle weakness will show abnormal flow volume loop on spirometry.
- Interstitial lung disease will show decreased transfer factor.
- Interstitial lung involvement is very common in the context of anti-Jo-1 anti-synthetase syndrome and anti-PM-scl overlap syndromes.
- High resolution CT early features are organizing pneumonia and non-specific interstitial pneumonia (NSIP). These can be reversed with appropriate immunosupression.

Laboratory
- Raised CK typical, but may be normal.
- Raised ALT from muscles, rather than liver in context of raised CK.
- Raised CRP and ESR common.
- *Anti-Jo-1 antibodies:* 30–40% of adult inflammatory myositis.
- *Anti SRP antibodies:* 5–10% of adult inflammatory myositis.

Imaging
- Modality of choice is MRI.
- Oedema on STIR sequences demonstrates active inflammation.
- Fat infiltration is a late sign and is not reversible.

EMG
- Low amplitude and early recruitment pattern.
- Spontaneous activity present.

Biopsy
- Infiltration of lymphocytes.
- Muscle fibre necrosis.

Management
- *Systemic glucocorticoids:* normally high dose oral prednisolone or pulsed intravenous methylprednisolone.
- Intravenous cyclophosphamide if lung involvement.
- Methotrexate as steroid sparing agent, but avoid if lung involvement.
- Azathioprine and mycophenolate mofetil are alternative steroid sparing agents.
- High dose iv immunoglobulin is effective especially in context of suspected infection where immunosupression would be inappropriate.

Autoimmune inflammatory disorders: systemic vasculitis

Systemic vasculitis incorporates a wide spectrum of conditions that cause inflammation in blood vessels. Vasculitis can be a primary disease or be secondary to other autoimmune diseases, such as RA and SLE. The traditional classification criteria for primary vasculitis was based on the size of the vessels involved. More recent classification criteria taking into account the presence of ANCA antibodies and the histological features of the inflammatory lesions are under development. Also the nomenclature has recently changed adding to the confusion.

This section will cover large vessel vasculitidies (giant cell arteritis (GCA) and Takayasu's arteritis) and small/medium vessel primary vasculitis taking into account the role of ANCA antibodies.

Large vessel vasculitis

Takayasu's

- This disease is more common in Japan, Southeast Asia, India and Mexico. The female to male ratio is approximately 9:1, and it presents in those under 40. In the USA, the incidence is 2–3 cases/million.
- The presentation is usually with ischaemic symptoms of claudication or organ ischaemia (e.g. stroke). Clinical features include bruits and diminished peripheral pulses.
- PET (positron emission tomography) scanning is useful to detect occult disease. MRI is useful to monitor disease progression.
- Treatment is with high dose glucocorticoids. Immunosuppressant agents are used but there is little trial evidence. There are also reports of successful use of TNF-α blockers in particular Infliximab.

GCA

- GCA is the most common form of vasculitis in Europe with an incidence rate of up to 18/100,000. The female to male ratio is approximately 2:1. It presents almost exclusively in those over the age of 55.
- The commonest presentation is temporal headache with raised systemic inflammatory markers. Other features also include jaw claudication, myalgia (see next bullet point) and cranial neuropathies, in particular visual loss.
- There is an association with polymyalgia rheumatica (PMR). This is a condition presenting with proximal muscle pain and marked stiffness in the same age group. The systemic inflammatory markers are also raised. PMR is much more common than GCA. Half of patients with GCA have PMR symptoms. It has been reported that up to 20% of patients with PMR have GCA features, although that may be an over-estimation.
- There are no gold standard investigations. A positive biopsy confirms GCA, but a negative biopsy does not exclude disease as there can be skip lesions. The diagnosis remains clinical. The effectiveness of ultrasound in the diagnosis of GCA is an area of ongoing research.
- Treatment is with prolonged high dose glucocorticoid use. There is little evidence for other immunosuppressant agents, but there are reports of successful treatment with monoclonal antibodies against IL-6.

Small/medium vessel vasculitis

Anti-neutrophil cytoplasmic antibodies (ANCA) were discovered in 1985 and have been a very useful clinical tool for the diagnosis of vasculitis. We now also know that these antibodies are pathogenic and activate neutrophils that cause tissue damage through the release of reactive oxygen species. Two staining patterns are described—cytoplasmic (c-ANCA) and perinuclear (p-ANCA). c-ANCA is most closely associated with granulomatosis with polyangiitis (formerly Wegner's granulomatosis) while p-ANCA is typically associated with eosinophillic granulomatosis with polyangiitis (formerly Churg–Strauss) and microscopic polyangiitis.

Proteinase 3 (PR3) and myeloperoxidase (MPO) are now known to be the targets for c-ANCA and p-ANCA, respectively, and can be measured using immunoassay techniques. ANCA immunofluorescence is now used as a screening tool in most laboratories and, if positive, immunoassay is used to confirm the presence of MPO or PR3. A positive immunofluorescence ANCA with negative MPO and PR3 is known as a 'non-specific ANCA' and is a common finding in other non-vasculitic autoimmune rheumatic conditions and chronic infection.

Granulomatosis with polyangiitis (GPA) (formerly Wegner's granulomatosis)

- This is a rare systemic necrotizing vasculitis, which can affect multiple systems.
- The classic triad involves the upper airways, lungs, and kidneys.
- The skin, joints, nerves, and eyes are also commonly affected.
- PR3 (c-ANCA) is found in 67–90% of cases. The diagnosis is otherwise made on histology. Raised systemic inflammatory markers are common.
- Treatment is with immunosuppressive agents:
  - Glucocorticoids and methotrexate for mild single organ disease.
  - Cyclophosphamide for severe cases.
  - Rituximab also increasingly used in severe cases (trials ongoing).
  - Plasma exchange in life-threatening cases.

Eosinophillic granulomatosis with polyangiitis (EGPA) (formerly Churg-Strauss)

- The key distinguishing feature is the presence of a peripheral eosinophilia, and a previous history of asthma or allergic rhinitis is found in most patients.
- Skin and nerve lesions are common. Renal involvement is less common than GPA. (50% vs. 90%). Gut involvement can also occur with colitis.
- Histology often shows a necrotizing arteritis with eosinophillic infiltration.
- MPO (p-ANCA) is present in 60–70%. Systemic inflammatory markers are often raised. The eosinophilia can be quite marked.
- Treatment is similar to GPA, but EGPA tends to be more sensitive to high dose glucocorticoids and has a better prognosis.

Microscopic polyangiitis (MPA)

- This condition predominantly affects the kidneys and is associated with an MPO (p-ANCA), but without eosinophilia.
- Pulmonary, joint, and skin involvement occurs in around half of patients.
- There is no granuloma formation on histology.
- Treatment is along the same lines as GPA.

Drugs used in the treatment of rheumatological conditions

For drugs used to treat Rheumatological conditions, see Table 9.6.

Table 9.6 Drugs used in the treatment of rheumatological conditions

Drugs used in the treatment of gout			
Drug: main indication(s)	**Mechanism of action**	**Side effects**	**Interactions**
Colchicine: used for acute attacks. Also licenced for familial Mediterranean fever	Inhibits mitosis by binding to tubulin	Diarrhoea, nausea, vomiting, and abdominal pain. Hepatic and renal impairment. Rarely myopathy	Increased colchicine toxicity with amiodarone, macrolides, anti-fungals, anti-virals, grapefruit juice
Allopurinol: long-term therapy to reduce uric acid levels	Xanthine oxidase inhibitor	Rash, can worsen renal impairment, GI disturbance. May trigger acute attacks, ∴ do not start during attack and administer prophylactic colchicine or NSAID for at least first month	Enhances effects and increases toxicity of azathioprine and mercaptopurine
Febuxostat: same indication as allopurinol	Xanthine oxidase inhibitor. Different binding site from allopurionol	GI disturbance, rash, abnormal LFTs. Caution if eGFR <30 mL/min. Contraindicated in ischaemic heart disease (IHD) and congestive cardiac failure (CCF). Prophylactic colchicine for first 6 months	Manufacturer advises similar caution with azathioprine and mercaptopurine
Uricosuric drugs: e.g. probenecid and sulfinpyrazone	Increase uric acid excretion in the urine	GI disturbance. Avoid if eGFR <30 mL/min. Contraindicated in acute porphyria	Reduces excretion of methotrexate, antibacterials, e.g. penicillins, cephlasporins, meropenem, and ciprofloxacin
Anti-inflammatories			
Class	**Role in rheumatic diseases**	**Side effects**	**Interactions**
Glucocorticoids: e.g. prednisolone oral or depo-medrone im	Used for short-term symptom control. Low-dose prednisolone used early in RA has been shown to slow progression of joint erosions	Weight gain, diabetes, osteoporosis, mood disturbance, hypertension (see Chapter 15, 'Endocrinology')	Liver enzyme inducer: reduces effect of liver metabolized drugs
Classical NSAIDs: e.g. diclofenac and naproxen	Symptomatic benefit, but do not alter disease progression	Reflux and GI bleed, renal toxicity. Hypertension, rash	Increase risk of GI bleed with anticoagulants and increased risk of renal impairment with any other drug capable of causing renal impairment
Nabumatone *COX II inhibitors:* e.g. eterocoxib		Like classical NSAIDs, but less GI toxicity	
Diseases modifying anti-rheumatic drugs (DMARDS)			
Drug: main indication(s)	**Mechanism of action**	**Side effects and monitoring**	**Interactions and special notes**
Hydroxychloroquine: add-on therapy in RA and used as single agent in SLE	Anti-malarial, possibly interferes with antigen processing and evidence of TLR7 and TLR9 inhibition	Retinopathy. *Patients advised to have annual eye checks*	Increased risk of arrhythmias with amiodarone and moxifloxacin *Relatively safe in pregnancy*
Methotrexate: RA, peripheral SpA, PsA, vasculitis, and connective tissue disease (CTD) maintenance	Anti-metabolite, interferes with folate synthesis	Liver toxicity, bone marrow toxicity, nausea, acute pneumonitis and/or fibrosis. *Monthly FBC and LFT*	Increased risk of bone marrow toxicity with trimethoprim & co-trimoxazole. *Discontinue at 3-6 months in men and women prior to conception*

Table 9.6 Drugs used in the treatment of rheumatological conditions (*continued*)

Drug: main indication(s)	Mechanism of action	Side effects and monitoring	Interactions and special notes
Sulfasalazine: RA, SpA, PsA	Anti-inflammatory and antimicrobial	Liver toxicity, bone marrow toxicity, GI symptoms, hypersensitivity reactions. *Monthly FBC and LFT initially, then 3-monthly after 6 months if stable*	Increased risk of leucopenia with azathioprine and mercaptopurine *Relatively safe in pregnancy*
Leflunomide: RA, SpA, PsA, maintenance in vasculitis	Anti-metabolite	Liver toxicity, bone marrow toxicity, hypertension, diarrhoea *Monthly FBC and LFT*	Very long half-life *Discontinue after 6 months in men and in women prior to conception*
Azathioprine: RA, vasculitis, and CTD maintenance	Purine-synthesis inhibitor	Liver toxicity, bone marrow toxicity, GI side effects. *Monthly FBC and LFT Check thiopurine methyltransferase (TPMT) enzyme activity prior to starting*	Allopurinol interaction (see also in this table). Increased toxicity risk if low TPMT activity. *Relatively safe in pregnancy*
Immunosupressants			
Drug: main indication(s)	Mechanism of action	Side effects and monitoring	Interactions and special notes
Cyclophosphamide: induction therapy in severe vasculitis and CTD	Alkylating agent	Myelotoxicity, renal toxicity, nausea, and vomiting. Susceptibility to opportunistic infections especially *Pneumocystis jorvecii.* Hair loss at high doses. *FBC and U&Es 10–12 days after IV infusion*	Liver enzyme inducers accelerate metabolism of cylophosphamide into active metabolites increasing toxicity. Liver enzyme inhibitors reduce therapeutic effects. *Increased risk of bladder malignancy and infertility*
Mycophenolate mofetil: induction therapy in moderate vasculitis and used for maintenance after cyclophosphamide	Purine-synthesis inhibitor	Liver toxicity, bone marrow toxicity. Diarrhoea and GI side effects. *Monthly FBC & LFT*	Nil significant
Biologics			
Target cytokine or molecule	Licence	Side effects	Pregnancy
Anti TNF-α monoclonal antibodies: infliximab, adalimumab, certolizumab, golimumab	RA, PsA, AS	Severe infections particularly in first 6 months. Re-activation of TB. Injection site reactions. Contraindicated if previous history of malignancy, but 10-year registry data has not demonstrated increased risk	Insufficient data in pregnancy and for men trying to conceive, therefore not recommended
TNF-α decoy receptor: etanercept	RA, PsA, AS		
Anti-CD20 B-cell surface marker monoclonal antibody: rituximab	RA	Severe infection, hypogammaglobulinaemia, reactivation of viral hepatitis	
CD80/86 co-stimulatory molecule decoy receptor: abatacept	RA	Severe infection	
Anti-IL-6 monoclonal antibody: tocilizumab	RA	Severe infection, neutropenia, elevated cholestrol	

Drug-induced rheumatic effects

Drugs causing hyperuricaemia

- Diuretics.
- Low-dose aspirin.
- Cyclosporin.
- Pyrazinamide.
- Ethambutol.
- L-dopa.
- Nicotininc acid.

Drug-induced lupus

Many drugs are known to trigger a drug-induced lupus illness (see following list). The development of positive lupus auto-antibodies, mainly ANA is common. At-risk patients tend to have a genetic deficiency of N-acetyltransferase (slow acetylators). In the majority of cases, the illness resolves on withdrawal of the offending drug. There is no contraindication to using these drugs in patients with classical SLE.

Medications most commonly associated with drug-induced lupus

- Hydralizine.
- Procainamide.
- Isoniazid.
- Minocycline.
- Sulfasalazine.
- Quinidine.
- Chlorpromazine.
- Methyldopa.

Drug-induced vasculitis

Several drugs can cause drug-induced vasculitis. Patients often develop a milder vasculitis limited to the skin, but organ involvement can also occur. Drug-induced vasculitis is often associated with the development of ANCA antibodies PR3 and MPO. After withdrawal of the offending drug, patients may need immunosuppressive therapy, depending on the severity, but treatment duration is short compared with idiopathic ANCA-associated vasculitis.

Medications most commonly associated with drug-induced vasculitis

- Prophythiouracil.
- Carbimazole.
- Anti-TNF agents (Infliximab, Etanercept, Adalimumab).
- Clozapine.
- Minocyline.
- Allopurinol.
- d-penicillamine.

Multiple choice questions

1. The following disorders are all associated with the development of pseudogout apart from:

A. Wilson's disease.
B. Haemochromatosis.
C. Primary hyperparathyroidism.
D. Diabetes insipidus.
E. X-linked hypophosphataemic rickets.

2. Which of the following diseases is most associated with gout?

A. Psoriasis.
B. Rheumatoid arthritis.
C. Cutaneous lupus.
D. Systemic lupus erythematosus.
E. Sjogren's syndrome.

3. Which of the following *HLA* genotypes are associated with the development of RA?

A. *HLA B27.*
B. *HLA B51.*
C. *HLA DR4.*
D. *HLA DR3.*
E. *HLA DQ6.*

4. Which statement best describes rheumatoid factor?

A. It is an IgG molecule directed against the Fc portion of human IgM.
B. It is an IgM molecule directed against the Fc portion of human IgG.
C. It is an IgM molecule directed against the Fc portion of human IgE.

D. It is an IgG molecule directed against the Fc portion of human IgE.
E. It is an IgA molecule directed against the Fc portion of human IgM.

5. Each of the following are known to be associated with the development of anti-nuclear antibodies except:

A. Silicon breast implants.
B. Smoking.
C. Increasing age.
D. Haemochromatosis.
E. Drug induced lupus.

6. Which of the following is a marker of poor prognosis in RA?

A. Male sex.
B. Acute onset.
C. Rheumatoid factor negative.
D. Smoking.
E. *HLA B27* inheritance.

7. What percentage of patients with reactive arthritis go on to develop recurrent episodes after 6 months of the initial onset?

A. 5%.
B. 10%.
C. 15%.
D. 20%.
E. 80%.

8. Which of the following is *not* included in the American College of Rheumatology classification criteria for systemic lupus erythematosus?

A. Malar rash.
B. Raynaud's.
C. Arthralgia.
D. Serositis.
E. Oral ulcers.

9. Which of the following conditions is most associated with a positive anti-proteinase 3 (PR3) ANCA?

A. Eosinophillic granulomatosis with polyangiitis (formerly Churg–Strauss).
B. Microscopic polyangiitis.
C. Granulomatosis with polyangiitis (formerly Wegner's granulomatosis).
D. Cryoglobulinaemia.
E. Anti-synthetase syndrome.

10. Which of the following antibiotics increases the risk of bone marrow toxicity if prescribed alongside methotrexate?

A. Rifampicin.
B. Gentamicin.
C. Chloramphenicol.
D. Linezolid.
E. Trimethoprim.

For answers, please see Appendix: Answers to multiple choice questions, page 313.

CHAPTER 10

Cardiology

Cardiac anatomy

The heart is a four-chambered, conical-shaped muscular pump in the mediastinum with its apex located in the 5th intercostal space in the mid-clavicular line in the healthy adult. The heart is fist-sized and lies obliquely within the thorax, such that its anterior surface is formed largely of the right ventricle and right atrium, while the left atrium and the left ventricle are orientated posteriorly. The right and left sides of the heart effectively operate as two pumps arranged in series, sending blood through the pulmonary and systemic circulations. Dilation of the left ventricle (such as in severe aortic or mitral regurgitation) results in displacement of the apex beat to the axilla, while hypertrophy of the left ventricle (such as in severe in aortic stenosis) results in a hyperdynamic, thrusting apex beat, which is not displaced. Dilation of the right ventricle (as occurs with pulmonary hypertension) results in lifting of the anterior chest wall at the left sternal edge during diastole, known as a right ventricular heave.

The heart is located within the pericardium—a double-layered sac that completely surrounds the heart apart from the points where the great vessels enter and leave. Pericardial sinuses are formed by the reflection of the pericardium around the heart. These sinuses are small, blind-ending spaces between the heart and the great vessels (oblique sinus), and around the aorta and pulmonary trunk posterior to the heart (transverse sinus). The external fibrous pericardium prevents excessive distension of the heart. It is lined on its internal face by a parietal layer of serous pericardium, which is continuous with the visceral layer of serous pericardium (epicardium) forming the pericardial cavity. This contains a thin layer of fluid permitting the heart to move within the pericardial sac. The fibrous pericardium is able to gradually stretch but a rapid increase in pericardial fluid, e.g. due to sudden bleeding, will cause ventricular compression and compromise pump function resulting in cardiac tamponade.

The wall of the heart is made up of three layers—the epicardium, the muscular myocardium, and endocardium. The orientation of the muscle fibres change between these layers, such that the contracting ventricle rotates in a corkscrew fashion between the apex and aortic outflow tract. Atria and ventricles are separated by the annulus fibrosum, such that electrical activity is usually only able to pass between the chambers via the atrioventricular (AV) node. This fibrous skeleton also supports the cardiac valves at the base of the cusps.

The systemic circulation drains into the right atrium via the superior and inferior venae cavae, while the hearts venous drainage enters the right atrium via the coronary sinus. The right atrium is separated from the left atrium by the inter-atrial septum within which can be found the fossa ovalis, a remnant of the foramen ovale, which permits shunting of blood between atria in the foetus. Right atrial contraction forces blood into the right ventricle through the tricuspid valve. Papillary muscles arising from the ventricular wall attach to the loose edges of the cusps of the valve via chordae tendinae, which maintain the direction of the cusps. Right ventricular contraction forces blood into the pulmonary trunk via the infundibulum. The inter-ventricular septum separates the right and left ventricles and bulges into the right ventricle because of higher pressures in the left ventricle. The pulmonary valve prevents regurgitation of blood from the pulmonary circulation into the right ventricle. This comprises three semilunar cusps.

Blood returns from the pulmonary circulation to the left atrium via four pulmonary veins (two inferior and two superior). The mitral valve of the left atria comprises only two cusps (anterior and posterior) and is also anchored with the help of papillary muscles. The wall of the left ventricle is approximately twice as thick as the right ventricle. It pumps blood into the aorta via the left ventricular outflow tract. The aortic valve comprises of a left, right, and non-coronary cusp. Aortic sinuses are formed behind the cusp from which the left coronary artery arises from the posterior sinus and the right coronary artery from the anterior sinus.

The coronary circulation

The coronary arteries must meet the high metabolic requirements of the constantly contracting myocardium, and be able to match the increase in demand during stress and exercise. As ventricular wall contraction effectively arrests flow in the coronary circulation, the majority of coronary

Table 10.1 The innervation of the heart

Type	Nerve	Innervated site	Function
Parasympathetic (efferent)	Vagus nerve	SA node. AV node. Coronary arteries	Decreases heart rate. Dilation of coronary arteries. A small reduction in contractility
Sympathetic (efferent)	Cervical and upper thoracic spinal nerves via sympathetic ganglia	SA node. AV node. Cardiac muscle fibres. Coronary arteries	Increases heart rate. Increases force of contraction. Constriction of larger coronary arteries
Sensory (afferent)	Follows sympathetic ganglia via white rami communicantes and spinal nerves	Myocardium	Pain from myocardium ischaemic

blood flow occurs during diastole. The myocardium contains a high capillary density to reduce the diffusion distance of metabolites, as well as a high myoglobin content such that total oxygen extraction from the coronary circulation is high. As the coronary arteries are functional end arteries with little collateralization between them, flow limitation secondary to atherosclerosis, or obstruction when a plaque ruptures and thrombus forms can lead to stable angina and myocardial infarction, respectively.

The right coronary artery passes from the anterior aortic sinus in the atrioventricular groove to the inferior border of the heart. Seventy per cent of people have a right dominant circulation, where the posterior descending artery arises from the right coronary artery and runs in the inferior inter-ventricular groove, whereas in 10%, this branch arise from the left circumflex artery (left dominant system). It is possible for both the right coronary artery and left circumflex to both supply the posterior descending artery in a co-dominant system (20% of people). A branch of the right coronary artery supplies the AV node in 90% of people.

The left main stem passes from the posterior aortic sinus and divides to give the left anterior descending artery and left circumflex artery. The left anterior descending supplies the septum (via septal branches), apex, and anterior wall (via diagonal branches) of the left ventricle. The left circumflex supplies the lateral wall (via oblique marginal branches) and the inferior wall is supplied by either the left circumflex or right coronary artery depending on which artery is dominant.

The epicardial venous drainage of the heart empties into the coronary sinus, which runs in the posterior atrioventricular groove and receives blood from the great cardiac vein (anteriorly), posterior lateral cardiac veins, and the middle cardiac vein (from the inferior inter-ventricular groove). Posterior lateral cardiac veins and branches of the middle cardiac vein are common sites for left ventricular lead placement of cardiac resynchronization devices. The smaller cardiac venous system is the Thebesian venous network. This system is responsible for draining the subendocardium particularly of the right ventricular and portions of the inter-ventricular septum directly into the right ventricle itself via small orifices <0.5 mm in diameter.

Innervation of the heart

The heart receives innervation from parasympathetic, sympathetic, and sensory fibres, which together form superficial and deep cardiac plexi below the aortic arch (Table 10.1).

Sensory fibres run in close proximity to cervical and thoracic spinal nerves, and explains the phenomenon of referred cardiac pain to the chest arms and neck during myocardial ischaemia.

Cardiac physiology

Electrical excitation and conduction

Action potentials are generated intrinsically within the heart at the primary pacemaker, the sino-atrial node, modulated by the autonomic nervous system. The sino-atrial node lies on the posterior wall of the right atrium between the crista terminalis and the superior vena cava. Other tissue (such as the atrioventricular node and purkinje network) are able to act as secondary pacemakers in the heart as they display a slower intrinsic rate of depolarization. However, they become important during complete heart block when they produce a slow, but often insufficient rate of ventricular contraction. The maximum diastolic membrane potential of a sinoatrial node cell is –55 to –60mV and a combination of voltage-gated ion channels carrying sodium and calcium ions (such as I_f, the 'funny' current, a t-type calcium current and a background sodium leak) known as the voltage clock, and stimulation of sodium–calcium exchange and other voltage gated ion channels by release of calcium from intracellular stores, known as the calcium clock, then depolarizes the cell until an action potential is fired at about –40 mV. The upstroke of the action potential in an SA node cell is a result of the influx of Ca^{2+} ions through voltage-gated L-type Ca^{2+} channels and repolarization via delayed rectified K^+ channels.

Usually the atrioventricular node is the only way by which electrical excitation can spread from atria to ventricles. From here, the bundle of His transmits depolarization along the inter-ventricular septum. The bundle of His divides into the left and right bundle branches, which pass down the inter-ventricular septum and transmit impulses initially to the endocardial regions of the left and right ventricles, respectively. The left bundle divides into an anterior and posterior fascicle, and these together with the right bundle branch transmit impulses to Purkinje fibres, which rapidly conduct the wave excitation across the endocardium. Excitation then spreads from endo- to epicardium via gap junctions between ventricular myocytes (see Fig. 10.1).

The function of the pacemaker and conducting system of the heart can be modulated by autonomic nervous system activity. Sympathetic nerve activity to the sino-atrial increases the magnitude of the funny current, thereby decreasing the time taken for depolarization to occur and increasing heart rate (positive chronotropic effect). This is mediated by catecholamines binding to β_1-receptors, leading to an increase in intracellular cAMP, which increases I_f. Similarly, sympathetic activity decreases the time taken for conduction through the AV node. Parasympathetic (vagal) nervous activity slows heart rate (bradycardia) by slowing the rate of depolarization of the pacemaker potential in SA node cells. Furthermore, pacemaker cells are hyperpolarized increasing the time required to reach threshold for an action potential. Both of these effects are the result of acetylcholine binding to muscarinic (M_2) receptors. Reduced pacemaker potential is the result of reduced intracellular cAMP concentration, and hyperpolarization is the result of activation of K^+-channels (I_{KACh}).

Cardiac action potentials

The key events in cardiac action potentials (see Fig. 10.2):

- *Phase 0:* at threshold, voltage-dependent Na^+ channels open, leading to rapid depolarization in ventricular and atrial myocytes.
- *Phase 1:* Na^+ channels only remain open for a few milliseconds, and quickly in-activate when the cell is depolarized, leading to a partial re-polarization (absent in sinoatrial node cells).
- *Phase 2:* voltage-gated L-type Ca^{2+} channels are then activated, allowing an influx of Ca^{2+}, which maintains depolarization (the main depolarizing current in the sinoatrial node). In atrial and ventricular myocytes, the plateau phase of the action potential is maintained by closing of inward rectifier potassium channels and an inward current from the electrogenic $3Na^+/Ca^{2+}$ exchanger. Depolarization of atrial cells is of shorter duration (200 msec) than that of Purkinje fibres and ventricular myocytes, where a longer plateau phase occurs and action potentials last for 300–400 msec.
- *Phase 3:* delayed outwardly rectifying K^+ channels (as well as other potassium channels) open to allow an efflux of K^+, ultimately repolarizing the cell.
- *Phase 4:* no sooner have pacemaker cells repolarized than they start to depolarize again on account of the pacemaker potential pacemaker cells tend to have a less polar 'resting' membrane potential than ventricular myocytes (–60 mV, as opposed to ~–80 mV for most cells) because of their inherent leakiness to Na^+.

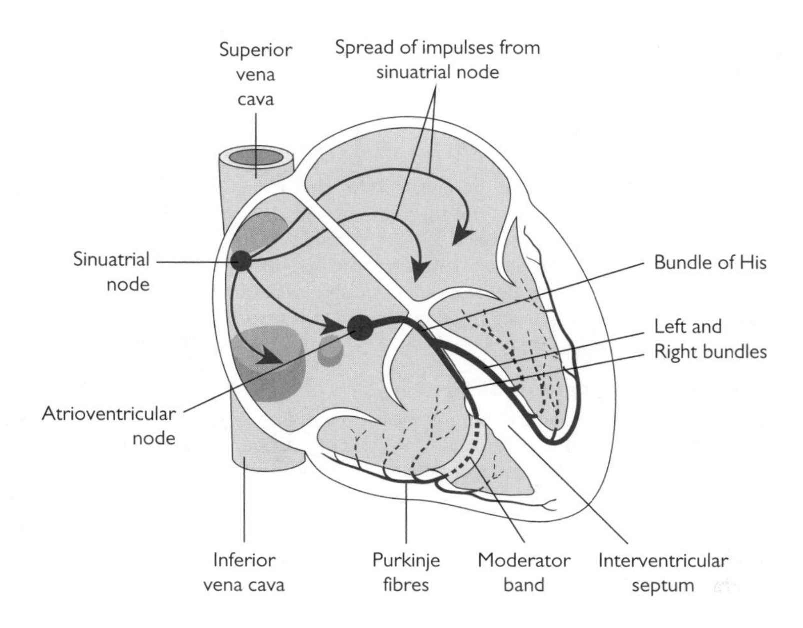

Fig. 10.1 The conducting system of the heart. The fibrous skeleton of the heart separates the muscle of the atria from that of the ventricles, which are connected only by the bundles of His.

Reproduced from P MacKinnon and J Morris, *Oxford Textbook of Functional Anatomy: Volume 2 Thorax and Abdomen*, 2005, Figure 5.4.15, p. 77, by permission of Oxford University Press

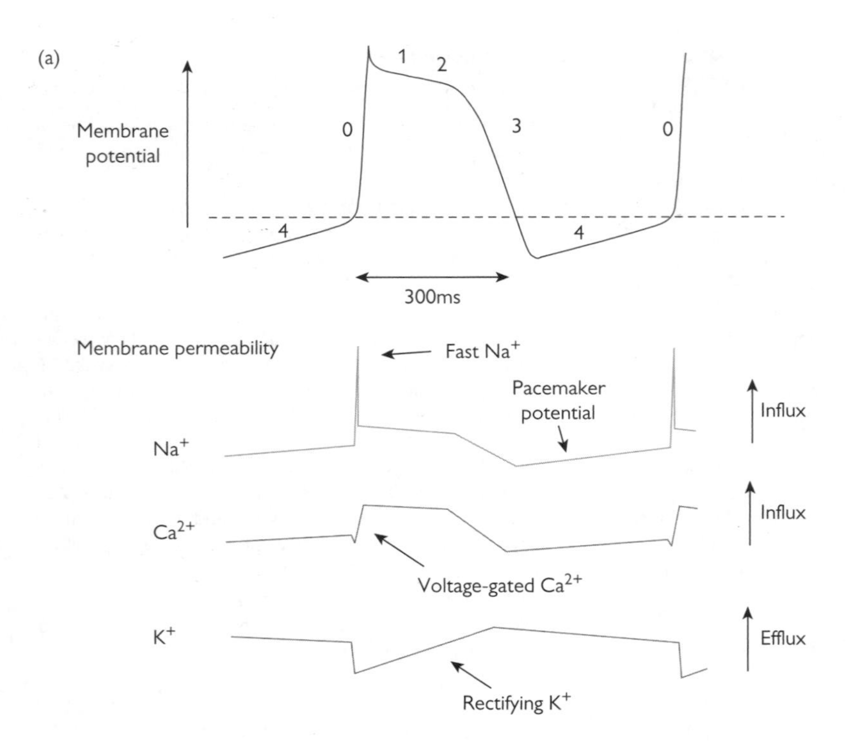

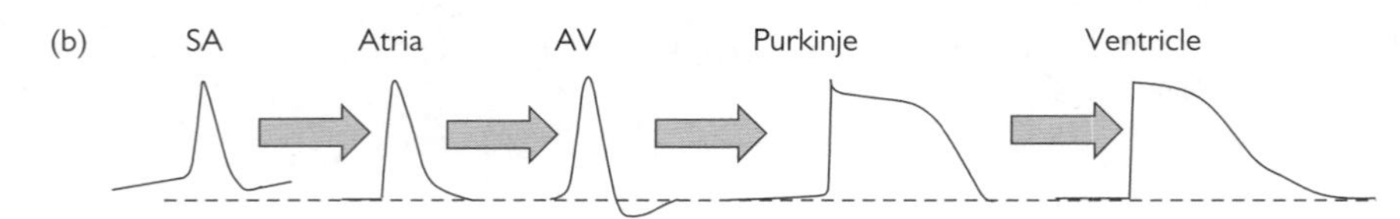

Fig. 10.2 (a) Cardiac action potential and membrane permeability; (b) change in action potential response profile across cardiac tissue–longer depolarizations correspond to protracted Ca2+ channel opening.

Refractory period

Following the cardiac action potential, a further action potential cannot be initiated until the Na^+ channels have recovered from inactivation during depolarization. This ensures that the action potential is propagated in one direction only within healthy tissue, and cannot double-back on itself to create a self-sustaining re-entrant circuit into tissue that has recently depolarized.

The electrocardiogram (ECG)

The ECG is a recording of the electrical events associated with myocardial depolarization and repolarization, measured as changes in potential difference at the body surface. Certain features are common in healthy subjects (see Fig. 10.3A):

- *The P wave* is the first event of the cardiac cycle and arises from depolarization of the atria and lasts around 0.08 sec.
- *The PR interval* is the period from the start of the P wave to the first negative deflection of the QRS complex (it should more logically be known as the PQ interval). A large proportion of the PR interval is flat (after the P wave) and this represents the time taken for conduction through the AV node—the heart is essentially isoelectric during this period. The PR interval lasts 0.12–0.2 sec.
- *The QRS complex* is a record of ventricular depolarization and, as such, is analogous to the P wave reflecting depolarization of the atria. It lasts for only a short time, less than 0.12 sec.
- *The ST segment* corresponds to the plateau phase of the ventricular action potential and, like the major part of the PR interval, represents the heart in an isoelectric state.
- *The T wave* is a record of ventricular repolarization. As the action potential duration is shorter in the epicardium than the endocardium, repolarization occurs in the opposite

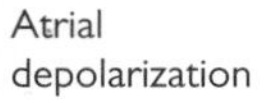

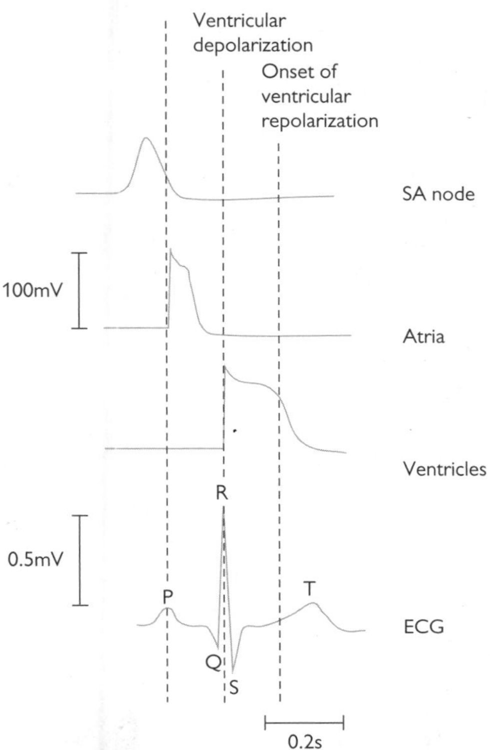

Fig. 10.3A The relationship between the onset and duration of the action potentials of cardiac cells during a single cardiac cycle and the ECG trace.

direction to that of depolarization. The T wave is, therefore, normally in the same orientation as the QRS complex.

- *The QT interval* or time between ventricular depolarization and repolarization is an indication of the average ventricular action potential duration. This varies with heart rate as sympathetic stimulation shortens the ventricular action potential (positive lusiotropic effect) by increasing voltage gated delayed rectifier potassium currents. QT interval is therefore corrected to the RR interval using Bazett's formula:

$$QTc = QT/\sqrt{RR} \text{ interval } (sec)$$

where *QTc* is usually 0.35–0.45 sec.

The orientation of the waves of the ECG varies according to the position of the lead used to record it. The ECG was first recorded using three electrodes—one on each arm and one on the left leg. Together, these three points make up *Einthoven's triangle*. An ECG trace is generated by resolving the electrical vector arising from the movement of charge within the myocardium onto one of the three leads connecting the above three electrodes. Each of the three leads is in a different orientation and emphasize different features of the ECG:

- *Lead I:* right arm (–) to left arm (+) – horizontal.
- *Lead II:* right arm (–) to left leg (+) – 60° below horizontal.
- *Lead III*—left arm (–) to left leg (+) – 120° below horizontal.

The standard leads are, therefore, designed such that a positive deflection results movement of positive charge points towards left the arm (Lead I) or the left leg (Lead II or III). The 12-lead ECG also combines the augmented limb leads (aVR, aVL, aVF) and the unipolar chest leads (V1–6). This way changes in the pattern of the ECG in specific leads can help localize pathology to a particular area of the heart. For example, ST elevation due to right coronary artery occlusion can often be seen in the inferior leads (II, III, aVF), left circumflex occlusion in the lateral leads (V5, 6, I, and aVL) and left anterior descending occlusion in the anteroseptal leads (V1–4). Occlusion of the left main stem can produce ST elevation in aVR in addition to wide spread changes (ST elevation or depression with T wave inversion) throughout the precordial leads (See Fig. 10.3B).

Normal cardiac rhythm and arrythmias

The spread of controlled spread of electrical excitation throughout the myocardium allows for co-ordinated mechanical activity of the pumping chambers and is designed to only allow electrical waves to travel in one direction, and to prevent their arriving too close together, making for inefficient contraction of cardiac muscle. Abnormalities in cardiac rhythm can arise from a number of mechanisms.

Conduction block

Infarction, inflammation or fibrosis of the AV node can prevent the conduction of P waves through to the bundle branches (Box 10.1).

Slowing of conduction can also occur lower down the conduction network to produce trifasicular block, right bundle branch block, left bundle branch block (where the QRS duration is greater than 0.12 sec), left anterior fasicular block or left posterior fasicular block. Tri-fasicular block,

BOX 10.1 DEGREES OF AV NODAL BLOCK

- First degree (prolongation of the PR interval beyond 0.2 sec).
- Second degree, mobitz type 1 (or Wenkebach), where the PR interval gradual prolongs until a P wave is not conducted through to the ventricles.
- Second degree, mobitz type II, where there are 2 or more P waves for every QRS (2:1 or 3:1 block or higher).
- Complete heart block where there is no relationship between P waves and the QRS, which may be narrow if pacemaker activity is junctional or broad if it arise from the bundle branches themselves.

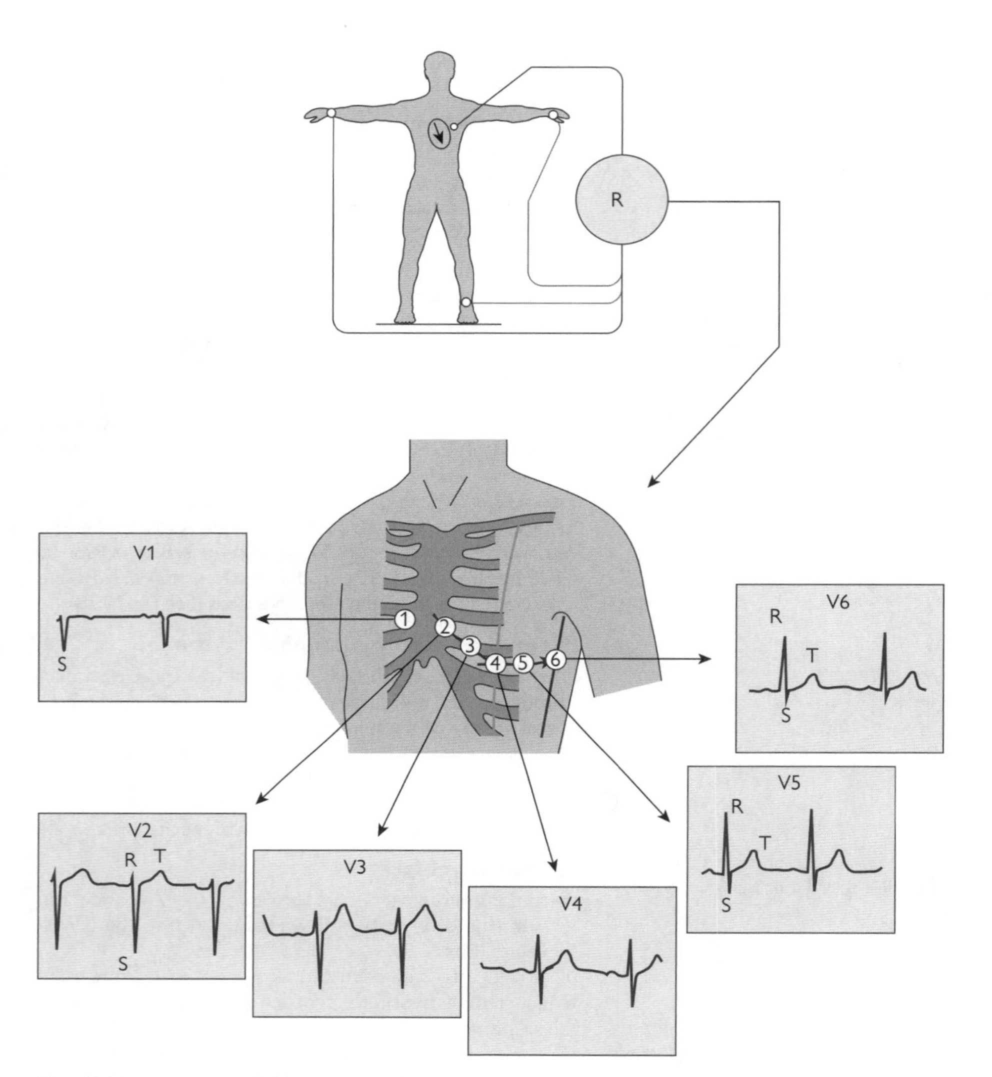

Fig. 10.3B Unipolar recording of the ECG with the standard chest leads. The limb leads are connected together to provide a virtual earth as shown in the inset figure at the top. The exploring electrode is then placed in one of six positions on the chest (leads V1 to V6) as shown. Recordings from leads V1 and V2 usually show a pronounced S wave, while leads V5 and V6 show a large R wave. Lead V1 is placed at the right margin of the sternum in the fourth intercostal space. Lead V2 is placed at the left margin of the sternum in the fourth intercostal space. Lead V3 is placed midway between leads V2 and V4. Lead V4 is placed on the mid-clavicular line (shown here in light purple) in the fifth intercostal space. Lead V5 is placed at the same level as lead 4 in the anterior axillary line. Lead V6 is also placed at the same level as lead 4 but in the mid-axillary line (shown here in dark purple).

second degree, mobitz type II, and complete heart block are often associated with inadequate heart rates or ventricular pauses, which can cause syncopy, heart failure, and even asystolic arrest, which can be prevented by implantation of a permanent pacemaker.

Re-entry

The refractory nature of cardiac muscle immediately after depolarization normally ensures that the impulse wave only travels in one direction. Re-entry applies to a circuit of cardiac tissue, which can be either anatomically or functionally distinct from the surrounding tissue. If conduction velocity around part of the circuit is slow enough or refractory period short enough then the wave of excitation can re-enter the same circuit and cycle continuously (see Fig. 10.4). Examples include:

- *Atrioventricular re-entrant tachycardia* (AVRT or Wolff–Parkinson–White syndrome) where an accessory pathway other than the AV node exists between the atria and ventricles such that a wave of excitation can conduct through the AV node and back-up the accessory pathway (anterograde conduction), or down the accessory pathway and back up the AV node (retrograde conduction) in a circuit. The accessory pathway can often be treated by percutaneous catheter ablation.
- *Atrioventricular nodal re-entrant tachycardia* (AVNRT), where the AV node is able to conduct via a slow pathway, as well as its usual fast pathway and is in itself able to sustain re-entry. This can be treated with vagal manoeuvres (such as the valsalva manoeuvre, i.e. exhaling against a closed glottis or carotid sinus massage), AV node slowing drugs or slow pathway modification of the AV node by catheter ablation in refractory cases.
- *Typical atrial flutter* occurs due to a re-entrant circuit around the right atrium via the cavotricuspid isthmus, lateral wall, roof, and septum. It can be rate controlled with AV node slowing drugs, pharmacologically- or electrically-cardioverted, or treated by catheter ablation to produce conduction block along the cavotricuspid isthmus. Sustained atrial flutter carries the same risk as atrial fibrillation of left atrial appendage thrombus formation due to blood stasis and, therefore, thromboembolic stroke.
- *Atrial fibrillation* often occurs as multiple re-entrant circuits around the four pulmonary veins of the left atria, although the pulmonary veins also have a role in initiating and sustaining AF via generating abnormal automaticity. Like atrial flutter it can be rate controlled with AV node slowing drugs, pharmacologically-, or electrically-cardioverted, or treated by left atrial catheter ablation.
- *Ventricular tachycardia* can arise from an anatomical inexcitable gap/area of slow conduction within the ventricles, such as the scar of an old myocardial infarction, areas of fibrosis (arrhythmogenic right ventricular cardiomyopathy), or myocardial disarray (with hypertriophic cardiomyopathy). Regions of slowed conduction velocity and short refractory period can also be generated by ischaemia or inherited channelopathies (such as Long QT and Brugada's syndrome). VT is treated using pharmacological or electrical cardioversion, over-drive pacing of the ventricle (either via a temporary pacing wire or an implantable cardiac defibrillator) or in refractory cases by catheter ablation.

Normal tissue — Functionally or anatomically distinct 'ring' of tissue

- Free transmission in both directions around the ring from the point of stimulation—circus movement not possible
- Depolarization wave transmitted to downstream cardiac tissue

Damaged tissue

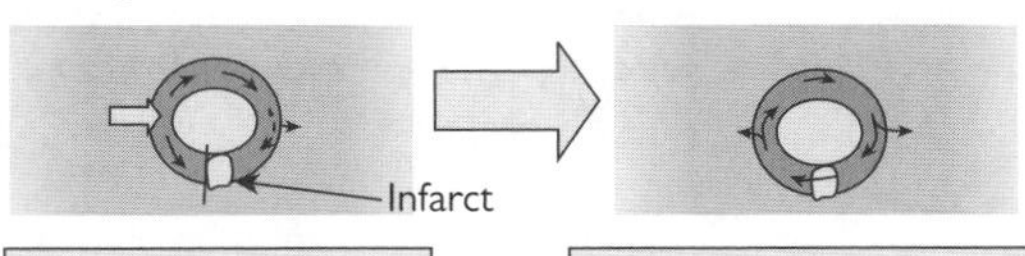

Infarcted tissue blocks anterograde transmission

Retrograde transmission via infarcted area generates circus movement and retrograde transmission

Fig. 10.4 Circus movement caused by re-entry in cardiac tissue.

Reproduced from R Wilkins et al., *Oxford Handbook of Medical Sciences, Second Edition*, 2011, Figure 6.29, p. 429, by permission of Oxford University Press.

Abnormal automaticity

Heart rate is normally determined by the pacemaker cells of the sinoatrial node. However, in atrial tachycardia another area within the atria can generate rhythmic firing of action potentials at a faster rate. Atrial tachycardia can be pharmacologically- or electrically-cardioverted, rate controlled with AV node slowing drugs or directly catheter ablated.

Atrial fibrillation is also often initiated and also sustained by ectopic activity within the pulmonary veins that produce multiple waves of excitation often centred around the pulmonary veins themselves. This leads to chaotic asynchronous contractile activity of the atria. Atrial stasis can lead to diastolic heart failure and also the development of a thrombus in the left atrial appendage (and the risk of a thromboembolic stroke). The recurrent bombardment of the AV node also leads to fast irregular contraction of the ventricles, which can lead to palpitations, chest pain, and breathlessness. For these reasons, AF is treated with thromboprophylactic drugs, such as aspirin or warfarin (or, more recently, percutaneous left atrial appendage occlusion devices). AF can be pharmacologically- or electrically-cardioverted or rate controlled with drugs aimed at slowing AV node conduction. Cardioversion to sinus rhythm can also be achieved in symptomatic patients refractory to treatment with catheter ablation treatment centred around the pulmonary veins and left atria.

Cardiac physiology

The cardiac cycle

The synchronized contraction of the heart's chambers in response to the propagation of electrical activity together with the appropriate opening and closing of the heart's valves, allows the organ to function as an efficient mechanical pump. The Wiggers diagram represents the phases of the cardiac cycle and correlates the pressure and volume changes in the main chambers with the heart sounds and the ECG (Fig. 10.5).

- *In early diastole*, the atria and ventricles are relaxed, and the pressure in the heart chambers is low. Blood from the large systemic veins (superior and inferior vena cava), and that returning from the lungs (pulmonary veins) flows into the right and left atria respectively. The atrioventricular (AV) valves are open at this stage of the cycle, so the majority of blood passes passively from the atria to the ventricles, which can sometimes be heard as a quiet third heart sound.
- *In late diastole*, depolarization from the sinoatrial node causes atrial depolarization and the P wave of the ECG. Atrial contraction provides little ventricular filling in the healthy heart at rest, but becomes more important during exercise when diastole shortens. Arial contraction also becomes important when the left ventricle becomes hypertrophied, and does not relax and passively fill as

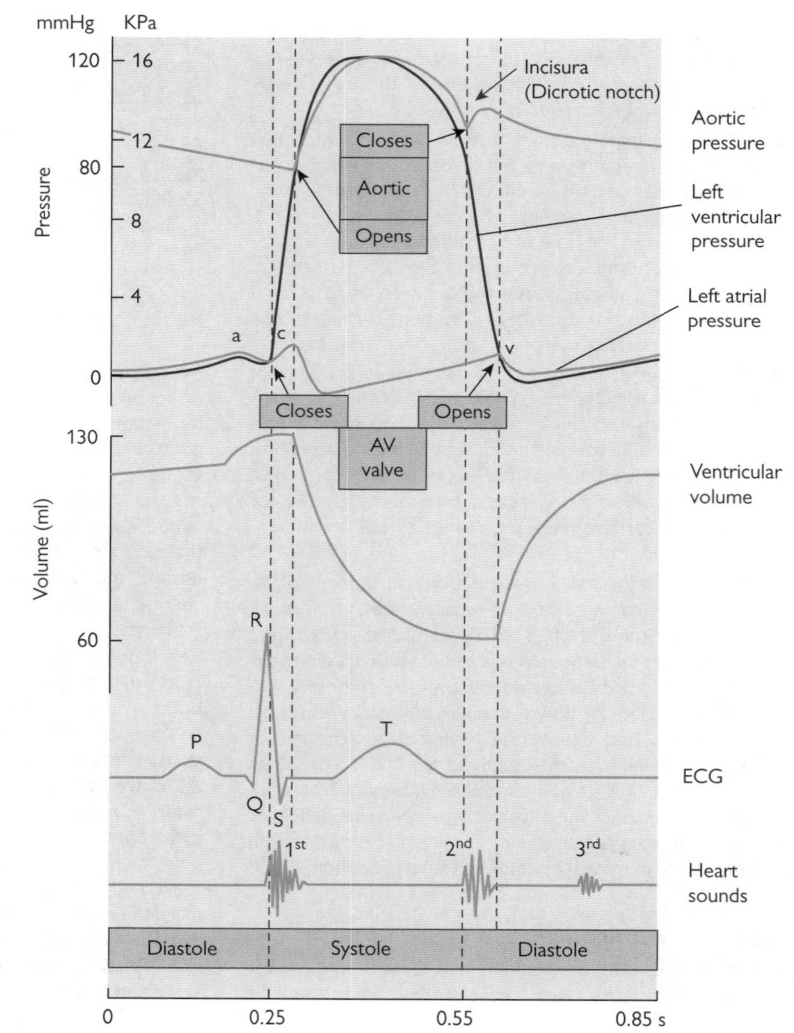

Fig. 10.5 The major mechanical and electrical events of the cardiac cycle. The pressure changes shown are for the left side of the heart and reflect the underlying mechanical events. The heart sounds are also shown. It is particularly important to note the relative timing of the various events. For example, the QRS complex (which reflects ventricular depolarization) largely precedes ventricular contraction, while the first heart sound is heard as the AV valves close following the start of the rise in intraventricular pressure. See text for further explanation.

Reproduced from G Pocock and CD Richards, *Human Physiology: The Basis of Medicine, Third Edition*, 2006, Figure 15.14, p. 274, by permission of Oxford University Press

efficiently. In such conditions, a quiet fourth heart sounds can sometimes be heard associated with atrial contraction and passing of blood into the ventricles. The volume of the ventricles increases as they fill (to a maximum of about 130 mL under resting conditions). Atrial contraction is represented by the A wave seen in the jugular venous pulse as there are no valves between the right atria and superior vena cava.

- Shortly after the QRS and ventricular depolarization, contraction of the ventricles causes the pressure to rise and the AV valves snap shut causing the first heart sound. This is reflected in a small C wave in the jugular venous pulse before the *x* descent. There is then a brief period of isovolumetric contraction as ventricular pressure continues to rise eventually exceeding that in the aorta/pulmonary artery (80/15 mmHg, respectively), at which point the artic and pulmonary valves open at the start of the ejection phase (0.3 sec). During the ejection phase, the atria fill which is seen as the V wave of the jugular venous pulse. After ventricular contraction reaches a peak (120 mmHg systemic, 30 mmHg pulmonary) and left ventricular pressure falls below aortic pressure, the aortic (and pulmonary) valves close causing the loud second heart sound. Bulging of the aortic valve and the rocking motion of the relaxing ventricle at this point can sometimes cause a dicrotic notch in the aortic pressure trace. This is followed by a brief phase of isovolumetric ventricular relaxation as the pressure eventually falls below that of atrial pressure and the atrioventricular valves open again to start ventricular filling. Pressure in the aorta (and pulmonary artery) falls more slowly as recoil of the elastic arterial wall adds kinetic energy to the passage of blood.

Each stroke of a healthy adult human heart under resting conditions ejects around 70 mL into the systemic circulation via the aorta. This volume is known as the 'stroke volume'. The heart rate under the same conditions is usually around 70 beats/min. Knowing these two parameters, we are able to calculate the amount of blood that is pumped out of the heart every minute (the cardiac output):

$$\text{Stroke volume} \times \text{heart rate} = \text{Cardiac output}$$
$$70\ \text{mL} \times 70\ \text{beats/min} = 4.9\ \text{L/min}$$

Preload and the Frank–Starling mechanism

The force generated by contraction of cardiac myocytes is dependent on their resting length – just as it is for skeletal muscle fibres. The 'length–tension' relationship for skeletal muscle, therefore, bears some similarity to the relationship between the end diastolic volume when the ventricle is fully relaxed and the stroke volume of cardiac muscle. As end diastolic volume increases and the ventricular muscle is stretched, the muscle responds up to a point, by increasing its contractile force and stroke volume. Beyond a certain level of filling, dilation of the muscle, leaking valves, and the law of Laplace (inefficient conversion of circumferential tension into radial pressure in large spheres) means stroke volume eventually falls. Under normal physiological conditions, the heart is on the ascending limb of the Frank–Starling graph as seen in Fig. 10.6. This way it can respond to an increase in venous filling pressure, or preload, by passing on the volume of blood to the arterial side of the circulation, thereby matching right- and left-sided cardiac output and preventing congestion. Sympathetic nervous stimulation shifts the Frank–Starling relationship to produce greater contractility at a given end diastolic volume and also changes the shape of the curve itself.

The cellular mechanisms behind the Frank–Starling relationship are still an area of research, but seem to involve an increase in the sensitivity of the myofilaments and troponin C to calcium as the sarcomere is stretched.

Valvular disease

Effective valves in the heart are essential for optimal pumping because they allow efficient passage of blood between chambers, but prevent backflow. There are a number of potential causes of narrowing or leaking of heart valves:

- *Stenosis:*
  - Excessive calcification.
  - Congenital malformation (e.g. bicuspid aortic valve).
  - Rheumatic fever (autoimmune damage to valve tissue).
- *Regurgitation:*
  - Poorly supported valves (due to papillary muscle of chordae tendonae dysfunction).

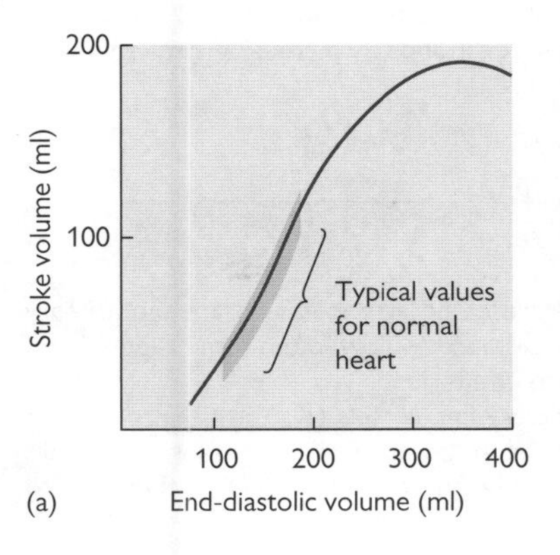

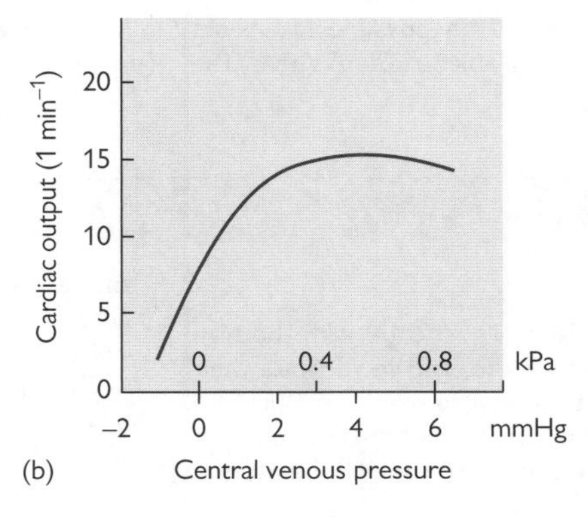

Fig. 10.6 (a)The relationship between end-diastolic volume and stroke volume determined using an isolated heart–lung preparation. (b) The relationship between cardiac output and central venous pressure in the intact heart.

Table 10.2 Murmurs arising from valvular and structural cardiac defects

Valvular lesion	Murmur	Radiation	Signs of severity
Aortic stenosis	Ejection systolic	Aortic area (second intercostal space, left sternal edge) to the carotids	Loss of second heart sound, thrusting apex beat, slow rising pulse, narrow pulse pressure
Aortic regurgitation	Early diastolic	Lower left sternal edge	Short murmur, displaced apex, collapsing pulse, wide pulse pressure
Mitral stenosis	Late systolic with opening snap	Axilla	Atrial fibrillation, tapping apex, malar flush, pulmonary hypertension (right ventricular heave, palpable P2, tricuspid regurgitation, giant V waves in JVP, pulsatile liver, peripheral oedema)
Mitral regurgitation	Pansystolic	Axilla	Displaced apex, pulmonary hypertension (right ventricular heave, palpable P2, tricuspid regurgitation, giant V waves in JVP, pulsatile liver, peripheral oedema)
Pulmonary stenosis	Ejection systolic	Left sternal edge, second intercostal space	Right ventricular heave, palpable P2, tricuspid regurgitation, giant V waves in JVP, pulsatile liver, peripheral oedema
Pulmonary regurgitation	Early diastolic	Lower left sternal edge	Often associated with pulmonary hypertension
Tricupsid regurgitaion	Pansystolic	Lower left sternal edge	Often associated with pulmonary hypertension
Atrial septal defect	Pulmonary flow murmur, fixed splitting of second heart sound with respiration	Left sternal edge	Associated right heart failure
Ventricular septal defect	Pansystolic murmur is large	Left sternal edge	More quiet with increasing severity. Associated right heart failure

- Damaged valve leaflets (due to endocarditis, rheumatic fever or connective tissue disease).
- Annular dilation.

The physiological impact of heart valve disease is a loss of effective pumping in the heart resulting in signs and symptoms of reduced cardiac output, such as breathlessness, angina, and syncopy, particularly on exertion.

Murmurs

The movement of blood past defective heart valves can cause murmurs, in addition to the physiological heart sounds on auscultation (see Table 10.2). Where the murmur occurs in the cardiac cycle, its duration, where the sound radiates, too, and its effects on the aortic pressure wave and apex beat all give clue to the which heart valve is involved and the severity of the defect. As a rule murmurs associated with right-sided valvular lesion become louder on inspiration as negative intrathoracic pressure encourages venous return to the heart and flow of blood through the right heart. Murmurs associated with left-sided valvular lesions become louder on expiration as intrathoracic pressure increases and an increase in afterload transiently reduces cardiac output before the Frank–Starling mechanism responds by increasing stroke volume as preload increases.

Vascular physiology

Vascular anatomy

Arteries have thick, muscular walls to cope with the high pressures that they are exposed to, and to facilitate their constriction and dilatation to modulate blood pressure and flow distribution. Arteries becomes progressively smaller, but more numerous with distance from the heart; the smallest arteries are called arterioles and are the primary determinant of resistance to flow, often termed peripheral vascular resistance or afterload.

Capillaries are very fine vessels (<50 μm) that distribute blood from the arterioles throughout tissues. The walls of capillaries are only one endothelial cell in thickness to facilitate easy diffusion of O_2 and glucose necessary for cellular respiration down the concentration gradient from the incoming blood, in to the tissues. Waste metabolites (CO_2, urea) diffuse in the opposite direction. An exception to this basic rule applies in the lungs (pulmonary circulation), where capillaries come into close contact with alveolar air to facilitate gaseous exchange, with the loss of CO_2 to the atmosphere and the uptake of O_2 into the red blood cells, where it is transported bound to haemoglobin.

Venules and veins carry blood away from tissues and back to the heart. They have some vascular smooth muscle, but not as much as arteries. As a result, they can contract and relax, but the changes in diameter are far less dramatic than in arteries. Blood leaving the capillaries enters venules, which often run side-by-side with the feed arteriole. In this way, metabolites produced by the tissue being supplied can affect the feed arteriole smooth muscle by counter-current exchange. Venules progressively converge, pooling blood into increasingly large vessels. There is little pressure difference across the venous circulation, meaning that unaided flow of blood would be very slow. As a result, veins contain valves to prevent retrograde flow (backflow) and the venous return of blood to the heart runs superficial to deep and is aided by contraction of the surrounding skeletal muscles. This is particularly important in humans, where our upright stance means that the effects of gravity have to be overcome to ensure the return of blood to the heart from our feet. The amount of blood returning to the atria of the heart determines preload.

Modulators of vascular tone

An important feature of our blood vessels is that they contract and dilate in response to numerous signalling molecules in the body. The cellular mechanisms by which these effects occur are illustrated in Fig. 10.7.

Systemic vasoconstriction

The primary stimulus for vascular smooth muscle contraction is activation of the sympathetic nervous system that innervates blood vessels. Increased sympathetic drive results in release of noradrenaline (NA) from sympathetic nerve terminals, which activates α_1 and β_2-adrenoceptors on the smooth muscle cells. Most arteries and arterioles (although not those in the coronary circulation) have α_1-receptors and contract in response to NA; α_2-adrenoceptors are also found in these arteries, but they are probably stimulated by circulating adrenaline rather than by sympathetic nerve derived NA. Arteries that supply skeletal muscle and some veins have a predominance of β_2-adrenoceptors, which causes them to dilate in response to NA and circulating adrenaline. The net effect of increased sympathetic nervous system activity is to redistribute blood flow away from the internal organs to the skeletal muscles to prepare for 'fight or flight'.

ATP and neuropeptide Y are co-transmitters that are often released with NA to cause rapid or long lasting vasoconstrictor effects respectively. Stimulation of β-receptors in the kidney also increases the amount of renin available to catalyse the first step in the renin-angiotensin-aldosterone system. One of the products of this system is angiotensin II, which is a powerful vasoconstrictor through stimulation of angiotensin (AT) receptors on the smooth muscle (primarily AT_1 receptors).

Local vasoconstrictors

The endothelins (ET_1, ET_2, ET_3, of which ET_1 is the most abundant) are endothelium-derived vasoconstrictor peptides, acting through ET_A and ET_B receptors on the smooth muscle. However, the action of ET_1 is modulated through stimulation of ET_B receptors on the endothelium, which leads to the release of an endothelium-derived vasodilator, nitric oxide (NO).

Thromboxane A_2 (TXA_2) is a prostanoid synthesized in platelets in response to vascular injury. As well as stimulating platelet activation, TXA_2 is a powerful local vasoconstrictor, which helps to reduce blood loss after injury.

Local vasodilators

Adenosine is primarily produced as a by-product of ATP breakdown, and can either be seen as a local or systemic vasodilator through stimulation of A_2 receptors on the smooth muscle (except in the kidney, where stimulation of A_1 receptors causes vasoconstriction). Adenosine is important in the heart, where it blocks AV conduction and reduces the force of contraction; adenosine release might be partly responsible for the pain associated with heart attacks. Adenosine is also a neuromodulator (A_1 receptors), a bronchoconstrictor (A_1), and a pro-inflammatory mediator (A_3).

Nitric oxide (NO) is one of a number of endothelium-derived vasodilators that are generated to cause local vasodilatation. Stimuli for NO generation include shear stress (the lateral stress experienced by endothelial cells due to blood flow), hypoxia, and circulating neurohormonal factors (e.g. substance P, bradykinin) that act to increase endothelial intracellular Ca^{2+}. Endothelium-derived NO also acts as a powerful inhibitor of platelet activation and inflammatory cell adhesion. Dysfunction in NO production has been implicated in many cardiovascular diseases, including atherosclerosis. NO is the most important endothelium-derived relaxing factor in large arteries.

Prostacyclin (PGI_2) is a product of arachidonic acid metabolism, stimulated in response to many of the same mediators as NO. PGI_2 acts synergistically with NO (the effect of combined release is greater than the sum of the two parts).

Endothelium-derived hyperpolarizing factor (EDHF) is the dominant endothelium-derived factor in small (resistance) arteries. Its identity is still an unresolved issue, but K^+ ions appear to play a prominent role.

Signal integration and intracellular contractile processes

The extent of constriction of any artery depends on the balance of vasoconstrictor and vasodilator stimuli. The signals from the different mediators are almost exclusively channelled through modulating the concentration of cytoplasmic

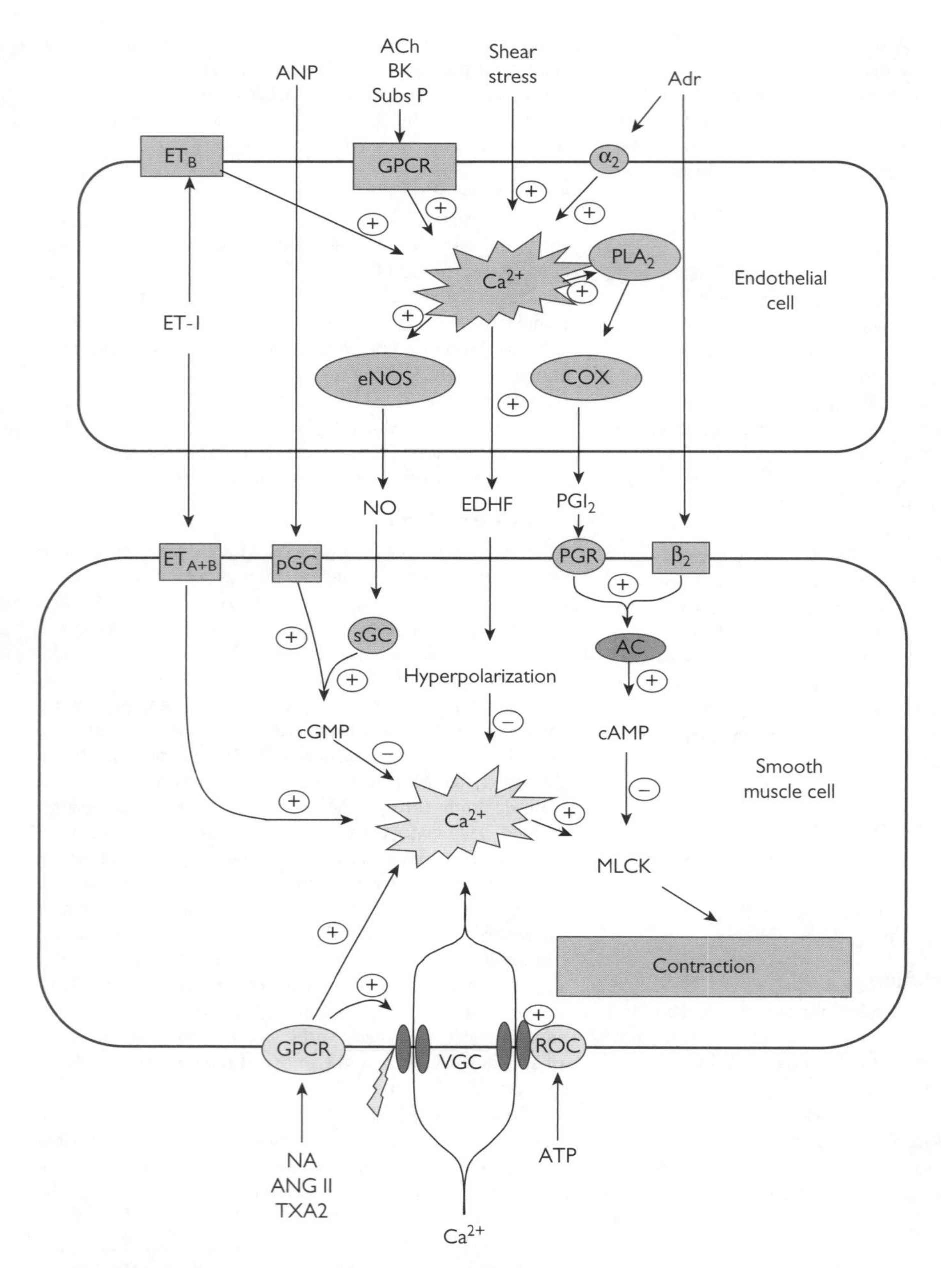

Fig. 10.7 Some of the cellular mechanisms underlying vascular smooth muscle contraction and dilation in response to endogenous signals. Ach, acetylcholine; ANP, atrial natriuretic peptide; Adr, adrenaline; A2, A2 adrenoceptor; AC, adenylate cyclase; Ang II, angiotensin II; BK, bradykinin; B2, B2 adrenoceptor; ETA and ETB, endothelin receptors A and B; ET-1, endothelin-a; eNOS, endothelial nitric oxide synthase; COX, cyclo-oxygenase; EDHF, endothelium-derived hyperpolarizing factor; GPCR, G-protein-coupled receptor; MLCK, myosin light chain kinase; sGC/pGC, soluble and particulate guanylate cyclase; NA, noradrenaline; PLA2, phospholipase A2; PER, prostaglandin receptor; PGI2, prostacyclin; ROC, receptor-operated channel; Subs P, substance P; TXA2, thromboxane A2; VGC, voltage-gated channel.

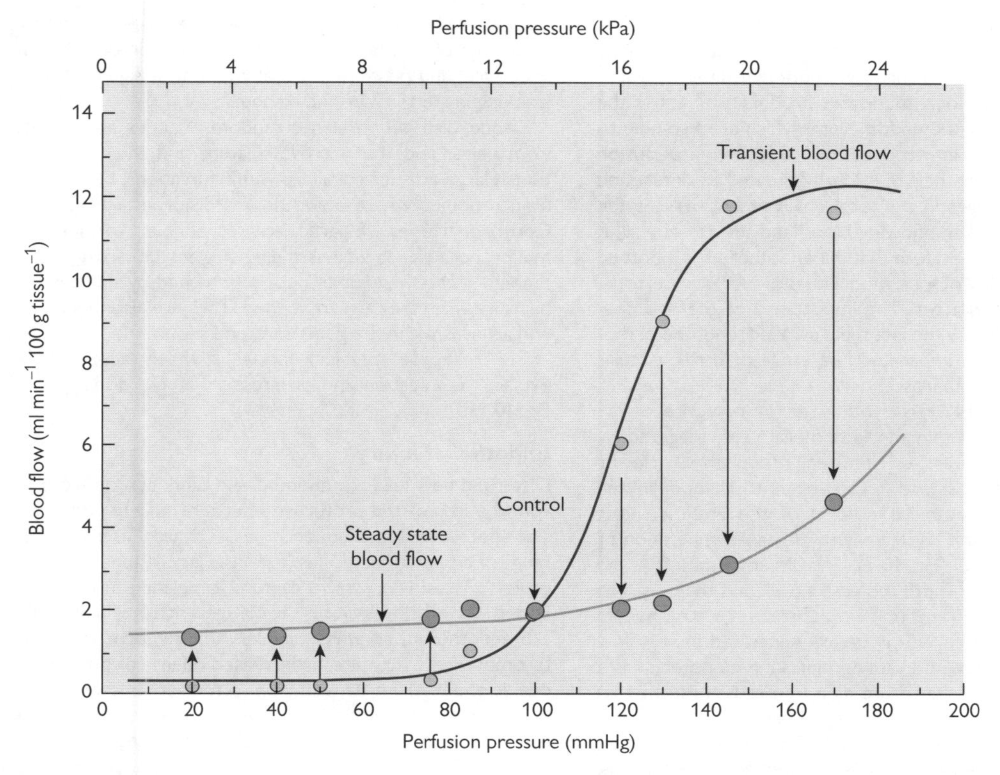

Fig. 10.8 Graph showing the autoregulation of blood flow in an isolated perfused skeletal muscle of the dog. The white circles represent the blood flow measured immediately after the perfusion pressure had been raised or lowered from the control level. As perfusion pressure is altered, there is a transient rise or fall in blood flow but autoregulatory mechanisms quickly restore blood flow to levels close to control (shown by the dark purple circles.).

calcium (Ca^{2+}_i), or through altering the phosphorylation status of the myofilaments, through myosin light chain kinase and phosphatase (mainly vasodilators). Ca^{2+}_i derived from intracellular stores in the sarcoplasmic reticulum and through voltage-gated Ca^{2+} channels binds to calmodulin, which stimulates myosin light chain kinase (MLCK) to phosphorylate myosin—an essential step in the interaction of smooth muscle myosin with actin. The integration of signaling pathways is summarized in Fig. 10.7.

Regional blood flow is under local control

Although there is some modification of the pattern of blood flow upon sympathetic stimulation, determined by the distribution of α- and β-adrenoceptors in blood vessels of different tissues, there is also the capability for responding to the specific needs of a particular organ or tissue. Therefore, superimposed on these systemic mechanisms that control overall blood pressure, are local control mechanisms that react to the immediate metabolic requirements of a given tissue. This way blood flow through the capillary bed is sufficient to provide for metabolic need, but never two high as cause capillary rupture. This phenomenon is known as autoregulation (see Fig. 10.8).

Myogenic vasoconstriction

At high perfusion pressures, stretch of vascular smooth muscle cells can open stretch activated, non-selective cation channels that cause depolarization and opening of voltage-gated calcium channels. This mediates arteriole vascular smooth muscle contraction to opposes the rise in perfusion pressure and bring flow to the capillary bed back to normal. The transient increase in blood flow may also 'wash out' metabolic vasodilators produced by the perfused tissue.

Metabolic vasodilation

Hypo-perfusion of arteriole vascular smooth muscle can directly cause vasodilation by opening ATP responsive potassium channels. As ATP levels in the cell lower, opening of K_{ATP} channels hyperpolarizes the membrane and reduces calcium entry through voltage-gated calcium channels. A reduction in pH can also lead to a conformational change in the myofilaments making them more difficult to activate.

There are also local mediators produced by either the perfused tissue or the endothelium, which are also able to cause vasodilation in response to a reduction in perfusion pressure. The endothelium is ideally situated to detect and respond to changes in the local environment, as it is the interface between the flowing blood and the vessel wall. It is not surprising, therefore that the endothelium is a hotbed for the production of local modulators of blood vessel tone, particularly vasodilators. The importance of the endothelium is highlighted by the fact that so-called 'endothelial dysfunction' has been implicated in a range of cardiovascular disease, including atherosclerosis.

Nitric oxide (NO) is synthesized in response to an increase in Ca^{2+} within the endothelial cells, triggered by ischaemia, shear stress, or circulating modulators, including bradykinin and substance P. Ca^{2+} binds to calmodulin and stimulates the endothelial isoform of the enzyme, nitric oxide synthase (eNOS), leading to increased generation of the free radical NO (Fig. 10.7). This is a small molecule and diffuses rapidly into both the vessel wall, and the lumen to cause vasodilatation and inhibition of platelet and monocyte function. Endothelial NO is usually generated in very low concentrations (low nM range), indicating its potency as a signalling molecule. Its nature as a free radical means that it is highly reactive, with a biological half-life of only a few seconds. Most of the effects of NO are cGMP-mediated, but there is evidence of cGMP-independent mechanisms, particularly when NO is generated in higher concentrations. Organic nitrates that are often used in angina undergo tissue-mediated metabolism to release NO.

NO is also known to be the non-adrenergic, non-cholinergic (NANC) neurotransmitter found in specific nerves and an inducible isoform of the enzyme (iNOS) is expressed in response to inflammatory stimuli; local concentrations of NO from iNOS are believed to be ~1000 times higher than those from eNOS, reflecting its change in function from a highly controllable local mediator to a cytotoxic agent for use by the immune system.

Prostacyclin (PGI_2) acts synergistically with NO and is generated in response to similar stimuli. It has a relatively short half-life (<5 min), but its dilution in flowing blood reduces its activity as it is washed away from its site of production. PGI_2 is synthesized from arachidonic acid by a three-step process involving phospholipase A_2, cyclo-oxygenase 1 (COX-1) and prostacyclin synthase. PGE_2 is a closely related prostanoid that also causes vasodilatation.

Atherosclerosis: coronary artery disease, cerebrovascular disease, and peripheral vascular disease

Atherosclerosis is a complex disease process that results in the deposition of lipids in discrete lesions (plaques) found in the walls of large conduit arteries. Although early atherosclerotic lesions or fatty streaks are found in almost all of us from an early age, their prevalence is greatly increased by a number of risk factors, including genetic predisposition, sex (male, and post-menopausal women), a high lipid diet, smoking, hypertension, and diabetes.

Plaque distribution is not random. Plaques are absent from veins, and the microvasculature and their distribution in large arteries coincides with bifurcations, bends, and branch points, where blood flow is disturbed (turbulent). Coronary arteries are particularly susceptible to plaque formation because, as well as their being tortuous and highly branched, the flow is particularly disturbed by the beating heart in which they are embedded. They are also functional end arteries without a good collateral supply.

The response to injury model is widely accepted to explain the initiation and progression of the disease (see Fig. 10.9):

Endothelial injury

Disturbed flow leads to endothelial dysfunction or erosion, with the loss of the protective effects of NO in particular. The affected endothelium becomes 'activated', expressing a range of adhesion molecules (e.g. vascular cell adhesion molecule 1; VCAM-1), which 'capture' circulating monocytes. Endothelial erosion exposes the collagen-rich prothrombotic sub-endothelium, to which platelets adhere, forming microthrombi. There may also be increased release of pro-atherogenic endothelium-derived ET-1. A further consequence is the generation of the oxidizing free radical, superoxide, from NAD(P)H oxidases in the endothelial membrane.

Inflammation

Captured monocytes infiltrate through the endothelium, where they differentiate into macrophages in response to growth factors, cytokines and chemo-attractants generated by infiltrating T-lymphocytes (e.g. granulocyte colony stimulating factor; G-CSF), which go on to generate high concentrations of several pro-oxidant species (superoxide, nitric oxide, peroxynitrite) designed to kill pathogens. The inflammatory process is exacerbated by adherent platelets, which degranulate, releasing a number of pro-inflammatory mediators (e.g. platelet-derived growth factor). Neighbouring smooth muscle cells begin to proliferate and migrate to form the 'neo-intima' in response to growth factors and in the absence of anti-mitogenic NO. The smooth muscle cells of the neointima conform to a non-contractile, secretory phenotype, generating extracellular matrix to stabilize the developing plaque (fibrosis).

Lipid accumulation

Normally, circulating lipids, in the form of low-density lipoproteins (LDL), diffuse readily in and out of the vessel wall without consequence. However, in the highly oxidizing environment of a developing atherosclerotic lesion, LDL is rapidly oxidized (forming OX-LDL), which is recognized by scavenger receptors on macrophages, prior to phagocytosis. The OX-LDL is trapped in the vessel wall in macrophages (now called foam cells), which ultimately die, releasing their contents to form the lipid-rich core of the plaque.

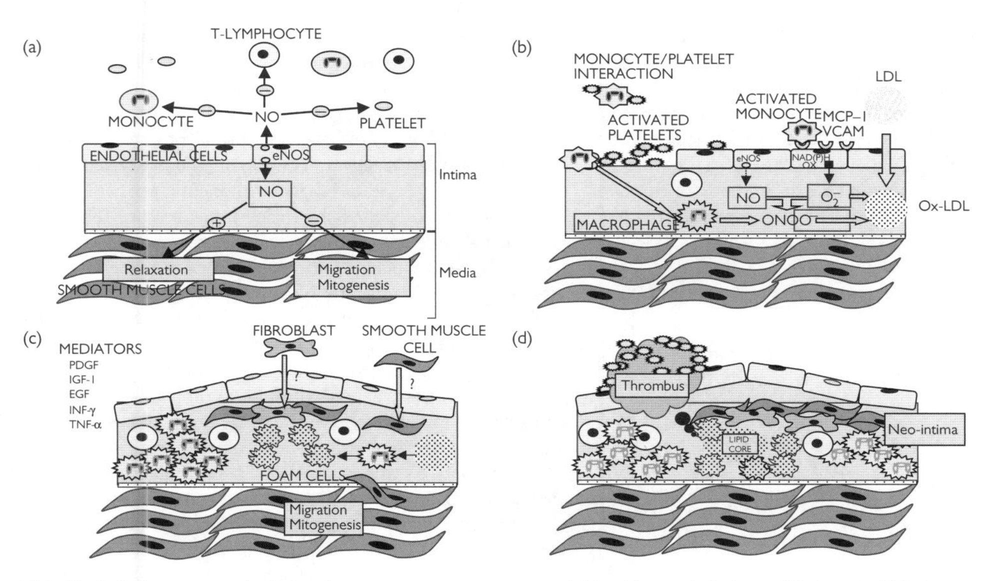

Fig. 10.9 Pathogenesis of atherosclerosis—response to injury: (a) healthy endothelium; (b) damaged/dysfunctional endothelium; (c) inflammatory phase; (d) unresolved inflammation; plaque rupture; thrombosis.

Calcification is also a feature of mature plaques in humans. It is this stage of the atherosclerotic process for which the most effective treatments have been targeted. First, lowering plasma LDL levels is known to reduce mortality in patients with atherosclerosis-related conditions—moderate benefits can be seen with improved diets, but the recent introduction of the drug class known as statins, which inhibit *de novo* synthesis of cholesterol in the liver, have shown dramatic improvements in lipid lowering and are routinely prescribed to 'at risk' patients. It has since transpired that statins also have a range of other benefits, particularly with respect to the restoration of a healthy endothelium, antiplatelet effects, and plaque stabilization. Other primary prevention is aimed at reducing the prevalence of pro-oxidant species by stopping smoking, and treating diabetes and hypertension.

Most atherosclerotic plaques stabilize at this point, as inflammation is resolved. A stable plaque will partially occlude the lumen of the artery and the extent and site of the occlusion (or 'stenosis') will determine whether the subject suffers from symptoms. Stable angina pectoris is caused by restricted blood flow through a stenosed coronary artery. Patients with angina therefore suffer severe chest pain caused by hypoxia associated with insufficient blood supply to part of the myocardium in response to increased demand (e.g. exercise). Symptoms can be successfully managed using organic nitrate drugs (glyceryl trinitrate spray or sublingual tablet). Sufferers are also recommended to take low dose aspirin daily to reduce the chance of thrombosis, as well as β-blockers to reduce the work rate and oxygen demand of the heart. Severe cases may be treated with balloon angioplasty and stenting, or bypass surgery, particularly if the lesion is located proximally in an epicardial coronary artery so that a large area of myocardium is threatened, or refractory to medical treatment. Although both procedures are better at treating symptoms than medical therapy, they carry risks including that of re-occlusion (due to restenosis or thrombosis). Stenoses in the large conduit arteries of the leg (e.g. femoral arteries) can lead to ischaemia (lack of oxygen) to the affected limbs, leading to severe pain and, in some cases, infection or gangrene. Treatments for peripheral vascular disease also include angioplasty and stenting, or bypass grafting. Very severe cases require amputation to prevent sepsis and gangrene.

Plaque rupture

Plaques that remain inflamed can become unstable (prone to rupture). The mechanism that determines the stability of atherosclerotic plaques is not yet fully understood, but the consequences of plaque rupture can be devastating. Material from the core bursts through the weakened neo-intima, where it comes into contact with the blood. This material is highly thrombogenic, leading to rapid platelet adhesion and aggregation, with the associated activation of the coagulation cascade. The resulting thrombus can either completely occlude the artery at the site of the plaque or become dislodged, forming an embolus that passes further down the arterial tree before occluding a smaller vessel. The result is an acute ischaemic event; in the heart (coronary arteries), this causes myocardial infarction, in the brain (carotid arteries), a stroke, and in the leg, acute limb ischaemia. All are extremely serious and require emergency treatment, although the severity of the event is entirely dependent on the site of the thrombus, the size of the ischaemic area and the speed at which the correct medical attention is provided. Treatment in all cases involves anti-thrombotic therapy (such as aspirin, clopidogrel and heparin) and, in the case of myocardial infarction, percutaneous coronary intervention (PCI) either urgently (non-ST elevation myocardial infarctions and unstable angina) or in the case of ST elevation myocardial infarctions that meet criteria, immediate primary PCI (or thrombolysis if not available). A mortality benefit has been proven in these cases.

Capillary fluid exchange

The movement of fluid across a capillary barrier is described by the Starling equation as a balance between the hydrostatic forces, and the oncotic forces due to the osmotic pressure exerted by proteins on each side of the barrier.

$$J_v = K_f A [(P_c - P_i) - \delta(\pi_c - \pi_i)]$$

where J_v is the net fluid movement, K_f is the filtration coefficient (a property of the barrier that depends on its surface area, thickness and permeability), A is the area of filtration, P is hydrostatic pressure, and π oncotic pressure in the capillary (c) and interstitial (*i*) respectively, and δ is the reflection co-efficient of the barrier for proteins.

While P_c is autoregulated as described earlier, other values vary depending on the type of vascular bed. Hepatic sinusoids have a reflection co-efficient close to 0, while glomerular capillaries are very tight and have a reflection co-efficient of 1 and an oncotic pressure in Bowman's capsule of 0. As glomerular filtration occurs and fluid leaves the capillary, proteins are trapped and the oncotic pressure in the capillary rises to oppose the hydrostatic pressure. The main driving force behind glomerular filtration is therefore P_c that is tightly autoregulated with the help of tubuloglomerular feedback (see Chapter 16, Nephrology).

The Starling equation also helps us understand why fluid accumulates in body cavities under certain pathological conditions and why measuring the protein content of the fluid helps in the diagnosis. If fluid accumulates because of an increase in P_c (such as in the lungs during left ventricular failure) or a decrease in π_c (such as in nephrotic syndrome, or with poor synthetic function in liver failure) then the accumulating fluid would be expected to have a low protein content or π_i (assuming lymphatic drainage is not impaired) and this is known as a transudate. In the case of an infection or malignancy, the interstitial protein content or π_i, is raised and this is known as an exudate.

Cardiovascular physiology and control of the circulation

Blood pressure detection

Blood pressure is constantly monitored by baroreceptors. There are 'high pressure receptors' in the aortic arch, pulmonary artery, and carotid sinus, and 'low pressure receptors' in the atria and adjacent large veins. Signals from both high and low pressure receptors are integrated in the 'cardiovascular centres' in the upper medulla and respond by appropriate stimulation of the parasympathetic (to slow the heart in response to high blood pressure) or sympathetic (to accelerate heart rate, constrict blood vessels, and increase blood volume in response to low blood pressure) branches of the autonomic nervous system (Fig. 10.10).

Blood pressure determination

In the short term, the cardiovascular system can be considered a closed circuit and the pressure within the system

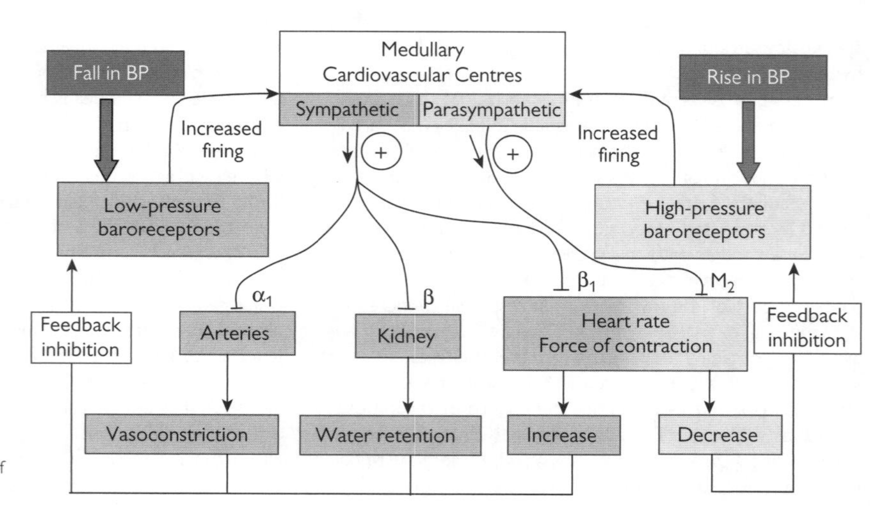

Fig. 10.10 Baroreceptor reflex responsible for blood pressure homeostasis.

Reproduced from R Wilkins et al., *Oxford Handbook of Medical Sciences, Second Edition*, 2011, Figure 6.37, p. 449, by permission of Oxford University Press.

is determined by the reflex control of cardiac output and total peripheral resistance. In the longer term, the role of the kidney in determining blood volume becomes increasingly important for blood pressure control.

Blood volume

Pressure natriuresis and hormonal control of sodium and water reabsorption by the renin-angiotensin-aldosterone system, antidiuretic hormone, and natriuretic peptides are essential to regulate effective circulating volume. This becomes increasingly important with age as blood vessel stiffness increases and the circulation is less able to dampen fluctuations in blood volume.

Cardiac output

This is determined both by heart rate and stroke volume modulated by both branches of the autonomic nervous system in response to baroreceptor and brainstem control.

Vascular resistance

While a reduction in compliance of the major arteries can influence particularly systolic blood pressure with aging (the Windkessel effect), the main resistance vessels of the circulation are arterioles. Poiseuille's Law describes the relationship between the resistance of a circular tube being inversely proportional to its radius raised to the fourth power. Arteriolar resistance is influenced by the sympathetic nervous system in response to baroreceptor and brainstem control.

Blood pressure and heart rate have a diurnal variation being higher during waking hours driven by the levels of sympathetic drive, renin-angiotensin-aldosterone system activity, cortisol, and antidiuretic hormone levels.

Reflex responses

The rapid and integrated response to changes in blood pressure in humans is best illustrated with the example of what happens when we stand up.

- *The action of standing* leads to a rapid pooling of venous blood in the legs due to gravity, leaving less blood in the large central veins for return to the heart. More than 0.5 L of blood is redistributed in this way upon standing.
- *The reduction in preload* leads to a reduction in stroke volume (Frank–Starling law) and, consequently, cardiac output. Arterial pressure falls momentarily. Baroreceptors in the large veins and atria detect the fall in central venous pressure.
- *Signals from the low-pressure baroreceptors* are processed in the cardiovascular centres of the medulla and the sympathetic nervous system is stimulated (Fig. 10.10).
- *Heart rate increases, peripheral vascular resistance increases, central veins contract*, all of which returns arterial and venous pressure to near-normal levels within a few seconds.

The importance of the sympathetic nervous system in this process is highlighted by the fact that a major side-effect of inhibitors of the synthesis of noradrenaline (NA), is postural hypotension (low blood pressure on standing, which can cause syncopy)

Exercise

During exercise, the arterial baroreflex needs to be reset to a higher operating pressure to allow for a rise in heart rate and mean arterial pressure via sympathetic stimulation and vagal withdrawal in order to maintain adequate perfusion to exercising muscle. This occurs via two interacting pathway—anticipatory central command from higher centres, and peripheral feedback from the exercising muscles themselves.

Descending signals from higher brain centres, termed 'central command', exist that vary in relation to an individual's perception of effort during physical exertion, and is independent of the actual workload or force production. This provides a feedforward, anticipatory response to exercise that is presumably calibrated to ones own conscious and subconscious experiences during previous motor activity. The 'pressor' reflex from exercising muscles also makes an important contribution during exercise by providing afferent feedback to influence autonomic control of arterial pressure. This is based on the actual work done by the muscle in relation to the blood supply it is receiving. The feedback mechanism, while being important during a single bout of exercise, may also act to calibrate feedforward control for future exertion in a continuously dynamic process.

The resultant increase in perfusion to exercising muscle is therefore maintained by:

- Increased heart rate and stroke volume through stimulation of β_1-adrenoceptors.
- Vasoconstriction of blood vessels supplying the major organs, and the gut through α_1-adrenoceptors.
- Vasodilatation of arteries that supply exercising skeletal muscle through β_2-adrenoceptors (partly mediated by the endothelium) and activation of local mediators in response to any hypoxia that rapidly develops during exercise.

These processes combine to cause a considerable increase in cardiac output to account for the massive increase in oxygen consumption, and a prioritization of blood distribution to favour muscles at the expense of other tissues. In a trained athlete, heart rate can easily treble (from ~50 beats/min to >150 beats/min), stroke volume can more than double (80 – >160 mL/min), resulting in an increase in cardiac output from ~4 L/min to up to ~40 L/min in world class athletes. If peripheral resistance were to remain constant, systolic blood pressure under these conditions would rise above 1000 mmHg, which would clearly exceed the limits of blood vessel strength. In the event, blood pressure usually only reaches approximately double the normal values (~200 mmHg), indicative of an overall decrease in peripheral resistance.

Hypertension

Hypertension is characterized by chronically elevated blood pressure and is a risk factor for other cardiovascular diseases, including coronary artery disease, myocardial infarction, stroke, and heart failure. The majority of hypertension is primary or 'essential' in that no clear cause can be identified.

BOX 10.2 SECONDARY CAUSES OF HYPERTENSION

- *Vascular causes:* e.g. coarctation of the aorta, renal artery stenosis.
- *Renal disease:* any cause of chronic renal failure.
- *Endocrine diseases:* e.g. Cushing's, Conn's syndromes, and phaeochromocytoma.
- *Others causes:* such as drugs and pregnancy.

These people are assumed to have a genetic predisposition, perhaps in combination with, as yet, unidentified environment factors that has lead to abnormal long-term renal, autonomic, or vascular control of effective circulating volume and blood pressure. However, in around 5% of cases, a secondary cause can be identified, especially when hypertension develops in younger patients (Box 10.2).

Due to the labile nature of blood pressure in response to the environment, defining hypertension and making a reliable diagnosis can be difficult. In reality, an artificial limit is defined, based on the level of risk and cost of treating the condition. Blood pressure should be assessed with two different readings on at least two different clinic visits (and 24 hour blood pressure recording used if necessary). Drug treatment, as well as lifestyle advice and risk factor modification should be offered to patients with blood pressure greater than 160/100 mmHg, or if the 10-year cardiovascular risk (as estimated using tools such as the Frammingham or Q-risk calculator) is greater than 20%, drug treatment should also be offered to those with blood pressures over 140/90, but less than 160/100 mmHg. If the 10-year cardiovascular risk is less than 20%, then this later group of patients should be treated with lifestyle advice and risk factor modification alone, but carefully monitored.

Heart failure

The inability of the heart to meet the supply needs of the body is known as heart failure. It is characterized by a flattening of the Frank–Starling curve such that the heart is not able to respond to an increase in venous return by passing it on to the arterial side of the circulation through increasing cardiac output.

Regardless of the cause of heart failure, inadequate cardiac output leads to the following chain of events (see Fig. 10.11 and Box 10.3). Blood pressure falls and is sensed by the baroreceptors and through a fall in renal perfusion pressure.

Signals from the baroreceptors result in the stimulation of the sympathetic nervous system, which restores blood pressure to normal levels by increasing heart rate (via cardiac β_1-adrenoceptors), vascular resistance (α_1-receptors in arterioles) and also blood volume (via β-adrenoreceptors in the kidney, accompanied by an increase in the renin-angiotensin-aldosterone system and antidiuretic hormone levels).

The shortfall in cardiac output is therefore compensated for at the expense of increased heart rate, peripheral vascular resistance (afterload) and blood volume (preload) although

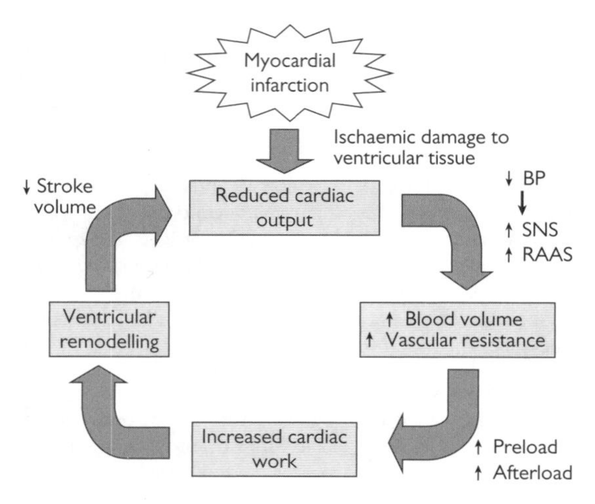

Fig. 10.11 The vicious cycle of heart failure is triggered by ischaemic damage to the ventricle. SNS, sympathetic nervous system; RAAS, renin–angiotensin–aldosterone system.

Reproduced from R Wilkins et al., *Oxford Handbook of Medical Sciences, Second Edition,* 2011, Figure 6.33, p. 439, by permission of Oxford University Press.

BOX 10.3 CAUSES OF HEART FAILURE

- *Systolic (inadequate contraction):* myocardial infarction, dilated cardiomyopathy [which can be ischaemic, viral/infectious, toxic (e.g. alcohol, doxorubicin), metabolic (e.g. haemochromotosis, hyperthyroidism), or secondary to nutritional deficiencies (e.g. thiamine, vitamin D, selenium), autoimmune, tachycardia mediated, peripartum, genetic, catecholamine mediated (stress-induced, sub-arachnoid haemorrhage, phaeochromocytoma)].
- *Diastolic (inadequate relaxation and filling):* hypertension (especially in combination with AF), hypertrophic cardiomyopathy, restrictive cardiomyopathy.
- *Pericardial disease:* pericardial effusions/tamponade, constrictive cardiomyopathy.
- *Rate dependent:* both extremes of brady- and tachycardia.
- *Valvular disease.*

persistent stretch of cardiomyocytes leads to the expression and release of BNP, as well as ANP as part of a compensatory response to limit the increase in blood volume.

Unfortunately, this short-term maintenance of blood pressure has long-term consequences. Following a myocardial infarction, the increased work rate of the heart, coupled with the increased resistance against which it has to pump blood, leads to the thickening of the non-infarcted ventricular walls (remodelling). Simultaneously, the reduction in renal perfusion activates the renin-angiotensin-aldosterone system, leading to sodium and water retention, and oedema, which can be particularly catastrophic in the lungs where it impedes oxygenation and will therefore worsen cardiac function. The increase in central venous pressure constitutes an increase in cardiac preload, which might be predicted to improve cardiac contractility, according to the Frank–Starling law. However, the sympathetic compensation that has already taken place means that increasing the preload fails to increase contractility. Instead, the heart becomes increasingly dilated leading to further pump failure. The combination of stretch and remodelling makes the heart more able to sustain re-entrant ventricular arrhythmias initiated by the high level of sympathetic drive to the myocardium.

Treatment of heart failure

The aim of treatment of heart failure is to treat the underlying cause where possible and slow the progression of the disease and prolong the life of sufferers. ACE inhibitors, angiotensin-receptor antagonists, and aldosterone antagonists are aimed at limiting the amount of sodium and water retained by the kidneys and reducing the level of angiotensin II-mediated vasoconstriction. ACE inhibition may also slow the process of cardiac remodelling. Veno- and vaso-dilatation by these drugs, as well as long-acting nitrates and hydralazine reduce cardiac workload through reducing preload, although they may have some impact on afterload as well. In chronic stable heart failure β-blockers also help reduce the work of the heart and prevent sympathetically-induced arrhythmias. All of these drugs have been shown to improve mortality. Treatment of ventricular arrhythmias in those with poor ejection fractions and prolonged QRS duration using an implantable cardiac defibrillator has also been shown to improve mortality. Cardiac resynchronization devices can also improve symptoms and produce a degree of reverse remodelling in symptomatic patients with poor ejection fractions and broad left bundle branch blocks. In these cases, the delay in conduction between the septum and lateral wall worsens pump function and combined pacing of the septum (via a right ventricular pacing lead) and the lateral wall (via a left ventricular lead positioned via the coronary sinus) can partly correct this.

Loop diuretics, particularly in combination with thiazides, while useful in rapidly reversing pulmonary oedema, may ultimately worsen renal function and in the long term are not known to confer a mortality benefit. Positive inotropes, such as dobutamine and milrinone (a phosphodiesterase inhibitor) are also sometimes given intravenously in acute cardiogenic shock. They increase cardiac output at the expense of increasing myocardial oxygen demand and potentially worsen the underlying cause of the condition.

Digoxin has been used in chronic heart failure as a positive inotrope, particularly when atrial fibrillation is present, which it can help rate control by blocking the AV node. Digoxin acts primarily by inhibiting the Na^+/K^+ pump, leading to an increase in intracellular Na^+, which exchanges with calcium through the Na^+/Ca^{2+} exchange. Ultimately, the extra Ca^{2+} is taken up into the sarcoplasmic reticulum, meaning that more Ca^{2+} is released by calcium-induced calcium release at the arrival of the next action potential. However, digoxin has a narrow therapeutic window and an overload of intracellular calcium in ventricular myocytes can predispose to self-sustaining calcium-induced calcium release, which may drive the electrogenic Na^+/Ca^{2+} exchange in reverse and cause after depolarizations and ectopic activity, which may precipitate arrhythmia. While digoxin reduces the rate of hospitalization in heart failure patients, it has not been shown to improve mortality.

Drugs used in the treatment of cardiovascular disease

For drugs used in the treatment of cardiovascular disease, see Table 10.3. See Box 10.4 for common drug-induced cardiovascular reactions.

Table 10.3 Drugs used in the treatment of cardiovascular disease

Anti-thrombotics			
Class	Example/major efficacy trial	Common side effects	Interactions
Cyclo-oxygenase inhibitors	Acetylsalicylic acid (aspirin) inhibits COX1 and COX2 to prevent thromboxane action on platelet aggregation	Peptide/duodenal ulceration, bleeding, exacerbation of asthma, angio-oedema	Other NSAIDS
Thienopyridine P_2Y_{12} receptor inhibitors	Platelet ADP receptor antagonists, which prevent aggregation (e.g. Clopidogrel CURE trial, Prasugrel TRITON-TIMI38 trial)	Bleeding, neutropenia, TTP, bradycardia (caution with Prasugrel in those under 60 kg or over 75 years old)	Cytochrome P-450 2C19 poor metabolizers have lower levels of the active metabolite of clopidogrel. NSAIDS, some PPIs, other anticoagulants, phenytoin, tamoxifen

(continued)

Table 10.3 Drugs used in the treatment of cardiovascular disease (*continued*)

Class	Example/major efficacy trial	Common side effects	Interactions
Non-thienopyridine $P2Y_{12}$ receptor inhibitors	Platelet ADP receptor antagonists, which prevent aggregation (e.g. Ticagrelor—PLATO trial)	Bleeding, shortness of breath, bradycardia	Inhibitors of CYP3A4, (ketoconazole), inducers of CYP3A4 (rifampicin, St. John's wort), digoxin, cyclosporin
Glycoprotein IIb/IIIa inhibitors	Platelet Gp IIb/IIIa inhibitor to prevent aggregation (e.g. abciximab—EPIC trial)	Bleeding, thrombocytopenia	Other anticoagulants
Direct thrombin (III) inhibitors	Bivalent (bivalirudin, iv, ACUITY or HORIZONS-AMI), univalent (dabigatran, oral, RE-LY)	Bleeding	Other anticoagulants
Factor Xa inhibitors	*Via antithrombin III:* low molecular weight heparin (ESSENCE), fondaparinux (OASIS5). *Direct Factor Xa inhibition:* rivaroxaban (ROCKET-AF), apixiban (ARISTOTLE)	Bleeding, heparin-induced thrombocytopenia (not fondaparinux)	Other anticoagulants
Coumarins	Vitamin K antagonist inhibiting production of clotting factors II, VII, IX and X (e.g. warfarin)	Bleeding, warfarin necrosis, osteoporosis	Other anticoagulants, antibiotics (e.g. macrolides, metronidazole), statins, amiodarone, alcohol, cranberry juice, St John's wort, ginseng, gingko
Thrombolytics			
Class	**Example/major efficacy trial**	**Side effects**	**Interactions**
Plasminogen activators	E.g. streptokinase (ISIS2), recombinant-tPAs (e.g. tenecteplase, alteplase)	Haemorrhage, hypersensitivity reaction (streptokinase)	Other anti-coagulants
Anti-anginals			
Drug	**Mechanism of action**	**Common side effects**	**Interactions**
Nitrates	E.g. glyceryl trinitrate, isosorbide mononitrate, coronary vasodilation via release of nitric oxide	Hypotension, headaches	Sildenafil, other anti-hypertensives
β-blockers	Reduction in heart rate and cardiac metabolic demand, e.g. atenolol (ISIS1)	Bronchospasm, bradycardia, hypotension, depression, type II diabetes, Raynauds syndrome, erectile dysfunction	Salbutamol/salmeterol, other antihypertensive, or bradycardic drugs
Calcium channel blockers	Reduction in heart rate (especially non-dihydropridines: diltiazem/verapamil), cardiac metabolic demand, coronary vasodilation (dihydropridines: amlodipine)	Bradycardia, hypotension	Other antihypertensive, bradycardic or negatively inotropic drugs. Drugs metabolized via CYP3A4, CYP2C9 and CYP2D6
Nicorandil	Vascular smooth muscle potassium channel opener causing coronary vasodilation (IONA trial)	Hypotension, headaches, mouth and peri-anal ulcers	Other antihypertensives
Ivabradine	Inhibition of the pacemaking current I_f to reduction heart rate (BEAUTIFUL trial)	Bradycardia, AV block, luminous phenomenon	Inhibitors of CYP3A4 (e.g. ketoconazole, macrolides)
Ranolazine	Sodium channel blocker reduces myocardial oxygen demand (MERLIN-TIMI36 trial)		Inhibitors of CYP3A (diltiazem, ketoconazole, macrolides, grapefruit juice), digoxin, simvastatin, cyclosporin

Table 10.3 Drugs used in the treatment of cardiovascular disease (*continued*)

Heart failure drugs			
Drug	**Example/main efficacy trial**	**Side effects**	**Interactions**
ACE inhibitors	Enalapril (SOLVD), ramipril (AIRE)	Hypotension, angio-odema, cough (from kinase II inhibition and accumulation of bradykinin), renal impairment (especially in renal artery stenosis)	Other hypotensive or nephrotoxic drugs
Angiotensin receptor blockers	Losartan	Hypotension, renal impairment, angio-oedema	Other hypotensive or nephrotoxic drugs
β-blockers	*Short acting:* metoprolol (MERIT-HF). *Long acting:* bisoprolol (CIBIS II).α–*blocking properties:* carvedilol (CAPRICORN)	See under anti-anginals	See under anti-anginals
Ivabradine	SHIFT trial in patients already on a β–blockers with a resting pulse above 70 beats/min	See under anti-anginals	See under anti-anginals
Aldosterone antagonists	Spiranolactone (RALES), eplerenone (EPHESUS)	Hyperkalaemia, renal impairment, hypotension, gynaecomastia (not eplerenone)	Other hypotensive or nephrotoxic drugs. Antidepressants (reduces their effectiveness). CYP3A4 inhibitors (e.g. ketoconazole, macrolides)
Hydralazine	Vascular smooth muscle vasodilation and NO donor (useful in combination with isosorbide dinitrate in black African Americans: A-HeFT)	Hypotension, headache, reflex tachycardia, drug-induced lupus	Other hypotensive drugs
Nitrates	Isosorbide dinitrate (A-HeFT)	See under anti-anginals	See under anti-anginals
Loop diuretics	Furosemide, bumetanide	Hypotension, hypokalaemia, hyponatraemia hypomagnesaemia, renal impairment, gout, ototoxicity	
Thiazide diuretics	Metolazone	Hypotension, hypokalaemia, hyponatraemia, hyperglycaemia, gout, hypercalcaemia, metabolic alkalosis, agranulocytosis, thrombocytopenia, pancreatitis	Loop diuretics, other antihypertensives
Digoxin	(DIG trial)	AV block, ventricular tachycardia, gynaecomastia, xanthopsia, nausea, diarrhoea	Hypokalaemia potentiates the effects of digoxin. Hydroxychloroquine increases plasma levels
Lipid lowering drugs			
Drug	**Mechanism of action/major efficacy trial**	**Side effects**	**Interactions**
Statins	HMG Co-A reductase inhibition, e.g. simvastatin (4S trial), atorvastatin (PROVE-IT), rosuvastatin (JUPITER)	Myopathy, rhabdomyolysis, headache, hepatitis, rash	Increased risk of myopathy with CYP3A4 inhibitors, e.g. cyclosporine, erythromycin, diltiazem, grapefruit juice
Fibrates	PPAR-α agonists that modulate fat metabolism, e.g. fenofibrate	Dyspepsia, myopathy, gallstones	Increased risk of myopathy when combined with statins
Cholesterol absorption inhibitors (ezetimibe)	Blocks internalization of the NPC1L1/ cholesterol complex	Diarrhoea, myalgia, headache, hepatitis, hypersensitivity reaction, gallstones, pancreatitis	Increased risk of myopathy with CYP3A4 inhibitors

(*continued*)

Table 10.3 Drugs used in the treatment of cardiovascular disease (*continued*)

Drug	Mechanism of action/major efficacy trial	Side effects	Interactions
Nicotinic acid	Blocks fat break down in adipose tissue lowering very low density lipoprotein (VLDL, an LDL precursor) and increasing high density lipoprotein (HDL)	Facial flushing, vomiting, headache, gout, hyperglycaemia	Increased risk of myopathy when combined with statins
Omega-3-fatty acids/fish oils	After MI: GISSI-prevenzione	Bleeding (if more than 3 g/day consumed)	
Bile acid sequestrants	Ion exchange resin, which binds bile acids and promotes conversion of plasma cholesterol to bile acid, e.g. cholestyramine	Constipation, tooth discoloration, cholesterol gallstones	Decreased absorption of lipophilic drugs such as warfarin, digoxin, spiranolactone
Anti-arrhythmic drugs			
Drug	**Mechanism of action**	**Side effects**	**Interactions**
Vaughan Williams Class I	Use dependent block of the voltage-gated sodium channel (NaV1.5) to prolong refractory period/slow conduction velocity. Ia (fast kinetics), e.g. procainamide, Ib, e.g. lignocaine, mexiletine, Ic (slow kinetics), e.g. flecainide (see CAST trial), propafenone	Pro-arrhythmic in context of ischaemic heart disease, negatively inotropic, hypersensitivity reactions	May raise defibrillation threshold of ICDs/pacemakers. Cytochrome P450 2D6 inhibitors, e.g. amiodarone, digoxin, cimetidine
Vaughan Williams Class II	β-blockers	See under anti-anginals	See under anti-anginals
Vaughan Williams Class III	Potassium channel blockers prolong refractory period, e.g. amiodarone or dronedarone (also have Class I, II and IV properties), sotalol (Class II properties – see SWORD trial)	QTc prolongation, hepatitis, thyroid imbalance (amiodarone), hypersensitivity reactions	Other QTc prolonging drugs, may raise defibrillation threshold of ICDs/pacemakers
Vaughan Williams Class IV	Calcium channel blockers slow conduction velocity	See under anti-anginals	See under anti-anginals
Vaughan Williams Class V	Other mechanisms, e.g. AV node blocking agents (e.g. adenosine, digoxin), magnesium sulphate	Adenosine (bronchospasm, heart block, flushing, hypotension)	
Anti-hypertensive drugs			
Drug	**Mechanism of action**	**Side effects**	**Interactions**
ACE inhibitors/ATR1 antagonists	See under heart failure drugs	See under heart failure drugs	See under heart failure drugs
β-blockers	See under anti-anginals	See under anti-anginals	See under anti-anginals
Calcium channel blockers	See under anti-anginals	See under anti-anginals	See under anti-anginals
Thiazide diuretics	See under heart failure drugs	See under anti-anginals	See under anti-anginals
α-blockers	E.g. doxazosin	Hypotension	Other antihypertensives or vasodilators
Centrally acting anti-hypertensives	E.g. methyl-dopa and clonidine (α_2 and imidazoline-I_1 agonist reduces brainstem sympathetic outflow), moxonidine (imidazoline I_1 agonist), guanethidine (inhibition of neuronal noradrenaline re-uptake—NET_1), reserpine (inhibition of vesicular mono-amine transporter VMAT)	Hypotension, dry moth, constipation, rebound hypertension on withdrawal	Other antihypertensives. Tricyclic antidepressants

Table 10.3 Drugs used in the treatment of cardiovascular disease (*continued*)

Drugs used in pulmonary hypertension			
Drug	**Mechanism of action**	**Side effects**	**Interactions**
Calcium channel blockers	See under anti-anginals	See under anti-anginals	See under anti-anginals
Prostaglandins	E.g. Iloprost	Hypotension, flushing, congestive heart failure	Other antihypertensive drugs or vasodilators
Endothelin antagonists	E.g. bosentan	Hypotension	Other antihypertensives or vasodilators
Phosphodiesterase V inhibitors	E.g. sildenafil	Hypotension, dry mouth, constipation, rebound hypertension on withdrawal	Other antihypertensives

BOX 10.4 COMMON DRUG-INDUCED CARDIOVASCULAR REACTIONS

- *Hypertension:* steroids, MAO inhibitors, NSAIDS, clonidine/methyldopa withdrawal.
- *Worsening heart failure:* β-blockers, Ca-channel blockers, any drugs worsening renal function.
- *Worsening angina:* α-blockers, vasopressin, oxytocin, excess levothyroxine.
- *Direct myocardial toxicity:* halothane, alcohol, chemotherapy agents (e.g. doxorubicin).
- *Long QTc:* Class 1a/III anti-arrhythmics, tricyclic antidepressants, hypocalcaemia, hypokalaemia (see www.azcert.org).

Multiple choice questions

1. The following findings are obtained during a right and left heart catheterization in a 40-year-old woman. *Pressures (mmHg):* right atrial = 9 (mean), right ventricle = 36/2, pulmonary artery = 35/13, pulmonary capillary wedge pressure = 10 (mean), aortic = 125/75. *Saturations (%):* superior vena cava = 65, right atrial = 75, right ventricle = 76, pulmonary artery = 75, aortic = 97. The most likely diagnosis is:

A. Tricuspid regurgitation.
B. Ventricular septal defect.
C. Tetralogy of Fallow.
D. Atrial septal defect.
E. Sinus venosus defect.

2. Select the correct pairing of voltage-driven ion currents with the phase of the cardiac action potential it is mainly responsible for:

A. *Phase 0:* I_{Na} (fast sodium current).
B. *Phase 1:* I_{NCE} (sodium calcium exchange current).
C. *Phase 2:* I_f (hyperpolarization activated current).
D. *Phase 3:* I_{CaL} (L-type calcium current).
E. *Phase 4:* I_{Na} (fast sodium current).

3. A 40-year-old woman presents with a history of frequent fast irregular palpitations, which are occasionally accompanied by syncopy. She drinks around 40 units of alcohol a week, but minimal caffeine. Transthoracic echocardiography confirms normal left ventricular systolic function and no significant valvular defects but a severely dilated left atrium-measuring 4.8 cm. 12-lead ECG demonstrates sinus rhythm with a short PR interval and delta waves that are positive in the inferior and anterior leads. The most appropriate treatment would be:

A. Amiodarone.
B. Flecainide.
C. Sotalol.
D. Slow pathway modification of the AV node with radiofrequency ablation.
E. Radiofrequency ablation of a left lateral accessory pathway.

4. A 35-year-old man presents with breathlessness at rest. On examination, his blood pressure is 150/90 mmHg, pulse 110 beats/min and he has a raised jugular venous pressure. On palpation of the precordium he has a parasternal heave and palpable second heart sound. Auscultation reveals a systolic murmur loudest at the left sternal edge. All of the following should be included in the differential diagnosis except:

A. Pulmonary embolism.
B. Left ventricular aneurysm.
C. Primary pulmonary hypertension.
D. Left to right shunt.
E. Mitral valve disease.

5. Which of the following vaso-active substances are *not* peripheral vasoconstrictors?

A. Endothelin.
B. Phenylephrine.
C. Adenosine.
D. Thromboxane A2.
E. Angiotensin II.

6. A 35-year-old man is found on a routine medical check to have a blood pressure of 180/100 mmHg. On examination, he has radio-femoral delay, but no radio-radial delay. Auscultation reveals an ejection systolic murmur with a normal pulse character and apex beat. The most likely diagnosis is:

A. Renal artery stenosis.
B. Essential hypertension.
C. Conns syndrome.
D. Aortic co-arctation with a bicuspid aortic valve.
E. Phaeochromocytoma with a rheumatic aortic valve.

7. Which of the following drugs do not impact on mortality in heart failure?

A. Nitrates and hydralazine.
B. ACE inhibitors.
C. Eplerenone.
D. Furosemide.
E. β-blockers.

8. Which of the following is a direct thrombin inhibitor?

A. Bivalirudin.
B. Rivaroxiban.
C. Warfarin.
D. Abciximab.
E. Prasugrel.

9. Which of the following drugs is a Class Ib anti-arrhythmic?

A. Propafenone.
B. Mexilitine.
C. Procainamide.
D. Dronedarone.
E. Verapamil.

10. Which of the following drugs do *not* lower plasma lipids?

A. Nicotinic acid.
B. Fenofibrate.
C. Cholestyramine.
D. Ezetimibe.
E. Dabigatran.

For answers, please see Appendix: Answers to multiple choice questions, page 313.

CHAPTER 11

Respiratory medicine

Anatomy

The thoracic cage and diaphragm

The thoracic cage comprises of pairs of ribs, costal cartilage, the sternum, thoracic vertebrae, and intercostal muscles. The diaphragm is attached to the inferior margins of the thoracic cage and separates the thoracic cavity from the abdomen. Together the diaphragm and thoracic cage participate in ventilation, and protect the thoracic organs. During inspiration, the ribs move upwards and outwards like bucket handles lifting upwards. This increases the thoracic diameter in all directions. During expiration, the ribs sink back down and the volume of the thoracic cage thoracic cage shrinks. The diaphragm moves downwards with inspiration by contraction at the central tendon, and upwards with expiration with relaxation. Several other muscles attach to the thoracic cage including the accessory muscles of respiration, such as sternocleidomastoid and some of the scalene muscles.

Sternum

The sternum comprises three fused bones (manubrium sternum, the sternal body, and the xiphisternum), which articulate anteriorly with the ribs via costal cartilage. The manubrium articulates with the clavicle and the first two ribs. At the superior end is found the suprasternal notch, as well as two notches either side of this where the head of the clavicle articulates. The sternal angle (or angle of Louis) is the point where the manubrium fuses with the body of the sternum. The body articulates with the cartilage of ribs 2–7. The xiphisternum is found inferiorly and is the smallest sternal bone. Ribs 1–7 are therefore vertebra-sternal ribs in that they are fused anteriorly to the sternum via costal cartilages. Ribs 8–10 are vertebra-chondral ribs as the rib is fused to the costal cartilage of the rib above and Ribs 11–12 are not fused to the sternum at all. 0.5% of the population have a cervical rib, since it articulates with the seventh cervical vertebra. Sometimes this can cause lower brachial plexus compression.

Intercostal muscles

The intercostal muscles are made up of three layers of muscle between each rib. Anteriorly, the external intercostals run obliquely downward and medially, and posteriorly they run downward and laterally to elevate the ribs in inspiration. The internal intercostals also run obliquely, but in the opposite direction to the external intercostals and are involved in forced expiration. The internal intercostals contain the intercostal neurovascular bundle and separate the thoracic cage from the parietal pleura.

The intercostal neurovascular bundle consists of the intercostal vein, artery, and nerve, and runs under the rib in the costal groove. The anterior roots from each thoracic spinal nerve form the intercostal nerves, which give off muscular and cutaneous branches to supply the muscular walls of the thorax and abdomen, and the corresponding dermatome.

The thoracic cage

The thoracic cage blood supply is via the anterior and posterior intercostal arteries. The 1st to 6th anterior intercostal arteries are branches from the internal thoracic artery from the subclavian artery. The musculophrenic artery supplies the 7th to 9th anterior intercostal arteries. The 10th and 11th intercostal arteries only have a posterior supply. A branch of the subclavian artery supplies the 1st and 2nd posterior intercostal arteries while the thoracic aorta supplies the 3rd to 11th. All posterior arteries run forward and anastamose with the corresponding anterior intercostal artery. Veins follow the course of the corresponding artery. Generally, anterior and posterior intercostal veins anastomose to drain into the internal thoracic and then azygous vein, which drains into the superior vena cava.

Diaphragm

The diaphragm is a muscular dome like structure, consisting of a peripheral muscular part and a central aponeurosis. The diaphragm attaches to the inside of the xiphisternum and the lower six costal cartilages and ribs. The right crus attaches to the front of the upper three lumbar vertebrae, and the left to the 1st and 2nd lumbar vertebrae.

Central tendon

The central tendon formed by the insertions of the muscular attachments partially fuses with the base of the pericardium. The inferior vena cava and the right phrenic nerve pierce the diaphragm at the level of the 8th thoracic vertebrae. The oesophagus, the left and right vagus nerves, and the left gastric artery and vein pierce the diaphragm at the level of the 10th thoracic vertebrae. The aorta, azygous vein, and thoracic duct pierce the diaphragm at the level of the 12th thoracic vertebrae. The sympathetic chain and greater and lesser splanchnic nerves also pierce the diaphragm.

The phrenic nerve from the 3rd, 4th, and 5th cervical roots supplies the diaphragm. Since sensory innervation to the diaphragm is via the phrenic nerve, when the diaphragm is inflamed pain is referred to the shoulder tip, which is the cutaneous portion of the phrenic nerve.

The lungs and pleura

The thoracic cage contains two lungs either side of the mediastinum. The mediastinum can be divided into superior (containing the thymus) and inferior areas by the sternal angle of Louis. The inferior area is subdivided into the anterior, middle (contains the heart and great vessels), and posterior areas. The lungs are divided into lobes by the visceral fissures. The right lung comprises of the superior, middle, and inferior lobes. The middle and inferior lobes are separated by the oblique fissure and the horizontal fissure separates the superior and middle lobes. The left lung comprises of the superior and inferior lobes divided by the oblique fissure. The lingula forms a projection of the lower left upper lobe and may be an embryological remnant of the left middle lobe lost through evolution. Posteriorly, the lungs start at T12 moving laterally to the 10th rib at the mid-axillary line. It reaches the 8th costal cartilage at the mid-clavicular line and ends at the 4th costal cartilage anteriorly, although the left lung contains the cardiac notch.

The hilum is the point where all the pulmonary vessels, lymph drainage, and nerves enter and leave. The left and right pulmonary arteries return mixed venous blood to the lungs for gas exchange in the alveoli, while re-oxygenated blood returns to the left atria via the four pulmonary veins. The lungs themselves receive oxygenated blood from branches of the descending aorta known as bronchial arteries.

At the root of the lung is a pulmonary nerve plexus comprised of parasympathetic fibres from the vagus nerve and sympathetic fibres from the sympathetic chain. Parasympathetic fibres innervate airway smooth muscle, pulmonary vessels, and secretory glands of the airways. Parasympathetic fibres also carry sensory feedback from stretch receptors in the airways, baroreceptors in the pulmonary arteries, and chemoreceptors in the pulmonary veins. Sympathetic fibres also innervate airway smooth muscle, pulmonary vessels, and secretory glands.

The lungs are surrounded by membranous pleura, which are made up of an inner visceral pleura that is adherent to the surface of the lungs, and an outer parietal pleura, adherent to the inside of the thoracic cavity. Visceral and parietal pleura are continuous with each other at the hilum of the lung and, at this point, a double layer of parietal pleura extends inferiorly, forming the pulmonary ligament, which provides space for the pulmonary vessels to move during ventilation.

Between the two layers of pleura exists a potential space, the pleural cavity, which is normally filled with a few millilitres of pleural fluid. This aids the movement of the pleural layers against each other during inspiration and expiration. At the end of a normal expiration, intrapleural pressure is negative relative to atmospheric pressure (–5 cmH_2O). This is because of the inherent mechanical tendancy of the lungs tend to collapse inwards and the chest wall to recoil outwards. During inspiration, the muscles of chest wall and diaphragm expand the chest well, and increase intrathoracic volume thus reducing intrapleural pressure further. In this way, alveolar pressure is reduced (by up to 5 cmH_2O in normal subjects) and inspiration is initiated. Conversely, during normal expiration, the muscles of chest wall and diaphragm relax, decreasing intrathoracic volume, increasing alveolar pressure above atmospheric pressure and causing expiration. A forced expiration, during which contraction of certain chest wall muscles results in an even higher increase in intrapleural pressure, which obviously increases expiratory rate further. Intra-oesophageal pressure is approximately equal to intrapleural pressure and can be recorded by introducing a pressure transducer into the oesophagus. If air enters this space, the lungs collapse in a condition known as a pneumothorax.

The pleural space can also become filled with transudative or exudative fluid in some conditions, and this is visible on a chest X-ray as a blunting of the angles of, for example, the costodiaphragmatic recess (Box 11.1). When fluid needs to be drained from the pleural cavity, it is usually done by inserting a needle into the intercostal space, over the border of the lower rib to avoid damage to neurovascular bundle.

Intercostal and phrenic nerves innervate the parietal pleura and inflammation of this layer can result in localized pleuritic pain, as the two layers of pleura rub during breathing. Pleural pain can also be referred—inflammation of the diaphragmatic pleura can result in abdominal wall pain, while inflammation of mediastinal pleura can be referred to the neck and shoulder. In contrast visceral pleura receives no sensory innervation.

BOX 11.1 CAUSES OF PLEURAL EFFUSIONS

- *Transudates (pleural:serum protein <0.5, pleural:serum* lactate dehydrogenase *(LDH) <0.6):* left ventricular failure, liver cirrhosis, nephrotic syndrome.
- *Exudates (pleural:serum protein >0.5, pleural:serum LDH >0.6):* bacterial pneumonia, empyaema (low pH), malignancy (low pH), pulmonary emboli, connective tissue disease (rheumatoid arthritis, SLE, Wegener's, etc.), traumatic (oesophageal rupture—raised amylase, haemothorax, chylothorax).
- *Rare causes:* Meigs syndrome (with ascites due to a benign ovarian tumour), Asbestos exposure, Mediterranean fever, yellow nail syndrome, post-thoracotomy syndrome.

The airways

The upper airways comprise those parts of the respiratory tract above the trachea. They are lined by respiratory epithelium, which is characteristically pseudostratified and ciliated. Frequent goblet cells secrete mucous, which absorbs smaller inhaled particles not excluded by the nose. The continuous beating motion of cilia prevents these particles from entering the lungs by shifting mucous upwards and out of the respiratory tract, where it is swallowed or expectorated (mucociliary escalator; Box 11.2). This is an important defence against the entry of foreign, potentially pathogenic, particles.

The upper airways start with the oral cavity, nose, and sinuses, naso-oropharynx, laryngopharynx, and larynx. The larynx plays important roles in producing speech and sound, allowing for ventilation, and protecting the trachea and bronchial tree during swallowing. The epiglottis is an elastic flap of cartilage, which lies behind the tongue and forms the entrance to the larynx. During swallowing, elevation of the hyoid bone draws the larynx upward and, as a result, the epiglottis folds down to a more horizontal position. This prevents food from going into the trachea and instead directs it posteriorly to the oesophagus.

The thyroid cartilage is V-shaped and forms the prominence in the neck called the 'Adam's apple' in men. Below this, the cricoid cartilage is the only complete ring of cartilage in the respiratory system. The cricothyroid membrane runs between the thyroid and the cricoid anteriorly, and in an emergency can be pierced to provide an airway during laryangeal obstruction (a tracheostomy).

The intrinsic muscles of the larynx (such as thyroarytenoid, posterior and lateral cricoarytenoid, interarytenoid, aryepiglottic and cricothyroid muscles) control movements within the larynx, and the tension on the vocal cords. All the intrinsic muscles of the larynx are supplied by the recurrent laryngeal nerve, a branch of the vagus, which loops under the arch of the aorta and ligamentum arteriosum on the left, and under the sub-clavian artery on the right. It can be damaged by thyroid surgery as it runs posteriorly to the gland.

The trachea starts just below the cricoid cartilage. It has c-shaped cartilaginous rings, with a fibrous muscular band (trachealis) over the cartilage-deficient area posteriorly. The trachea bifurcates into right and left main bronchi at the angle of Louis, and as the right main bronchus is wider, and more vertical, foreign bodies more likely to lodge in this tract. The right upper lobe bronchus is given off, before the right main bronchus enters the hilum of the lung. The main bronchi then enter each lung at the hilum and inside the lungs bronchi divide into lobar bronchi. The lobar bronchi continue to divide and after approximately four divisions form bronchioles, which each supply a single lobule. Each bronchiole divides into 5–7 terminal bronchioles, which then form 2–5 respiratory bronchioles (characterized by the presence of sporadic alveoli). Distally, respiratory bronchioles form 2–11 alveolar ducts from which most alveoli lead via alveolar sacs. The airways divide 20–25 times before reaching the alveoli (where most gas exchange occurs), and between each division become smaller in length and diameter than more proximal segments. In healthy subjects, the upper airways contribute most to total pulmonary resistance because their total cross-sectional area is markedly less than for more distal segments.

The alveoli form the major compartment specialized for gas exchange between blood and air. There are approximately 300 million alveoli in the two lungs with a combined surface area of 80–140 m^2. This, coupled with their proximity to pulmonary capillaries, enhances the rapid exchange of gases between blood and air. The blood–air barrier separates the alveoli and capillary blood. This comprises the thin, single-layered alveolar epithelial cells, the fused basal laminae of the epithelial layer and capillary endothelial cells, and the endothelial cells themselves. Together, these three layers are only about 1.5 μm thick and greatly facilitate diffusional gas exchange.

Type II alveolar cells are more rounded and account for the remaining 5% of alveolar surface area. They secrete surfactant, which is mainly dipalmitoylphosphatidylcholine (DPPC) and other phospholipids, from about 30 weeks gestation. By adsorbing to the air-water interface of alveoli with the hydrophilic head groups in the water and the hydrophobic tails facing towards the air, surfactant reduces surface tension (T) at the liquid-air interface. From Laplace's Law, a lower pressure (P) is required to hold open small alveoli (approximately 50 μm in radius, r)

$$P = 2T/r$$

Surfactant therefore maintains the stability of alveoli and minimizing the work required inflating the lungs. Insufficient surfactant is believed to account for infant respiratory distress syndrome in premature babies. Type I alveolar cells comprise about 95% of the alveolar surface and are characteristically squamous. Type I cells are involved in gas exchange and the absorption of surfactant, promoting its turnover.

BOX 11.2 CYSTIC FIBROSIS

Autosomal recessive condition caused by mutations in the gene *CFTR* (cystic fibrosis transmembrane conductance regulator) on chromosome 7. The most common mutation is ΔF508 resulting in the loss (Δ) of a phenylalanine (F) at position 508. The protein controls a chloride channel in the apical membrane of epithelial cells. In the airways there is reduced secretion of chloride into the surface mucus with subsequent sodium and water reabsorption into the cells causing dehydration of the surface mucus which is then much more viscid and is not cleared by the mucociliary escalator. This leads to recurrent respiratory infections (particularly with organisms, such as *Pseudomonas aeruginosa*) and bronchiectasis. However, epithelial dysfunction can also lead to pancreatic insufficiency and male infertility.

Respiratory physiology

Ventilation and diffusion

Ventilation

Ventilation is the process by which inspired gases reach and expired gases are removed from the alveoli. Alveolar ventilation is dependent on the rate and depth of ventilation and the resistance to the flow of air (i.e. the interrelationship between depth and rate).

$$\dot{V}_A = (V_T - V_D).r$$

where $\dot{V}_A$ is alveolar ventilation rate, V_T is tidal volume, V_D is dead space volume and *r* is respiratory rate.

In a healthy individual the conducting airways are approximately 150 mL and this volume is frequently referred to as dead space, i.e. the volume of each breath, which does not ventilate the exchange zones. Anatomical dead space refers to the volume of the lung that is not alveoli; physiological dead space is the volume of the lung that does not exchange gases with the pulmonary circulation. In healthy individuals, these values are approximately equal, however, during lung disease physiological dead space may be significantly increased as a result of reduced efficiency of pulmonary gas exchange. Normal tidal volume is approximately 500 mL and respiratory rate 15 breaths/min. Total ventilation is, therefore, 7500 mL/min. However, the physiological dead space volume of the lungs is approximately 150 mL, and therefore only 5250 mL/min is useful alveolar ventilation. 2250 mL/min is simply ventilation of the dead space.

Lung volumes

The measurement of lung volumes using spirometry, and how lung volume can change with respect to time are important clinical tests of lung function. They vary between individuals and are influenced by age, gender, size and posture. However, standard values are available and variations from this can be useful in the diagnosis of lung pathology. The most important examples, illustrated in Fig. 11.1 are given in Table 11.1.

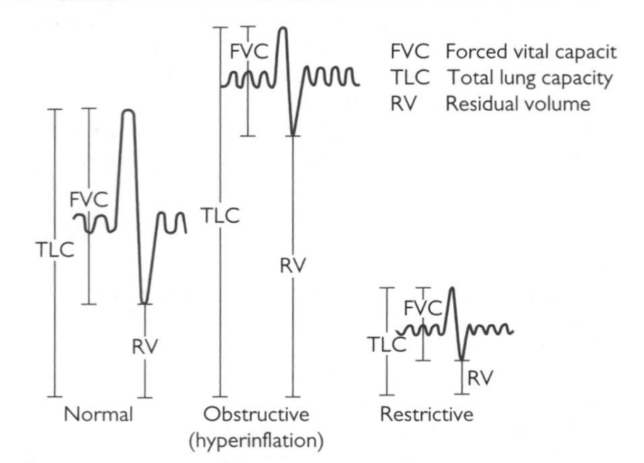

Fig. 11.1 Lung volumes: physiological and pathological.
Reproduced from M Longmore et al., *Oxford Handbook of Clinical Medicine, Eight Edition,* 2010, p. 159, by permission of Oxford University Press

Of the lung volumes described in Table 11.1, residual capacity (and any other lung volumes which incorporate it) cannot be directly measured with spirometry, since this is the volume that cannot be exhaled). In order to assess these volumes an alternative technique, for example, helium dilution, is required. Helium dilution involves allowing a known concentration of helium in a known volume to equilibrate in the lungs (a second volume) over several breathes. The concentration of helium in the circuit is then re-measured. As the pulmonary circulation does not absorb helium, the initial amount of helium and the final amount of helium can

Table 11.1 Different measures of lung volume using spirometry and their definitions

Name (abbreviation)	Description
Residual volume (RV)	Volume of gas in the lungs after a maximal expiration
Functional residual capacity (FRC)	Volume of gas in the lungs after a normal expiration
Inspiratory reserve volume (IRV)	Volume of extra gas that can be inhaled at the end of a normal inspiration by a maximal inspiratory effort
Expiratory reserve volume (ERV)	Volume of extra gas that can be exhaled at the end of a normal expiration by a maximal expiratory effort
Inspiratory capacity (IC)	Volume of gas that can be inhaled following a normal expiration by a maximal inspiratory effort
Tidal volume (V_T)	Amount of gas inhaled or exhaled during one normal breath
Vital capacity (VC)	Amount of gas that can be inhaled by a maximal inspiratory effort following a maximal expiration
Total lung capacity (TLC)	The total volume of the lungs at the end of a maximal inspiratory effort

be equated (concentration × each respective volume), and from this total lung volume calculated.

Restrictive lung diseases restrict lung expansion and result from small lung volumes. Examples include:

- *Extrinsic conditions:* neuromuscular disease (e.g. Guillain Barré), obesity, kyphosis.
- *Intrinsic conditions:* pulmonary fibrosis, infant respiratory distress syndrome (from lack of surfactant), pleural effusions.

The change in lung volume with respect to time is an indication of airway resistance and obstruction to flow. *In vivo*, the uppermost parts of the bronchiolar tree contribute most to the total resistance because, although individually their radius is large, small bronchioles, and terminal bronchioles are much greater in number and therefore have a larger combined surface area. About one-third of total airway resistance arises from the nose, pharynx, and larynx—mouth-breathing (for example, during exercise) significantly reduces this value. Of the lower bronchial tree the greatest resistance to airflow occurs in medium-sized bronchi.

During a forced expiration intrapleural pressure rises to positive levels as described previously. While this increases the driving force for air to exit the lungs, it also causes compression of the airways, which increases their resistance and decreases airflow. Since the effect on airways resistance is greater, there is a certain peak expiratory flow rate (measurable using a peak flow meter) above which increases in expiratory effort do not result in increases in expiratory rate. This peak flow rate decreases as airway resistance increases. Obstructive airway disease (for example, asthma) reduces peak flow rate and also the proportion of vital capacity that can be expired in 1 sec (see Fig. 11.2). FEV1/FVC of less than 70% is therefore used to define obstructive lung disease, which can be fixed (chronic obstructive airways disease, emphysema, and chronic bronchitis) or variable (such as asthma where measuring diurnal variation in peak flow may be more useful).

Airway obstruction can cause turbulent flow in the airways, which can be heard as wheezing under certain pathological conditions. Whether airflow in a given tube is laminar or turbulent is determined by the ratio of inertial to viscous forces (the Reynolds number). When inertial forces

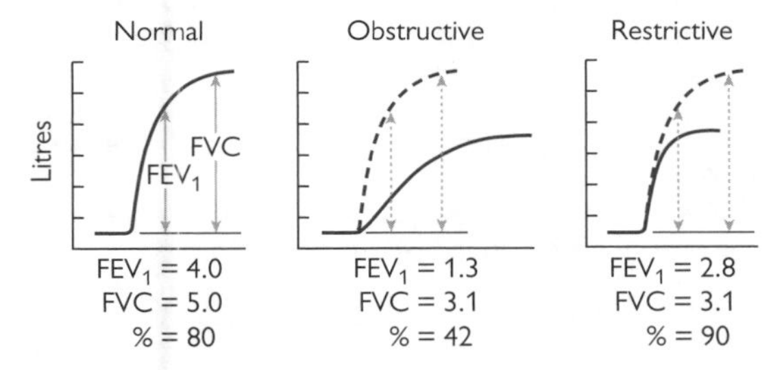

Fig. 11.2 Examples of spirograms.

Reproduced from M Longmore et al., *Oxford Handbook of Clinical Medicine, Eight Edition*, 2010, p. 157, by permission of Oxford University Press

dominate (at high Reynolds number), such as when airways become narrowed, flow becomes turbulent. Wheeze that is inspiratory in nature tends to originate from obstruction in the upper airways, whereas expiratory wheeze tends to come from obstruction of the lower airways.

Another way to assess lung function is by recording a maximum flow/volume loop. For this, a subject inspires rapidly from residual volume to total lung capacity and then exhales as hard as possible back to residual volume. Resistance to flow is greatest at low volumes in lower airway obstruction (e.g. COPD), while resistance to expiratory flow is greatest at higher lung volumes for upper airway obstruction, as shown in Fig. 11.3.

Diffusion

Under normal conditions the process of ventilation continuously fills the alveoli with (a mixture approximating to) atmospheric air while mixed venous blood enters the pulmonary circulation. The gases in these two compartments are brought into close contact with each other and O_2 and CO_2 move in opposite directions between them across the blood–gas barrier by simple diffusion. The blood–gas barrier is formed of the alveolar epithelium, the capillary endothelium, and their fused basement membranes and associated structures.

The rate at which gas moves from a region of high partial pressure to a region of low partial pressure is proportional to the partial pressure difference and solubility of the gas concerned and the surface area of the barrier to be traversed, and inversely proportional to the thickness of the barrier and the square root of the molecular weight of the gas under consideration (Fick's law). The total surface area of the alveoli taking part in gas exchange in the lungs is large (50–100 m^2) and the thickness of this barrier is only 0.3 μm. The structure of the blood–gas barrier is therefore optimized for rapid gas exchange. At 37°C, CO_2 is some 20 times more soluble in water than O_2 and, since they are of similar molecular weight, the rate of diffusion of CO_2 is much greater, even though the partial pressure gradient for CO_2 is not so great. It must be remembered that the mechanisms that exist in red blood cells for increasing the solubility of O_2 and CO_2 do not exist in the blood–gas barrier and do not speed up the rate of diffusion.

On average, one cardiac cycle is more than enough time for rapidly diffusing gases (for example, CO_2, normally O_2) to equilibrate across the blood–gas barrier and they are said to be 'perfusion limited'. In other words, the level of perfusion in the capillary limits the amount of the gas that can cross the blood–gas barrier and the alveoli are in equilibrium with the blood at the end of the capillary. More slowly diffusing gases (CO, O_2 under certain pathological conditions) are said to be 'diffusion limited'. That is to say that the level of diffusion limits the uptake of the gas into the blood.

At altitude (when the partial pressure gradient for O_2 is reduced) or during diseases, which lead to thickening of the alveolar wall, the transport of O_2 can become diffusion limited. Exercise significantly reduces the length of time taken for blood to traverse the length of a pulmonary capillary,

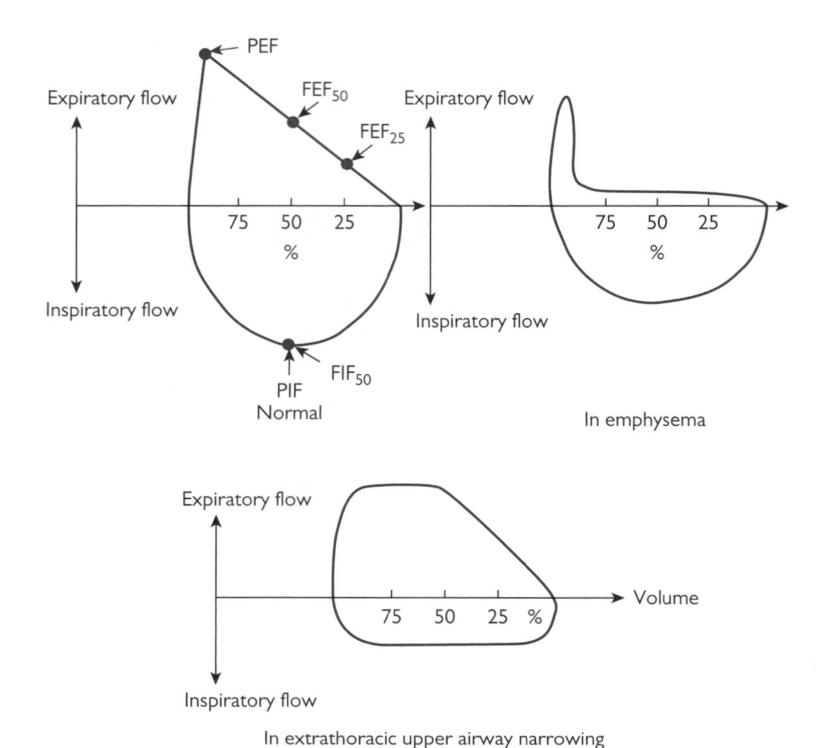

Fig. 11.3 Flow volume loops.

PEF=peak expiratory flow; FEF_{50}=forced expiratory flow at 50% TLC; FEF_{25}=forced expiratory flow at 25% TLC; PIF=peak inspiratory flow; FIF_{50}=forced inspiratory flow at 50% TLC.

although in healthy subjects the rate of diffusion of O_2 is still sufficiently high to prevent its transport from becoming diffusion limited.

The transport of CO across the blood–gas interface is always diffusion limited and as it binds haemoglobin tightly, it is therefore used to measure the properties of the blood–gas interface. The amount of CO disappearing from an inhaled sample over 10 sec is measured and, assuming that the amount of starting CO in the blood is negligible, reflects the area and thickness of the blood–gas barrier. From this the CO transfer co-efficient can be calculated (K_{CO}) and when multiplied by alveolar volume (V_A), this gives a transfer factor (TL_{CO}), which is reduced in interstitial lung disease, and in chronic thromboembolic disease or pulmonary hypertension where pulmonary perfusion is limited. It can appear to be supra-normal in conditions, such as pulmonary haemorrhage where haemoglobin in the alveolar space facilitates the uptake of CO. Owing to its high solubility, the transport of CO_2 is rarely diffusion limited.

In an ideal lung with no dead space the partial pressure of CO_2 at the end of expiration (end tidal CO_2 or $PeCO_2$) would approach that of arterial CO_2 ($PaCO_2$). Conversely, if no diffusion of CO_2 occurred as the entire lung was dead space, the end tidal CO_2 would be the same as inspired CO_2 (P_ICO_2) which is ~0. The Bohr equation uses this logic to produce an estimate of the volume of dead space (V_{DS}) in the lung as a ratio of tidal volume (V_T) using the following equation:

$$V_{DS}/V_T = PaCO2 - PeCO2/PaCO2$$

Composition of alveolar gases

The partial pressure of O_2 or CO_2 in an ideal alveolus is determined by the content of the gas in the inspired air and rate at which the gas is removed or added to the alveolus in proportion to the rate at which the alveolus is ventilation. It follows from this that an increase in ventilation will be accompanied by an increase in alveolar O_2 and a decrease in alveolar CO_2.

The composition of alveolar gases can be calculated from the alveolar gas equations, which are given by;

$$PAO_2 = P_IO_2 - (\dot{V}O_2 / \dot{V}_A) \cdot P_{Atm\cdot} \text{ and}$$

$$PACO_2 = P_ICO_2 + (\dot{V}CO_2 / \dot{V}_A) \cdot P_{Atm\cdot}$$
$$= (\dot{V}CO_2 / \dot{V}_A) \cdot P_{Atm\cdot} \left(\text{as } P_ICO_2 \text{ is} \sim 0\right)$$

Rearranging the later equation to make $\dot{V}_A$ the subject and substituting into the first equation gives us:

$$PAO_2 = P_IO_2 - PACO_2/R$$

where PAO_2, P_IO_2 and $PACO_2$ are the partial pressures of oxygen in alveolar (A) and inspired air (I), and carbon dioxide in alveolar air respectively. R is the respiratory quotient, which is the ratio of CO_2 production ($\dot{V}CO_2$) to O_2 utilization ($\dot{V}O_2$). R is dependent upon dietary status and other factors, but is normally about 0.8.

PAO_2 can be calculated for an individual patient knowing the percentage of inspired oxygen (P_IO_2), measuring $PaCO_2$ (which is approximately equal to $PACO_2$) from an arterial blood gas and assuming R to be 0.8.

An arterial blood gas will also give PaO_2, and so an average alveolar-arterial (Aa) oxygen gradient for the lungs can be calculated which is usually less than 3 kPa (Box 11.3).

Ventilation and perfusion matching

Both ventilation and perfusion vary throughout the lung and even in the physiological situation they are not perfectly matched.

Regional differences in ventilation

In upright subject the apices of the lungs are ventilated less efficiently than the bases. This can be observed by analysing the distribution of inhaled radioactive gas (for example, ^{133}Xe). The apex of the lung must support the lungs weight due to gravity and is, therefore, more distended and less compliant. The base of the lung undergoes a larger volume change during ventilation because at the beginning of inspiration it is relatively less inflated and thus more compliant as the diaphragm moves downwards. This effect is gravity dependent and in the supine position anterior regions of the lung become the best ventilated.

Pulmonary perfusion

Considerable inequality of perfusion exists within the lung. Radioactive technetium macro aggregated albumin (Tc99m-MAA) can be used together with a gamma camera to visualize this. In the upright human lung blood flow decreases linearly from the base to apex. This is affected by changes to posture and activity. Gravity is the major determinant of perfusion since the hydrostatic pressure in significantly lower than in the systemic circulation. The mean pressure within the pulmonary system is 9–18 mmHg, with systolic and diastolic pressures usually less than 30 and 15 mmHg, respectively. As right- and left-sided cardiac outputs are matched then it also follows that pulmonary vascular resistance is significantly smaller than systemic vascular resistance.

In addition, increased pressure within the pulmonary circulation (for example, from increases in either right-sided cardiac output or pulmonary venous pressure) lowers pulmonary vascular resistance even further. This is due to *recruitment* of normally closed vessels towards the apices of the lungs, as well as *distension* of already open vessels. Recruitment and distension normally occur together.

The lung is divided into zones according to the perfusion pattern seen in the upright lung from apices to base (see Fig. 11.4);

- *Zone 1:* alveolar pressure greater than pulmonary arterial pressure—no flow, i.e. dead space.
- *Zone 2:* pulmonary arterial pressure is greater than alveolar pressure—blood flow is therefore determined by arterial alveolar difference (not arterial venous difference because venous pressure is so low and much lower than alveolar pressure).
- *Zone 3:* venous pressure exceeds alveolar pressure (flow determined by arterial venous pressure difference in usual way). As one moves down this zone perfusion increases due to distension of blood vessels.

Ventilation–perfusion relationships

The matching of ventilation and perfusion in all regions of the lung is a critical determinant of healthy gas exchange. The ventilation–perfusion ratio is a useful measure of this. Regions of the lung that are under-perfused (resulting in an increased $\dot{V}/\dot{Q}$ ratio, and an increase in dead space) exhibit a gas composition approaching that of inspired air, and similarly, under-ventilated areas (decreased $\dot{V}/\dot{Q}$ ratio, and increased right to left shunt) result in decreased PO_2 and increased PCO_2 in pulmonary venous blood; in other words, the gas composition approaches that of mixed venous blood. For an individual alveolus, the partial pressure of oxygen could be considered as being dependent on the local $\dot{V}/\dot{Q}$ ratio by modifying the alveolar gas equation as follows:

$$PAO_2 = P_IO_2 - (\dot{Q}/\dot{V}_A)\cdot P_{Atm}.$$

The effect of a regional mismatch in ventilation and perfusion on whole lung function is to reduce its efficiency as a gas exchanger (increase $PaCO_2$ and decrease PaO_2). However, *in vivo*, the raised $PaCO_2$ results in an increase in ventilation. While this can help to eliminate extra CO_2, it is a far less efficient mechanism for compensating for reduced O_2 transfer. This is because, whereas the CO_2 dissociation curve is linear, the O_2 dissociation curve is flat at high PaO_2 values. Consequently, while it is possible to increase the excretion of CO_2 by increasing ventilation, it is more difficult to increase O_2 loading into blood.

There is a greater increase in perfusion from the apex of the lung to its base than there is for ventilation (in the upright lung). This is primarily because the density of blood

BOX 11.3 INCREASED Aa GRADIENT

An increased Aa gradient is the result of:

- Impaired diffusion (e.g. pulmonary fibrosis/oedema).
- Mismatching of ventilation to perfusion (e.g. increased shunt or dead space).

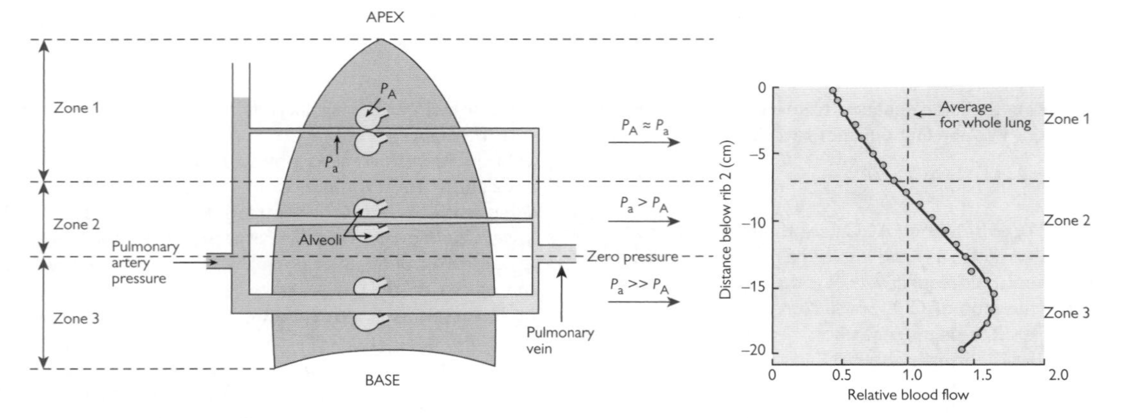

Fig. 11.4 The influence of the hydrostatic and alveolar pressures on the distribution of blood flow in the upright lung. Blood flow depends on the perfusion pressure (here assumed to be proportional to the pressure Pa in the pulmonary arteries for simplicity) and on the vascular resistance. When the perfusion pressure exceeds the alveolar pressure PA, vascular resistance is low and blood flow is high (zone 3). When perfusion pressure is low and is similar in value to the alveolar pressure, the pulmonary vessels will be compressed and vascular resistance will be increased (zone 1).

Reproduced from G Pocock and CD Richards, *Human Physiology: The Basis of Medicine, Third Edition,* 2006, Figure 16.21, p. 389, by permission of Oxford University Press

is greater than inspired air. The $\dot{V}/\dot{Q}$ ratio is, therefore, greatest at the apex of the lung and least at its base (see Fig. 11.5).

An uneven $\dot{V}/\dot{Q}$ ratio results in a decrease in the oxygenation of the blood for two reasons;

- The apical regions of the lung are proportionately better ventilated, than they are perfused and, therefore, the basal regions, which are proportionately better perfused than they are ventilated, dominate the PO_2 of blood leaving the lung.

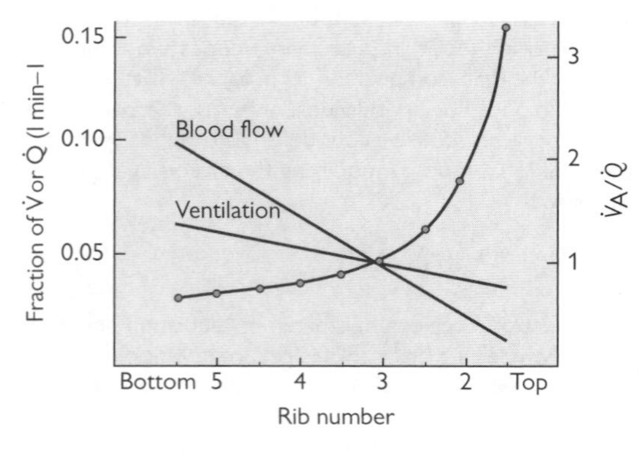

Fig. 11.5 The distribution of ventilation, blood flow, and the ventilation–perfusion ratio in the normal upright lung. Straight lines have been drawn through the data for ventilation and blood flow (data shown in Fig. 11.4). Note that the ventilation–perfusion ratio rises slowly at first, and then rapidly towards the top of the lung.

Reproduced from G Pocock and CD Richards, *Human Physiology: The Basis of Medicine, Third Edition,* 2006, Figure 16.22, p. 330, by permission of Oxford University Press

- The Hb–O_2 dissociation curve is flat at high PO_2 values. Therefore, although well-ventilated regions of the lung can increase PO_2, they do not increase the concentration by a corresponding amount, and can certainly not compensate for under-ventilated regions of the lung. The CO_2 dissociation curve is linear in the physiological range and, therefore, under-ventilated regions of the lung do not contribute to the elevation of total CO_2 in blood leaving the lungs.

In healthy upright subjects, the depression of PO_2 in blood leaving the lung by $\dot{V}/\dot{Q}$ mismatch is trivial producing an Aa gradient of less than 3 kPa. It can become far more significant in disease where the degree of mismatch is far greater. $\dot{V}/\dot{Q}$ mismatching is limited physiologically as hypoxic regions of the lungs undergo vascular vasoconstriction. The precise mechanism underlying this is unknown, but it occurs in isolated lung and may be at least in part related to the production of cADP ribose, which causes the release calcium from intracellular stores in pulmonary vascular smooth muscle in response to hypoxia, and/or oxygen sensitive potassium channels which close during hypoxia, depolarise the cell membrane and cause calcium influx via voltage gated calcium channels. It is believed that this response directs blood flow away from under-ventilated (hypoxic) areas of the lung. At high altitude global hypoxic pulmonary vasoconstriction can greatly increase pulmonary vascular resistance and cause right heart failure. If the hypoxic pulmonary vasoconstriction is not evenly distributed, it can direct flow to less constricted vessels and cause high altitude pulmonary oedema (HAPE).

Oxygen and carbon dioxide transport

Oxygen transport in the blood

Oxygen is transported in the blood in two distinct forms; dissolved in solution and complexed to haemoglobin (Hb). Hb is packaged in red blood cells (erythrocytes) to prevent its filtration by the glomerulus and to limit the rises in blood viscosity, which would arise, were Hb dissolved in plasma. The amount of oxygen dissolved in the blood is proportional to its partial pressure (Henry's law). At 37°C only 15 mL O_2 can be delivered per minute at a partial pressure of 13 kPa (100 mmHg) assuming complete extraction of all oxygen, which even then is inadequate to meet resting O_2 consumption, which is 300 mL/O_2 min. However, dissolved O_2 represents the major pathway for transport of O_2 across capillary walls to respiring cells, and the only pathway from the alveoli to red blood cells.

Haemoglobin (Hb) is a 64.5 kDa tetramer made up of 2α (141 amino acids) and 2β (146 amino acids) subunits (although a number of physiological and pathological variants exist). Each protein subunit is bound to a haem- group containing a porphyrin ring with four pyroles and a central ferrous (Fe^{2+}) ion at the centre (see Chapter 7, 'Haematology'). Each molecule of haemoglobin may therefore bind up to four O_2 molecules. The amount of O_2 bound to a sample of Hb can be expressed either as a concentration (normally mL O_2/100 mL blood) or, alternatively, as a percentage saturation of maximal O_2 capacity. The reaction between Hb and O_2 is both rapid and reversible. Binding of O_2 to Hb is cooperative such that the binding of each O_2 molecule to the Hb tetramer facilitates the binding of the next. This positive co-operativity is a particular property of tetrameric Hb. The hill co-efficient for Hb is, therefore, 2.8, rather than 4 (see Chapter 8, 'Clinical Pharmacology'). The Hb dissociation curve compared to that of myoglobin can be seen in Fig. 11.6.

Increases in H^+, CO_2 and temperature each shift the Hb-O_2 dissociation curve to the right and favour the unloading of O_2. This is clearly of physiological benefit in metabolically active muscle, which will have a high demand for O_2 and where pH will be decreased, CO_2 production raised and at an increased temperature. The effects of pH and CO_2 on the Hb-O_2 dissociation curve are known collectively as the Bohr effect. 2,3-diphosphoglycerate (2,3-DPG) produced by erythrocytes during glycolysis, binds to Hb and reduces its affinity for O_2. The production of 2,3-DPG is raised during hypoxic conditions also favouring the delivery of O_2 to the tissues.

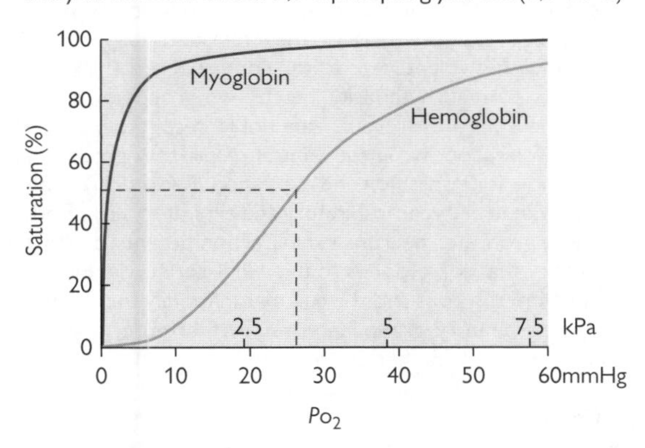

Fig. 11.6 A comparison between the oxygen dissociation curves for myoglobin and hemoglobin. Myoglobin has a P50 value of about 0.13 kPa (1 mmHg) while hemoglobin has a P50 of 3.46 kPa (26 mmHg).

Reproduced from G Pocock and CD Richards, *Human Physiology: The Basis of Medicine, Third Edition,* 2006, Figure 13.8, p. 235, by permission of Oxford University Press

Many variants and modified forms of haemoglobin have been described, only a few of which will be detailed here;

- *Sickle haemoglobin* (HbS) results from a mutation of the β-globin polypeptide. HbS polymerizes, especially under conditions where O_2 is low or acidity is high (for example, in respiring tissues). The polymerized protein distorts the shape of the erythrocyte, making it sickled-shaped, and causes it to obstruct small capillaries triggering sickling crises (see Chapter 7, 'Haematology').
- *Foetal haemoglobin* (HbF) has a raised affinity for O_2 compared with adult haemoglobin. This facilitates delivery of O_2 to the foetus from maternal uterine blood, which is at a lower partial pressure than normal arterial blood. HbF tends to disappear from foetal red blood cells a few months after birth.
- *Myoglobin* is a monomeric form of haemoglobin expressed in striated muscle fibres. It has a much higher affinity for O_2 than haemoglobin and does not demonstrate cooperativity in its binding of O_2. Myoglobin acts as a store of O_2 available in hypoxic conditions, and also allows O_2 to be delivered to respiring cells when muscle is contracted and perfusion reduced.
- *Carboxyhaemoglobin* CO has an affinity for Hb approximately 200 times that of O_2. Consequently, inhaling even a low concentration of CO causes anaemia by reducing the amount of Hb available to bind O_2. Carboxyhaemoglobin is red in colour, so patients suffering from CO poisoning do not appear anaemic.
- *Methaemoglobin* contains Fe^{3+} ions in its haem groups, rather than Fe^{2+}. Oxidizing agents like nitrites and sulphonamides can cause this to occur. Methaemoglobin does not carry O_2 efficiently. Erythrocytes contain an enzyme, methaemoglobin reductase, which can catalyse the reduction of the Fe^{3+} ion back to its Fe^{2+} form.

Carbon dioxide transport in the blood

Carbon dioxide is transported in the blood in three forms, namely dissolved CO_2, HCO_3^- and complexed to blood proteins as carbamino CO_2. In arterial blood HCO_3^- makes up 90% of total CO_2 carried, dissolved CO_2 5% and carbamino CO_2 5%. In venous blood the equivalent proportions are 60, 10%, and 30%.

- *Dissolved CO_2:* obeys Henry's law and, since it is 20 times more soluble in blood than O_2, accounts for a significant proportion of total CO_2 transported by blood.
- *Bicarbonate:* is formed by the hydration of dissolved CO_2 to form carbonic acid, which subsequently dissociates into H^+ and HCO_3^-. The hydration reaction is accelerated 13,000-fold by the enzyme carbonic anhydrase, which is found within erythrocytes, both intracellularly and on their surface.

$$CO_2 + H_2O \leftrightarrow H_2CO_3 \leftrightarrow H^+ + HCO_3^-$$

CO_2 diffuses across red blood cell membranes into the cytosol where the hydration reaction to form carbonic acid proceeds. The carbonic acid generated subsequently dissociates into $H^+ + HCO_3^-$. In order to allow this reaction to proceed HCO_3^- is transported out of the erythrocyte in exchange for extracellular Cl^- ions on AE1 (anion-exchanger isoform 1) and protons are buffered by intracellular buffers (primarily Hb, whose deoxygenated form is a more powerful proton buffer than its oxygenated form). The erythrocyte intracellular chloride concentration is, therefore, higher for venous erythrocytes for than arterial erythrocytes (chloride shift):

- *Carbamino CO_2*: CO_2 can bind to the terminal amine groups of blood proteins, either intracellularly or extracellularly. Hb is the most significant protein for carrying CO_2 in this way and, deoxygenated Hb binds CO_2 more readily than oxygenated CO_2.

The carbon dioxide dissociation curve is right-shifted (promoting offloading of CO_2) by the presence of oxyhaemoglobin. This is known as the Haldane effect and is analogous to the Bohr effect for O_2 carriage (see Fig. 11.7A, B). The Haldane effect arises because deoxyhaemoglobin is a weaker acid than oxyhaemoglobin and more readily binds either H^+ (allowing the dissociation of carbonic acid to proceed) or the weak acid CO_2 (allowing the formation of carbamino CO_2). Similarly, under acid conditions the offloading of O_2 from oxyhaemoglobin is promoted (Bohr effect). The Haldane effect and the Bohr effect both arise because deoxygenated haemoglobin is a weaker acid (better proton acceptor) than oxygenated haemoglobin.

Control of breathing

The act of breathing is largely automated and is regulated to meet the body's requirements for O_2 uptake and CO_2 excretion. It can be voluntarily over-ridden for short periods and certain activities (such as sneezing, coughing, swallowing, or speech) also require short-term adjustments to breathing pattern.

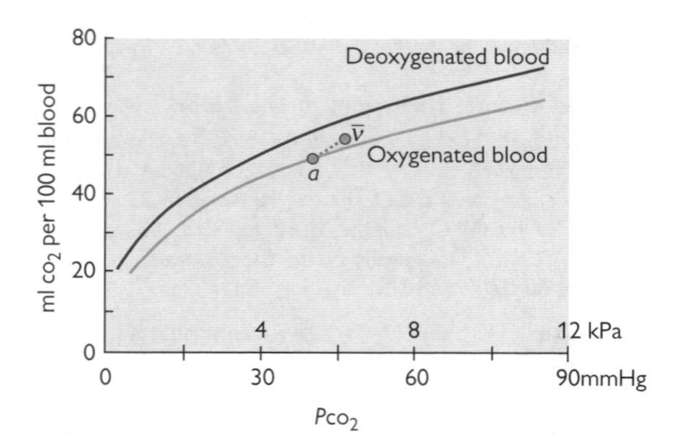

Fig. 11.7A The carbon dioxide dissociation curve for whole blood and the Haldane effect. *a*, arterial blood; $\bar{v}$, mixed venous blood.

Reproduced from G Pocock and CD Richards, *Human Physiology: The Basis of Medicine, Third Edition*, 2006, Figure 13.10, p. 236, by permission of Oxford University Press

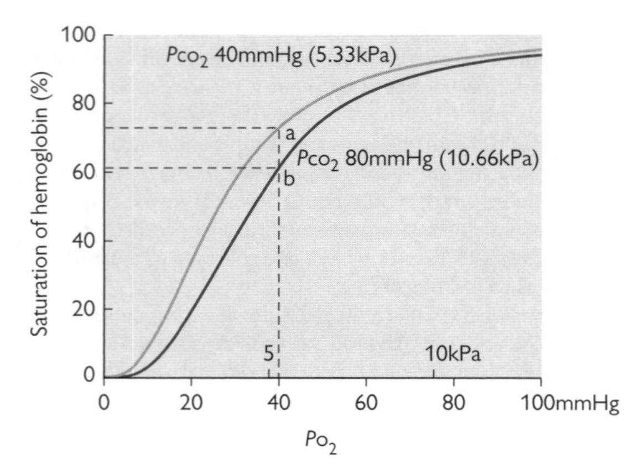

Fig. 11.7B The effect of increasing PCO_2 on the oxyhemoglobin dissociation curve. As PCO_2 increases the P50 value for the dissociation curve is shifted to the right. This is known as the Bohr shift. The dissociation curve is affected in a similar manner by a fall in pH or an increase in 2,3-DPG or temperature. The effect of the rightward shift is to decrease the affinity of hemoglobin for oxygen. This is shown by the difference in hemoglobin saturation when PO_2 is 5.33 kPa (40 mmHg) as PCO_2 increases from 5.33 kPa (40 mmHg) (point a) to 10.66 kPa (80 mmHg) (point b).

Reproduced from G Pocock and CD Richards, *Human Physiology: The Basis of Medicine, Third Edition*, 2006, Figure 13.7, p. 234, by permission of Oxford University Press

Central control

The respiratory rhythm is generated in respiratory centres in the medulla. Sectioning of the brainstem above these areas abolishes voluntary (cortical) control of breathing, but leaves its normal rhythmicity intact. Two groups of upper motor neurons are relevant—the dorsal respiratory group initiate inspiration, while the ventral respiratory group are responsible for inspiration and expiration. Reciprocal inhibition is evident between inspiratory and expiratory cells. Both of these groups of neurons exhibit action potentials with a frequency that corresponds to the ventilatory cycle. Higher inputs from the pons and the cortex can modify the rhythm of the respiratory group neurons. Furthermore, afferent fibres (largely from chemoreceptors, see 'Chemoreceptor control of breathing') can also regulate their activity.

Certain reflex responses from the lungs modify breathing behaviour. The Hering-Breuer reflex describes the inhibition of inspiration as the lungs are stretched. This reflex pathway limits the depth of inspiration, particularly during heavy breathing.

Irritant receptors in the nasal mucosa and other airways result in a reflex sneeze or cough. This response helps to clear the airways of the original irritant. J-receptors, located in the lung interstitium, respond if the lungs become congested, and limit the rate and depth of breathing.

Chemoreceptor control of breathing

The most important function of the lungs is to regulate the levels of CO_2 and O_2 within the blood. PCO_2 is the main factor control respiration in healthy individuals, and is sensed by central chemoreceptors located in the ventral surface of the medulla and peripheral chemoreceptors in the carotid body, and in the wall of the aortic arch. Sensing of PO_2 is via the peripheral chemoreceptors only. These organs are able to respond to changes in blood gases and initiate rapid changes in respiratory rate in response. An increase in ventilatory rate will tend to increase PaO_2 and have the reverse effect on $PaCO_2$.

Central chemoreceptors are responsive to changes in the pH of the extracellular fluid of the brain. In turn, the pH of this compartment is determined by the pH of blood and CSF. The blood–brain barrier and the CSF–brain barrier are relatively impermeably to charged proton equivalents (for example H^+ or HCO_3^-) and, therefore, it is PCO_2 that is the major determinant of pH of the brain interstitium. Increases in CO_2 shift the equilibrium:

$$CO_2 + H_2O \leftrightarrow H^+ + HCO_3^-$$

to the right and thus decrease pH. Central chemoreceptors respond to this by increasing action potential frequency in their afferent nerve, which results in an increase in ventilatory rate, which will reduce PCO_2. It is important to note that the pH of the CSF is more sensitive to changes in PCO_2 than the pH of the brain interstitium. This is because the proton-buffering capacity of the CSF is lower. Consequently, ventilatory rate is most sensitive to the composition of this compartment.

Peripheral chemoreceptors are small (7 × 5 mm) encapsulated organs, which receive a high blood supply and, in contrast to central chemoreceptors sense PO_2, pH and PCO_2 in arterial blood. The afferent nerve fibres of peripheral chemoreceptors fire more frequently in response to lowered PaO_2 or arterial pH, or raised $PaCO_2$. They are the only part of the respiratory system, which is able to elicit an increase in ventilation in response to reduced PaO_2. The exact cellular mechanism by which they sense O_2 is unknown, but may involve mitochondrial cytochromes, the metabolic sensor AMP-activated protein kinase (AMPK), and/or oxygen/pH sensitive potassium channels. The firing rate of the afferent nerve shows a large increase as PO_2 is lowered below about 13 kPa (100 mmHg)—above this value the peripheral chemoreceptors are relatively insensitive to changes in oxygen tension. Although peripheral chemoreceptors are responsive to alterations in PO_2, this effect is quantitatively less important than their response to PCO_2. This is important in patients with COPD who are chronic CO_2 retainers. In these patients, the main factor determining respiratory drive becomes PaO_2. Administering high concentrations of inhaled oxygen to these patients therefore risks reducing respiratory rate further and worsening their respiratory acidosis. The percentage of oxygen administered therefore needs to be carefully controlled with on-going monitoring of arterial blood gases to ensure adequate oxygenation without worsening CO_2 retention.

The carotid bodies (although not the aortic arch chemoreceptors) are also responsive to decreases in pH not elicited by an alteration to PCO_2. This response explains the hyperventilation observed in patients suffering from, for example, diabetic ketoacidosis (Kussmaul breathing).

Whole-body regulation of gas tensions

In general, CO_2 tensions are a more important determinant of ventilatory rate than O_2 tensions. This can be demonstrated experimentally by precisely controlling the composition of inspired gas, while simultaneously recording ventilatory rate. Until a threshold value is reached (about 13 kPa/100 mmHg) reducing oxygen tensions have only a minor effect on ventilation. In contrast, even small increases in CO_2 tensions dramatically increase ventilatory drive. Hypoxia does increase the sensitivity of ventilatory rate to PCO_2.

Drugs used in the treatment of respiratory disease

For drugs used in the treatment of respiratory disease, see Table 11.2. See Box 11.4 for drug-induced respiratory reactions.

Table 11.2 Drugs used in the treatment of respiratory disease

Bronchodilators			
Class/mechanism	Example	Common side effects	Interactions
Short acting β2 agonists	Salbutamol (inhaled or nebulized)	Tremor, headache, dry mouth, flushing, tachycardia/arrhythmia, hypokalaemia, paradoxical bronchospasm	β-blockers, diuretics (hypokalaemia), digoxin

(continued)

Table 11.2 Drugs used in the treatment of respiratory disease (*continued*)

Class/mechanism	Example	Common side effects	Interactions
Long-acting β2 agonists	Salmeterol	As for short-acting β2 agonists	As for short-acting β2 agonists
Short-acting muscarinic antagonists	Ipratropium (inhaled or nebulized)	Dry mouth, sedation, flushing, tachycardia, constipation, urinary retention, acute angle glaucoma	Other anticholinergic medications (tricyclic antidepressants, anti-Parkinsonian drugs)
Long-acting muscarinic antagonists	Tiotropium	As for short-acting muscarinic antagonists	As for short-acting muscarinic antagonists
Phosphodiesterase inhibitors/adenosine receptor antagonists	Aminophylline, theophylline (oral or iv)	Tachycardia/arrhythmias, nausea, diarrhoea, seizures	Inhibitors and inducers of cytochrome P450 (phenytoin, cimetidine, erythromycin, ciprofloxacin)
Bronchial smooth muscle calcium channel blocker	Magnesium sulphate (iv)	Flushing, sweating, hypotension, muscle weakness, hypothermia	Sedatives, antihistamines, tricyclic antidepressants
Anti-inflammatories			
Class	**Example**	**Common side effects**	**Interactions**
Inhaled steroids	Beclomethasone	Cough, oral candidiasis	
Systemic steroids	Prednisolone	See Chapter 15, 'Endocrinology'	See Chapter 15, 'Endocrinology'
Leukotriene antagonists	Montelukast	Indigestion, thirst, dry mouth, diarrhoea, agitation, hallucinations, depression, tremor	Rifampacin, phenobarbitone
Mast-cell stabilizers	Sodium cromoglycate	Cough, headache,	
Mucolytics			
Drug	**Mechanism of action**	**Side effects**	**Interactions**
Carbocisteine	Reduces the viscosity of mucous in COPD and bronchiectasis		Cough linctus or suppressants
Oxygen therapy			
Therapy	**Method**		**Role**
Percentage controlled oxygen	*Via a venture mask (colour coded:* blue 24%, white 28%, yellow 35%, red 40%, green 60%)		To provide oxygenation while avoiding excessive CO_2 retention in COPD
Long-term oxygen therapy	Given at home for at least 15 hr/day		Chronic hypoxaemia <7.3 or <8 kPa, where there is right heart failure or secondary polycythaemia
Continuous positive airway pressure (CPAP)	Tight fitting full-face mask and machine to blow air/oxygen at a prescribed pressure (4–20 cmH_2O). Some machines can auto-titrate the level of positive pressure on a breath-by-breath basis to maintain an open airway.		To splint the tongue and pharynx in obstructive sleep apnoea. Respiratory failure due to COPD or left ventricular failure
Bi-level positive airway pressure (BiPAP)	Provides variable control of inspiratory and expiratory positive airway pressure, either on detection of inspiration (spontaneous) or a given timing. Can be non-invasive via a securely fitting full-face mask, as well as via endotracheal intubation/tracheostomy		*Non-invasive:* respiratory failure due to COPD, left ventricular failure. *Invasive:* respiratory failure, multi-organ failure, reduced consciousness, paralysis of respiratory muscles (e.g. Guillain-Barré)

Table 11.2 Drugs used in the treatment of respiratory disease (*continued*)

Respiratory stimulant			
Drug	Mechanism of action	Side effects	Interactions
Doxapram	Stimulates peripheral chemoreceptors. Increases tidal volume and respiratory rate	Hypertension, tachycardia, seizures, tremor, sweating, vomiting	Decongestants, MAO inhibitors

BOX 11.4 DRUG-INDUCED RESPIRATORY REACTIONS

- *Bronchospasm:* aspirin, adenosine, beta-blockers, sodium chromoglycate, N-acetyl cysteine, antibiotics (e.g. amphotericin, erythromycin, sulfonamides, and aminoglycosides).
- *Cough:* angiotensin-converting enzyme inhibitors, inhaled medications, mycophenolate, mofetil, nitrofurantoin, propofol, beta-blockers.
- *Pulmonary fibrosis:* amiodarone, sulfasalazine, methotrexate, gold, nitrofurantoin, bleomycin, cyclophosphamide.
- *Pleural reactions:* methotrexate, bromocriptine, drug induced lupus.

Multiple choice questions

1. Which of the following conditions is likely to produce a higher carbon monoxide transfer co-efficient (K_{CO})?

A. Pulmonary fibrosis.
B. Alveolar haemorrhage.
C. Anaemia.
D. COPD.
E. Pulmonary oedema.

2. You are concerned that a 30-year-old man on the intensive care unit may have ARDS (acute respiratory distress syndrome). Which of the following would be consistent with this diagnosis?

A. Elevated K_{CO} (carbon monoxide transfer co-efficient).
B. Reduced lung compliance.
C. A pulmonary wedge pressure of 30 mmHg.
D. Unilateral infiltration on CXR.
E. PaO_2:FiO_2 ratio of 50 kPa (375 mmHg).

3. Concerning pulmonary anatomy, which of the following is correct?

A. The left lung has a larger volume than the right.
B. Terminal bronchioles lead to alveolar ducts.
C. The lingual forms part of the left upper lobe.
D. The glottis narrows on inspiration.
E. Posteriorly the lungs extend to the level of T10.

4. Which of the following measurements would best help distinguish upper airway obstruction from asthma?

A. Flow/volume loop.
B. Peak expiratory flow rate (PEFR).
C. FEV1/FVC.
D. TLC.
E. K_{CO}.

5. Concerning the haemoglobin-oxygen dissociation curve:

A. Low pH shifts the curve to the left.
B. 2,3-DPG shifts the curve of the left.
C. High temperature shifts the curve to the left.
D. Low PCO_2 shifts the curve to the left.
E. The shift of the curve to the left due to high PCO_2 called the Haldane effect.

6. Which of the following most commonly cause a transudative pleural effusion

A. Pneumonia.
B. Pulmonary embolism.
C. Malignancy.
D. Rheumatoid arthritis.
E. Nephrotic syndrome.

7. **A raised Aa gradient secondary to a high V/Q ratio is most likely due to:**

   A. Pulmonary embolism.
   B. Pneumothorax.
   C. Pulmonary fibrosis.
   D. Right- to left-sided shunt.
   E. Pulmonary oedema.

8. **Which of the following are indications for long-term oxygen therapy (LTOT)**

   A. PaO_2 = 8.5 kPa, $PaCO_2$ = 3.5 kPa.
   B. PaO_2 = 6 kPa during an infective exacerbation of COPD, PaO_2 = 8.5 kPa when stable.
   C. PaO_2 = 7.0 kPa, $PaCO_2$ = 7.0 kPa.
   D. PaO_2 = 7.5 kPa and mean pulmonary artery pressure of 15 kPa.
   E. PaO_2 = 8.5 kPa and Hb=19 g/dL with a red cell mass of 40 mg/kg (normal < 35 mg/kg).

9. **Which of the following drugs are NOT associated with causing pulmonary fibrosis?**

   A. Amiodarone.
   B. Sulfasalazine.
   C. Methotrexate.
   D. Bosentan.
   E. Nitrofurantoin.

10. **Regarding haemoglobin, which of the following statement is true?**

   A. Hb has a lower affinity for O_2 than Hb (O_2).
   B. Mb has a lower affinity for O_2 than Hb.
   C. HbF has a lower affinity for O_2 than HbA.
   D. Hb has a lower affinity for O_2 than Hb(CO).
   E. Hb has a lower affinity for O_2 than metHb.

For answers, please see Appendix: Answers to multiple choice questions, page 313.

CHAPTER 12

Neurology

Neuroanatomy

Together, the peripheral nervous system (PNS) and central nervous system (CNS) comprise an integrated network of neurons that allow rapid transmission and processing of information as nervous impulses. In conjunction with the endocrine system, this network is responsible for homeostasis of an organism, as well as for its behavioural patterns. In man this includes higher-level functions, such as thinking and memory, as well as more basic activities.

Nervous tissue comprises two basic cell types:

- Neurons (excitable cells that transmit nervous impulses long distances).
- Glial cells (non-neural support cells that are closely associated with neurons).

Neurons

There are approximately 10^{20} neurons in the human nervous system, of which 10^{11} are in the brain. All neurons, whether central or peripheral, include three separate parts:

- *Dendrites:* multiple long processes, specialized for receiving external stimuli from other cells.
- *Cell body (perikaryon):* containing the cell nucleus.
- *Axon:* conducts a nervous impulse to other cells. Axons form synapses with other cells (neurons and non-nerve cells) via swellings called terminal boutons.

Glial cells

From the Greek word for glue, since it was originally thought that their role was simply to 'stick' the brain together, 'glia' is an umbrella term for all the non-neuronal cell types in the CNS. There are 10 times more glial cells than neurons in the brain and they have many important functions. They insulate neurons, provide structural support and help maintain the surrounding environment, play a role in repair of neurons, and form part of the blood–brain barrier. Several different types of glial cell exist, and these differ between the PNS and CNS.

- *Astrocytes* are star-shaped cells with many processes. Their most important function is to form the blood–brain barrier. In so doing, they control metabolic exchange with the extra-cellular fluid and blood, thus controlling the extracellular environment of the brain.
- *Microglia* are small cells with multiple processes and dense drawn-out nuclei. They are the mononuclear phagocytic arm of the immune system within the CNS. They are important in inflammation and repair. When activated, the morphology of the cell changes to resemble that of the macrophage, and they perform the same functions, namely phagocytosis and antigen-presentation.
- *Oligodendrocytes* are cells found only in the CNS. They produce myelin to insulate neuronal axons and increase the speed of conduction. They can each insulate more than one neuron, unlike peripheral myelin-producing cells (Schwann cells) and wrap around their axons. Modified membrane layers with raised lipoprotein content make up the myelin that insulates the axons.
- *Schwann cells* myelinate axons in the PNS. The Schwann cell wraps its membrane around the axon. The membranes of the cell merge to form myelin (a lipoprotein). More than one cell is required to insulate each axon. There are gaps between the Schwann cells, called nodes of Ranvier, with an internodal gap of 1–2 mm (the length of the Schwann cells).
- *Unmyelinated axons* are of smaller diameter. Unmyelinated cells still have a covering of Schwann cells, but each Schwann cell can cover many unmyelinated axons. The Schwann cells lie adjacent to one another to form a continuous sheath; hence, there are no nodes of Ranvier. In the CNS, there are many unmyelinated axons, which have no sheath whatsoever.

Peripheral nervous system

The PNS is composed of all nervous tissue outside of the brain and the spinal cord. It functions as both an efferent system, conducting signals from the CNS to the periphery, and as an afferent system, transmitting sensory information to the CNS. The PNS is composed of nerves, ganglia, and nerve endings.

It can be broadly subdivided into:

- Somatic nervous system.
- Autonomic nervous system (ANS).

Somatic nervous system

The somatic nervous system is responsible for efferent signals controlling skeletal muscle, and transmitting afferent peripheral sensory information from the skin, joints, and body wall.

Dermatomes

The cutaneous distribution of somatic sensory nerves is segmental (Fig. 12.1). This results in an ordered pattern of dermatomes—regions of skin whose somatic sensory

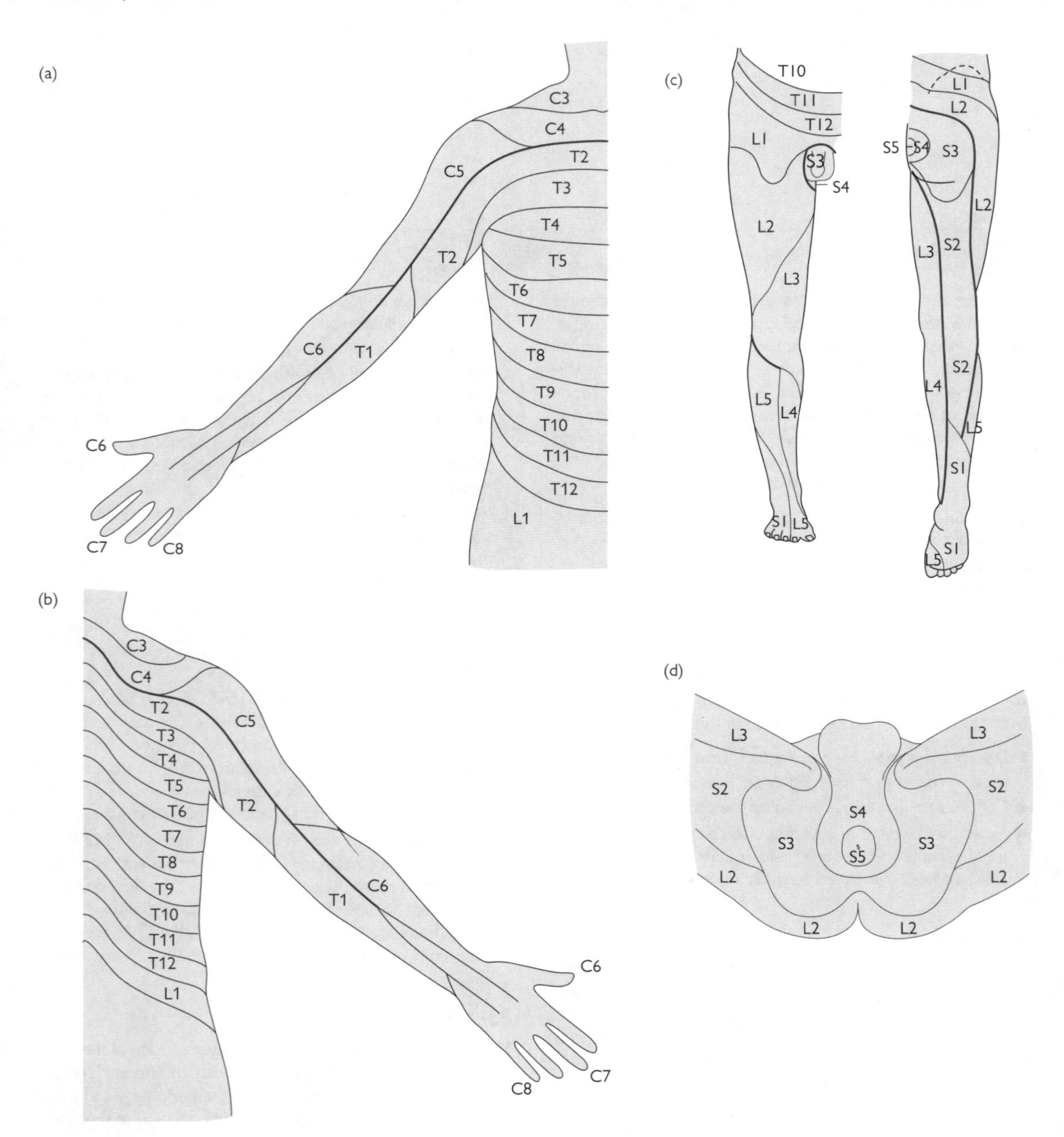

Fig. 12.1 Approximate distribution of dermatomes. (a) On the anterior aspect of the upper limb. (b) On the posterior aspect of the upper limb. (c) on the lower limb; (d) on the perineum.

Reprinted from *Aids to the examination of the Peripheral Nervous System*, 4th edition, 2000, pp. 56–59, with permission from The Guarantors of Brain

supply originates from branches of the same spinal nerve. The distribution of dermatomes is crucial to localizing the level of nerve root compression or spinal cord trauma. However, there is considerable overlap in sensory supply between adjacent dermatomes, and loss of a single nerve root, therefore, rarely produces distinguishable effects. Autonomous zones with minimal overlap that are frequently tested for loss of sensation include:

- *C5:* lateral arm and proximal forearm.
- *C6:* regions thumb and index finger.
- *C7:* middle and index finger.
- *C8:* small digit and hypothenar area.
- *L1:* inguinal region.
- *L2:* lateral thigh.
- *L3:* inferior medial thigh.
- *L4:* medial aspect of great toe.
- *L5:* medial aspect of digit II.

Myotomes

Myotomes refer to muscle groups innervated by the same spinal nerve root. Peripheral nerve damage can produce severe weakness and atrophy. Damage to a single nerve root yields detectible, but not complete weakness, due to overlap in supply. Myotomes are assessed using isometric resistive muscle testing as follows:

- *C4:* shoulder elevation.
- *C5:* upper limb abduction.
- *C6:* elbow flexion.
- *C7:* wrist flexion.
- *C8:* thumb extension.
- *T1:* digit abduction/adduction.
- *L1–L2:* hip flexion.
- *L3:* knee extension.
- *L4/L5:* ankle dorsiflexion.
- *S1/S2:* ankle plantar flexion.

Reflexes

Reflex movements are involuntary and occur independent of a command from the brain. The reflex arcs mediating these movements are composed of sensory and motor components. Reflex responses usually occur within 20 ms following specific sensory stimuli. These movements are typically defensive and involve withdrawal.

Rapid monosynaptic reflexes are mediated by a synaptic connection between a sensory neurone and an α-motor neuron in the ventral horn of the spinal cord (e.g. knee-jerk reflex; see Fig. 12.2(a)). Marginally slower polysynaptic reflexes relay on spinal interneurons between the sensory input and motor output neurons to mediate their effect (Fig. 12.2(b)). Frequently, polysynaptic reflexes act to modulate efferent motor activity on the basis of proprioceptive information provided by sensory afferents.

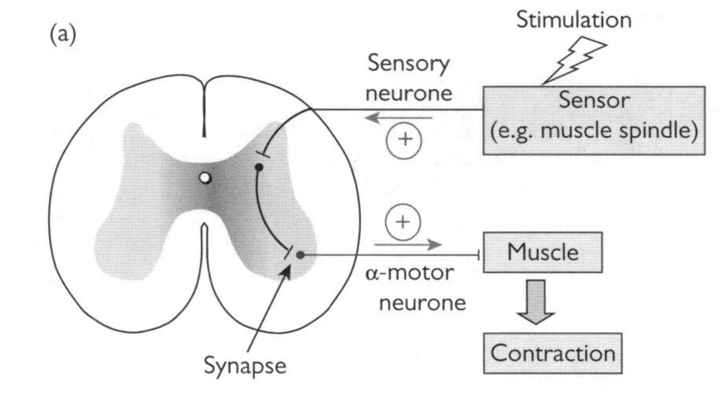

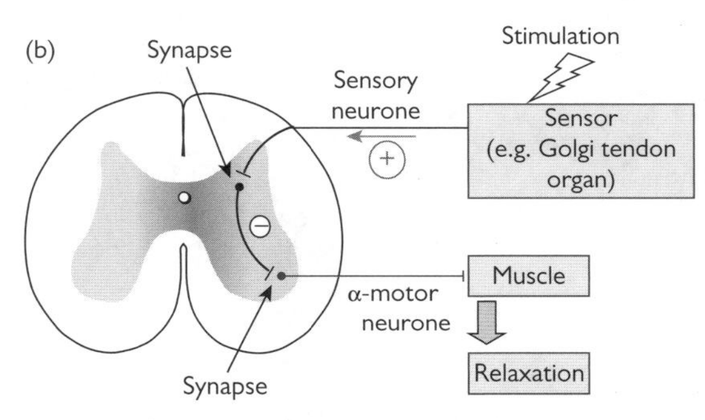

Fig. 12.2 (a) Monosynaptic reflex arc. (b) Polysynaptic reflex. An interposed inhibitory interneurone results in reduced stimulation of the α-motor neuron, leading to muscle relaxation.

The following reflexes can be used to assess the level of damage in the nervous system:

- *Ankle:* S1, S2.
- *Knee:* L3, L4.
- *Supinator:* C5, C6.
- *Biceps:* C5, C6.
- *Triceps:* C7.

Autonomic nervous system

The ANS broadly consists of pathways composed of preganglionic and post-ganglionic neurons supplying a peripheral organ (excluding the sympathetic supply to the adrenal medulla).

There are a number of similarities between the sympathetic and parasympathetic nervous systems (see Table 12.1):

- Both feature a single synapse, found in ganglia positioned between the spinal cord and the target organ or issue. The neurones that stretch between the spinal cord and the ganglia are called preganglionic, those between the ganglia and the target are post-ganglionic. The sympathetic nerves that supply the adrenal medulla are an exception to this rule, as they do not feature ganglia.

Table 12.1 Differences between the parasympathetic and sympathetic nervous systems

	Parasympathetic	Sympathetic
Spinal outflow	Cranial (nerves III, VII, IX, X) and sacral	Thoracic and lumbar
Position of ganglia	Near (or in) target tissue	Near spinal cord (paravertebral sympathetic chain)
Primary neurotransmitter at target	ACh	Mainly noradrenaline (ACh in sweat glands and at adrenal medulla)
Primary receptors at tissue	ACh muscarinic receptors (M_1, M_2, M_3)	Adrenoceptors (α_1, α_2, β_1, β_2, β_3)
Co-transmitters	Nitric oxide (NO), vasoactive intestinal peptide (VIP)	ATP, neuropeptide Y

- The neurotransmitter released by the preganglionic neurone at the ganglionic synapse is exclusively ACh, which acts on nicotinic ACh receptors on the post-ganglionic neurone to propagate the signal.
- A cocktail of neurotransmitters is often released at the synapse with the tissue. Cotransmitters often have different functions and durations of action.

There are also important differences as can be seen in Table 12.1.

Sympathetic division

The sympathetic division is known as the thoracolumbar outflow (T1–L2/3). Preganglionic cell bodies are located in the lateral horn of the thoracic spinal cord. Preganglionic neurons synapse on:

- *Paravertebral ganglia:* cervical (3), thoracic (12), lumbar (2/3), and pelvic.
- *Prevertebral ganglia:* coeliac, aorticorenal, superior mesenteric, inferior mesenteric (see Enteric division below).
- *Adrenal medulla:* chromaffin cells.

Parasympathetic division

The parasympathetic division is known as the craniosacral outflow. Preganglionic cell bodies originate in the brainstem (see 'The cranial nerves') and in the sacral spinal cord. These synapse on their corresponding post-ganglionic neurons close to their target organ.

Enteric division

A subdivision of the ANS forms a complex visceral parasympathetic/sympathetic network supplying the GI tract, with cell bodies contained in the intramural plexus of the intestine wall (see Fig. 12.3).

Central nervous system

The CNS broadly refers to the structures of the brain and the spinal cord, but can be further divided into:

- The telencephalon
- The diencephalon.
- The mesencephalon.
- The rhombencephalon.
- The spinal cord.

The eye and ear will also be considered as important sensory organs associated with the CNS.

Telencephalon

The telencephalon consists of the cerebral cortices, nucleus accumbens, caudate, putamen and globus pallidus.

Cerebrum

The cerebrum comprises the two cerebral hemispheres, separated by the longitudinal fissure, but connected by the corpus callosum, a large white matter structure. Each hemisphere extends from the frontal bones rostrally to the occipital bones caudally. The hemispheres lie in the anterior and middle cranial fossa, above the tentorium cerebelli. The falx cerebri extends into the longitudinal fissure.

The outermost layer of the cerebrum is the cerebral cortex, a gray matter structure composed of neuronal cell bodies, dendritic structures, and synaptic connections. The deeper white matter component of the cerebrum is composed of heavily myelinated nerve fibres (see Fig. 12.4), which can be classified as follows:

- *Projection fibres:* connections from cerebral cortex to subcortical structures such as brainstem and thalamus (e.g. corona radiata).
- *Commisural fibres:* connections from one cerebral hemisphere to the other.
- *Association fibres:* connections between different areas of cerebral cortex.

The cerebral cortex is subdivided into various regions (see Figs 12.5–12.8). The frontal lobe is the largest component, and is separated from the parietal lobe by the central sulcus. The lateral sulcus separates the temporal lobe from the parietal and frontal lobes. The parietal lobe is separated from the most caudal cerebrum, the occipital lobe, by the parieto-occipital sulcus.

- *Frontal lobe lesions may cause:* disinhibited behaviour, personality change, perseveration, difficulty planning tasks, anosmia, Broca's (expressive) dysphasia.
- *Parietal lobe lesion may cause:* apraxias, visuospatial neglect, homonymous hemianopias (typically inferior quadrantinopias).
- *Temporal lobe lesions may cause:* Wernicke's (receptive) dysphasia, memory impairment, cortical deafness, homonymous hemianopias (typically superior quadrantinopias).

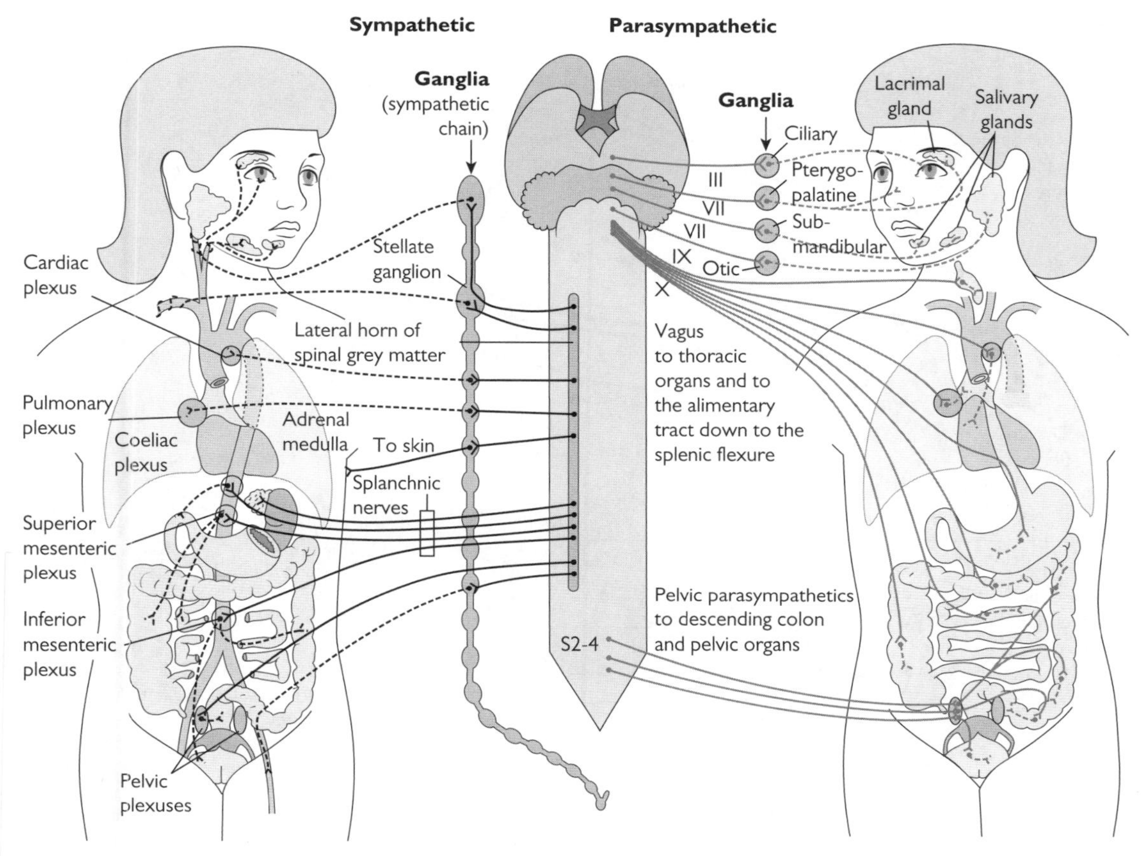

Fig. 12.3 Diagrammatic overview of the sympathetic (left) and parasympathetic (right) components of the autonomic nervous system.

Reproduced from P MacKinnon and J Morris, *Oxford Textbook of Functional Anatomy: Volume 3*, 2005, Figure 6.11.2, p. 168, by permission of Oxford University Press

- *Occipital lobe lesions may cause:* homonymous hemianopias, cortical blindness, visual agnosia.

Chronic cognitive impairment can result from a variety of diseases of the cortex (as well as other brain areas; see Box 12.1).

Basal ganglia

Within the subcortical white matter lie various clusters of gray matter, known as the basal ganglia. The major components are:

- Striatum (telencephalon).
  - Caudate nuclei.
  - Putamen.
- Globus pallidus (telencephalon).
- Nucleus accumbens (telencehalon).
- Sub-thalamic nuclei (diencephalon).
- Substantia nigra (mesencephalon).

The basal ganglia receive extensive cortical sensory and motor input and output to cortical areas responsible for the higher order processing of movement, such as prefrontal cortex and supplementary motor areas. This link is thought to coordinate planning and control of complex behaviour by suppressing some movements and activating others.

Pathology: Parkinsonism

Parkinsonism refers to symptoms of resting tremor (usually 4-6Hz), bradykinesia and rigidity, which have a wide variety of causes, the most common of which is Parkinson's disease (see Box 12.2). This is a neurodegenerative condition of the dopaminergic cells of the pars compacta of the substantia nigra, a key part of the basal ganglia. The neurodegeneration is characterized by an abnormal accumulation of the protein alpha-synuclein bound to ubiquitin in the damaged cells. This insoluble protein accumulates inside neurons forming inclusions called Lewy bodies. The exact link of these inclusions to the pathophysiology of Parkinson's

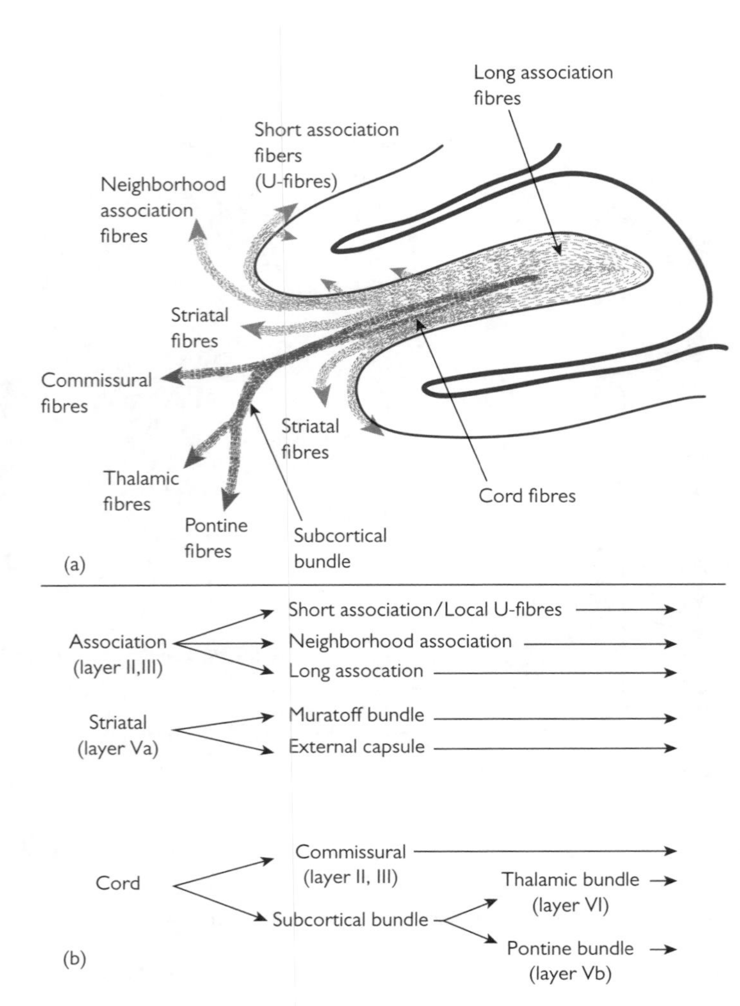

Fig. 12.4 White matter organization. Diagrammatic representation of the organization of white matter fibre pathways emanating from a given area of the cerebral cortex in the coronal plane (a). Schema of the principles of organization of the white matter fibre pathways arising from any given area of the cerebral cortex (b).

Adapted from JD Schmahmann et al., *Fiber Pathways of the Brain*, 2010, Figure 5.2, p. 84, by permission of Oxford University Press

disease and its underlying causes is still an area of research. A variety of pharmacological agents targeting dopaminergic neurotransmission are used to treat Parkinson's disease and are summarized at the end of the chapter. More recently, neurosurgical techniques, such as deep brain stimulation, have been used with good effect in those where medications are unable to control tremor and motor fluctuations associated with the condition. This technique makes use of a precisely located stimulating electrode targeted at the thalamus, globus pallidus, or subthalamic nuclei connected to a lead and pulse generator located subcutaneously, in a similar way to a cardiac pacemaker.

Diencephalon

The diencephalon is composed of four components:

- Hypothalamus (ventral-most).
- Subthalamus.
- Thalamus.
- Epithalamus (dorsal-most).

The hypothalamus is located between the optic chiasma and the caudal border of the mammillary bodies. It is composed of the hypothalamic nuclei, which can be further divided into the supraoptic and paraventricular nuclei.

The thalamus is a gray matter structure and is expanded at its posterior end as the pulvinar. The subthalamus contains cranial parts of the substantia nigra and red nucleus. The epithalamus contains the habenular nuclei and the pineal gland.

Mesencephalon/midbrain

The midbrain connects the forebrain and hindbrain, and contains the cerebral aqueduct of the ventricular system. Dorsal to the aqueduct is the tectum, which includes the four raised structures of the superior and inferior colliculi.

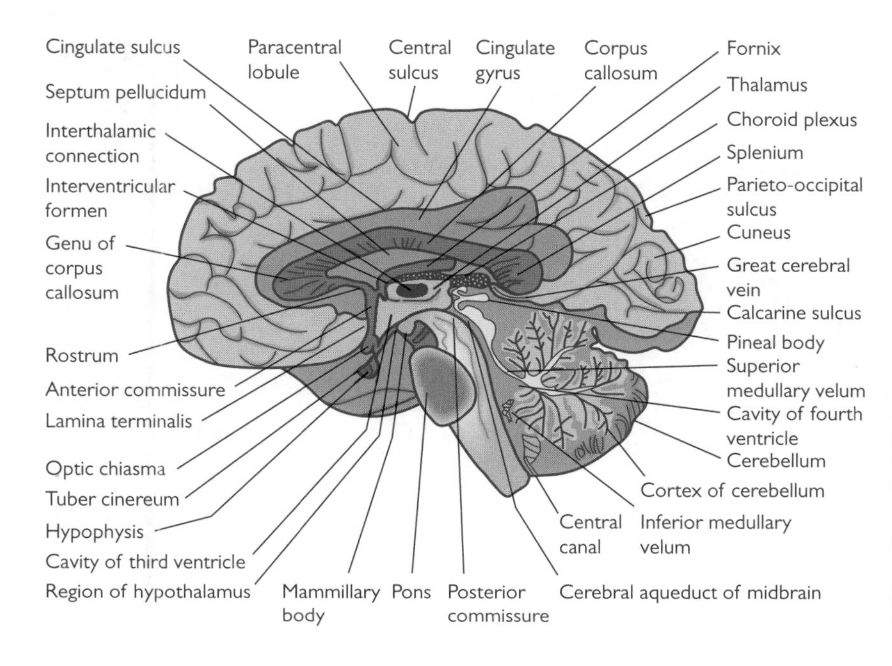

Fig. 12.5 Median sagittal section of the brain to show the third ventricle, the cerebral aqueduct, and the fourth ventricle.

Reproduced from R Wilkins et al., *Oxford Handbook of Medical Sciences, Second Edition*, 2011, Figure 11.36, p. 711, by permission of Oxford University Press

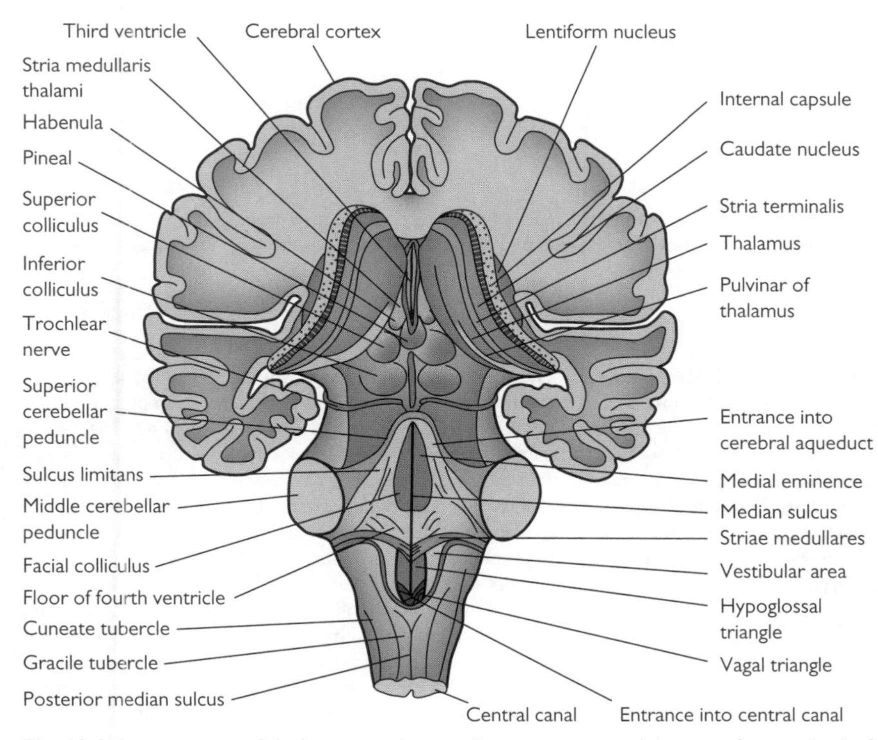

Fig. 12.6 Posterior view of the brainstem showing the two superior and the two inferior colliculi of the tectum of the midbrain.

Reproduced from R Wilkins et al., *Oxford Handbook of Medical Sciences, Second Edition*, 2011, Figure 11.37, p. 711, by permission of Oxford University Press

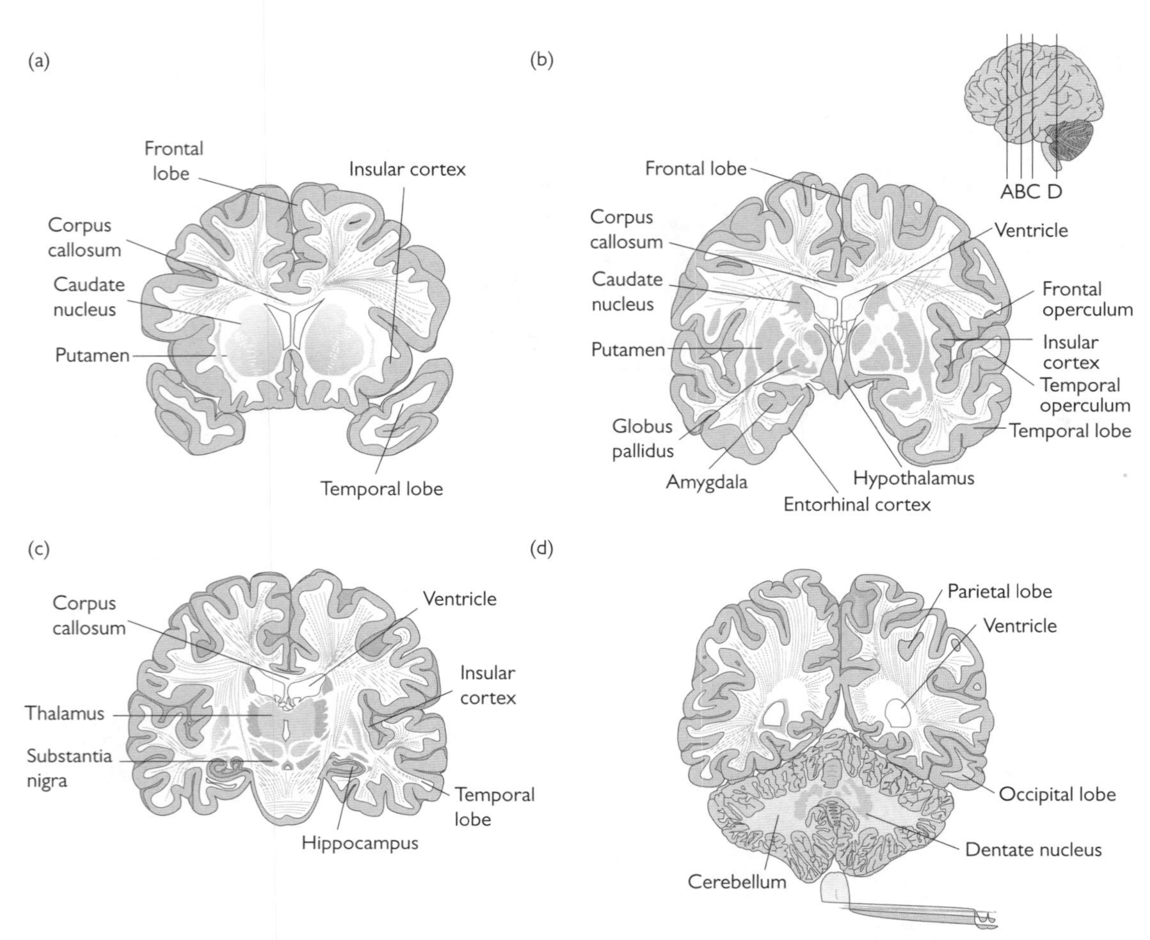

Fig. 12.7 Several brain regions are shown in these sections of the human brain. The sections are from rostral (a) to caudal (d) and the approximate location of these sections are shown on the lateral surface view of the brain shown in the top right corner of the figure.

Ventral to the aqueduct are the cerebral peduncles which comprise the crus cerebri and posterior tegmentum. The anterior and posterior components of the midbrain are separated by the substantial nigra. The midbrain also contain small number of visual fibres running from the optic tract which terminate in the pretectal nucleus. The ventral periaqueductal gray matter contains the trochlear and oculomotor nuclei. The central tegmentum also contains the red nucleus at the level of the superior colliculus.

Rhombencephalon/Hindbrain

The hindbrain is comprises:

- The cerebellum.
- The pons.
- The medulla oblongata.

The cerebellum lies in the posterior cranial fossa, dorsal to the medulla and pons. The structure is composed of two hemispheres, each with a highly convoluted and ridged cortex of gray matter, and deeper layers of white matter. The two hemispheres are connected by a midline vermis. Within the deep white matter lie gray matter nuclei: the dentate, emboliform, globose, and fastigial. The cerebellum is connected to the midbrain via the superior and middle cerebellar peduncles, whilst the inferior cerebellar peduncle provides connections to the medulla. The cerebellum acts in combination with motor cortex and basal ganglia to compare motor intention versus actual performance. This allows for the calculation of fine adjustments to correct for error. Cerebellar pathology therefore manifests in an inability to coordinate complex motor tasks, or simple tasks with an element of timing.

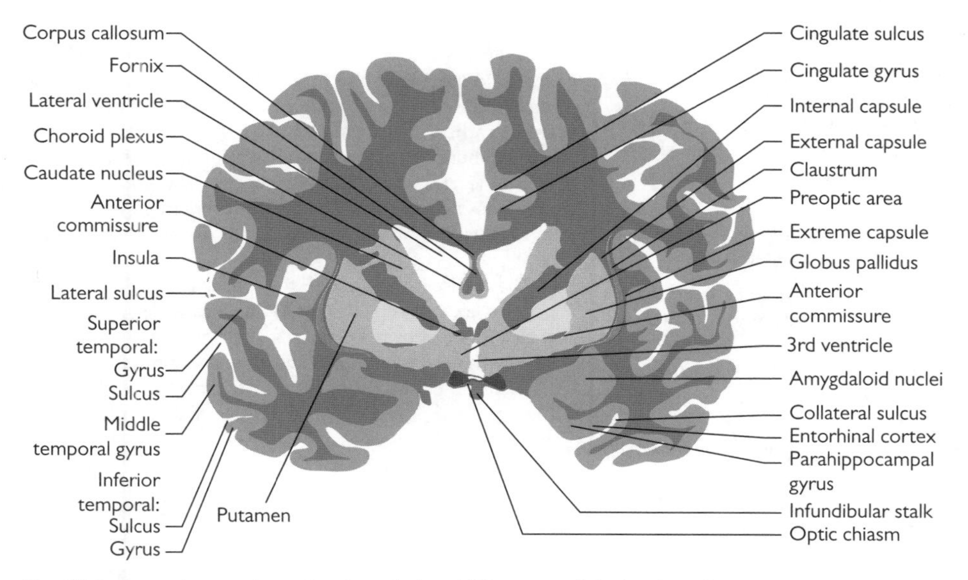

Fig. 12.8 Coronal anatomic section through the middle region of the basal ganglia.
Reproduced with permission from http://www.brains.rad.msu.edu, and http://brainmuseum.org, supported by the US National Science Foundation

BOX 12.1 CONDITIONS THAT CAN EFFECT THE CORTEX AND LEAD TO CHRONIC COGNITIVE DECLINE

Dementia and progressive cognitive impairment
- Alzheimer's disease.
- Lewy body dementia.
- Multi-infarct dementia.
- Rarer causes:
  - Huntingdon's disease.
  - Pick's disease (fronto-temporal dementia).
  - Progressive supranuclear palsy.
  - AIDS-associated dementia.
  - Creutzfeldt–Jacob disease.

Reversible causes of chronic cognitive impairment
- Drug intoxication.
- Hypothyroidism.
- Thiamine or Vitamin B12 deficiency.
- Normal pressure hydrocephalus.
- Intracranial mass/tumour.
- Depression.

The pons (metencephalon) lies caudal to the midbrain and rostral to the medulla. Positioned on the anterior surface of the cerebellum, the pons contains transverse fibres connecting the two hemispheres of the cerebellum.

BOX 12.2 CAUSES OF PARKINSONISM

- Parkinson's disease.
- Drug induced (neuroleptics).
- Diffuse Lewy Body disease.
- Progressive supranuclear palsy.
- Multisystem atrophy.
- Normal pressure hydrocephalus.
- Wilson's disease.
- Toxins eg. carbon monoxide, MPTP (1-methyl-4-phenyl-1,2,3,6-tetrahydropyridine).

The medulla oblongata (myelencephalon) connects the caudal pons to the rostral spinal cord. On the ventral aspect lie the medullary pyramids, separated by the median fissure. Posterior to the pyramids on the ventral surface lie the olivary nuclei (olives).

The eye

A sphere, approximately 2.5 cm in diameter, with the cornea bulging forwards. The anterior chamber is situated between the cornea and the iris. The iris defines the pupil, which leads to the posterior chamber between the muscular iris and lens. The anterior and posterior chambers contain aqueous humor. The vitreous chamber behind the lens contains vitreous humor.

In coronal section, three layers can be discerned:

- The sclera, which anteriorly gives rise to the transparent cornea covered by stratified epithelium.
- The pigmented choroid, lining the posterior eyeball, which becomes the iris and in the posterior chamber establishes a ciliary body from which ciliary processes, which secrete aqueous humor the retina.
- The innermost layer, comprising a pigmented epithelium under which lie receptor cells—rods and cones.

These cells contain photosensitive pigment made up of a light-absorbing molecule called retinal, bound to a membrane protein called opsin. Each cell type, rods, and the three types of cone, contains a different visual pigment, made up of retinal and a different opsin molecule, each of which has a different peak light absorption energy. Colour vision relies on the three types of cone, which are maximally excited by light with short (blue, 437 nm), middle (green, 533 nm), and long (red, 564 nm) wavelengths. In contrast, the rod system is achromatic, since there is only one visual pigment, known as rhodopsin, with a peak absorbency at 498 nm. Transduction occurs via a cascade of events triggered by the absorption of a photon by the pigment molecule. In rods the retinal usually exists as the 11-cis isomer. Excitation of the rhodopsin by a photon causes a series of conformational changes in the retinal, ending ultimately in the all-trans state. Rhodopsin is unable to bind all-trans retinal, so the retinal becomes detached. A semi-stable intermediate configuration called metarhodopsin II activates transducin, a G-protein, which in turn activates phosphodiesterase to convert cyclic GMP (cGMP) to 5'GMP. The lowered cGMP concentration decreases Na^+ influx through a cGMP-gated channel. Thus in the dark, cGMP concentrations are raised, and so there is a constant Na^+ current, known as the dark current. The resting membrane potential is therefore relatively depolarized, at around 40 mV, and light causes a hyperpolarization to around-70 mV. A similar cascade operates in cones. Detached retinal is recycled in the pigment epithelium by converting the all-trans retinal to all-trans retinol (vitamin A). All-trans retinol is the precursor for 11-cis retinal, and is not synthesized in the body. Dietary vitamin A deficiency can therefore cause night-blindness or, if severe, even total blindness. The dynamic range of photosensitivity of cones is maintained through light adaptation. The transduction cascade also inactivates a cGMP-gated Ca^{2+} channel. Ca^{2+} inhibits guanylate cyclase (GTP $\rightarrow$ cGMP); thus a negative feedback loop operates to maintain a fairly constant cGMP concentration through a range of absolute levels of brightness, and so keep the cell maximally sensitive to changes in light level.

Neuronal ganglion cells from the rods and cones converge on the optic disc where these axons pass through the retina. The area where there are no photoreceptors results in a small scotoma known as the blind-spot. Retinal arteries and veins, derived from the central artery of the retina and associated veins, also pass with the optic nerve, and run on the vitreous aspect of the retina.

The optic nerves from each eye meet at the optic chiasm. Fibres arising from the nasal retinae from each eye cross, so that when the fibres continue as the optic tract, each tract carries information about left and right hemifields, rather than from left and right retinae. The optic tract continues to the lateral geniculate nucleus (LGN), when the ganglion cell fibres synapse. The visual pathway continues from the LGN as the optic radiation, which passes back to the primary visual cortex at the occipital pole, as shown in Fig. 12.9.

The intrinsic muscles of the eye sphincter and dilator pupillae control pupil diameter. The lens is suspended from the ciliary body by the circular suspensory ligament; the tension of the ligament and, hence, the curvature of the lens, is determined by the ciliary muscle. The macula lies lateral to the optic disc; it is the site of sharpest vision—the fovea—and contains only cones.

Two folds of skin constitute the eyelids, separated by the palpebral fissure. The inner surface of the eyelids is covered by a mucosal layer— the conjunctiva—which is continuous with the surface of the eyeball to form the conjunctival sac. The fibrous orbital septum acts as a framework for the eyelid and is thickened at the margins to form tarsal plates, and medial and lateral palpebral ligaments. Lacrimal gland secretions (tears) enter the conjunctival sac at the lateral upper eyelid. Tears drain into the lacrimal puncta, through canals to the lacrimal sac and then via the nasolacrimal duct to the nose.

Eye movements are controlled by cranial nerves with the lateral rectus muscle being supplied by the VI cranial nerve, the superior oblique muscles being supplied by the IV cranial nerve, and all other muscle being supplied by the III cranial nerve. Sympathetic pupilomotor fibres responsible for pupillary constriction are also carried with the III cranial nerve, and lesions of this nerve or of the sympathetic fibres along their entire course (e.g. brainstem, apex of the lung, thyroid lesions, carotid artery dissections, cavernous sinus lesions) can cause a Horner's syndrome (miosis, ptosis, and sometimes anhydrosis on the side of the lesion).

The ear

The ear is divided into three structures.

Outer ear

This comprises the auricle, a fold of skin reinforced by cartilage, from which the external auditory meatus made of cartilage and then bone extends to the tympanic membrane.

Middle ear

This lies within the petrous temporal bone, comprising the vertical tympanic cavity, which is fluted at its upper end as the epitympanic recess. Pathology of the middle ear can lead to conductive deafness (see Box 12.3).

The oval and round windows (fenestra ovale and rotundum) provide connections with the inner ear. Three articulated bones—the ossicles—are present. The malleus (hammer), connected to the tympanic membrane

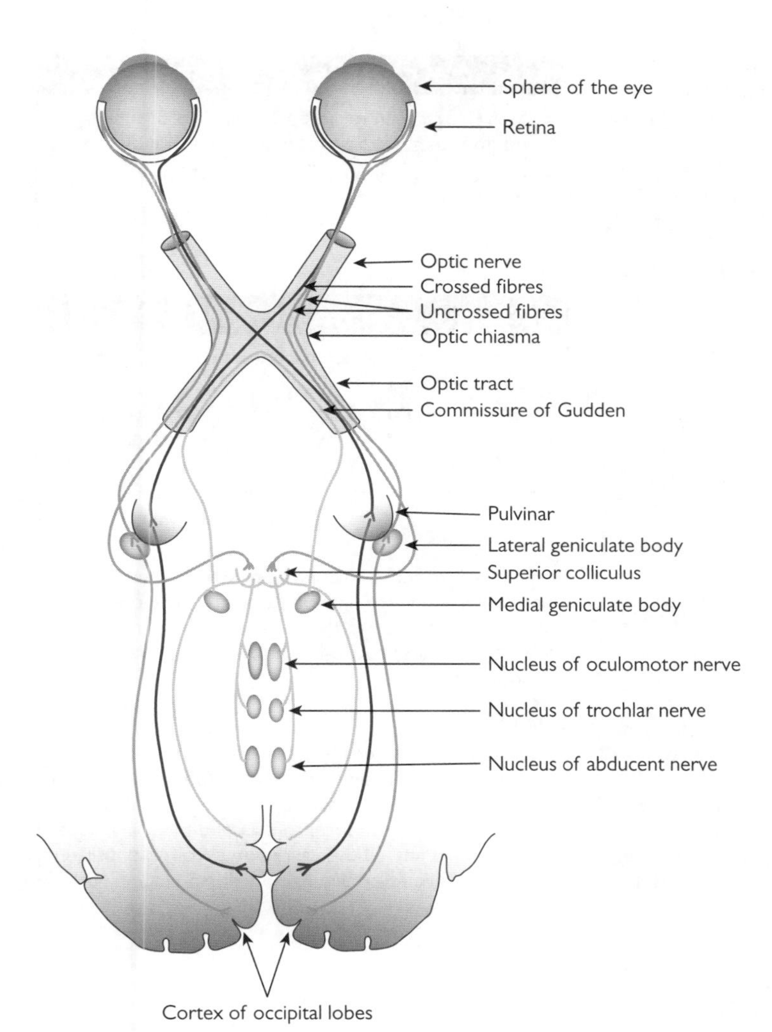

Fig. 12.9 Processing of visual information via the retina, optic nerves, optic chiasma, and optic tract to the occipital lobes in a human brain.

This figure was published in Gray, *Anatomy of the Human Body*, Twentieth edition, throughly revised and re-edited by Warren H. Lewis, plate 722, Elsevier. Copyright the editors, 1918.

articulates with the incus (anvil), which in turn articulates with the stapes (stirrup), attached to the oval window.
The chain of synovial joints transmits vibration from the tympanic membrane to the oval window. The tensor tympani muscle dampens vibrations of the tympanic membrane; stapedius limits vibration of the stapes.

The tympanic cavity is continuous with the nasal cavity through the bony and then cartilaginous auditory tube, which is lined by mucosa. This connection equalizes the pressure in the middle ear with atmospheric pressure.

Inner ear

This lies within the petrous temporal bone, which comprises a bony labyrinth lined with endosteum and filled with perilymph (continuous with CSF through the perilymphatic duct, the aqueduct of the cochlea).

Within the bony labyrinth lies a membranous labyrinth, filled with endolymph, which resembles intracellular fluid. The bony labyrinth comprises:

- The cochlea, containing the organ of hearing.
- The vestibule and semicircular canals, for perception of orientation.

The cochlea makes 2.5 turns around the central modiolus in which the cochlear nerve travels. The vestibule is continuous with the cochlea and with the three semicircular canals, which lie perpendicular to each other. The aqueduct of the vestibule reaches the posterior cranial fossa at the internal auditory meatus.

The membranous labyrinth forms a series of ducts and sacs.

The spiral cochlear duct (scala media) is wedge-shaped. It defines two channels: the vestibular and tympanic canals, which meet at the tip of the cochlea. The vestibular membrane separates the duct from the vestibular canal; the basilar membrane separates the duct from the tympanic membrane.

Vibrations of the oval window initiate vibrations of the perilymph in the canals and then of the endolymph in the duct. The organ of Corti lies on the basilar membrane and detects these vibrations.

The semicircular canals contain three semicircular ducts, which are enlarged to form ampullae where they join with a sac-like structure, an otolith organ termed the utricle. The utricle is continuous with the other otolith organ, the saccule, which in turn is continuous with the cochlear duct.

Endolymph within this network is reabsorbed to the bloodstream from the endolymphatic duct within the aqueduct of the vestibule.

Pathology of the cochlea can lead to sensorineural deafness (see Box 12.3) whilst pathology relating to the vestibule can cause vertigo (see Box 12.4).

BOX 12.3 CAUSES OF DEAFNESS

- *Sensorineural:* central lesions, acoustic neuroma, head trauma, drugs/toxins (aminoglycosides, lead).
- *Conductive:* ear wax, middle ear infection, otosclerosis.

BOX 12.4 CAUSES OF VERTIGO

- *Labyrinthine:* viral, bacterial otitis media, Meniere's disease, trauma.
- *Central:* acute vestibular neuronitis, vascular disease space occupying lesions, multiple sclerosis, drugs/ toxins (e.g. alcohol).

Spinal cord

The spinal cord arises from the caudal medulla and runs via the foramen magnum, extending to the border of the first lumbar vertebra. The spinal cord runs in the vertebral canal, surrounded by the structures of the vertebral column. The outer layer of the cord is composed of white matter columns or tracts, which surround the inner core of gray matter. The gray matter has a characteristic cross shape, with dorsal and ventral horns.

Enlargements of the spinal cord are present at C7–8 and L4–5, the points at which the cervical and lumbosacral plexuses, respectively, arise. The spinal cord tapers to the conus medullaris at its caudal extremity. There is a deep anterior median fissure and a shallower posterior median sulcus along the longitudinal length of the cord. Thirty-one pairs of spinal nerves arise along the cord as anterior (motor) and posterior (sensory) roots. Posterior roots display a posterior root ganglion.

Central pathways

All sensory fibres enter the spinal cord through the dorsal roots, with their cell bodies lying just before the dorsal root in the dorsal root ganglia (see Fig 12.10). Axons from mechanoreceptors and proprioceptors ascend the spinal cord in the dorsal columns. These carry fibres from the ipsilateral side of the body, and continue to the dorsal column nuclei at

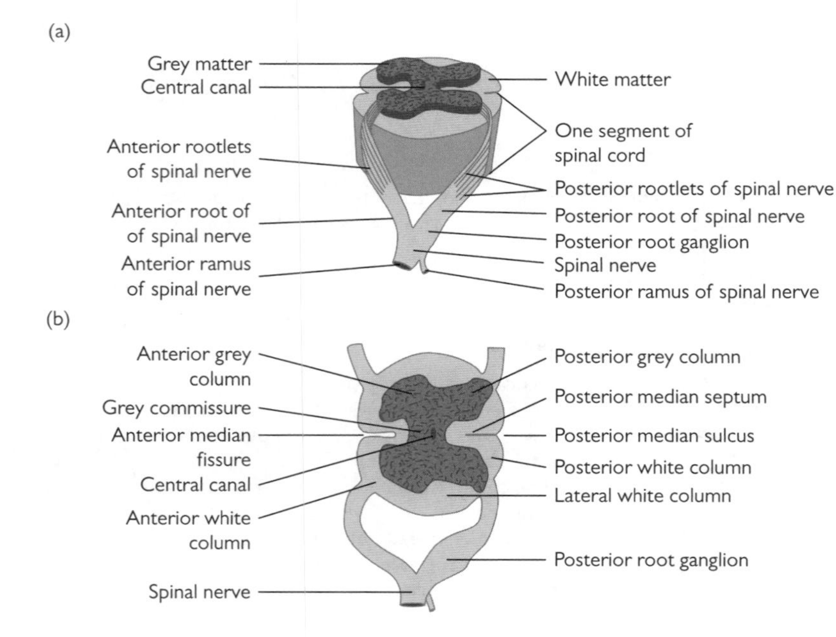

Fig. 12.10 Transverse section through lumbar part of spine: (a) oblique view; (b) face view, showing anterior and posterior roots of a spinal nerve.

BOX 12.5 BROWN-SEQUARD SYNDROME

Lateral hemisection of the spinal cord, which damages the:

- Corticospinal tracts causing *ipsilateral* upper motor neurons weakness below the level of the lesion.
- Ascending dorsal column fibres causing *ipsilateral* loss of proprioception and vibration sense.
- Crossing ascending spinothalamic tract fibres causing *contralateral* loss of pain and temperature sensation.

the level of the medulla. Nociception and temperature sensation are carried by the anterolateral system. Axons entering the spinal cord through the dorsal horns may ascend or descend one or two spinal segments in the tract of Lissauer, before synapsing onto secondary fibres and interneurons in the dorsal horn laminae. Referred pain is thought to be a result of cutaneous and visceral nociceptive afferents converging on the same secondary fibres through interneurons in the dorsal horn laminae. The secondary fibres decussate at the same spinal segment as they arise, and ascend in one of three tracts that form the anterolateral system on the contralateral side.

A hemisection of the spinal cord can cause Brown-Sequard syndrome and produce a characteristic pattern of sensory and motor symptoms (see Box 12.5).

Blood supply to the spinal cord

The spinal cord receives arterial supply from the anterior spinal artery, and two posterior spinal arteries. The anterior spinal artery supplies the ventral aspect of the cord, whilst supply to the dorsal aspect is split between the bilateral posterior spinal arteries. Segmental blood supply is also provided by radicular arteries, which provide anterior and posterior divisions supplying the cord. The largest radicular artery, the artery of Adamkiewicz, is variable, but typically found at the lower thoracic or upper lumbar level, reinforcing supply to two-thirds of the cord at the lumbosacral enlargement. Such radicular arteries can be compromised by aortic resections during surgical aneurysm repair.

Blood supply to the head and neck

Arterial supply to the central nervous system

The brain receives a dual blood supply bilaterally from the vertebral arteries and internal carotid arteries.

The vertebral arteries branch from the subclavian arteries and enter the skull via the foramen magnum. (see Fig 12.11) The two vertebral arteries unite in the midline at the lower border of the pons, forming the basilar artery. The basilar artery runs along the anterior median fissure of the pons, in the pontine cistern, with branches supplying the brainstem and cerebellum. The posterior cerebral arteries are the terminal divisions of the basilar artery. The posterior cerebral arteries also provide the posterior communicating arteries (see Fig 12.12) that anastamose with the internal carotid system (see Fig 12.13).

The internal carotid arteries branch from the common carotid arteries. They pass into the middle cranial fossa via the carotid canal and foramen lacerum, through the cavernous sinus. Each gives rise to the ophthalmic artery, the central artery of the retina and ciliary arteries bilaterally. The anterior and middle cerebral arteries are the major branches of the internal carotid, supplying the medial and lateral aspects of the cerebral hemispheres, respectively. The anterior communicating artery links the two anterior cerebral arteries, completing the anastomoses between the vertebral and carotid systems: the Circle of Willis (see Fig.12.12). Despite the interconnection of the two systems, there is minimal mixing of blood. However, in case of blockage, the anastomoses can provide collateral blood supply.

The external carotid also branches from the common carotid. This branches to supply structures of the head and neck other than the brain:

- Superior thyroid.
- Ascending pharyngeal.
- Superficial temporal.
- Lingual, facial.
- Occipital.
- Posterior auricular.
- Superficial temporal.

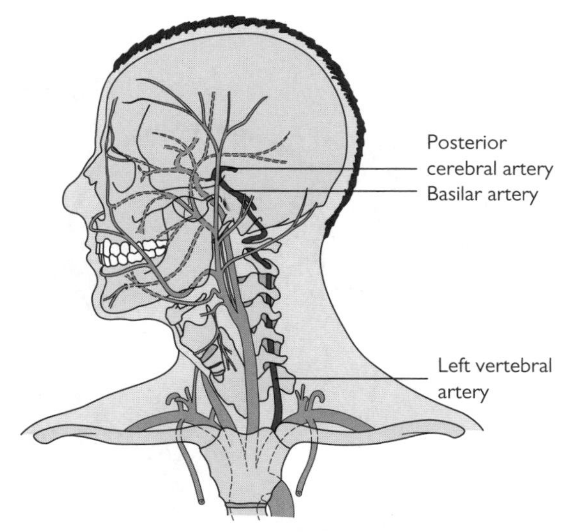

Fig. 12.11 Vertebral artery and its main branches.

Reproduced from P MacKinnon and J Morris, *Oxford Textbook of Functional Anatomy: Volume 3*, 2005, Figure 6.10.3, p. 155, by permission of Oxford University Press

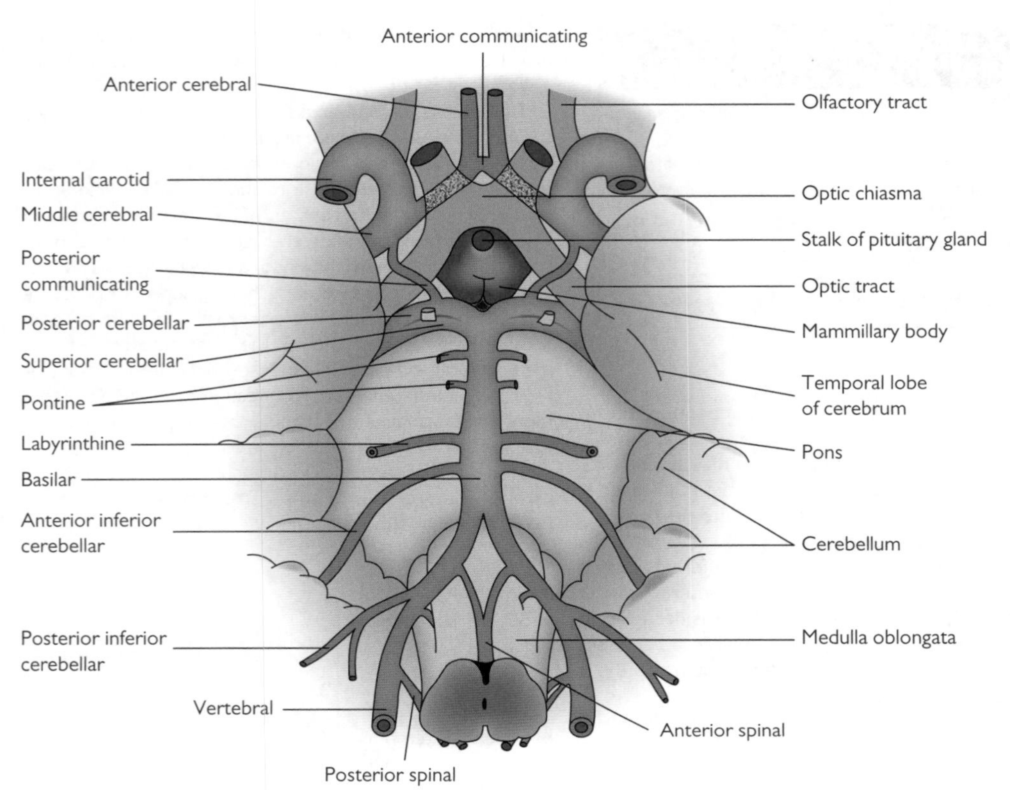

Fig. 12.12 Intracranial branches of the vertebral artery; circle of Willis.

Reproduced from P MacKinnon and J Morris, *Oxford Textbook of Functional Anatomy: Volume 3*, 2005, Figure 6.10.4, p. 155, by permission of Oxford University Press

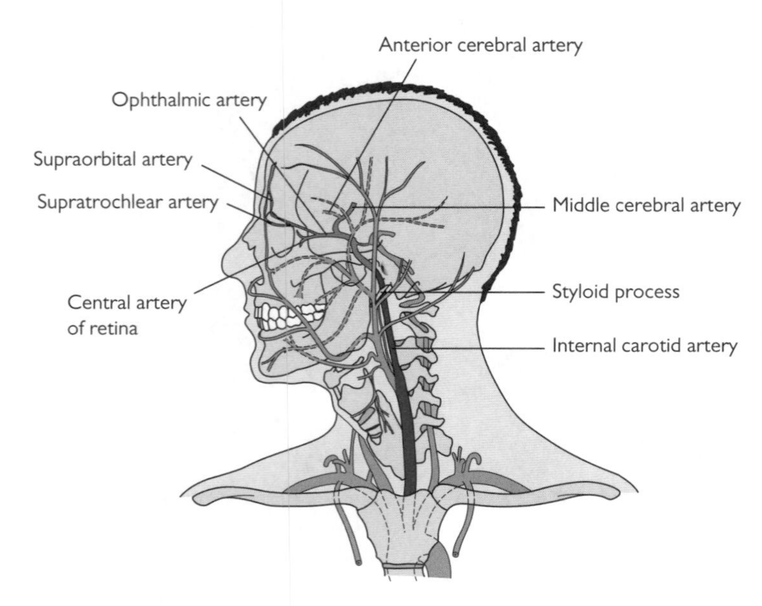

Fig. 12.13 Common and internal carotid arteries and their main branches.

Reproduced from P MacKinnon and J Morris, *Oxford Textbook of Functional Anatomy: Volume 3*, 2005, Figure 6.10.6, p. 156, by permission of Oxford University Press

It has two terminal branches which arise within the parotid gland:

- The maxillary artery, giving rise to three groups of branches that supply the temporal fossa, infratemporal fossa, cranial dura, nasal cavity, oral cavity, and pharynx.
- The superficial temporal artery.

Arterial supply to the cerebral hemispheres

Anterior cerebral artery supply

- Medial aspects of frontal and parietal lobes.
- Extreme dorsolateral aspect of hemisphere.
- Corpus callosum.
- Includes regions of sensory and motor cortex relevant to lower limb.

Middle cerebral artery supply

- Lateral surfaces frontal and parietal cortex.
- Lateral surface of temporal cortex excluding inferior temporal gyrus.
- Lenticulostriate branches to basal ganglia and internal capsule.

Posterior cerebral artery supply

- Occipital lobe.
- Inferior temporal gyrus.

Venous drainage

Between the periosteum and dura mater lie the intracranial venous sinuses (see Fig 12.14). These run in grooves of the underlying bones and drain tributary veins from the brain, eye, and skull interior, diploic veins from the marrow of the cranial bones, and CSF from the subarachnoid space.

The superior sagittal sinus runs in the attached margin of the falx cerebri, with lacunae along its length containing arachnoid granulations to reabsorb CSF. The sinus drains into:

- The transverse sinus, which runs along the attached margin of the tentorium cerebelli, then turns inferiorly to become the sigmoid sinus.
- The inferior sagittal sinus runs in the free margin of the falx cerebri.
- The straight sinus forms from the unification of the inferior sagittal sinus and the great cerebral vein.
- The intercommunicating cavernous sinuses are positioned either side of the sphenoid, pituitary gland and drain into:
    - The superior and inferior petrosal sinuses, which drain into the transverse and sigmoid sinus, respectively.
    - The sigmoid sinus, which drains into the internal jugular vein.

There are also extracranial veins:

- The supratrochlear vein and supraorbital vein drain the forehead.
- The facial vein, superficial temporal vein, and posterior auricular veins drain the face and scalp.
- The superior temporal vein unites with the maxillary vein to form the retromandibular vein, which bifurcates to unite with:
    - The facial vein (anteriorly) as it enters the internal jugular vein.
    - The posterior auricular vein to establish the external jugular vein.

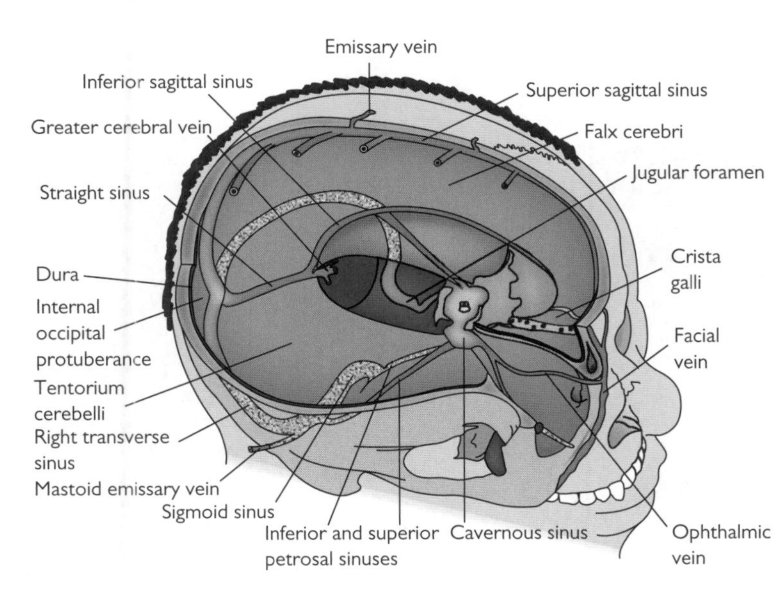

Fig. 12.14 Dural venous sinuses.

Reproduced from P MacKinnon and J Morris, *Oxford Textbook of Functional Anatomy: Volume 3*, 2005, Figure 6.9.2, p. 144, by permission of Oxford University Press

In the neck:

- The external jugular vein receives the anterior jugular vein, which has drained the superficial chin and neck, then itself drains into the subclavian vein.
- The internal jugular vein receives tributaries from the neck then unites with the subclavian vein to establish the brachiocephalic vein.

Lymphatic drainage

Superficial vessels accompanying superficial veins drain into a collar of nodes around the neck, including submental, submandibular, parotid, mastoid, and occipital groups. The nodes, in turn, drain to deep cervical nodes draining deeper structures. These nodes drain through jugular trunks into the venous circulation at the junction of the internal jugular and subclavian veins.

The lingual and palatine tonsils, together with the retropharyngeal lymphatic tissue form a ring of lymphatic tissue in the mucosa and submucosa of the nose, pharynx, and mouth.

The meninges

Three connective tissue layers surround the brain and spinal cord—dura mater, arachnoid mater, and pia mater.

The inelastic dura mater composed of:

- *Outer endosteal layer:* the periosteum, which lines the bones of the cranium and at openings of the skull is continuous with that on outer surface.
- *Inner meningeal layer:* continuous with that of the spinal cord.

At some points, the meningeal layer is doubled-back on itself to form folds of dura. These produce four septa:

- *Falx cerebri:* a midline septa between the cerebral hemispheres, which meets the tentorium cerebelli.
- *Tentorium cerebelli:* a horizontal septa on the roof of the posterior fossa, which separates the cerebrum from the cerebellum.
- *The falx cerebelli*: a vertical septa that descends from the tentorium and separates the cerebellar hemispheres.
- *The diaphragm sellae:* the roof of the turnica sella.

The middle layer, the arachnoid mater follows the folds of the meningeal layer of dura mater, to which it is loosely attached.

The innermost layer, the pia mater closely envelopes the brain and spinal cord. It is separated from the arachnoid mater by the subarachnoid space, filled with CSF, which cushions the brain.

Meningeal spaces

The three layers of the meninges yield three meningeal spaces:

- *Epidural (extradural) space:* a potential space between skull bones and periosteal layer of dura. Location of epidural haemorrhage, frequently following trauma to pterion and damage to mid-meningeal artery.
- *Subdural space:* space between dura and arachnoid mater. Bridging veins cross this space, draining to venous sinuses, and can be torn following head trauma or a sudden change in velocity.
- *Subarachnoid space:* space between arachnoid and pia mater containing CSF. Subarachnoid haemorrhage frequently results from rupture of berry aneurysms or trauma.

Cerebrospinal fluid

CSF is secreted by the choroid plexus , a vascularized epithelial structure, into each of the ventricles of the brain. CSF flows from the fourth ventricle of the brain into the subarachnoid space (see Fig 12.15). CSF exchanges freely

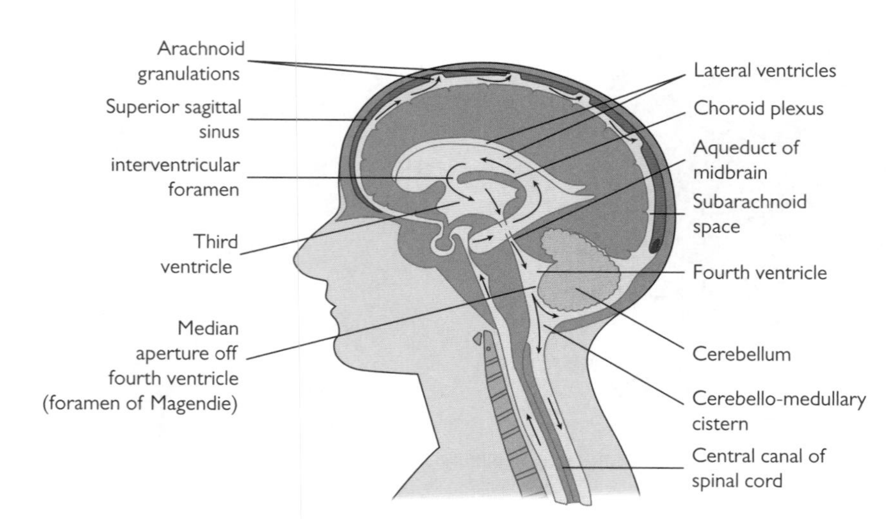

Fig. 12.15 Circulation of cerebrospinal fluid.

Reproduced from P MacKinnon and J Morris, *Oxford Textbook of Functional Anatomy: Volume 3*, 2005, Figure 6.9.3, p. 144, by permission of Oxford University Press

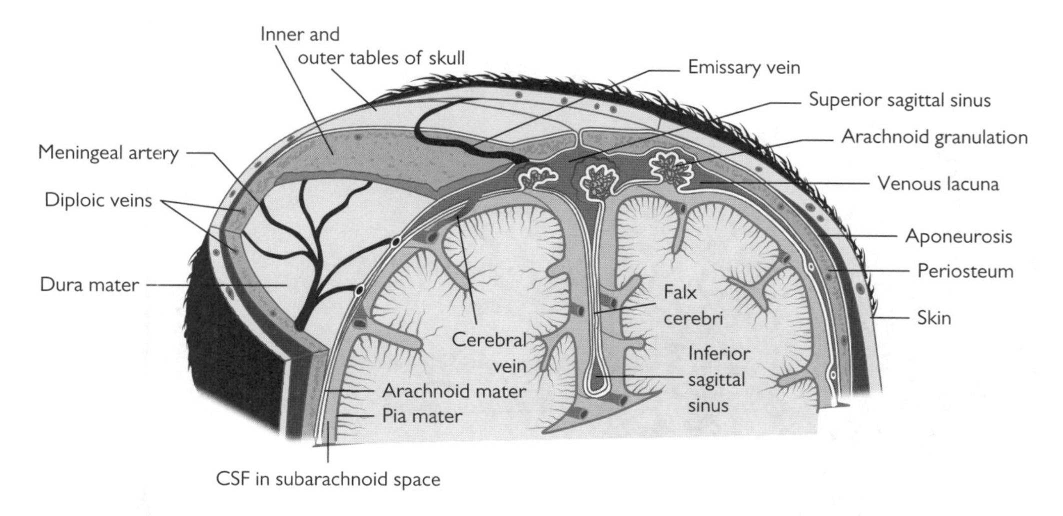

Fig. 12.16 Coronal section through cranium to show scalp, meninges, and arachnoid granulations.

Reproduced from P MacKinnon and J Morris, *Oxford Textbook of Functional Anatomy: Volume 3*, 2005, Figure 6.9.4, p. 145, by permission of Oxford University Press

with the extracellular fluid surrounding neurones across the pia mater covering the surface of the brain and across the epithelial lining (ependyma) of the ventricles (see Fig 12.16). In the choroid plexus, the epithelial cell barrier dictates the composition of CSF, insulates it from the blood. Elsewhere, the capillary endothelium prevents free diffusion from the blood into the brain extracellular fluid. In these ways, the blood–brain barrier is established. CSF can be sampled using the technique of lumbar puncture. This is usually carried out in the adult recumbent patient lying on their side, by introducing a spinal needle between the lumbar vertebrae at the level of L3/4, L4/5 or L5/S1 under local anaesthetic. The needle passes through the ligamentum flavum and dura into the sub-arachnoid space at the level of the cauda equine so that the cord itself is not damaged. An opening pressure is measured with a manometre (usually 6–150 mm of CSF) and samples can be taken to measure protein (0.2–0.4 g/L), and glucose (usually more than 2/3 of blood glucose), perform microscopy for a cell count (usually less than 5 white cells/mm^3 CSF and no red cells), and Gram stain, as well as to perform viral PCR and measure oligoclonal bands (see Box 12.6 for a list of abnormal findings).

BOX 12.6 ABNORMAL CSF FINDINGS

- *Elevated protein:* infection (bacterial, viral, or fungal), sub-dural haematoma, malignancy, Guillain–Barré syndrome.
- *Low glucose:* bacterial (including TB) meningitis, fungal meningitis, mumps meningitis, Herpes simplex encephalitis.
- *Polymorphs:* bacterial meningitis.
- *Lymphocytes:* viral meningitis/encephalitis, TB, Lyme disease, HIV associated malignancy (lymphoma/leukaemia), vascultitis, SLE.
- *Xanthochromia:* red cell break down indicative of sub-arachnoid haemorrhage, but may only be visible 12 hr after the event.
- *Oligoclonal bands:* multiple sclerosis, Guillain–Barré syndrome, lymphoma, SLE, neurosarcoidosis.

Nerves of the head and neck

The cranial nerves

There are twelve cranial nerves (see Fig 12.17). The cranial nerves originate from the CNS as follows:

- *Forebrain:*
  - *I*—olfactory.
  - *II*—optic.
- *Midbrain:*
  - *III*—occulomotor.
  - *IV*—trochlear.
- *Pons:*
  - *V*—trigeminal.
  - *VI*—abducent.
  - *VII*—facial.
  - *VIII*—vestibulocochlear.

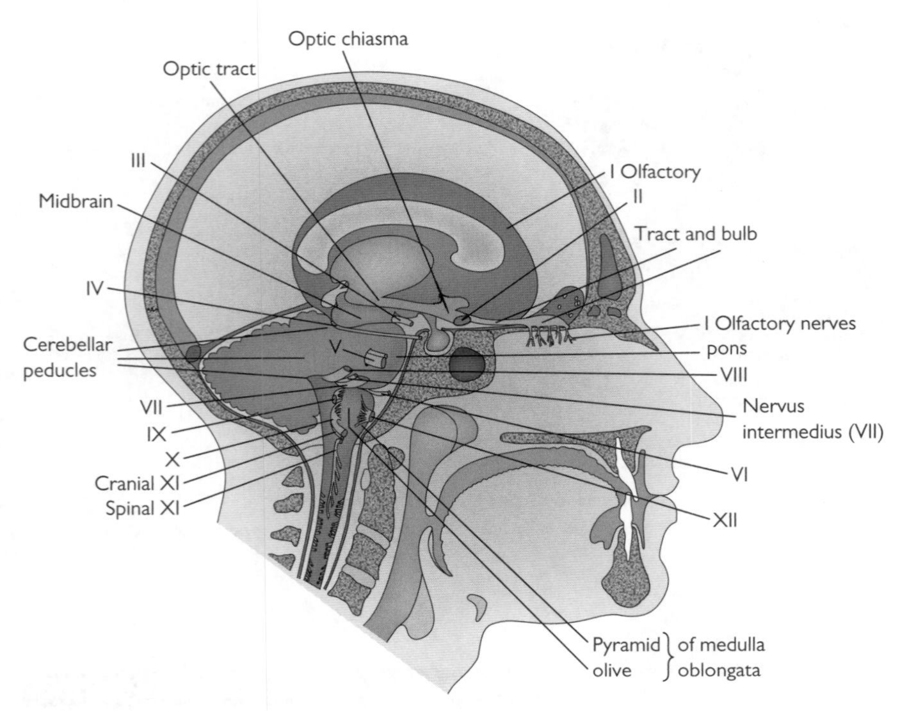

Fig. 12.17 Origin of the cranial nerves from the brainstem.

Reproduced from P MacKinnon and J Morris, *Oxford Textbook of Functional Anatomy: Volume 3*, 2005, Figure 6.11.1, p. 167, by permission of Oxford University Press

- *Medulla:*
  - *IX*—glossopharyngeal.
  - *X*—vagus.
  - *XI*—accessory.
  - *XII*—hypoglossal.

Sensory functions

These are performed by:

- I: olfaction.
- II: vision.
- VIII: balance and hearing.

Motor functions

These are performed by:

- IV: eye.
- VI: eye.
- XI: pharynx, larynx, shoulder, neck.
- XII (tongue).

Mixed sensory, motor and autonomic (parasympathetic: III, motor; VII and IX, secretomotor) functions are performed by the remaining five nerves.

The cranial nerves are summarized in Table 12.2. Causes of defects are summarized in Box 12.7.

The cervical plexus

- Formed from anterior rami of C1–C5, and located behind the carotid sheath. C1 emerges above the atlas, with C2–4 pass through the intervertebral foramina above the corresponding cervical vertebra (see Fig 12.18).
- Segmental branches supply the prevertebral muscles. In addition, the ansa cervicalis supplies the strap muscles though upper (C1) and lower limbs.
- Sensory fibres carried in C2–C4 are arranged as the lesser occipital nerve C2, the great auricular nerve C2,3, the transverse cutaneous nerve C2,3 and the supraclavicular nerve C3,4.
- The phrenic nerve formed from C3–5 passes to the diaphragm to provide motor supply and sensory supply to the overlying pleura and peritoneum.

Table 12.2 Cranial nerves

Origin	Cranial nerve	Component fibres	Structures innervated	Functions
Forebrain	I Olfactory II Optic	Sensory Sensory	Olfactory epithelium Retina	Olfaction Vision
Midbrain	III Oculomotor	Motor Parasympathetic	Superior, medial and inferior rectus, inferior oblique and levator palpebrae eye muscles Pupillary constrictor and ciliary muscle of the eye	Movement of the eyeball Pupil constriction and accommodation
	IV Trochlear	Motor	Superior oblique eye muscle	Movement of the eyeball
Pons	V Trigeminal	Sensory Motor	Face, scalp, cranial dura mater, nasal and oral cavities, cornea Mastication muscles, tensor tympani muscle	Sensation Opening and closing the mouth, mastication, tension on tympanic membrane
	VI Abducens	Motor	Lateral rectus eye muscle	Movement of the eyeball
	VII Facial	Sensory Motor Parasympathetic	Anterior 2/3 tongue Muscles of facial expression, stapedius muscle Salivary and lacrimal glands	Taste Movement of the face, tension on middle ear bones Salivation and lacrimation
	VIII Vestibulocochlear	Sensory	Vestibular apparatus of ear Cochlea	Position and movement of head Hearing
Medulla	IX Glossopharyngeal	Sensory Motor Parasympathetic	Pharynx, posterior 1/3 of tongue Eustachian tube, middle ear Carotid body and sinus Stylopharyngeus muscle Parotid salivary glands	Sensation and taste Sensation Chemo- and baroreception Swallowing Salivation
	X Vagus	Sensory	Pharynx, larynx, oesophagus, external ear Aortic bodies, aortic arch	Sensation Chemo- and baroreception
		Motor	Thoracic and abdominal viscera	Visceral sensation
		Parasympathetic	Soft palate, pharynx, larynx, and upper oesophagus Thoracic and abdominal viscera	Speech and swallowing Control of gastrointestinal, cardiovascular, and respiratory systems
	XI Accessory	Motor	Trapezius and sternomastoid muscles	Head and shoulder movement
	XII Hypoglossal	Motor	Intrinsic and extrinsic muscles of the tongue	Movement of the tongue

BOX 12.7 CAUSES OF CRANIAL NERVE DEFECTS

- Any cause of a motor or sensory mono- or polyneuropathy (see Box 12.8 and 12.9).
- Special anatomical sites where compression/lesions can alter groups of cranial nerves:
  - *Jugular foramen syndrome*—IX/X/XI.
  - *Lateral medullary syndrome*—ipsilateral Horners, V (pain/temp), VII, IX/X, cerebellar peduncle, and contralateral loss of pain and temperature (spinothalamic tracts).
  - *Cerebellopontine angle*—e.g. acoustic neuroma; VIII, V, VII (late).
  - *Cavernous sinus syndrome*—e.g. thrombosis, internal carotid aneurysm; III/IV/VI, opthalmic division of V, sympathetic carotid plexus.

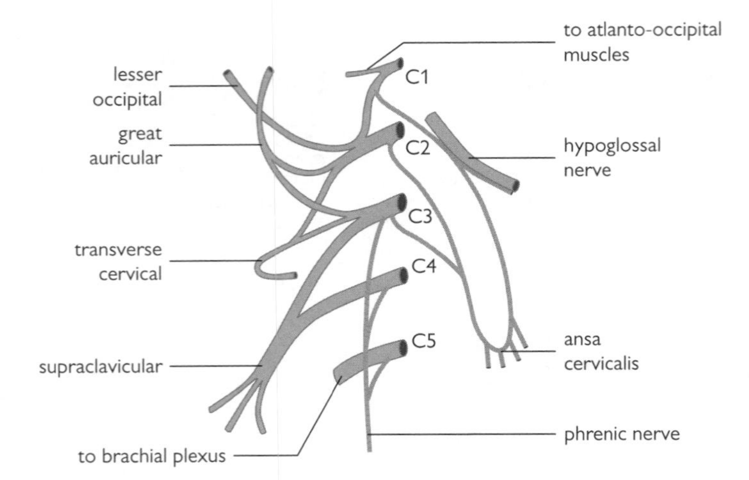

Fig. 12.18 Cervical plexus. The ansa cervicalis has been deflected medially; it normally lies anterior to the plexus.

Reproduced from P MacKinnon and J Morris, *Oxford Textbook of Functional Anatomy: Volume 3*, 2005, Figure 6.12.1, p. 189, by permission of Oxford University Press

- Posterior primary rami of cervical nerves segmentally supply extensors of the neck.

Skull and spine

The bones of the skull form the cranium and facial skeleton.

The cranium contains the brain and immediate relations, and is divided into the upper vault, comprising four flat bones (see Fig 12.19):

- The frontal bone anteriorly.
- The occipital bone posteriorly.
- Two lateral parietal bones.
- The lower base, characterized by stepped fossae (see Fig 12.20 and Fig 12.21):
  - *Anterior*—containing the frontal lobes of the brain, formed from the orbital plates of frontal bone, cribriform plate of the ethmoid bone, lesser wing of the sphenoid bone.
  - *Middle*—containing the temporal lobes of the brain, formed from the greater wing and body of the sphenoid bone, (vertical) squamous, and (horizontal) petrous parts of temporal bone
  - *Posterior*—containing cerebellum, pons. medulla oblongata, formed from the petrous part of temporal

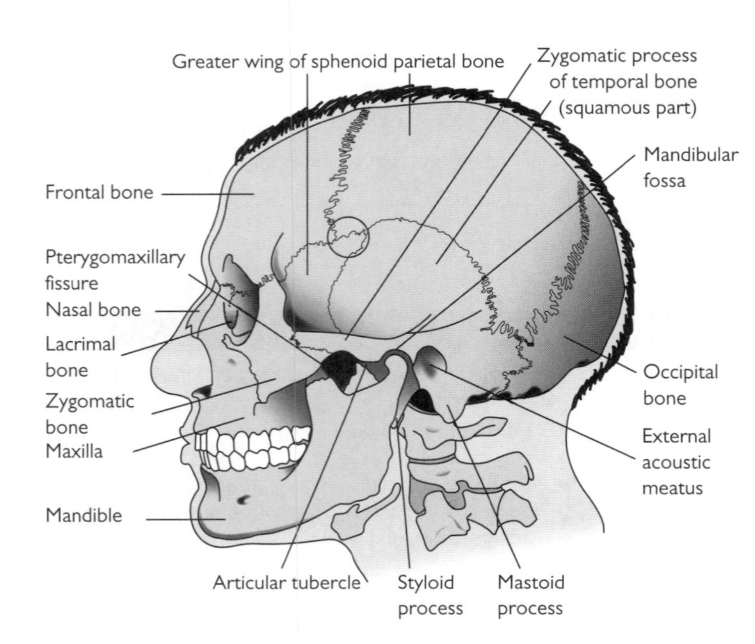

Fig. 12.19 Lateral aspect of skull, pterion circled.

Reproduced from P MacKinnon and J Morris, *Oxford Textbook of Functional Anatomy: Volume 3*, 2005, Figure 6.1.11, p. 47, by permission of Oxford University Press

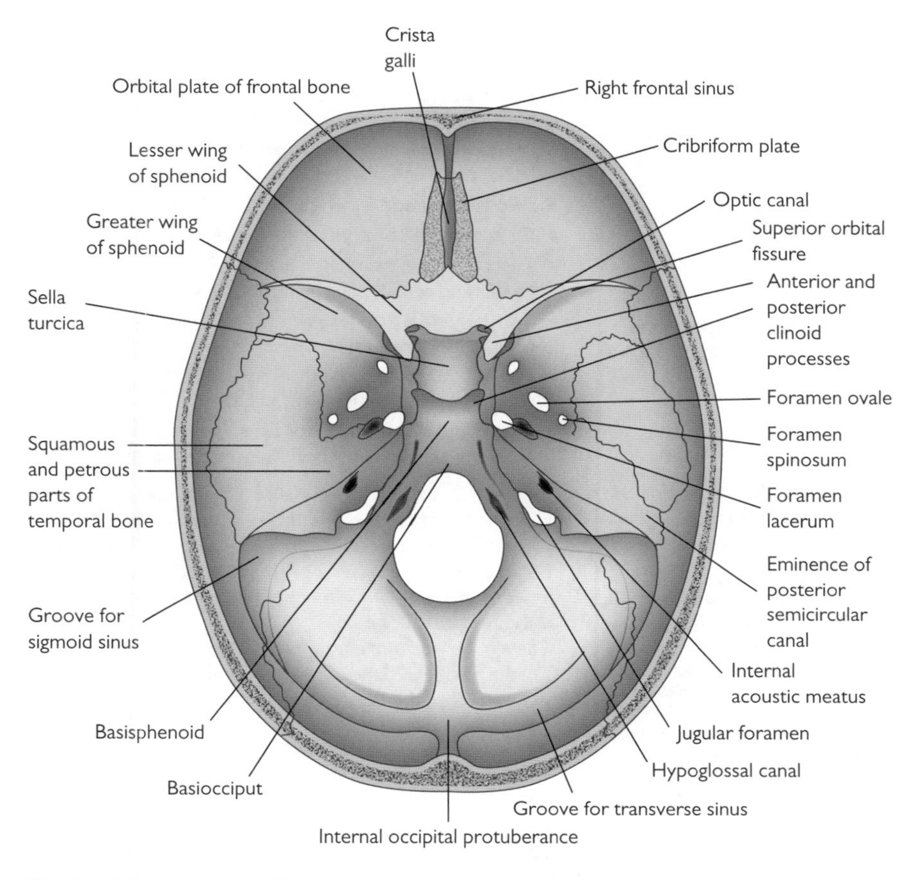

Fig. 12.20 Interior of skull. The foramen rotundum is hidden by the anterior clinoid process.

Reproduced from P MacKinnon and J Morris, *Oxford Textbook of Functional Anatomy: Volume 3*, 2005, Figure 6.1.14, p. 48, by permission of Oxford University Press

bone, squamous part of occipital bone and body of the sphenoid bone.

There are a number of important features in the base of the skull.

The anterior fossa

In the cribriform plate of the ethmoid bones foramina and conveys the olfactory nerve I.

The middle fossa

- In the greater wing of the sphenoid bone the foramen ovale conveys the mandibular division of trigeminal nerve VII and the lesser petrosal nerve
- The foramen rotundum conveys the maxillary division of trigeminal nerve VIII.
- The foramen spinosum conveys the middle meningeal artery and vein at the medial edge of the petrous part of the temporal bone.

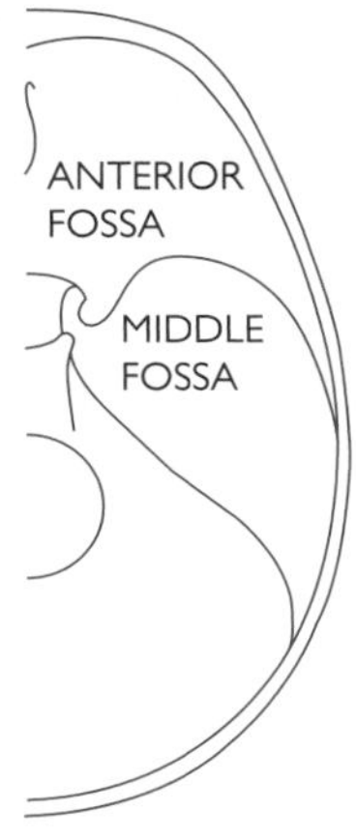

Fig. 12.21 Cranial fossae.

Reproduced from P MacKinnon and J Morris, *Oxford Textbook of Functional Anatomy: Volume 3*, 2005, Figure 6.1.3, p. 48, by permission of Oxford University Press

- The upper part of the foramen lacerum conveys the internal carotid artery (from the carotid canal) between the body and less wing of the sphenoid bone and the optic canal conveys the optic nerve II, ophthalmic artery between the greater and lesser wings of the sphenoid.
- The superior orbital fissure conveys the occulomotor nerve III, trochlear nerve IV, ophthalmic branch of trigeminal nerve VI, and abducent nerve VI in the body of the sphenoid.
- The sella turnica is a depression in which sits the pituitary gland.
- The junction of the frontal, parietal, and temporal bones, the pterion, is the thinnest and weakest point of the lateral skull.

The posterior fossa

- The foramen magnum in the occipital bone conveys the medulla oblongata, spinal part of accessory nerve XI, upper cervical nerves, and vertebral arteries, anterior to which the brainstem lies on the clivus.
- The hypoglossal canal conveys the hypoglossal nerve XII
- The internal acoustic meatus in the petrous temporal bone conveys the facial nerve VII, vestibulocochlear VIII nerves, and labyrinthine artery.
- The jugular foramen between the petrous temporal bone and the occipital bone conveys the glossopharyngeal nerve IX, vagus nerve X, accessory nerve XI, and sigmoid sinus.

The pyramidal pterygopalatine fossa is defined by the sphenoid, palatine, and maxilla bones: it contains the maxillary division of the trigeminal nerve, maxillary artery, and accompanying veins and lymphatics.

The bones that comprise the facial skeleton are suspended below the anterior cranium and comprise:

- Two nasal bones, joined to form the ridge of the nose.
- Two maxillary bones, which form the floor of orbit, lateral wall of the nose, floor of nasal cavity, and carry upper teeth.
- Two lacrimal bones, which form medial wall of orbit.
- One ethmoid bone, which forms the roof of the nose.
- The cribriform plate of the ethmoid, together with the vomer and septal cartilage forms the nasal septum.
- Two zygomatic bones, which form lateral wall of the orbit, cheek bone.
- Two palatine bones, with a perpendicular plate, which contributes to lateral wall of orbit.
- A horizontal plate that, together with the palatine processes of the maxillary bones, form the hard palate.

There are four paired paranasal air sinuses, contained within the frontal, maxillary, ethmoid, and sphenoid bones.

The mandible carries the lower teeth. It articulates with the cranium at the temporomandibular joint, which is between the head of the mandible and the mandibular fossa of the temporal bone

Seven cervical vertebrae form the skeleton of the neck. C1 (the atlas), C2 (the axis) and C7 are atypical. The long spine of C7 is the vertebra prominens, the superior-most process, which can be palpated.

The lateral masses of the C1 vertebra articulates with condyles on the occipital bone at the alanto-occipital joint, a loosely encapsulated synovial joint, which permits flexion and extension (nodding movements). Lateral masses of the atlas articulate with superior facets of the axis at alanto-axial joints to permit rotation. In addition, the odontoid process or dens makes a midline articulation with an anterior facet.

Neurophysiology

Neurons, typically made up of a soma (or the cell body), dendrites, and axon, are integral to the transmission of information throughout the nervous system. By inducing changes in the electrical voltage differences across the cell membrane (the action potential), neurons are able to produce electrical signals that that travel quickly and reliably over long distances. The information encoded in this electrical signal can then be transferred to another neuron or lead to the desired outcome, such as muscular contraction. In order to understand how the action potential is generated and propagated, one must first consider what happens under rest conditions.

Resting membrane potential

The neuron is surrounded by a semi-permeable phospholipid bilayer, which maintains a different concentration of ions in the extra- and intracellular compartments (Table 12.3). This concentration difference is crucial to the function of excitable cells and is maintained by an array of ion pumps.

Table 12.3 Different concentration of ions in the extra- and intracellular compartments

Ions	Extracellular concentration	Intracellular concentration
Sodium	140 mM	5-15 mM
Potassium	4 mM	140 mM
Calcium	2.4 mM	0.1 μM
Chloride	110 mM	5 mM
Bicarbonate	24 mM	10–20 mM
Hydrogen	40 nM	70 nM

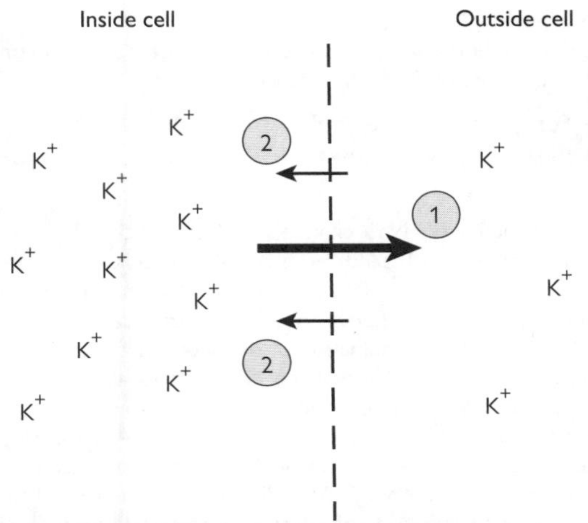

Fig. 12.22 The movement of potassium ions across the semi-permeable membrane. 1 Represents the movement down the concentration gradient and 2 represents the movement of potassium ions down the electrical gradient.

The Na^+/K^+ ATPase is the most important of these and is responsible for the active transport of three intracellular sodium ions out of the cell in exchange for two potassium ions being pumped into the cell.

Fig. 12.22 is a pictorial depiction of the movement of potassium ions across the cell membrane. The differential concentration of ions inside and outside the cell results in the movement of potassium out of the cell. In the case of uncharged particles, diffusion would results in the movement of particles continuing until the concentrations on both sides of the membrane are equal. However, as the potassium ions are positively charged, as more of them move out of the cell, the inside of the cell becomes negatively charged. Therefore, as potassium ions move down the concentration gradient, they generate an electrical gradient in the opposite direction. A steady state is reached when the electrical gradient prevents any further movement of potassium ions down the concentration gradient. The potential at which there is no net flux of ions across the membrane is called the equilibrium, or Nernst, potential. In the case of potassium this is approximately –95 mV.

As the phospholipid membrane is also permeable to ions other than potassium, the overall resting potential of the membrane must also depend on the concentrations of these ions and how easily they cross the cell membrane (the permeability). The resting membrane potential can be expressed in the form of the Goldman equation:

$$E_m = 58 \log \{(p_k[k^+]_o + p_{Na}[Na^+]_o + p_{Cl}[Cl^-]_i) / (p_k[K^+]_i + p_{Na}[Na^+]_i + p_{Cl}[Cl^-]_o)\};$$

where E_m is the resting potential and p is the permeability of each ion. Since, at rest, the membrane is most permeable to potassium ions, the actual membrane resting potential (~ –70 mV) lies closest to the potassium equilibrium potential.

Generation and propagation of the action potential

An action potential is a short, typically lasting approximately 1 ms, change in the membrane potential that allows a signal to be sent down the length of a neuron (Fig. 12.23).

In order for an action potential to be triggered the cell membrane must first be depolarized—this may occur either as an effect of neurotransmitter action at the synapse or as a direct consequence of a previous action potential. Once sufficient depolarization of the membrane has occurred and the threshold potential is reached, voltage-gated sodium channels open, leading to an influx of sodium ions into the cell. As the permeability of sodium increases, the membrane potential shifts nearer the equilibrium potential of sodium (+60 mV) and the cell membrane depolarizes completely. Thus, the action potential is triggered. Since the action potential is only triggered once the threshold potential has been reached, the signal sent down the neuron is all-or-nothing.

The opening of the sodium channels is short lived and, as they inactivate, the membrane potential starts to fall again. This phase of the action potential is also associated with the opening of voltage-gated potassium channels making the membrane even more permeable to potassium channels than at rest. This can result in the membrane potential coming even closer to the equilibrium potential of potassium, a phenomenon called after-hyperpolarization. The ion fluxes occurring in this sequence are very small in comparison with the number of ions present in the extra- and intracellular solutions, and the Na^+/K^+ ATPase restores the ion homeostasis to its resting conditions, preparing the membrane for the next action potential. There is a refractory period during which the neuron is resistant to firing another

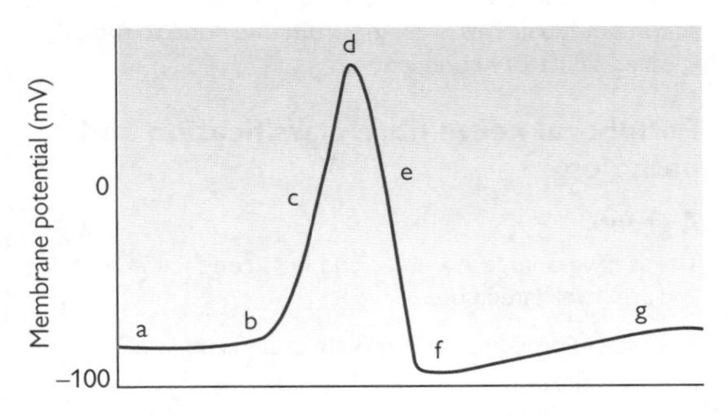

Fig. 12.23 The action potential. (a) Resting potential. (b) Opening of sodium ion channels. (c) Influx of sodium ions. (d) Closing of the sodium ion channels and opening of potassium ion channels. (e) Efflux of potassium ions. (f) After-hyperpolarization as a consequence of increased membrane permeability to potassium ions. (g) Closing of the potassium ion channels as the membrane returns to its resting condition.

action potential. The absolute refractory period is the time during which voltage-activated Na^+ channels recover from inactivation, and during which there are insufficient channels that can be recruited to initiate an up-stroke. The relatively refractory period correlates with the after-hyperpolarization, where larger stimuli are required to elicit a second action potential.

Each action potential leads to the generation of a passive and an active current in the neuron. The passive current represents the flow of charge along the length of the neuron, and the active current is the flow of sodium ions through the voltage-gated channels. As the passive current spreads along the length of the neuron, it depolarizes the membrane ahead and leads to the generation of a new action potential. Since each new action potential is regenerate in an all-or-nothing fashion, this process ensures that the amplitude and morphology of every action potential is identical, irrespective of where along the neuron it is recorded.

In small, unmyelinated neurons, voltage-gated sodium channels are found along the length of the axon allowing for continuous conduction of the signal. Although the transmission is effective, the conduction velocity of the signal is relatively slow. The speed of transmission is much improved in neurons with large diameter axons where the resistance within the axon is smaller and the flow of the passive current can be increased. However, this is not possible in peripheral nerves where fast conduction and relatively small diameter is required. In these situations, rapid conduction velocity is achieved by insulating nerve fibres with myelin. Myelin decreases capacitance and increases resistance across the cell membrane, thus helping to prevent the passive current leaking out of the axon. As ions cannot flow across the myelin layer, voltage-gated sodium channels are clustered in gaps in the myelin, called nodes of Ranvier. When an action potential is generated, the passive current flows to the next node of Ranvier, where it depolarizes the membrane and leads to the opening of voltage-gated sodium channels and generation of the next action potential. This 'skipping' from one node to the other is called salutatory conduction.

Peripheral nerve fibre classification and pathology

A group

These have a large diameter and high conduction velocity, and are myelinated fibres:

- A alpha fibres (mainly innervate skeletal muscle).
- A beta fibres (afferent or efferent fibres).
- A gamma fibres (efferent fibres).
- A delta fibres (afferent fibres).

B group

These are myelinated with a small diameter. Generally, they are the preganglionic fibres of the ANS and have a low conduction velocity.

C group

These are unmyelinated with a small diameter and low conduction velocity. These fibres include:

- Post-ganglionic fibres in the ANS.
- Nerve fibres at the dorsal roots carry sensory information.

Voltage-activated Na^+ channels can be blocked by local anaesthetics, which bind more readily to sodium channels in an activated state. This is referred to as use-dependent blockade. All nerve fibres are sensitive to local anaesthetics, but due to a combination of diameter, myelination, and activity, fibres have different sensitivities to local anaesthetic blockade. Type B fibres (sympathetic tone) are the most sensitive followed by type C (pain) and type A delta (temperature). Type A alpha (motor) fibres are least sensitive.

A variety of pathological conditions can influence peripheral nerve fibres, some of which demonstrate a preference for sensory A delta and unmyelinated C fibres (see Box 12.8), and some which are mainly motor neuropathies (see Box 12.9). Some pathology targets both the motor and sensory components of a particular nerve or individual nerves. This is known as a mononeuritis or a mononeuritis multiplex if several distinct nerves are involved (see Box 12.10). The pattern of peripheral nerve involvement can therefore give clues to the potential underlying cause.

BOX 12.8 CAUSES OF MAINLY SENSORY POLYNEUROPATHIES

- Diabetes mellitus.
- Vitamin B12 deficiency (especially dorsal columns).
- Alcohol.
- Uraemic neuropathy.
- Carcinomatous neuropathy.
- Amyloidosis.
- Leprosy.

BOX 12.9 CAUSES OF MAINLY MOTOR NEUROPATHIES (GENERALLY DEMYELINATING)

- Guillain–Barré syndrome and Miller Fisher (VII and oculomotor) syndrome.
- Hereditary sensory and motor neuropathy, e.g. Charcot–Marie–Tooth disease.
- Chronic inflammatory demyelinating polyneuropathy (CIDP).
- Lead poisoning.
- Porphyria.
- Multifocal motor neuropathy (association with IgM anti-GM1 antibodies).

BOX 12.10 CAUSES OF A MONONEURITIS MULTIPLEX

- Diabetes mellitus.
- Vasculitis.
- Amyloidosis.
- Polyarteritis nodosa.
- Rheumatoid arthritis.
- Systemic lupus erythematosus.
- Paraneoplastic syndrome.

Central nerve fibre pathology: multiple sclerosis

Multiple sclerosis (MS) is a chronic, demyelinating disease of the CNS. It typically presents between the ages of 20 and 40 years, with new cases rarely seen in young children or the elderly. The course of the disease can be extremely variable, with most patients initially experiencing relapses followed by complete or near-complete recovery. It is estimated that the disease affects approximately 2.5 million people worldwide, making it a leading cause of disability in young adults.

The aetiology of MS is unknown and is likely to represent a complex interaction between susceptibility genes and environmental triggers (Table 12.4).

In the vast majority of patients, a clinically-isolated syndrome (CIS) omens the onset of the disease, with the initial symptoms depending on the exact site of the responsible demyelinating lesion. Symptoms are typically transient, and resolve completely or partially within a few days or weeks. The common clinical manifestations of MS lesions include the following.

Table 12.4 The aetiology of multiple sclerosis

Evidence for genetic susceptibility	Evidence for environmental triggers
There is a female to male predominance (1.5:1)	There is an increase in the prevalence of MS with increasing distance from the equator
The *HLA-DRB1*1501* haplotype is associated with a 4-fold increase in the risk of MS	Children who emigrate before the age of 15 years acquire the MS prevalence rate of the new region they have moved to
There is a 20–40% increased risk of MS in first-degree relatives	There is an inverse correlation between sunlight exposure and the risk of MS (many believe this to be due to the immunomodulatory properties of vitamin D)
There is a 25–30% concordance in monozygotic, compared with 5% in dizygotic twins	Risk of MS is higher in individuals previously exposed to EBV

Optic neuritis

Characterized by unilateral visual loss that evolves over a period of few days, which may be associated with ocular pain exacerbated by eye movement. Clinical examination reveals a relative afferent pupillary defect, and swelling of the optic disc may be seen on fundoscopy. Resolution of acute optic neuritis often leads to optic atrophy.

Brainstem syndromes

May present as facial numbness or weakness, dysarthria, vertigo and ataxia, and motor or sensory symptoms. Ophthalmoplegia is common, with damage to the medial longitudinal fasciculus leading to internuclear ophthalmoplegia (the loss of movement of the adducting, but not the abducting eye when attempting to deviate the eyes to one side).

Transverse myelitis

May lead to weakness, sensory loss, paresthesia, and bladder or bowel dysfunction. Lesions in the cervical spine may lead to Lhermitte's sign, whereby the flexion of the neck leads to a sensation of an electrical shock radiating down the back and limbs. Uhthoff phenomenon refers to the transient worsening of neurological symptoms with elevation of temperature (e.g. during exercise or in a hot shower).

Cerebellar syndromes

May lead to gait ataxia, dysmetria, dysarthia, dysdiadochokinesia and an action tremor.

Patients may remain symptom free for months or years following the initial CIS. Most (approximately 85%) of cases then follow a relapsing-remitting form of the disease, with relapses interspaced by periods of clinical remission. Relapses may be triggered by infection and, in women, are more likely to occur in the first few months following childbirth. With time, incomplete recovery follows each relapse and patients begin to become increasingly disabled, with only around a third of patients remaining free of major disability 10 years after the onset of disease. After 25 years, approximately 90% of patients will have entered a secondary progressive course, characterized by a gradual progression of the disease. Approximately one in ten cases of MS follow a primary progressive course, with gradual progression of disability apparent from the disease onset.

The diagnosis of multiple sclerosis requires evidence of dissemination in space and time. In patients with relapsing-remitting MS, clinical diagnosis can be made on the basis of clinical signs of at least two lesions involving different regions of the central white matter at different times. In patients who have only had one clinical episode, contrast-enhanced MRI can be used to demonstrate subclinical lesions disseminated in space and time. CSF analysis, looking for evidence of oligoclonal bands, and neurophysiological methods, such as visual or brainstem auditory-evoked potentials, may be used to support the diagnosis.

Although they have no effect on the degree of recovery, high-dose corticosteroids shorten the duration of acute relapses. Due to the side-effect profile, steroids tend only be used for relapses that result in significant residual disability. Beta-interferons and glatiramer acetate are first-line disease modifying agents for relapsing-remitting MS. Although they have a modest effect on reducing the frequency of relapses, conclusive evidence for long-term benefit is lacking. Natalizumab is a humanized monoclonal antibody administered intravenously once a month. Although is seems to be more effective than beta-interferons and glatiramer acetate, it is associated with a small risk of progressive multifocal leuko-encephalopathy, and so tends to be used as a second- or third-line agent.

Synaptic function

Once an action potential has reached a synapse, further transmission may take an electrical or chemical form.

Electrical transmission

Electrical synapses, or gap junctions, mediate electrical transmission. They are made up of collections of paired ion channels, called connexons that allow ions and small molecules to flow between juxtaposed neurons. Gap junctions allow action potentials to spread between cells resulting in a very rapid form of neural transmission. The function of these synapses can be modulated my chemical signals that induce a conformational change in the proteins that make up the connexons, thus closing the junction. Gap junctions only make up a small minority of synapses and are typically found in areas requiring a high-degree of neuronal synchronization, such as the respiratory center in the medulla oblongata.

Chemical transmission

The majority of transmission within the nervous system is mediated via chemical synapses, which rely on excitation-secretion coupling. At rest, neurotransmitters can be found loaded inside synaptic vesicles tethered to cytoskeletal proteins, collectively known as the SNARE complex. As the action potential arrives at the synaptic terminal, depolarization of the membrane leads to the opening of neuronal voltage-gated calcium channels and a rise in the intracellular calcium concentration. In turn, these ions act on the calcium-binding domain on the SNARE complex, inducing a conformational change and fusion of the neurotransmitter vesicle with the presynaptic membrane. Consequently, the neurotransmitter is exocytosed into the synaptic cleft where it is able to act on receptors found on the post-synaptic membrane.

On reaching the post-synaptic membrane, the neurotransmitter can bind either ionotropic or metabotropic receptors. Ionotropic receptors are coupled to ion channels and, as the neurotransmitter binds, a conformational change allows ions to flow through a pore. The permeability of the activated channel to specific ions dictates the action of the neurotransmitter at the post-synaptic membrane. Ion channels, which allow the influx of sodium, bring the membrane closer to reaching threshold for the generation of an action potential. This small depolarization of the membrane is called an excitatory postsynaptic potential (EPSP). As a single EPSP is not large enough to result in sufficient depolarization, only the temporospatial summation of a large number of EPSPs will elicit an action potential. Conversely, an inhibitory post-synaptic potential (IPSP), which hyperpolarizes the membrane taking it further from the threshold necessary to trigger an action potential, is caused by an influx of chloride ions into the terminal.

Neurotransmitters may also bind to metabotropic receptors. These receptors influence intracellular signalling cascades, often through G protein-coupled mechanisms. Unlike ionotropic receptors, binding to these receptors has an indirect modulatory effect on the post-synaptic membrane.

Once they have exerted their action on their postsynaptic receptors, neurotransmitters need to be removed from the synaptic cleft. This may take a number of forms. In the neuromuscular junction, for example, acetylcholine is broken down by the enzymatic action of acetycholinesterase. The action of dopamine in the basal ganglia, on the other hand, is limited by its re-uptake into the presynaptic neuron where it can be used again. At some synapses, neurotransmitters can also bind to presynaptic autoreceptors, thus regulating their own release.

Pathology: botulism

Botulism is caused by the action of a potent neurotoxin produced by *Clostridium botulinum*, an anaerobic, Gram-positive, spore-forming rod. The neurotoxin acts by irreversibly binding to the SNAP-25 protein, a vital component of the SNARE complex, thus preventing the exocytosis of acetylcholine-loaded vesicles at the neuromuscular junction.

Sources of infection include:

- Wounds (especially associated with the injection of recreational drugs).
- Food-borne (may lead to small outbreaks associated with canned foods, such as fruit, fish, or vegetables).
- Honey (infant botulism).

Botulism is characterized by the absence of fever and is associated with early cranial nerve involvement and a progressive flaccid paralysis, often affecting the arms more than the legs. The weakness results in progressive respiratory impairment, ultimately leading to respiratory failure and death.

Blood and CSF examination is often unremarkable and detecting the toxin in the serum, wound site, stool, or food can confirm the diagnosis.

Management is largely supportive, but may include the administration of antitoxin or wound debridement. The return of synaptic transmission requires the sprouting of new nerve terminals and may take 6 months to occur.

Table 12.5 Different classes of small molecule neurotransmitters

Amino Acids	γ-Aminobutyric acid (GABA)
	Glycine
	Glutamate
Amines	Dopamine
	Noradrenaline
	Adrenaline
	Serotonin (5-HT)
	Histamine
Purines	ATP
Neuropeptides	Substance P
	Somatostatin
Acetylcholine	

Neurotransmitters

Neurotransmitters are molecules released by the presynaptic nerve terminal that carry information across the synaptic cleft. As the action of neurotransmitters is specific to the receptor they bind, they are responsible for differing effects at the post-synaptic membrane (see Table 12.5).

Glutamate

Glutamate is the most common excitatory neurotransmitter in the CNS. As most neurotransmitters, it is stored in vesicles at the presynaptic nerve terminal and released by exocytosis in response to an action potential. Glutamate can bind to four different receptors on the post-synaptic membrane, three ionotropic (AMPA, kainite, and NMDA) and one metabotropic. Unlike the other receptors, at resting potential, the NMDA receptor is blocked by magnesium ions and will only open in conjunction with depolarization produced by the AMPA or kainite receptors. As well as allowing the entry of sodium ions resulting in an EPSP, NMDA receptors allow the influx of calcium ions, which are involved in synaptic plasticity and excitotoxicity.

γ-Aminobutyric acid (GABA)

Along with glycine, GABA is one of the main inhibitory neurotransmitters in the CNS. It is synthetized from glutamate by the activity of glutamic acid decarboxylase (GAD).

GABA infers its effect through two main classes of receptors. The $GABA_A$-receptor is an ionotropic receptor, which allows a rapid influx of chloride ions, leading to an IPSP. The $GABA_B$-receptor, on the other hand, is a G-protein coupled metabotropic receptor, which inhibits voltage-gated calcium channels in nerve endings, thus reducing neurotransmitter release, and opens potassium channels leading to the hyperpolarization of the membrane.

The activity of GABA is terminated mainly by reuptake into the neuron.

Dopamine

Dopamine is most commonly found in the extrapyramidal motor system, as well as parts of the frontal cortex, limbic system, and the tuberohypophyseal system where dopamine release from the hypothalamus inhibits prolactin secretion from the anterior pituitary. Dopamine is of particular clinical relevance because of its involvement in a number of conditions, such as Parkinson's disease and schizophrenia.

To date, five types of metabotropic dopamine receptors have been identified (D_{1-5}). The D_2-family of receptors (D_2, D_3, and D_4) inhibit adenylate cyclase, thus reducing the influx of calcium ions and increasing the permeability to potassium ions. Conversely, the D_1-family of receptors (D_1 and D_5) have an excitatory action by stimulating adenylate cyclase.

Dopamine can be recaptured from the synaptic cleft and recycled into the presynaptic terminal by dopamine transporters. Its action can also be terminated through breakdown by monoamine oxidase (MAO) and catechol-O-methyl transferase (COMT).

Serotonin (5-HT)

The cell bodies of serotonergic neurons are grouped in the midline of the pons and upper medulla, and are often referred to as the raphe nuclei, projecting to many parts of the CNS. Serotonin is involved in many physiological processes, such as sleep, pain perception, thermoregulation, and appetite. Abnormal serotoninergic transmission has been implemented, amongst others, in depression, anxiety, schizophrenia, and migraine.

Seven classes 5-HT receptors have been identified with all but one, $5\text{-}HT_3$, acting through the G protein coupled-complex. The $5\text{-}HT_3$ receptor is a non-specific cation channel and is, therefore, excitatory.

Acetylcholine

Acetylcholine is widely distributed throughout the central and PNS. It is the principal neurotransmitter found in motor neurons in motor nuclei of the cranial nerves and ventral horn of the spinal cord, as well as the neuromuscular junction and the preganglionic neurons of the autonomic nervous system. In the brain, cell loss in the central cholinergic pathways, such as the nucleus basalis of Maynert, have been implemented in Alzheimer's disease.

Receptors for acetylcholine can be either ligand gated ion channels, nicotinic receptors (nAChR), or G protein-linked muscarinic receptors (mAChR). Nicotinic receptors are extremely rare in the CNS, but play a crucial role at the neuromuscular junction where they mediate transmission between peripheral motor neurons and skeletal muscle. A number of subtypes of the muscarinic receptor exist. The M_1-class (including the M_1, M_3, and M_5 subtypes) have an excitatory effect by blocking potassium channels. Conversely, the M_2 and M_4 subtypes of the receptor have an inhibitory effect through potassium channel activation and the inhibition of voltage-gated calcium channels. Muscarinic receptors also play an important role as autoreceptors on the presynaptic terminal of cholinergic neurons, inhibiting further release of acetylcholine.

The action of acetylcholine is terminated by enzyme degradation by acetylcholinesterase. Choline, a breakdown product of the reaction, is recovered back into the neuron, where it can be converted back into acetylcholine by choline acetyl transferase.

Pathology: Myasthenia gravis

Myasthenia gravis (MG) is an autoimmune disorder characterized by antibodies directed against the nicotinic acetylcholine receptor, thus impairing transmission at the neuromuscular junction. It is more common in women, and peaks in incidence in the second and third decade. There is a further peak in the sixth decade, when men are more commonly affected. IgG antibodies to nAChR are detectable in approximately three-quarters of patients with MG. Antibodies to muscle-specific kinase (MuSK), thought to activate complement-driven lysis of the post-synaptic membrane, can also be found in a large proportion of patients.

Most patients present with fatigue, diplopia, and weakness that typically worsens towards the end of the day. Only the ocular muscles are affected (ocular myasthenia) in approximately 15% of patients. The involvement of respiratory muscles may lead to respiratory failure. On clinical examination, fatigable weakness is the cardinal feature of MG—muscles become weaker with repetitive or sustained activity, e.g. sustained up-gaze leading to ptosis.

The diagnosis of MG can be supported by clinical, laboratory, and electrophysiological investigations. Although dramatic, the Tensilon test, where an iv injection of the short-acting acetycholinesterase inhibitor edrophonium is given, is rarely used and is contraindicated in patients with cardiac disease. Single fibre electromyography may be useful, with repetitive stimulation leading to a decrement in the amplitude of the recording.

Anticholinesterases (such as pyridostigmine) are the first line treatment in myasthenia gravis, preventing the breakdown of acetylcholine at the neuromuscular junction and improving muscle weakness. Corticosteroids are often used and have been shown to be effective at improving weakness and inducing remission. As steroids are associated with a significant risk of deterioration in proximal weakness in the first 2 weeks, treatment should be initiated in hospital. Remission can be maintained with azathioprine, allowing the steroid dose to be reduced. Intravenous immunoglobulin (IVIG) and plasma exchange significantly reduce antibody titres and produce short-term improvement in patients with a myasthenic crisis. Thymectomy also has a role in the management of MG, with almost a half of patients with thymic hyperplasia achieving full remission within 2 years.

Skeletal muscle

Skeletal muscles make up approximately 40% of the body's mass, and are responsible for everything from maintaining posture and perambulation to fine hand movements and blinking. Each muscle is made up of bundles of individual muscle fibres approximately 50 μm in diameter. The cell membrane of each muscle fibre encloses a number of myofibrils, each about 1 μm in diameter, composed of repeating units called sarcomeres (see Fig 12.24). Within each sarcomere are the interdigitated thin (mainly actin) and thick (mainly myosin) filaments. The thin filaments contain actin, tropomyosin and troponin, proteins integral to the functioning of the contractile mechanism. Thick filaments are formed from heavy and light chains of myosin attached to a titin protein core via myosin binding protein C. Titin anchors the thick filaments to the Z disc of the sarcomere

Excitation-contraction coupling in skeletal muscle is dependent on the release of a large intracellular store of calcium ions from the sarcoplasmic reticulum (SR). In order to facilitate this process, the plasma membrane of the muscle fibre (the sarcolemma) forms deep invaginations, known as transverse (T) tubules that extend deep into the fibre and are closely associated with the SR. The activation of the nicotinic acetylcholine receptors triggers an action potential that is propagated along the surface of the muscle membrane and down along the surface of the T tubules. Depolarization of the membrane induces a conformational change in the L-type voltage-gated calcium channels that, in turn, directly communicates with calcium channels, known as ryanodine receptors (RyR1 and RyR3), located on the surface of the SR. Opening of the RyRs by this 'voltage-induced-calcium-release' allows rapid entry of calcium into the cytoplasm.

Under resting conditions, tropomyosin covers the actin-binding sites on the thin filaments preventing the formation of cross-bridges with the myosin heads from the thick filament. As calcium binds to troponin, a conformational change is induced in tropomyosin, allowing the myosin head to bind to actin. This releases ADP and inorganic phosphate that was previously bound to the myosin, causing the myosin head to turn and results in a power stroke that shortens the sarcomere by approximately 10 nm. ATP then binds to the myosin where it is hydrolysed to ADP and inorganic phosphate. This releases the bond between actin and myosin, allowing the process to repeat as long as calcium and ATP are present. In the absence of repeated action potentials, calcium concentration in the cytoplasm falls rapidly as calcium ions are actively pumped back into the

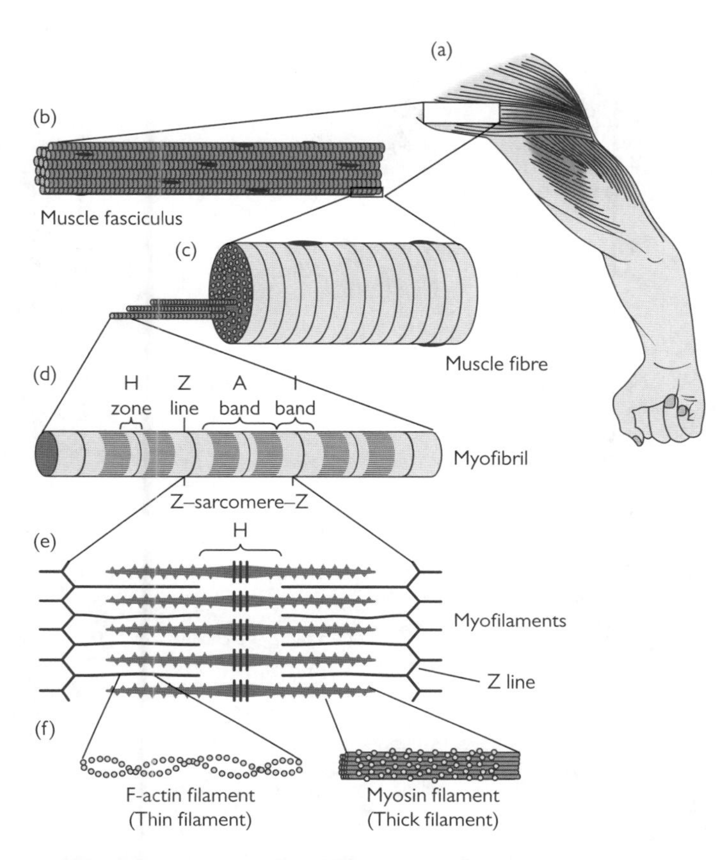

Fig. 12.24 The organization of skeletal muscle at various degrees of magnification. The appearance of the whole muscle (a); the appearance of a muscle fascicle (a bundle of muscle fibres; the nuclei of the muscle fibres are shown as the darker patches) (b); the appearance of a single muscle fibre (c); the structure of individual myofibrils (d); the arrangement of the protein filaments that make up the individual sarcomeres (e); the organization of actin and myosin in the thin and thick filaments (f). Note the absence of head groups in the central H zone which contains the tail region of the myosin molecules.

Reproduced from G Pocock and CD Richards, *Human Physiology: The Basis of Medicine, Third Edition*, 2006, Figure 7.2, p. 85, by permission of Oxford University Press

BOX 12.11 CAUSES OF MYOPATHIES

- Inflammatory (e.g. polymyositis).
- Metabolic (e.g. mitochondrial).
- Endocrine (e.g. hypo/hyperthyroidism, Cushing's syndrome).
- Drug induced (e.g. statins, steroids).
- Inherited dominant (myotonic dystrophy) or recessive (Duchenne's/Becker's dystrophy.

SR by the smooth endoplasmic reticulum calcium ATPase (SERCA) pump. As calcium is removed, tropomyosin once again prevents actin and myosin binding and contraction ceases.

Pathology: rigor mortis

ATP is necessary to break the bond between actin and myosin. This is seen in rigor mortis, where cross-bridges remain attached and muscles become stiff following death.

Drugs used in the treatment of Neurological disease

For drugs used in the treatment of neurological disease, see Table 12.6.

Table 12.6 Drugs used in the treatment of neurological disease

Antiepileptic drugs			
Drug	Mechanism of action	Side effects	Interactions
Benzodiazepines	Agonist at the benzodiazepine binding site on the $GABA_A$ receptor	Unwanted sedation, lightheadedness and confusion. May cause a paradoxical increase in seizures and aggression	*Reduced effect (liver enzyme inducers):* phenytoin, carbamazepine, barbiturates, rifampicin, chronic excess EtOH, sulphonylureas

(continued)

Table 12.6 Drugs used in the treatment of neurological disease (*continued*)

Drug	Mechanism of action	Side effects	Interactions
Carbamazepine	Inhibition of action potential generation by stabilizing the inactivated state of voltage-gated sodium channels	Vertigo, confusion, ataxia, and insomnia. May be associated with generalized erythematous rash	*Reduced effect (liver enzyme inducers):* phenytoin, barbiturates, rifampicin, chronic excess EtOH, sulphonylureas
Ethosuximide	Inhibition of action potential generation by blocking T-type calcium channels	Nausea, anorexia, headaches, and mood disturbance	*Reduced effect:* sodium valproate, carbamazepine, phenobarbital, phenytoin
Gabapentin	Mechanism unknown	Drowsiness, ataxia, nystagmus, and fatigue	
Lamotrigine	Inhibition of action potential generation by stabilizing the inactivated state of voltage-gated sodium channels. Inhibits glutamate release	Rash and hypersensitivity syndrome. Patients advised to seek immediate medical advice if a rash develops	*Increased effect:* sodium valproate
Levetiracetam	Mechanism unknown	Sleepiness, agitation, anxiety, and behavioural problems	
Phenobarbital	Agonist at the barbiturate site on the $GABA_A$ receptor	Sedation, respiratory depression, hypothermia, and hypotension	*Reduced effect (liver enzyme inducers):* phenytoin, carbamazepine, barbiturates, rifampicin, chronic excel EtOH, sulphonylureas. *Increased effect:* sodium valproate
Phenytoin	Inhibition of action potential generation by stabilizing the inactivated state of voltage-gated sodium channels	Dose-related vertigo, confusion, insomnia, and ataxia. Non-dose-related rashes, megaloblastic anaemia, teratogenesis, and gum hyperplasia	*Reduced effect (liver enzyme inducers):* carbamazepine, barbiturates, rifampicin, chronic excess EtOH, sulphonylureas
Sodium valporate	Multiple mechanisms, including enhancement of GABAergic transmission by inhibiting the breakdown and enhancing the synthesis of GABA, and the use-dependent blockade of voltage-gated sodium channels	Fatigue, nausea, tremor, weight gain, hair loss and teratogenesis	*Reduced effect (liver enzyme inducers):* carbamazepine, phenytoin, barbiturates, rifampicin, chronic excess EtOH, sulphonylureas
Topiramate	Multiple mechanisms, including blockade of voltage-gated sodium channels, acting as an agonist at the barbiturate site on the $GABA_A$ receptor, and antagonizing the NMDA receptor at the glutamate-binding site	Fatigue, sedation, impaired concentration, metabolic acidosis, glaucoma, and kidney stones	*Reduced effect (liver enzyme inducers):* carbamazepine, phenytoin, barbiturates, rifampicin, chronic excess EtOH, sulphonylureas
Vigabatrin	Enhancement of GABAergic transmission by inhibiting the breakdown of GABA	Sedation, mood disturbance, and loss of peripheral vision	
Anti-Parkinsonian drugs			
Drug	**Mechanism of action**	**Side effects**	**Interactions**
Levodopa	Metabolic precursor of dopamine that is able to cross the blood–brain barrier. Almost always co-administered with a peripherally-acting decarboxylase inhibitor	Nausea, vomiting, hallucinations, confusion, and postural hypotension. May lead to on/off phenomena and dyskinesias	*Increased effect:* non-specific MAO inhibitors—must be discontinued at least 14 days before starting levodopa (does not include specific MAO-B inhibitors)

Table 12.6 Drugs used in the treatment of neurological disease (*continued*)

Drug	Mechanism of action	Side effects	Interactions
Dopamine agonists, e.g. pramipexole and ropinirole	Agonists of striatal dopamine receptors (D_2 class sites)	Hallucinations, confusion, and orthostatic hypotension. Ergot derived agonists (e.g. pergolide) associated with valvular heart disease	
Catechol-O-methyltransferase (COMT) inhibitors, e.g. entacapone and tolcapone	Block the *O*-methylation of levodopa in the periphery, thus increasing delivery to the brain. Inhibit breakdown of dopamine in the synaptic cleft	Nausea, orthostatic hypotension, confusion and hallucinations. Tolcapone is associated with hepatotoxicity	
Selective MAO-B inhibitors e.g. rasagiline and selegiline	Inhibit breakdown of dopamine in the striatum	Nausea, GI symptoms, confusion and hallucinations	May lead to serotonin syndrome if used in conjunction with anti-depressants
Muscarinic receptor antagonists, e.g. benzhexol hydrochloride	Reduce the effects of the relative central cholinergic excess caused by dopamine deficiency	Constipation, dry mouth, and nausea and vomiting. May lead to confusion, hallucinations and impaired memory	
Amantadine	Antiviral agent, thought to alter dopamine release and have anticholinergic properties	Dizziness, lethargy, and anticholinergic effects	

Common drug-induced neurological reactions

- *Vertigo:* anticonvulsants (e.g. phenobarbital, phenytoin), aminoglycosides, furosemide, salicylates, alcohol and cocaine.
- *Retinopathy:* hydroxychloroquine, amiodarone, ethambutol, vigabatrin, chloromazine, and quinolones.
- *Optic neuritis:* phosphodiesterase type 5 inhibitors, amiodarone, linezolid, ethambutol, and isoniazid.
- *Extrapyramidal reactions:* antipsychotics, metoclopramide, and tricyclic antidepressants.
- *Idiopathic intracranial hypertension:* oral contraceptive pill, steroids, vitamin A, lithium, growth hormone, nitrofurantoin, phenytoin, thyroxine.
- *Peripheral neuropathy:* cisplatin, dapsone, metronidazole, amiodarone, thalidomide, cochicine, penicillamine.
- *Exacerbations of myasthenia gravis:* corticosteroids, local anaesthetics, antibiotics (e.g. aminoglycosides, quinolones, erythromycin, metronidazole), phenytoin, beta-blockers, calcium channel blockers, lithium, chlorpromazine, chloroquine.
- *Rhabdomyolysis:* alcohol, amphetamines, antimalarials, colchicine, corticosteroids, statins, zidovudine, isoniazid, diuretics.

Multiple choice questions

1. A 65-year-old woman with poorly controlled Type II diabetes mellitus complains of horizontal diplopia worse on looking to the right. On covering the right eye, the outermost image disappears. Which of the following cranial nerves is most likely responsible for the opthalmoplegia?

A. Left abducens.
B. Right abducens.
C. Left oculomotor.
D. Right oculomotor.
E. Right trochlear.

2. A 55-year-old man develops left-sided ataxia with Horner's syndrome and loss of pain and temperature sensation on his face. Which is the most likely artery to be occluded given this signs?

A. Basilar artery.
B. Posterior cerebral artery.
C. Posterior communicating artery.
D. Posterior inferior cerebellar artery.
E. Superior cerebellar artery.

3. A 40-year-old man who is a smoker has a 2-year history of deafness and tinnitus in his left ear. On examination, he has sensorineural hearing loss on the left, no nystagmus, and the left corneal reflex is absent. What is the most likely diagnosis?

A. Acoustic neuroma.
B. Multiple sclerosis.
C. Brainstem astrocytoma.
D. Basilar artery aneurysm.
E. Miller Fischer syndrome.

4. A 70-year-old female who is a smoker with high cholesterol and hypertension complains of progressive difficulty with writing and mental arithmetic. On examination, she has a right-sided homonymous inferior quadrantinopia, and right-sided visuospatial neglect. An MRI scan is most likely to demonstrate damage to which of the following structures?

A. Left frontal lobe.
B. Right subthalamic nucleus.
C. Left parietal lobe.
D. Right parietal lobe.
E. Left temporal lobe.

5. A 13-year-old girl is brought to clinic by her mother as she has recently developed a rash and appears to be stumbling a lot. On examination, she has bilateral ataxia and nystagmus, and a generalized erythematous rash. There is no family history of note, although her mother has epilepsy. She is otherwise well and has had no recent fevers or illnesses. The most likely diagnosis is?

A. Gliobastoma multiforme.
B. Miller Fischer syndrome.
C. Multiple sclerosis.
D. Friedreich's ataxia.
E. Carbamazepine overdose.

6. Which of the following concerning myasthenia gravis is correct?

A. It is caused by auto-antibodies against the muscarinic acetylcholine receptor.
B. Repetitive stimulation using single fibre electromyography leads to an increment in the amplitude of the recording.
C. The anticholinesterase pyridostigmine is typically the first line treatment for myasthenia gravis.
D. Thymectomy offers a cure to myasthenia gravis in all patients with thymic hyperplasia.
E. Diplopia that improves during the course of the day is a common feature.

7. Which of the following is not considered part of the basal ganglia?

A. Putamen.
B. Globus pallidus.
C. Nucleus accumbens.
D. Peri-aquaductal grey.
E. Sub-thalamic nuclei.

8. Which of the following CSF findings are *not* consistent with tubercular meningitis?

A. Low glucose.
B. Raised white cells, predominantly neutrophils.
C. Elevated protein.
D. Negative Gram stain.
E. Positive culture for acid-fast bacilli.

9. **Which of the following drugs used to treat Parkinson's disease inhibit catechol-o-methyltransferase?**

   A. Entacapone.
   B. Selegilline.
   C. Ropinirole.
   D. Benzhexol.
   E. Amantadine.

10. **Which of the following proteins do not form part of the thin filament in skeletal muscle?**

   A. Actin.
   B. Tropomyosin.
   C. Troponin C.
   D. Troponin I.
   E. Titin.

For answers, please see Appendix: Answers to multiple choice questions, page 313.

CHAPTER 13

Psychiatry

Introduction

Together, the peripheral and central nervous systems comprise an integrated network of neurons that allow rapid transmission and processing of information as nervous impulses. In conjunction with the endocrine system, this network is responsible for homeostasis of an organism, as well as for its behavioural patterns. In man, this includes higher-level functions, such as thinking, memory, and personality. An appreciation of how the major psychiatric illnesses manifest, and the current pathophysiological theories behind them aids understanding of how they are diagnosed and subsequently treated.

Schizophrenia: pathophysiological basis

Introduction

The term schizophrenia meaning literally 'split mind' is increasingly regarding as a term to describe a group of associated diseases, which have a number of different aetiological, neurobiological, and neurochemical processes, but which clinically present with 'psychosis', a final clinical picture where the sufferer is unable to distinguish between external reality, and their own internally generated thoughts and perceptions. As will be seen from the review of the evidence there is no single over-arching abnormality or pathological feature that can explain the clinical picture in schizophrenia. Consequently, several theories exist to explain the clinical picture observed.

Epidemiology

Schizophrenia has a prevalence of 0.5–1%, with slightly higher incidence in men. Onset occurs between 15–45 years of age. The course of schizophrenia is relapsing and remitting, lifelong, and characterized by acute episodes on the background of chronic progression of negative symptoms. Life expectancy is reduced, with suicide and cardiovascular disease making significant contributions.

Environmental risk factors

- Obstetric complications.
- Increased paternal age at conception.
- Maternal influenza during pregnancy.
- Maternal malnutrition.
- Winter birth.
- Abnormal early childhood developmental stages.
- Substance misuse, in particular 'skunk' cannabis.
- Lower social class over-representation.
- Exposure to early stressors and high familial expressed emotion.
- Increased risk in migrants.
- Personality factors.

Aetiology and pathophysiology

Schizophrenia is regarded as an illness with a multifactorial aetiology, which can be described along the Biological-Psychological-Social model more than any other psychiatric disorder (see 'Affective disorders: pathophysiological basis'). There are some factors that have become supported with significant evidence, and these are described.

Genetic factors

Schizophrenias show a strong genetic factor, with family, twin, and adoption studies suggesting greater than 50% and up to 80% heritability factors. There is significantly increased risk of schizophrenia in first degree relatives of probands of up to 15 times as compared with the general population. Twin studies have identified that monozygotic twins who may not show concordance in phenotype irrespectively confer increased risk to their offspring.

Molecular genetic studies have identified numerous genes associated with schizophrenia. Genome-wide linkage studies have provided evidence for association with 14 genes, including (amongst others).

- *DISC1:* 'disrupted in schizophrenia'—1q.
- *NRG1:* neuregulin—8p.
- *PCM1:* pericentriolar material—8p.
- *DTNBP1:* dysbindin—6p.
- *DAAO:* d-aminoacid oxidase—12q.

At a population level the associations may be modest, but it is argued that as schizophrenia is increasingly understood to be a spectrum of disorders there may be multiple gene-interactions and epigenetic effects influencing a final common pathway. It is interesting to note that the genes implicated in the pathogenesis of schizophrenia (listed above) are associated with cell division and not just neurotransmission.

Neuroanatomy

Neuroanatomical changes are observed at microscopic and macroscopic levels, as well as using neuroimaging studies.

- Gross neuroanatomy and structural imaging reveals decreased overall brain volume, enlarged third and lateral ventricles, and reduction in medial temporal lobe volume (especially the hippocampus). These associations are found in first-onset and pre-medicated patients with a diagnosis of schizophrenia irrespective of sub-type, and strongly supports it being a biological brain disease. There does remain overlap, however, with controls and are not diagnostically specific. Of note, first degree relatives tend to show changes in regional brain volume intermediate between patients and unrelated healthy controls.
- On a microscopic level, there are alterations in synaptic structure, and in cell density of neurons in the hippocampus, thalamus, and other areas of cortex.
- Using positron emission tomography (PET), single-photon emission computed tomography (SPECT), and functional magnetic resonance imaging (fMRI) cerebral blood flow has been shown to be disrupted with the finding of 'hypofrontality' through reduced frontal perfusion. This may relate to aberrant connectivity of brain regions.

Neurophysiology

There are a number of associated neurophysiological observations in schizophrenia:

- EEG shows increased that, fast and paroxysmal activity suggestive of 'noisy' or inefficient cortical processes.
- Sensory auditory-evoked potentials at 300 ms (P300—a measure of auditory processing) are reduced in amplitude. Similar P50-evoked potentials are deficient.
- Eye-tracking is abnormal in over 50% of individuals with schizophrenia.

Neurochemistry

- *Dopamine:* the most influential neurochemical theory of schizophrenia pathophysiology remains 'the dopamine hypothesis'. This describes that the symptoms of psychosis are a consequence of 'hyperdopaminergia', particularly within the mesolimbic system. This theory is supported by the following evidence:
  - All antipsychotics are D2 antagonists, with their potency being proportional to affinity.
  - Repeated amphetamine use (i.e. dopamine potentiation) can lead to a schizophrenia-like picture, as well as worsening psychotic symptoms in those with schizophrenia.
  - In patients with schizophrenia, injection of amphetamine causes a 2-fold greater decrease in [11C] raclopride (D2 receptor radioligand) than in control subjects. This corresponds to a 3-fold greater increase of synaptic dopamine release.
  - Deficiencies of dopaminergic regulation of the pre-frontal cortex are related to cognitive deficits.
- *Glutamate:* there is increasing interest in glutamatergic neurotransmission in schizophrenia. This is primarily based upon the following observations:
  - Antagonists of the NMDA glutamate receptor, such as ketamine and phenylcyclidine (PCP), can induce a schizophrenia-like psychosis.
  - NMDA receptor modulators, such as glycine have some antipsychotic effects.
  - Non-NMDA glutamate receptors are increased in frontal areas and reduced in the medial temporal lobe.
  - Role of glutamate in schizophrenia may be NMDA receptor hypofunction, aberrant glutamatergic regulation of dopamine function or a primary role of glutamate function itself (as most susceptibility genes are involved in glutamate transmission).
- *Serotonin:* interest in serotonergic neurotransmission abnormalities having a role in schizophrenia are supported by the following:
  - The hallucinogen, LSD is a 5-HT2A receptor agonist.
  - 5HT2 receptor antagonism is a consistent feature in the mechanism of action of the newer 'atypical' antipsychotics.
  - An allelic variation of the *5-HT2A* gene is a minor risk factor for schizophrenia.
  - Decreased expression of frontal cortex 5-HT2A receptors in schizophrenia.
- *GABA:* increase in the GABA synthetic enzyme, glutamic acid decarboxylase (GAD) in the cerebral cortex of schizophrenics.

Clinical diagnosis and symptoms

Paranoid schizophrenia is the most common, and is characterized by 'positive symptoms' during an acute episode and ongoing negative symptoms throughout the life of the individual.

Positive symptoms, which can respond well to pharmacological treatment, include:

- *Perceptual abnormalities:* hallucinations usually auditory in the form of 'voices', but can occur in any sensory modality (i.e. visual, olfactory, gustatory, somatic/tactile and visceral).
- *Disorder of thought content:* delusions. These are strongly held beliefs, despite evidence to disprove or to show that the contrary is true. These can be further categorized into a number of subtypes, but the most frequently elicited are persecutory, bizarre, grandiose, referential, love/jealousy, and nihilism.
- *Disorder of possession of thought/actions:* thought interference and passivity phenomena. This is the subjective experience and/or complaint of interference with thoughts, e.g. thoughts feel as though they are inserted or removed, or being broadcast, or that an external entity has taken control of ones thoughts or actions.
- *Disorder of the form of thought:* it is difficult to understand or follow what the individual is thinking, as manifested through the speech. This can be through responding to questions with inappropriate answers, seeming unconnectedness between themes discussed, or complete incomprehensibility of the thought processes. Associated behavioural disturbance and lack of insight.
- Schizophrenia has been shown to be associated with increased risk of violence.

First rank symptoms

Whilst lacking any specific diagnostic investigation, there are some specific positive symptoms that are traditionally regarded as suggestive of schizophrenia. These are known as 'first rank symptoms' and although are not exclusive to schizophrenia are associated with it. The validity has been questioned although in clinical practice they remain convincing:

- Audible thoughts (thought echo/'echo de la pensee').
- Running commentary (voice commenting on sufferers actions).
- Voices heard arguing.
- Passivity phenomena.
- Thought interference phenomena.
- Delusional perception (i.e. a normal sensory perception, such as seeing a red traffic light, leading to the individual immediately making an abnormal interpretation, such as deducing that this means that they have been made Head of State.

Negative symptoms describe the gradual longitudinal deterioration of the personality and development of cognitive deficits. These include avolition (lack of motivation), alogia (reduction in spontaneous speech), affect blunting (reduction in experience of mood), and associability (lack of interest in relationships). These symptoms are less responsive to pharmacological treatment.

There are a number of other forms of schizophrenia, including 'catatonic' (characterized by movement abnormality) and 'hebephrenic' (characterized by thought disorder problems).

Treatment

Treatment of schizophrenia can be physical, pharmacological, and psychosocial:

- *Physical treatments include electroconvulsive therapy (ECT):* as in the case of depression it is unclear how it has its main effect and is often reserved for chronic treatment-resistant cases.
- *Pharmacological treatments are listed at the end of this chapter:* they consist of antipsychotics (also known as 'major tranquillizers' or 'neuroleptics'). All of these medications share antagonism at the D2 receptor. First generation antipsychotics, such as haloperidol and chlorpromazine are characterized by strong D2 affinity and antagonism. They are associated with tardive dyskinesia with prolonged used at high doses. Second generation antipsychotics, such as olanzapine and amisulpride have the additional property of antagonism at the 5HT2A receptor. They demonstrate increased risk of development of 'metabolic syndrome', characterized by aberrant glucose tolerance, lipid dysregulation, and weight gain.
- Some antipsychotic medications are also available in slow-release injection form ('depot antipsychotics'). These may be used to increase compliance with medication should this be thought clinically relevant. It may also be a preferred route of administration for patients who do not wish to take oral medication on a daily basis.
- Clozapine (a second generation antipsychotic) is associated with agranulocytosis, and careful monitoring is a feature of its prescribing. It is also used in treatment-resistant and severe schizophrenia owing to its efficacy.
- *Psychological treatments and social interventions:* cognitive behavioural therapy, insight-focused, therapy, psychoeducation about medication and the illness, and social support, e.g. supported accommodation. The morbidity of schizophrenia is high and can be associated with considerable disability.

A note on tardive dyskinesia

A neurological consequence of long-term/high-dose antipsychotic treatment, in particular with more potent and first generation drugs (e.g. haloperidol). Characterized by repetitive involuntary movements with no purpose, akathisia, writhing movements, and sometimes orofacial dyskinesia (tongue protrusion, lip smacking, pursing, and other facial movements of which the sufferer is unaware). It can be minimized by reducing the dose of antipsychotic slowly and/or considering a second generation antipsychotic.

Affective disorders: pathophysiological basis

Introduction

The affective disorders involve a fundamental disturbance in *affect* or *mood*, from unipolar depression ('major depression'; depressive episodes only) to elation and irritability (manic episode, hypomania, or mania). In bipolar affective disorder ('BPAD', 'manic-depression', 'bipolar depression') there can be cycling between periods of low mood, and usually distinct periods of elation or irritably. This disturbance is usually accompanied by a collection of other biological, or somatic, and cognitive symptoms.

Unipolar depression

Epidemiology

Depression is predicted to be the largest cause of disability in the world by 2020 (Murray and Lopez, 1997) Lifetime prevalence is 3–20%, with women twice as likely to experience this as men (although this may be a reporting bias). The first episode often occurs during the 30s, with a second peak in 50s/60s. There is common comorbidity in neurological diseases and it is more common in cardiovascular disease compared with controls.

Risk factors for depression include:

- Female gender.
- Younger age of onset.
- Personal history of mental disorder.
- Positive family history.
- Urban residence.
- Lower socioeconomic status.
- Unmarried status.
- Physical illness.

The BioPsychoSocial model suggests that biological (e.g. neurobiological), psychological (e.g. thinking style), and social (e.g. lack of supportive relationships) factors all contribute to developing depression.

The diathesis-stress model suggests that there is a preexisting vulnerability, or 'diathesis' (e.g. genetic factors, factors in childhood development) towards developing depression, which is precipitated by later exposure to environmental factors, stressors or other trauma during later life.

Aetiology and pathophysiology

Depression is regarded as an illness with a multifactorial aetiology.

Genetic factors

Depression aggregates within families. The heritability estimate for major depression is between 33 and 48%. Individuals with unipolar disorder only show an excess of unipolar depression in relatives.

Molecular genetic studies show that genes for major depression overlap with those for anxiety and neuroticism. Therefore, it may be possible to understand the genetic basis of depression better by looking for loci that underlie neuroticism, and a recent study suggested a 'hotspot' on chromosome 12.

Genome-wide linkage studies suggest that in regions 15q, 17p, and 8p there may contributing genes to susceptibility in major depression. No candidate gene has been definitively identified but polymorphism in the human serotonin transporter gene (5-HTT or hSERT) located on 17q has been widely implicated. The serotonin transporter is a single transmembrane presynaptic protein responsible for serotonin re-uptake. The 5-HTT gene contains a common variable number tandem repeat (VNTR) polymorphism within one of its introns, as well as a common variant in the promoter region, shown to affect the level of gene expression. The 5-HTTLPR (long promoter region) polymorphism may be particularly implicated in the risk of developing depression, as well as the response to treatment.

The SERT/5HTT is a target for tricyclic antidepressants (TCAs) and selective serotonin re-uptake inhibitor (SSRI) antidepressants, which competitively bind to the 5HT binding site, thus reducing 5HT re-uptake.

Structural neurobiology

It is widely accepted that depression does not result from specific dysfunction within a single brain region or neurotransmitter system. The corticolimbic and corticostriatal networks are primarily most implicated.

- Neuropathological post-mortem studies have suggested cyto-architectural abnormalities in the anterior cingulate and prefrontal cortices, characterized by a decrease in glial cell density (in particular astrocytes). Structural brain changes have also been identified by MRI ,and are thought to be a consequence of chronic hypercortisolaemia, a frequent finding in depression. These include enlarged ventricles and prominent sulci, and reduced grey matter volumes in left hippocampal, frontal, and parietal association cortices.
- Functional imaging has suggested abnormalities in the (subgenual) ventromedial prefrontal cortex (an area connected to amygdala, nucleus accumbens and 5HT, noradrenergic (NA) and dopaminergic (DA) brainstem nuclei.

Neurochemistry: the monoamine hypothesis

The monoamine theory of depression has been the predominant neurochemical theory of depression for many years. Monoamine oxidase-A (MAO-A) metabolizes 5HT, DA, and NA, and it is suggested that MAO-A is increased in multiple brain areas in medication-free depressed subjects. (Meyer, 2006).

- *Evidence to support the role of 5HT in depression:*
  - Decreased plasma tryptophan (serotonin precursor) in depressed patients.

- Low CSF concentration of 5HIAA (serotonin metabolite), although this finding is not consistent and is also seen in those who have committed impulsive suicidal acts.
- Reduced 5HT and 5HIAA brain concentrations found post-mortem in depressed brain.
- Blunted endocrine responses found in hormones signalled by 5HT pathways (prolactin, growth hormone and cortisol).

- *Evidence to support the role of NA in depression:* blunted GH response seen to clonidine (NA-R agonist) in depression. This is a trait marker and does not resolve upon remission of the depressive episode.
- *Evidence to support DA in depression:*
  - In animal studies, antidepressants increase DA-R expression in *N. accumbens*.
  - Homovanillic acid (HVA, a DA metabolite) and lowered DA CSF levels are found in depressed patients.
  - Functional imaging shows increased binding to DA2/DA3 receptors in striatal areas in depressed patients.
- *Evidence for glutamate:* there is increasing evidence that glutamate transmission is altered in depressed patients.

Endocrine abnormalities

- *Hypothalamic–pituitary–adrenal (HPA) axis and cortisol:* the HPA axis is the primary stress axis in man. HPA hyperactivity, probably in response to CRH hypersecretion, occurs in individuals with severe mood disorder. The evidence for a role in depression is as follows:
  - About half of patients with Cushing's Disease suffer from depression, which resolves when the cortisol hypersecretion is corrected.
  - Around half of the individuals with major depression have an increased cortisol output.
  - Fifty per cent of depressed patients show non-suppression of cortisol in the dexamthasone suppression test (DST). However, this is not specific to depression and, therefore, cannot be used as a diagnostic test.

  The neurotoxic effects of high cortisol are thought to account for many of the structural brain changes seen on imaging in depressed patients.
- *Thyroid abnormalities:* abnormalities of the thyroid hormones are sometimes seen in depression, specifically:
  - Free tri-iodothyronine (T3) levels can be decreased in depressed patients.
  - Around a quarter of depressed subjects have a blunted TSH response to TRH.

Clinical diagnosis and symptoms

Clinically, unipolar depression can be divided into two subcategories—a single depressive episode and recurrent-depressive disorder, where an individual has experienced more than one episode. Episodes are characterized by core symptoms, which include a pervasive lowering of mood, anhedonia (an *inability* to experience enjoyment or pleasure), and a reduction in energy and activity. Associated 'biological' symptoms include sleep disturbance (too little or too much), early morning wakening (waking earlier than one would do normally), loss of appetite, diurnal mood variation (mood typically being worst in the morning), reduced libido, and psychomotor retardation (reduction of movement in line with low mood and motivation). Associated 'cognitive' symptoms include loss of concentration and motivation, poor self-esteem, ideas of guilt, hopelessness, and worthlessness. Depending of the number and severity of these associated symptoms, the acute depressive episode can be characterized as mild, moderate, or severe. There can also be symptoms of psychosis in severe depression, which are often congruent with the mood and may take the form of nihilistic delusions of death/rotting (e.g. Cotard's syndrome). In order to fulfil the clinical diagnosis a combination of these symptoms must have been present for at least 2 weeks.

Treatment

Treatment of unipolar depression can be physical, pharmacological, or psychological.

Physical treatments

These include electroconvulsive therapy (ECT) and occasionally transcranial magnetic resonance stimulation (tMRS). ECT has numerous physiological, biochemical, and neurobiological effects. It is unclear how it has its main effect, and is often reserved for more severe and intractable cases, unresponsive to augmented pharmacological treatments. It is administered under anaesthesia, and is thought to be associated with autobiographical memory loss with longer-term use. It remains, however, the single most effective way of treating depression. Psychosurgery is vanishingly infrequent.

Pharmacological treatments

These are listed at the end of this chapter. In unipolar depression, SSRIs are the treatment of choice, and are very effective with a number needed to treat (NNT) of approximately 5 or 6. These work by prolonging the presence of 5HT in the synapses through competitive binding at the 5HT re-uptake site of the re-uptake transporter. 5HT1A agonism is particularly implicated in recovery. Augmentation strategies are often used where there is treatment-resistance to monotherapy, e.g. use of second antidepressant from a different class, use of antipsychotic medication or lithium (mood stabilizer).

Psychological treatments

Cognitive behavioural therapy (CBT) has a strong evidence base in depressive disorder and, when used in conjunction with antidepressant, have a synergistic effect. The treatment consists of a 'course' of sessions with a trained CBT therapist, during which cognitions and behaviours are analysed and challenge, homework given, and new coping strategies developed.

Bipolar affective disorder

Epidemiology

Bipolar affective disorder is less common than unipolar depression, with a lifetime prevalence variously quoted as between 0.5 and 4%, with equal prevalence in men and women (unlike unipolar). The onset is most common in late adolescence/early adulthood.

Aetiology and pathophysiology

Bipolar affective disorder has a significantly greater contribution from genetic factors than unipolar depression, and its aetiology remains poorly understood.

Genetic factors

Twin studies demonstrate an estimated heritability of 40–70%. Family studies show an increased risk of both bipolar disorder and unipolar disorder in first-degree relatives of affected individuals (5–10% and 10–20%, respectively). The phenomenon of anticipation (intergenerational increasing severity and/or earlier age of onset) has been seen in bipolar disorder, in a similar way to that in Huntington's disease and Fragile X syndrome. Association studies indicate that, like the latter diseases, trinucleotide repeat sequences are significantly larger in bipolar patients than in controls.

Genome-wide association studies have not identified any specific gene that is highly implicated in BPAD. It is likely, as with unipolar depression, that inheritance is polygenic, with several genetic mechanisms that produce complex patterns of inheritance. Chromosomal regions that have been implicated include 4p16, 12q, and 18q.

There are a number of identified candidate genes—SLC6A4, TPH2, DRD4, SLC6A3, DAOA, DTNBP1, NRG1, DISC1, and BDNF (Serretti and Mandelli, 2008), although their interaction requires further study and understanding, and the variety of genes has led to some suggestion that the disorder may, in fact, represent a cluster of disorders with various pathophysiological processes resulting in a 'common' clinical picture. In particular, *CACNA1C* (alpha-1C subunit of the L-type voltage-gated calcium channel) has also been implicated in a genome-wide association study of several thousand people (Ferreira et al., 2008).

There is increasing evidence of overlap of genetic susceptibility with schizophrenia, most notably with DAOA, DISC1, NRG1, and COMT. Gene expression and molecular biological studies are likely to prove an increasingly important area in understanding the basis of BPAD.

Structural neurobiology

- Abnormal myelination has been observed in diffusion tensor imaging of the brains of sufferers of BPAD.
- Post-mortem studies of the brains of patients with bipolar disorder demonstrate reduced volume of non-pyramidal cell layers. In particular, loss of hippocampal interneurons is present in patients with bipolar disorder that might lead to hippocampal dysfunction.
- Neuroimaging studies suggest evidence of cell loss or atrophy in hippocampal brain regions. Thus, another suggested cause of bipolar disorder is damage to cells in the critical brain circuitry that regulates emotion.

Neurochemical

The neurochemical pathways involved in bipolar disorder are poorly understood, and based on a combination of clinical observation and response to medications. Multiple systems are thought to be implicated, including glutamatergic, dopaminergic, serotinergic, and noradrenergic. In particular, the role of calcium metabolism in glutamatergic transmission may have a significant role, and calcium channel blockers have been used to treat episodes of mania.

Clinical diagnosis and symptoms

Hypomania and mania are terms used to describe periods of elevated mood, which may include irritability, and associated behavioural disturbance and reduction in the need to sleep, which last for at least 4 days. In more severe cases, psychotic symptoms congruent with mood may be observed, e.g. grandiose delusions. There are often additional biological symptoms, such as increased libido and psychomotor agitation. Cognitive and perceptual symptoms include a subjective experience of racing thoughts and ideas, including jumping from topic to topic (flight of ideas) and speaking extremely rapidly (pressure of speech). Attention and concentration is usually extremely impaired and the behaviour of the individual is usually very chaotic.

Manic and/or episodes can be precipitated by, e.g. drugs, lack of sleep, stress. According to diagnostic criteria if a sufferer has previously experienced a depressive episode, or a previous manic or hypomanic episode a diagnosis of bipolar disorder is made. In the former situation, this is clear evidence of mood fluctuation in both directions; in the latter (i.e. previously elevated mood episode), although the depressive episode is absent, evidence exists that there is almost always a depressive episode for which help may not have been sought.

Treatment

The treatment of BPAD can be treated with physical, pharmacological, and psychological interventions.

Physical treatment

This may be in the form of ECT, during severe depressive episodes as described above. In addition, in intractable cases of mania, or when stupor occurs. Some patients may also prefer maintenance ECT to pharmacological treatment with mood stabilizer, although this is unusual.

Pharmacological treatment

Depressive episodes

The pharmacological treatments for bipolar depression are as for those in unipolar depression, although particular care must be taken not to precipitate a manic episode. Consequently antidepressants may be used in short periods rather than for the longer periods observed in unipolar depressive episodes.

Manic/hypomanic episodes

These episodes are treated with either an antimanic agent, such as lithium or sodium valproate. Increasingly, the antipsychotic medications are used to treat manic episodes, in particular olanzapine or haloperidol. This is for both pragmatic reasons in terms of being available in an intramuscular form, as well as demonstrating good clinical efficacy.

Mood stablilization

A number of agents are used as mood stabilizers. Lithium has strong evidence to support efficacy, and has many effects ranging from effects on cell membrane excitability, to transcription of genes. The definitive mechanism of action is unclear. Owing to the non-specificity of this drug, there are multiple side effects and careful monitoring is required. Sodium valproate and other anticonvulsants are also known to be of benefit in bipolar disorder. Similarly, the membrane stabilizing effect is thought to have an important role in their mechanism of action, although the mechanism of action is difficult to determine without a detailed understanding of the pathophysiology of BPAD. Antipsychotic medications are also efficacious as mood stabilizers. This may reflect a combination of the sedative effects, as well as having action on dopaminergic and serotonergic neurochemical systems, possibly reflecting some similarities between BPAD and psychotic disorders pathophysiological actions.

- *Psychological treatment:* cognitive behavioural therapy and insight-focused therapy is often of benefit in a similar way as that in unipolar depression.
- *Genetic counselling:* although not routinely carried out at present, it is possible that as the genetic risk in BPAD is increasingly understood, and in particular in large families with a strong history of BPAD, this may become increasingly important.

Alcohol and drugs of abuse

Clinical definitions of misuse

The International Classification of diseases defines the misuse of substances on the basis of the type of substance, clinical manifestations of use, and the severity/chronicity of intake. There are multiple theories regarding the basis of substance misuse, varying from genetic vulnerability factors (e.g. in alcohol misuse), self-medication in the context of psychotic symptoms (e.g. cannabis), as well as psychosocial factors (e.g. early exposure and observation of behaviour during childhood). The relationship between substance misuse is complex and in some cases controversial, e.g. there is a longstanding debate concerning whether the use of skunk cannabis is causative of psychotic mental illness, such as schizophrenia. The following definitions are used in practice to formulate substance misuse and its sequelae.

Acute intoxication

Physical, behavioural, and cognitive manifestations characteristic to the ingestion of a specific substance during a single episode of use.

- *Harmful use or abuse:* a pattern of use that is causing damage to health. The damage may be physical and/or mental.
- *Dependence:* 'A cluster of behavioural, cognitive, and physiological phenomena that develop after repeated substance use'. A definite diagnosis of dependence should be made only if at least three of the following have been present together in the past year:
  - Compulsion to take substance.
  - Difficulties controlling substance-taking behavior.
  - Physiological withdrawal state.
  - Evidence of tolerance.
  - Neglect of alternative interests.
  - Persistent use despite harm.

Substances of abuse can be graded according to their degree of potential psychological and physical dependent on a scale of 0–3 as seen in Table 13.1.

Table 13.1 Substances of abuse graded according to their degree of potential psychological and physical dependence on a scale of 0–3

Drug	Psychological dependence	Physical dependence
Heroin	3.0	3.0
Cocaine	2.8	1.3
Alcohol	1.9	1.6
Tobacco	2.6	1.8
Barbiturates	2.2	1.8
Benzodiazepines	2.1	1.8
Amphetamine	1.9	1.1
LSD	1.1	0.3
Cannabis	1.7	0.8
Ecstasy	1.2	0.7

Tolerance describes a state in which increasing doses of the same substance are required to produce the same effect.

Withdrawal states refers to a cluster of symptoms that occur upon the cessation or reduction of use of a psychoactive substance after persistent use of that substance. The onset and course of the withdrawal state are time-limited, and are related to the type of psychoactive substance and dose being used immediately before cessation or reduction of use. The withdrawal state may be complicated by convulsions.

Prevalence of illicit drug use

1 in 10 adults uses illicit drugs in any one year (Table 13.2).

Drugs used in the treatment of psychiatric disorders

For drugs used in the treatment of psychiatric disorders (see Table 13.3).

Table 13.2 Common instances of abuse, potential symptoms of intoxication and withdrawal and their various treatment options

Substance	Basis of effect	Clinical effects of intoxication	Signs of withdrawal	Associated psychiatric symptoms	Treatment options
Alcohol: physical dependence-forming substance	Action through alcohol binding sites of GABA-A receptors. *In withdrawal:* neuroadaptation of constant presence of alcohol in body suddenly being lowered		24–72 hr after last drink. Nausea and vomiting. Tremor (first symptom). Tachycardia. Sleep disturbance. Excessive sweating. Anxiety and agitation. Acute confusion. *Hallucinations:* typically tactile, visual and transient. *Seizures:* 'Delirium tremens' is a life-threatening medical emergency consisting of a triad of: • Clouding of consciousness. • Vivid hallucinations. • Marked tremor. Wernicke–Korsakoff syndrome	Depression. Anxiety. Change in personality. Suicidality. Pathological jealousy. Alcoholic hallucinosis. Wernicke–Korsakoff syndrome	*Psychosocial:* • Supportive drug and alcohol counselling to increase motivation for change (total abstinence versus controlled drinking). • *CBT:* social skills and relapse prevention strategies. • Alcoholics Anonymous *Pharmacological: detoxification* • Long-acting benzodiazepine (chlordiazepoxide), reducing dose over 5–7 days. • Parenteral thiamine (Wernicke–Korsakoff) to prevent mammillary body micro-infarction. • Multivitamins. • Anti-emetics
Maintenance and relapse prevention in alcohol dependence syndrome: • *Acamprosate (synthetic taurine analogue):* reduces craving by enhanced GABA transmission and reducing the excitatory effects of glutamate. • *Naltrexone:* opioid antagonist and thought to block the reinforcing effects of alcohol. • *Disulfiram:* blocks aldehyde dehydrogenase, causing toxic accumulation of acetaldehyde and side effects of headache, nausea, vomiting, flushing, and palpitations upon ingestion of small amount of alcohol, including, e.g. deodorants on skin.					

Table 13.2 Common instances of abuse, potential symptoms of intoxication and withdrawal and their various treatment options (*continued*)

Substance	Basis of effect	Clinical effects of intoxication	Signs of withdrawal	Associated psychiatric symptoms	Treatment options
Benzodiazepines	Agonism at the benzodiazepine receptor on the GABA receptor complex	Respiratory depression. Dependent upon whether short-acting ('hypnotics')/ long-acting ('anxiolytics'). *Hypnotics:* sedation and induction of sleep, amnesia. *Anxiolytics:* reduction of anxiety, agitation, and tension. 'Paradoxical Excitation' occurs in a sub-group	*NB:* physical dependence-forming substances. *Physical:* stiffness, weakness, GI disturbance, paraesthesia, flu-like symptoms, seizures, death	*Psychological:* anxiety, insomnia, nightmares, depersonalization, decreased memory, delusions, hallucinations, depression, visual disturbance ('Alice in Wonderland' micropsia or macropsia)	Confirmation of use (urine screen). Switch to diazepam (long half-life). Gradual dosage reduction in line with NICE guidance. Psychological therapy and/or self-help groups
Opioids: i.e. heroin, morphine, pethidine, codeine, methadone	Agonism at central and peripheral opioid receptors. Rapid receptor adaptation and associated neuro-modulation. High propensity for dependence	Euphoria. Analgesia. Respiratory depression. Sedation. Constipation. Reduced libido	Withdrawal symptoms peak at around 36 hr after last dose and can last up to 5 days Dysphoria. Muscle pain. Abdominal cramps, nausea and vomiting. Intense craving for more opioids. Lacrimation. Rhinorrhoea. Tachycardia. Sweating and pilo-erection. Shivering. Yawning. Dilated pupils. Restlessness. *NB:* Although unpleasant, opioid withdrawal is rarely, if ever, fatal	Not generally associated with psychosis	*Acute detoxification:* • *NB* This is a specialist intervention as methadone overdose can be fatal. • *Methadone:* synthetic opioid with long half-life (1–2 days). • Titrate dose against withdrawal symptoms (typically 10–40 mg daily). Rate of reduction guided by clinical circumstances. • Typically over 3 weeks or can be continued at low dose as maintenance. • *Lofexidine/clonidine:* centrally-acting $\alpha 2$ agonist. • Reduces withdrawal symptoms by reducing effect of rebound NA levels. Clonidine causes more hypotension than lofexidine. • Loperamide and antiemetics for GI symptoms. *Maintenance:* • Continue methadone at low dose. • Buprenorphine (partial opioid agonist), but can precipitate withdrawal. • Naltrexone (long-acting opioid antagonist)

(continued)

Table 13.2 Common instances of abuse, potential symptoms of intoxication and withdrawal and their various treatment options (*continued*)

Substance	Basis of effect	Clinical effects of intoxication	Signs of withdrawal	Associated psychiatric symptoms	Treatment options
Cannabis: hash, resin, skunk, weed	Agonism on centrally occurring cannabinoid receptors	Mild euphoria. Enhanced aesthetic experience. Distorted perception of time and space. Increased appetite. Red eyes. Respiratory irritation. Lack of co-ordination. Dry mouth. Tachycardia	*Discontinuation effects from high doses:* • Nausea. • Increased irritability. • Insomnia. *NB:* not strongly physical dependence-forming	*Intoxication:* • Anxiety. • Panic attacks. • Mild paranoia. *Longer-term sequelae:* • Psychosis. • Depression. • Amotivational syndrome	Nil specific. Drug counselling to increase motivation for change. Psychoeducational approach
Cocaine: coke, Charlie, snow, blow	Dopaminergic enhancement through inhibition of reuptake in synaptic cleft	Euphoria. Increased energy and confidence. Reduced need for sleep. Grandiosity. Over-talkativeness. Impaired judgement. Sexual disinhibition. Tachycardia. Hypertension. Dilated pupils	Dysphoria. Anxiety. Irritability. Hypersomnolence. Anhedonia. *NB:* not strongly physical dependence-forming	*During acute intoxication:* • Paranoia. • Hallucinations. • Formication. • Aggression. *Longer-term sequelae:* • Paranoid psychosis. • Depression. • Suicidal behaviour	*During acute intoxication:* • Benzodiazepines. • Antipsychotics if psychotic features develop +/− hospitalization and supportive physical monitoring. *Maintenance:* • Little evidence for pharmacological options. • Supportive drug counselling (advice, harm reduction, motivational interviewing). • CBT. • Narcotics Anonymous
Amphetamines: 'speed', crystal meth, 'tina' etc.	Enhancement of dopaminergic function	As for cocaine	Fatigue, listlessness, hunger. *NB:* not strongly physical dependence-forming	*Intoxication:* • *Psychosis:* paranoia, delusions and hallucinations. • Aggression. *Longer-term sequelae:* • Psychosis. • Depression and anxiety	As for cocaine
Ecstasy: MDMA		Euphoria. Heightened sense of perception. Anorexia. Tachycardia. Bruxism. Sweating	*NB:* not strongly physical dependence-forming	Depression. *Paranoid psychosis:* 'flashbacks' described by some users. Chronic use associated with neurotoxicity and cognitive impairment	*Supportive drug counselling:* advice, harm reduction, motivational interviewing

Table 13.2 Common instances of abuse, potential symptoms of intoxication and withdrawal and their various treatment options (*continued*)

Substance	Basis of effect	Clinical effects of intoxication	Signs of withdrawal	Associated psychiatric symptoms	Treatment options
Hallucinogens: e.g. LSD, psilocybins	Various	Effects can depend on both situation and expectation. Distorted sensory perception. Synaesthesia. Euphoria	*NB:* not strongly physical dependence-forming	*Acute intoxication:* • Dissociation. • Anxiety. • Unpredictable behavior. • Panic attacks. *Longer term:* • Flashbacks. • No clear evidence of link with psychosis	*Supportive drug counselling:* advice, harm reduction, motivational interviewing
Gamma-butaryl-lactone (GBL) and gamma-hydroxybutyrate (GHB)	Effects primarily mediated through action on GABA-B receptors	Reduced anxiety, disinhibition and sedation. Narrow therapeutic index, rapid onset. Can produce severe delirium and muscle rigidity	*GBL:* • Anxiety, sweating, fine tremor, resting tachycardia. • Untreated can proceed to delirium, severe tremors and muscle rigidity. • Rhabdomyolysis may occur with acute renal failure	• *Delirium with psychosis:* Visual and tactile hallucinations. • Paranoia. Post-withdrawal anxiety and insomnia	High dose benzodiazepines/ Baclofen (GABA_B agonist) to reduce risk of muscle rigidity. Titrated against response
Nicotine	Peripheral and central action of inhaled nicotine on nAChR	Nil specific, but longer-term effects on cytochrome function and metabolism of some drugs, e.g. clozapine	Irritability, insomnia, agitation, and restlessness		Opportunistic advice. Nicotine replacement therapy (NRT), *or* amfebutamone (Buproprion®/Zyban®). Atypical antidepressant with dopaminergic and noradrenergic actions, *or* Varenicline (Champix®) partial agonist to a4b2 nAChR

Table 13.3 Drugs used in the treatment of psychiatric disorders

Class/names	Mechanism of action	Indication	Side effects	Other issues
Antidepressants and anxiolytics				
Serotonin reuptake inhibitor (SSRI): e.g. fluoxetine, paroxetine, citalopram, sertraline	Competitive and/or allosteric binding to the 5HT re-uptake inhibitor. Increases synaptic concentration of 5HT	Depression. OCD. Bulimia nervosa. Anxiety	Headache. Nausea. Insomnia. Lightheadedness. Anxiety and agitation. Tremor. Sedation/somnolence. Hyponatraemia (caution in elderly)	*Very safe* (rarely lethal in overdose). *Rarely*, serotonin syndrome can occur particularly when swapping from one antidepressant to another: • MAOI> SSRI wait 2 weeks. • SSRI> MAOI wait at least 1 week (5 weeks if fluoxetine). • *Caution when using other drugs that are* seroton-ergic *such as* lithium *or* tryptophan. SSRIs can also inhibit the hepatic metabolism of other drugs (tricyclics, antipsychotics, anticonvulsants and increase the effect of warfarin)
Serotonin and norepinephrine reuptake inhibitor *(SNRI):* e.g. venlafaxine, duloxetine	Works as SSRI, but also has activity at NA transporter	Depression (2nd line)	Headache. Lightheadedness. Dry mouth. Nausea. Anxiety. Sexual dysfunction. Postural hypotension	Little effect on hepatic drug metabolism/ Do not give with MAOIs
Norepinephrine Reuptake Inhibitor (NRI) e.g. reboxetine		Depression	Dry mouth Constipation Insomnia Impotence and decreased libido at higher doses	
Benzodiazepines (see also drugs of abuse): lorazepam, diazepam, chlordiazepoxide, clonazepam	Agonist at benzodiazpine receptor as part of GABA-A receptor complex	Extreme agitation or rapid tranquillization. Anxiolytic. Alcohol withdrawal	Sedation. Dizziness. Amnesia	Tolerance, withdrawal, and dependence Paradoxical reaction (agitate, rather than sedate)
Azapirone, buspirone	5HT1a receptor partial agonist	Anxiety disorders. Augmentation of depression	Side effects worse early in treatment. Lightheadedness. Headache. Dysphoria. Galactorrhoea	Myaesthenia gravis. Acute closed angle glaucoma. Severely compromised liver and renal function. Concomitant treatment with MAOI (hypertensive crises)

Table 13.3 Drugs used in the treatment of psychiatric disorders (*continued*)

Class/names	Mechanism of action	Indication	Side effects	Other issues
β blockers: propranolol		Anxiety	Delayed ejaculation. Nocturnal enuresis. Induce myocardial depression and precipitate heart failure. Precipitation of asthma. Fatigue. Sleep disturbance with nightmares. Coldness of the extremities. Exacerbation of psoriasis	
Tricyclics: clomipramine, amitriptyline, imipramine	Act on multiple neurotransmitter pathway 5HT, NA, and ACh	Depression. OCD: clomipramine. Neuropathic pain	*Anticholinergic effects:* • Dry mouth. • Constipation. • Blurred vision. • Difficulty micturating and retention. • Worsening of glaucoma. • Confusion. *Adrenergic effects (blockade):* • Drowsiness. • Postural hypotension. • Sexual dysfunction. • Cognitive impairment. *Histamine H1 effects (blockade):* • Drowsiness. • *Weight gain.* *Cardiovascular effects:* • Tachycardia. • Hypotension. • Prolonged PR and QT segments. • ST depression and flattened T waves. • Negatively inotropic. • Heart block. • Arrhythmias. *Neurological:* • Fine tremor. • Poor coordination. • Headache. • Muscle twitching. • *Epileptic seizures (lowered threshold).* *Haematological:* • Agranulocytosis (rare). • Leucopenia. • *Eosinophilia.* *Dermatological:* • Rash. • Photosensitization	*See side effects:* ∴ **toxic in overdose!**

(*continued*)

Table 13.3 Drugs used in the treatment of psychiatric disorders (*continued*)

Class/names	Mechanism of action	Indication	Side effects	Other issues
Monoamine oxidase inhibitors *(MAOI)*: phenelzine, tranylcypromine	Inhibit monoamine oxidase	Depression	*CNS:* • Insomnia. • Drowsiness. • Headache. • Fatigue. • Tremor. • Mania. • Confusion. • Seizures (rare). *Autonomic:* • Blurred vision. • Difficulty micturating. • Sweating. • Dry mouth. • Postural hypotension. • Constipation. *Other:* • Sexual dysfunction. • Weight gain. • Peripheral neuropathy. • Oedema. • SLE type syndrome	MAOIs result in the accumulation of amine neurotransmitters, which can interact for up to 2 weeks after stopping medication with: *Tyramine contained in:* • Cheeses. • Meat and yeast extracts (marmite). • Smoked fish. • Hung poultry and game. • *Red wines, i.e.* Chianti *Drugs:* • Antidepressants, especially SSRIs will need a 2-week drug-free period when switching from MAOI to SSRI. • Adrenaline/noradrenaline. • L-dopa. • Opiates. • Alcohol. • Barbiturates. • Insulin and OHA
Reversible inhibitor monoamine oxidase (RIMA): moclobemide		Depression	As for MAOI	As for MAOI
Noradrenergic and specific serotonin antidepressant (NASSA): mirtazapine	Pre-synaptic antagonism at a2 adrenergic autoreceptor to enhance NA and 5HT release, thereby increasing 5HT1A agonism indirectly. Antagonist effects at various 5HT receptors, in particular 5HT2A and 2C	Depression. PTSD	Increased appetite. Weight gain. Sedation	*Cautions:* small risk of neutropenia and agranulocytosis
Serotonin agonist and reuptake inhibitor (SARI): trazadone	Weak 5HT reuptake inhibitor, antagonist at 5HT2R, metabolite is a 5HTagonist, blockade at postsynaptic α1R	Depression	Sedation. Cognitive impairment. Nausea. Dizziness. Postural hypotension. Priapism	

Table 13.3 Drugs used in the treatment of psychiatric disorders (*continued*)

Class/names	Mechanism of action	Indication	Side effects	Other issues
Lithium	Uncertain, although thought to relate at least partially to sodium-dependent intracellular second messenger systems; possible neuroprotective effects	Mania (NNT 6), mood stabilization and prophylaxis (NNT10-14)	Many side effects owing to potential to alter sodium-related processes: weight-gain, nephrogenic diabetes insipidus, increased appetite and thirst, polydipsia, nystagmus, tremor, nausea/ vomiting, diarrhea, ataxia and seizures with toxicity	Can cause hypothyroidism and renal failure due to accumulation; very low therapeutic index, and lethal in overdose; teratogenicity (Ebstein's anomaly). Requires periodic plasma monitoring of levels, as well as U&Es and TFTs in particular (6-monthly). Many drug-interactions e.g. ACE inhibitors can increase lithium levels with implications for toxicity NSAIDs – increase renal re-absorption of sodium and lithium. Diuretics – reduced renal clearance of lithium, particularly thiazide diuretics
Valproate	Complex action; inhibition of GABA catabolism, second messenger system-effects and possible genetic effects	Mania (NNT2-4); prophylaxis	Gastric irritation, hyperammonaemia and nausea, lethargy, tremor, hair loss with curly regrowth, thrombocytopaenia, leucopaenia, red cell hypoplasia and pancreatitis. Side effects usually dose-related	Major teratogen. During pregnancy consideration of risks of relapse versus risk of teratogenicity should be assessed, and supervised by psychiatrist or neurologist. Monitoring of BMI, FBC and LFTs only required. Interactions: Highly protein-bound and displaced by other protein-bound drugs e.g. aspirin, which can lead to toxicity. Also interaction with warfarin to increase warfarin levels. Hepatic metabolism – cytochrome-inhibitors can increase levels e.g. erythromycin and cimetidine

(continued)

Table 13.3 Drugs used in the treatment of psychiatric disorders (*continued*)

Class/names	Mechanism of action	Indication	Side effects	Other issues
Mood stabilizers and anti-manic *Antipsychotics ('Neuroleptics', 'Major tranquillizers')*				
First generation: e.g. haloperidol, chlorpromazine, flupentixol	Primary action antagonists at D2 receptors	Psychosis, acute phases, and prophylaxis	*Extrapyramidal side effects:* • Acute dystonias. • Akathisia. • Parkinsonism. • Tachycardia. • Torticollis. • *Through effects on tubero-infundibular dopaminergic pathway can cause hyper-prolactinaemia.* In prolonged use, tardive dyskinesia can occur: • Repetitive purposeless movements. • Orofacial movements. • Lip smacking. *Eye blinking*	Side effects can often be managed through using anti-cholinergic medication (e.g. procyclidine). Tardive dyskinesia must be managed initially through reduction of antipsychotic if appropriate/feasible. All antipsychotics produce prolongation of the QTc interval on the ECG and reduce the seizure threshold. Certain preparations available in slow-release injection 'depot' form. Monitoring of U&E, glucose, FBC, lipids, LFTs, and prolactin required in addition to weight, ECG, blood pressure. *Neuroleptic malignant syndrome (NMS):* an idiopathic reaction to FGA or SGA, usually in antipsychotic naïve (although not always), which results in muscle rigidity, confusion, hyperthermia and ataxia. Requires urgent supportive medical treatment with withdrawal of antipsychotic, treatment with benzodiazepines and sodium dantrolene. Monitoring of CK. Careful consideration to which antipsychotic to be used next. Can be used as mood stabilizers
Second generation: e.g.olanzapine, amisulpiride clozapine, risperidone	Second generation antipsychotics have D2 antagonism or partial agonist properties (e.g. aripiprazole), but also antagonism at 5HT2A receptor systems	Treatment of acute psychosis and prophylaxis in schizophrenia. May have effects on negative symptoms also. Certain preparations licensed for BPAD	Side effect profile regarding extra-pyramidal symptoms is preferable in SGAs, although present. Hypersalivation with clozapine There is an increased association with metabolic syndrome—hyperglycaemia, aberrant lipid metabolism, weight gain. Significantly increased risk of developing Type 2 diabetes mellitus	Considerably more expensive than first generation without significant evidence of greater efficacy (CATIE and CuTLASS trials). Monitoring of ECG, glucose, and lipids. Clozapine (third-line) associated with agranulocytosis requiring careful blood monitoring (initially weekly). NMS less likely with SGAs. Long-acting forms of SGAs are available for injection, but with different pharmacokinetic properties to FGAs

Reference: The Maudsley Prescribing Guidelines (2012). Wiley Blackwell.

Further reading

Ferreira MA, O'Donovan MC, Meng YA, Jones IR, Ruderfer DM, Jones L, et al. (2008). Collaborative genome-wide association analysis supports a role for ANK3 and CACNA1C in bipolar disorder. *Nature Genetics*, 40(9): 1056–1058.

Meyer JH, Ginovart N, Boovariwala A, Sagrati S, Hussey D, Garcia A, Young T, Praschak-Rieder N, Wilson AA, and Houle S. (2006). Elevated monoamine oxidase a levels in the brain: an explanation for the monoamine imbalance of major depression. *Archives of General Psychology*, 63: 1209–1216.

Murray CJ, and Lopez AD. (1997). Alternative projections of mortality and disability by cause 1990–2020: Global Burden of Disease Study. *Lancet*, 349: 1498–1504.

Serretti A, and Mandelli L. (2008). The genetics of bipolar disorder: genome 'hot regions,' genes, new potential candidates and future directions. *Molecular Psychiatry*, 13: 742–771.

Multiple choice questions

1. A 19-year-old heroin addict presents to the Emergency Department suffering from withdrawal symptoms and asking to be treated. Which of the following would be most appropriate?

(A) Lofexidine.
(B) Methadone.
(C) Bupronorphine.
(D) Diazepam.
(E) Diamorphine.

2. A 24-year-old man admits to experiencing auditory hallucinations and has persecutory delusions. A history from his partner reveals he has recently been experimenting with a drug of abuse. Which of the following is least likely to have precipitated a schizophrenic psychosis?

(A) Amphetamines.
(B) Cannabis.
(C) LSD.
(D) Heroin.
(E) Ketamine.

3. Which of the following are negative symptoms relating to schizophrenia?

(A) Auditory hallucinations.
(B) Persecutory delusions.
(C) Thought broadcasting.
(D) Thought interference.
(E) Avolition.

4. Which of the following drugs of abuse are least likely to produce physical dependence?

(A) Nicotine.
(B) LSD.
(C) Heroin.
(D) Diazepam.
(E) Alcohol.

5. A 40-year-old woman on long-term lithium for bipolar disorder presents feeling unwell. Which of the following symptoms are most likely to indicate lithium toxicity?

(A) Tremor.
(B) Nausea.
(C) Metallic taste.
(D) Ataxia.
(E) Polyuria.

6. A 50-year-old presents with agitation and headache after a visit to an Italian restaurant and is found to be in a hypertensive crisis. He takes a regular antidepressant. Which of the following antidepressants may be responsible for the crisis?

(A) Mirtazapine.
(B) Trazadone.
(C) Moclobemide.
(D) Amitryptilline.
(E) Citalopram.

7. Which of the following is a recognized treatment for schizophrenia?

(A) Clozapine.
(B) Depo-provera.
(C) Psychosurgery.
(D) Psychodynamic psychotherapy.
(E) Buspirone.

8. Imaging studies in schizophrenia have *not* demonstrated:

(A) An enlarged third ventricle.
(B) A reduced medial and temporal lobe volume.
(C) A grey matter volume deficit.
(D) Reduced frontal lobe blood flow.
(E) A correlation between ventricular enlargement and severity of symptoms.

9. A 25-year-old man being treated for schizophrenia presents with multiple episodes of sudden onset loss of consciousness whilst exercising. The most likely cause is

(A) Postural hypotension.
(B) Torsades-de-pointes.
(C) Nephrogenic diabetes insipidus.
(D) Carotid sinus hypersensitivity.
(E) Acute dystonia.

10. A 35-year-old man with depression presents with shivering and tremor. He has recently had a change in medication from sertraline to moclobemide. On examination he is hypertensive and tachycardic with dilated pupils and has a temperature of 38.5°C. The most likely diagnosis is:

(A) 1st presentation of a manic episode.
(B) Serotonin syndrome.
(C) Neuroleptic malignant syndrome.
(D) Munchausen's syndrome.
(E) Anaphylaxis.

For answers, please see Appendix: Answers to multiple choice questions, page 313.

CHAPTER 14

Gastroenterology

Anatomy

Oesophagus

Approximately 25 cm in length, the oesophagus conveys food from the mouth to the stomach. It is bounded by upper (striated muscle) and lower (smooth muscle) sphincters, and comprises three sections corresponding to vertebral levels.

The cervical oesophagus runs posterior the trachea and anterior to the cervical vertebrae and prevertebral fascia, with the common carotid arteries and recurrent laryngeal nerves running on either side. Blood is supplied from the inferior thyroid artery with venous drainage to the vertebral bracheocephalic and inferior thyroid veins. Lymphatic drainage is to the deep cervical nodes. Innervation is by the recurrent laryngeal nerve and the middle cervical ganglion (sympathetic).

The thoracic oesophagus is situated within the superior and posterior mediastinum, posterior to the trachea, left bronchus, and pericardial cavity. The thoracic vertebrae, thoracic duct, the azygous vein, and descending aorta are situated posterior to this section. It becomes the abdominal oesophagus after it penetrates the diaphragm. Oesophageal branches from the aorta and bronchial arteries supply the thoracic section, with venous drainage to the azygous and hemiazygous veins. Lymphatic drainage is to the tracheobronchial and posterior mediastinal nodes. The thoracic section is innervated by the vagus, sympathetic trunk, and greater splanchnic nerve.

The short retroperitoneal abdominal section starts at the point at which the oesophagus penetrates the right crus of the diaphragm (T10) and terminates at the cardia of the stomach. It is situated in the oesophageal groove on the posterior of the left lobe of the liver. Parietal peritoneum covers the anterior surface. Branches from the left inferior phrenic and left gastric artery supply the abdominal oesophagus, which is drained by the left gastric vein, which returns to the portal system. Lymph returns to the left gastric and coeliac nodes.

The oesophagus narrows at the cricopharangeal sphincter, at the points at which the aortic arch and left bronchus cross the oesophagus, and at the penetration of the diaphragm. These narrowings constitute locations at which foreign bodies can become lodged, and are also likely sites for carcinoma development.

The oesophagus is lined with stratified squamous epithelial cells. The lamina propria surrounds the epithelial layer and envelopes glands, which secrete mucus into the lumen. The muscularis mucosa, longitudinally-arranged smooth muscle, is apparent in the lower oesophagus. Blood vessels, nerves, and lymphatics are located within the submucosa. The muscularis externa comprises an external longitudinal layer and an internal circular layer, responsible for the propulsion of food. Striated muscle makes up the first third, with both striated and smooth muscle found in the middle third, and only smooth muscle present in the last third. The adventitia is an outer loosely supporting connective tissue layer, replaced after penetrating the diaphragm by the serosa.

Stomach

A J-shaped tube, the stomach, receives food from the oesophagus at the cardia (Fig. 14.1). Through secretions and muscular mixing of its contents, it continues the process of digestion initiated by secretion and mastication in the mouth, before presenting the partly digested chyme to the duodenum at the pyloric sphincter.

The anterior abdominal wall, diaphragm, and left lobe of liver lie anterior to the stomach. The lesser peritoneal sac separates the stomach from its posterior relations—the pancreas, left kidney and adrenal gland, spleen, aorta, coeliac trunk, and transverse mesocolon. The diaphragm lies superior to the stomach.

The stomach is characterized by numerous folds or rugae, and is lined by an invaginated columnar epithelial cell layer with gastric glands that project into the thin lamina propria that contains capillaries, nerve fibres, and lymphatics. The glands secrete gastric acid, digestive enzymes, mucus, and hormones. The submucosa, comprising connective tissue, capillaries, nerve fibres, and lymphatics envelops the epithelial tissue. There is a three-layered muscularis, comprising inner oblique, circular, and outer longitudinal fibres of smooth muscle, enveloped by a thin serosal membrane.

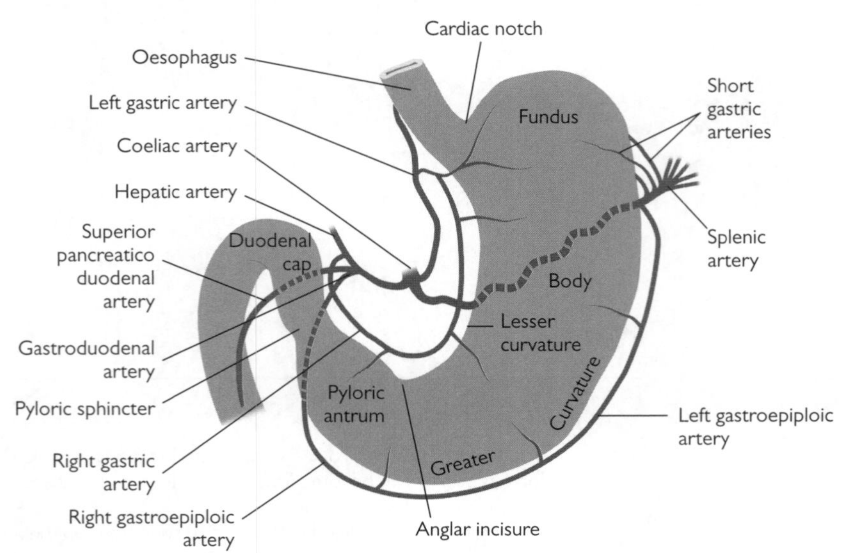

Fig. 14.1 Arterial supply to the stomach.

Reproduced from P MacKinnon and J Morris, *Oxford Textbook of Functional Anatomy: Volume 2 Thorax and Abdomen*, 2005, Figure 6.4.13, p. 138, by permission of Oxford University Press

The greater curvature forms the left border of the stomach, while the lesser curvature forms its right border. The narrow neck or cardia acts along with the lower oesophageal sphincter to prevent reflux. The upper section or fundus represents the gastric bubble on X-rays, and leads to the body or corpus. The pylorus forms the terminal section, connecting the stomach to the duodenum and is widest at the antrum. Transfer of chyme to the duodenum is regulated by the circular smooth muscle of the pyloric sphincter.

The omenta are double-layered folds of peritoneum that contain blood vessels and nerves supplying the stomach. The greater omentum runs from the greater curvature in front of the small intestines before reflecting towards the transverse colon. Part of the greater omentum, the gastrosplenic ligament connects the greater curvature with the spleen. The lesser omentum is attached to the lesser curvature and extends to the liver.

Blood supply

The stomach is supplied with blood by vessels derived from the coeliac artery or trunk, which branches from the aorta at the upper border of L1. The coeliac artery gives rise to the left gastric artery, hepatic artery, and splenic artery. The hepatic artery, in turn, divides into the right gastric artery and gastroduodenal artery. The left gastric artery supplies the left lesser curvature and the right gastric artery. Anastomoses of gastric arteries run in the lesser omentum. The splenic artery gives rise to short gastric arteries and to the left gastro-epiploic artery, which run in the gastrosplenic ligament to supply the upper part of the great curvature. The lower part is supplied by the right gastro-epiploic artery, which arises from the gastroduodenal artery. The right gastro-epiploic artery runs in the greater omentum in which it anastomoses with the left gastro-epiploic artery.

Venous drainage, for the most part, follows the course of the arteries, although there is no gastroduodenal or coeliac vein. The short gastric veins and left gastro-epiploic vein drain to the splenic vein, while the right gastro-epiploic vein returns blood to the superior mesenteric vein. The splenic and superior mesenteric veins unite to form the hepatic portal vein, which receives blood from the right and left gastric veins directly.

Lymph drainage

Lymph from the stomach drains to the coeliac nodes, via the splenic and pancreatic nodes (from the upper greater curvature), gastro-epiploic and pyloric nodes (from the lower greater curvature), and left and right gastric nodes (from the lesser curvature).

Nerve supply

Preganglionic sympathetic innervation of the stomach is from the thoracic splanchnic nerves (T6–9) via the coeliac plexus. Post-ganglionic fibres run along arterial branches to supply the stomach. Parasympathetic fibres from the vagus nerves supply the stomach via the oesophageal plexus, which forms the anterior gastric nerve (containing mainly left vagal fibres and providing the predominant innervation) and the posterior gastric nerve (mainly containing right vagal fibres).

Pancreas

The pancreas is a lobular retroperitoneal gland that runs across the posterior abdominal wall from duodenum to spleen. It can be anatomically divided into head, neck, body, and tail. The head is apposed to duodenum, anterior to the inferior vena cava, and posseses an uncinate process that extends leftwards and is separated from the neck by the superior mesenteric blood vessels (Fig. 14.2).

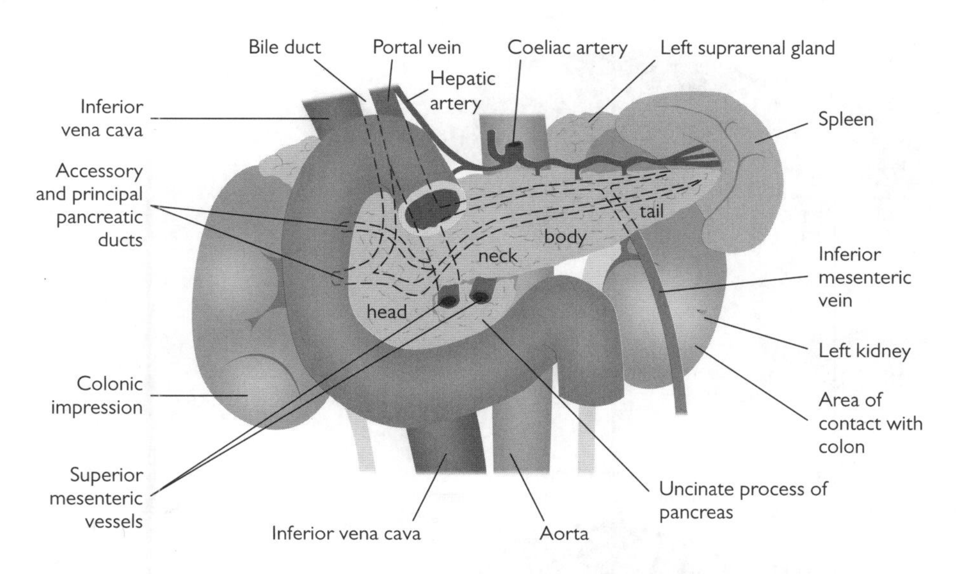

Fig. 14.2 Pancreas and its immediate relationships.

Reproduced from P MacKinnon and J Morris, *Oxford Textbook of Functional Anatomy: Volume 2 Thorax and Abdomen*, 2005, Figure 6.6.9, p. 164, by permission of Oxford University Press

The neck is situated immediately below the pylorus, and rests on the portal vein and common hepatic bile duct. The body curves in front of the aorta, and the left suprarenal gland and kidney. The tail passes in the lienorenal ligament to contact the spleen. The transverse mesocolon passes along the underside of the body and neck, and across the head.

The arterial supply to the head is from the superior and inferior pancreatico-duodenal arteries, which arise from the coeliac and superior mesenteric arteries, respectively. Other parts of the pancreas are supplied by branches of the splenic artery. Blood drains via counterpart veins to the portal vein, formed behind the neck. Lymph drains through vessels that follow blood vessels to end in the pancreatico-splenic nodes. Autonomic fibres from the coeliac plexus innervate the pancreas. Sympathetic fibres modulate vascular tone and convey pain, whereas parasympathetic vagal fibres induce both exocrine and endocrine secretion.

Microscopically, the pancreas is divided into exocrine and endocrine cells. In the exocrine tissue, acinar glands secrete alkaline digestive secretions containing enzymes. These secretions ultimately drain into the principal pancreatic duct, which unites with common bile duct to open into the duodenum, with an accessory duct draining the upper part of the head. The endocrine tissue comprises Islets of Langerhans, which possess different cell types that produce, store and secrete glucagon (α-cells), insulin (β-cells), and somatostatin (δ-cells).

Liver and biliary system

The largest internal organ, the wedge-shaped liver (Fig. 14.3) lies in the right upper quadrant of the abdomen. Its superior lies against the diaphragm, with its inferior at the costal margin. The parenchyma is enveloped by a thin fibrous capsule. The capsule is, for the most part, covered with peritoneum, with that on the upper surface reflected on to the diaphragm at coronary ligaments to leave a bare area. The falciform ligament divides the liver into right and left lobes, with the right being larger. The umbilical fissure, a cleft on the inferior surface, lodges the round ligament, which is an embryological remnant of the umbilical vein. Between the umbilical fissure and the gall bladder, which is attached to the under surface of the liver, is the quadrate lobe. Posterior to the quadrate lobe and separated by the portal vein, hepatic artery, and hepatic bile duct, lies the caudate lobe. The hilum of the liver, the porta hepatis, conveys the portal vein, hepatic artery, and hepatic bile duct. The inferior vena cava runs against the posterior of the liver.

Blood supply

Blood is supplied to the liver by right and left branches of the oxygen-rich hepatic artery arising from the coeliac axis of the aorta (20% of the total) and by the nutrient-rich portal vein. Blood perfuses endothelium-lined sinusoids, arranged between layers of hepatocytes, which possess phagocytic Kupffer cells. The peri-sinusoidal space (of Disse) separates

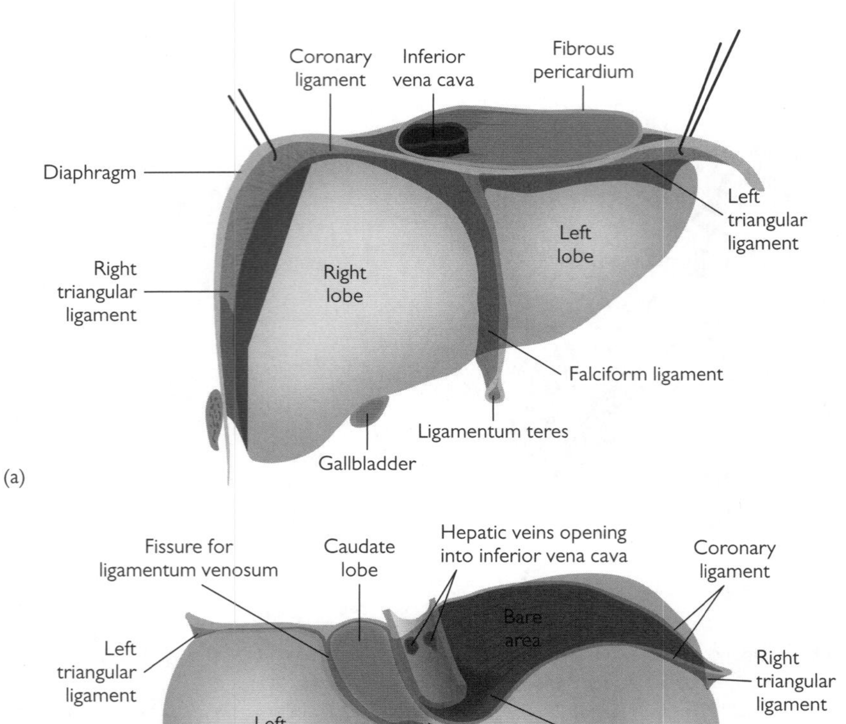

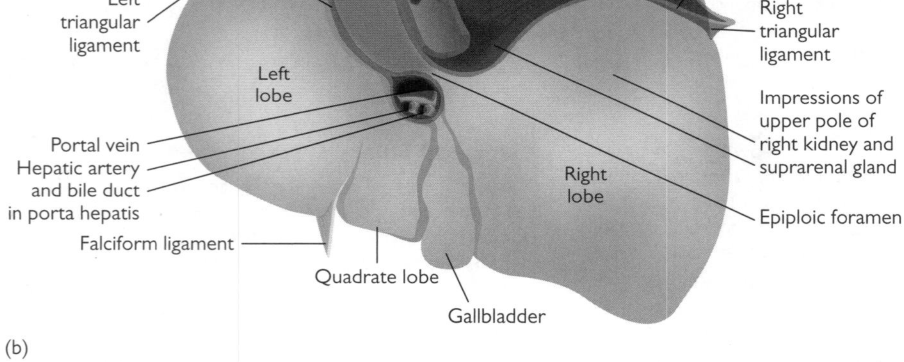

Fig. 14.3 (a) Anterior and (b) posterior views of the liver and its peritoneal reflections.

hepatocytes from the endothelial lining. Blood drains via three hepatic veins to the inferior vena cava. Anastomoses exist between tributaries of the portal venous system and tributaries of the systemic venous system; these provide collateral circulation during portal obstruction or hypertension. Oesophageal and rectal anastomosis can become varicose and the former is particularly prone to rupture causing life-threatening bleeding. Portal hypertension can also manifest as the umbilical vein becomes re-canalized and anastomoses with the systemic veins via engorged para-umbilical veins radiating from the umbilicus. This gives the appearance of *caput medusae* (latin for 'head of Medusa' from the similarity to Medusa's snake-like hair).

Protein-rich lymph formed in the peri-sinusoidal space drains predominantly via hepatic nodes at the porta hepatis. Sympathetic fibres from the coeliac plexus and parasympathetic fibres from the vagus enter the liver at the porta hepatis.

Bile

Hepatocytes secrete bile into microscopic canaliculi defined by the cells. The canaliculi drain into intrahepatic ductules, which unite to form the right and left hepatic ducts. These merge at the porta hepatis to form the common hepatic duct that runs in the lesser omentum. The gallbladder, an epithelial cell-lined sac with a smooth muscle wall, stores and concentrates bile; its cystic duct combines with the common hepatic duct to form the common bile duct. The common bile and pancreatic ducts form the ampulla of Vater, which conveys bile to the second part of the duodenum at the duodenal papilla, the opening of which is regulated by the sphincter of Oddi. Arterial blood to the biliary tree is supplied by the cystic artery—a branch of the right hepatic artery—and by the gastroduodenal artery. Venous drainage to the portal vein is via the cystic vein, with lymph draining to the hepatic nodes. Autonomic innervation of the gall bladder is largely by sympathetic and sensory fibres.

Spleen

A component of the reticulo-endothelial system, the fist-sized spleen is located beneath the 9th to 11th ribs. It has a convex outer surface, which rests under the left side of the diaphragm and a concave inner surface that is associated with the stomach, kidney, and splenic flexure of the descending colon. It comprises a vascular pulp enveloped by a fibrous capsule, covered by visceral peritoneum, except at the point at which blood vessels emerge, the hilum. The gastrosplenic ligament attaches the spleen to the greater curvature of the stomach, while the splenorenal ligament attaches the spleen to the left kidney.

The pulp is divided into white and red pulp. White pulp comprises lymphoid follicles, which are rich in cells of the immune system and can be enlarged in infections. This tissue is concentrated in peri-articular sheaths surrounding smaller arterioles. Red pulp comprises sinusoids engorged with blood (hence, the red colour) and splenic cords, which contain reticular cells and fibres, and a number of immune and blood cells, including granulocytes, macrophages, platelets, and erythrocytes. Blood cells exchange across an endothelial filter between the sinusoids and the splenic cords, with macrophages removing aged or damaged erythrocytes and particulate matter.

Blood supply

The splenic artery, which runs in the splenorenal ligament, gives rise to a number of branches at the hilum, which supply the spleen (with other branches supplying the stomach). A meshwork of trabeculae carries the trabecular arteries into the parenchyma. Trabecular veins draining the spleen follow the route and combine to form the splenic vein, which receives the inferior mesenteric vein before uniting with the superior mesenteric vein to form the portal vein. Lymph drains to the pancreatico-splenic nodes. The vascular smooth muscle of the spleen is supplied with sympathetic vasomotor fibres from the coeliac plexus, which follow the course of the branches of the splenic artery.

Small intestine

The small intestine continues the digestion of food, absorbs nutrients, adds secretions to the gastrointestinal tract and has an endocrine role. It comprises the duodenum, jejunum, and ileum (Fig. 14.4). A number of common properties are evident along the length of the small intestine. Folds in the mucosa and submucosa called plicae circulares, villi that possess simple tubular glands (intestinal glands or crypts of Lieberkühn) at their base, and the microvilli of the epithelial cell apical membranes all increase surface area to optimize absorptive and secretory processes.

In the lamina propria and submucosa there are aggregates of lymphoid material. These Peyer's patches sit under a specialized epithelial lining of M (microfold) cells, which abut antigen-presenting cells at their basolateral membrane. This apparatus acts to endocytose antigens from the lumen and initiate an immune response. Exocrine cells at the base of the crypts called Paneth cells secrete antimicrobial lysozyme.

Brunner's glands are deep, coiled glands extending into the muscularis mucosa, with extensive branching. These glands secrete alkaline mucous and distinguish the duodenum from the rest of the small intestine.

Duodenum

The first section of the small intestine is the *duodenum*, a C-shaped retroperitoneal organ that sits around the head of the pancreas. It receives chyme from the stomach along with bile from the gall bladder and pancreatic secretions. Alkaline secretions from the pancreas and crypts of Lieberkühn protect the duodenum against the acidity of the chyme.

The duodenum is divided into four parts:

- *The duodenal cap*, 5cm in length, starts at the gastroduodenal junction and is the only segment covered by peritoneum. The portal vein, common bile duct, gastroduodenal artery and inferior vena cava lie posterior to this segment, with the liver and gallbladder situated anteriorly.
- *A 7.5cm segment* that runs downwards around the head of the pancreas. It sits anterior to the hilum of the right kidney and right ureter and is crossed anteriorly by the transverse colon. The duodenal papilla is located in the posteriomedial wall of this segment, with the accessory pancreatic duct located just superior.
- *A 10-cm segment* that runs horiziontally to the left around the head of the pancreas. This segment is crossed anteriorly by the superior mesenteric vessels.
- *A short final segment,* 2.5 cm in length runs superiorly and to the left, terminating at the duodenal-jejunal junction, where the suspensory ligament of Treitz—a fibromuscular peritoneal fold arising from the right crus of the diaphragm—is attached. Contraction of the ligament facilitates progression of the duodenal contents along the small intestine. The inferior mesenteric vein passes on the left side of the duodenal–jejunal junction.

Blood supply

The duodenal blood supply reflects the embryological origins of the structure. The foregut is supplied by the coeliac axis, whereas the midgut is supplied by the superior mesenteric axis. The duodenal papilla defines this boundary and is the site of anastomoses between the superior pancreatico-duodenal artery (from the coeliac axis) and the inferior pancreatico-duodenal artery (from the superior mesenteric

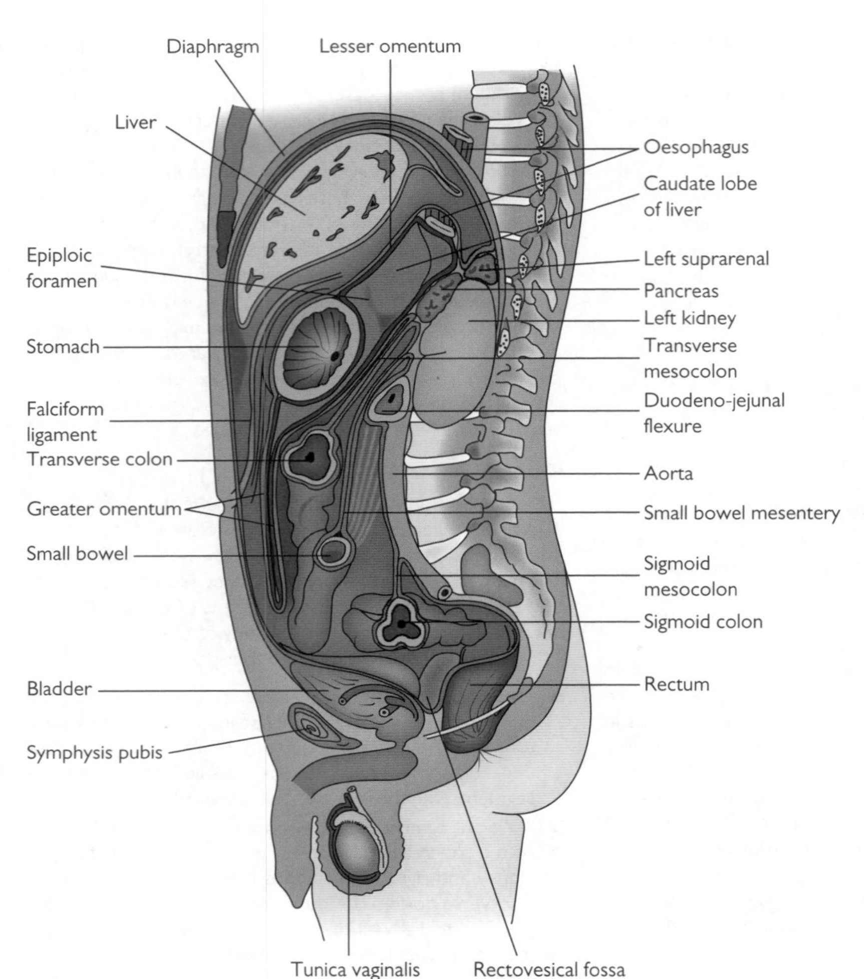

Fig. 14.4 Arrangement of peritoneum of the greater and lesser sacs in a parasagittal section of the abdominal cavity.

Reproduced from P MacKinnon and J Morris, *Oxford Textbook of Functional Anatomy: Volume 2 Thorax and Abdomen*, 2005, Figure 6.4.3, p. 134, by permission of Oxford University Press

axis). Venous drainage is through the superior pancreatico-duodenal vein to the hepatic portal vein, and through the inferior pancreatico-duodenal vein to the superior mesenteric vein. Duodenal lymphatic drainage is to the superior mesenteric and coeliac nodes. Sympathetic innervation is derived from the coeliac plexus and superior mesenteric plexus, with parasympathetic innervation via the vagus nerve. Nerve fibres to the duodenum accompany blood vessels.

Jejunem and ileum

The remainder of the small intestine, up to 10 m in length, comprises the *jejunum* (the upper two-fifths) and *ileum*. The jejunum is situated in the umbilical region, whereas the ileum resides in the hypogastrium and pelvis. A distinct junction between the two sections is not apparent, although the jejunum has a more pronounced mucosa, is more vascular and is of smaller diameter. The ileum, with a mesentery that contains more fat, terminates at the ileocaecal junction.

Starting at the duodenal–jejunal junction, the mesentery attaches the jejunum and ileum to the posterior abdominal wall. Its root originates from the left side of L2 and runs obliquely down to the right sacroiliac joint, crossing the abdominal aorta, inferior vena cava, psoas major muscle, right ureter, and right testicular/ovarian vessels (Fig. 14.5).

Blood vessels, nerve fibres, and lymphatic vessels are conveyed in the mesentery. Numerous branches of the superior mesenteric artery anastomose to form arterial arcades, which are shorter and more complex in the ileum. Vasa recta, straight arteries given off from the arcades, which anastomose within the intestinal wall, perfuse discrete sections of jejnum and ileum. Venous drainage occurs through the superior mesenteric vein, which unites with the splenic vein posterior to the neck of the pancreas to give rise to

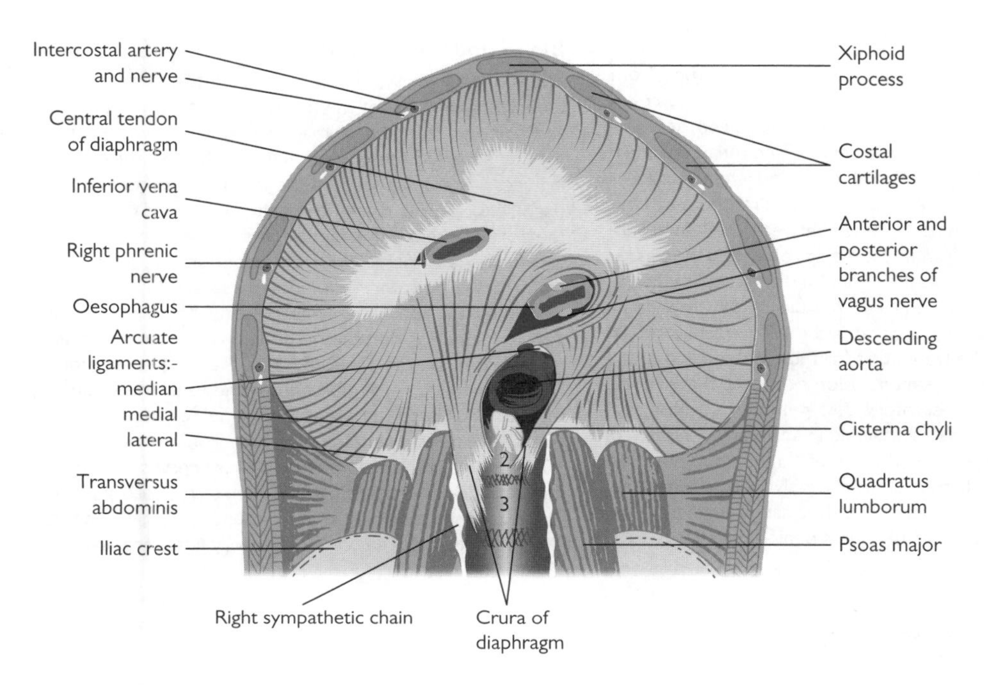

Fig. 14.5 The diaphragm forming the roof of the abdomen.

Reproduced from P MacKinnon and J Morris, *Oxford Textbook of Functional Anatomy: Volume 2 Thorax and Abdomen*, 2005, Figure 6.3.3, p. 122, by permission of Oxford University Press

the portal vein. With the exception of the terminal ileum, which drains into the ileocolic nodes, lymphatic drainage of the jejunum and ileum is to the mesenteric nodes, which feed the superior mesenteric lymph nodes. Parasympathetic nerve fibres from the vagus nerve via the coeliac plexus and sympathetic nerve fibres from the greater and lesser splanchnic nerves form the myenteric and submucosal plexi within the intestinal wall.

Large intestine

The most distal part of the gastrointestinal tract, the large intestine, completes the absorption of electrolytes and water and stores faeces prior to defecation. The large intestine comprises four sections: the caecum and appendix, colon, rectum, and anal canal (Fig. 14.4). The caecum and colon are characterized by taenia coli, three longitudinal bands of smooth muscle on the outside of the caecum. The taenia act like drawstrings to cause the formation of furrows of mucosa, called haustra. The outer surface of the colon exhibits fat filled pouches, the epiploic appendices.

Caecum

This is a pouch that connects the ileum with the colon. Covered in peritoneum, but lacking mesentery, it is situated distal to the ileocaecal junction in the right iliac fossa and lies over iliacus and psoas.

Appendix

The appendix, which unlike the caecum and colon, lacks taenia coli, is a blind-ending tube connected to the caecum that is around 10 cm in length and, in most cases, sits in a retrocaecal position. Its position within the right iliac fossa corresponds to McBurney's point, a surface location one-third along a diagonal line from the right anterior superior iliac spine to the umbilicus. This is the point to which pain ultimately localizes in cases of appendicitis when the parietal peritoneum surrounding the appendix becomes inflamed. A triangular mesentery that is a continuation of the mesentery of the terminal ileum, the meso-appendix, conveys branches of the ileocolic artery and vein, and lymph nodes that drains to the ileocolic nodes. The caecum and appendix receive sympathetic and parasympathetic innervation from the superior mesenteric plexus, with fibres accompanying blood vessels in the meso-appendix.

Colon

The colon is divided into four sections: ascending, transverse, descending, and sigmoid (Fig. 14.6). The caecum gives rise to the ascending colon, which is retroperitoneal (covered on its anterior, lateral, and medial surfaces), lacks mesentery and makes contact with the posterior abdominal wall. The ascending colon runs upwards on the right side of the abdomen and turns medially under the liver at the right colic (hepatic) flexure to become the transverse colon. Covered in peritoneum, with mesentery that runs from the inferior border of the pancreas, the transverse colon runs to the left colic (splenic) flexure at the spleen, at which point it becomes the descending colon. The retroperitoneal descending colon (covered on anterior and lateral surfaces) passes down the left lower abdominal quadrant to reach the sigmoid colon. Peritoneal recesses between the lateral surfaces of the ascending and descending colon, and the posterior abdominal wall form the right and left paracolic gutters. The phrenicocolic ligament, which attaches the diaphragm to the left colic flexure, separates the left paracolic gutter from the spleen. The translation from the descending colon to the intraperitoneal sigmoid colon occurs at the level of the pelvic brim. The mesentery, the sigmoid mesocolon, is a fold of peritoneum that is attached in an inverted V-shaped curve with the apex at the division of the left common iliac artery. The left limb runs along the pelvic brim, while the right limb ends at the level of the third sacral segment. The left ureter runs down into the pelvis behind the apex.

Blood and nerve supply

Blood and nerve supply to the large intestine reflects the embryological origin of the sections. The caecum, appendix, ascending colon, and proximal transverse colon are supplied by the superior mesenteric artery, whereas the remaining sections are supplied by the inferior mesenteric artery (Fig. 14.6). Blood drains through corresponding veins to the portal system—the inferior mesenteric vein and splenic vein unite and merge with the superior mesenteric vein to form the portal vein. Inferior mesenteric lymph nodes drain the right side of the large intestine. These nodes drain into the superior mesenteric nodes, which directly collect lymph from the left side, and into the para-aortic nodes. Parasympathetic nerve fibres from the vagus nerve supply the sections up to the distal transverse colon, with subsequent structures innervated by fibres from sacral segments S2–4 running in splanchnic nerves. These nerves also convey sympathetic nerve fibres derived from spinal cord segments T10–L2, which synapse in the mesenteric ganglia and run along the vascular tree. Visceral sensory fibres are conveyed

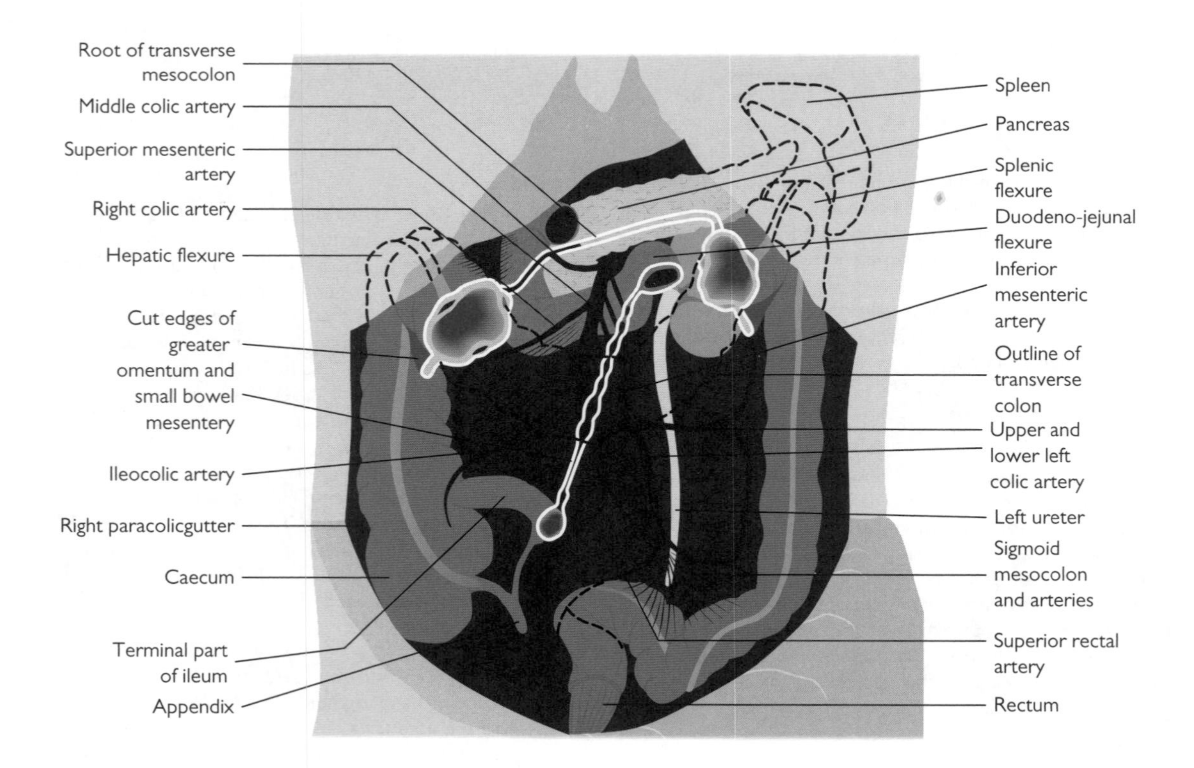

Fig. 14.6 Arterial supply to the small and large bowel derived from the superior and inferior mesenteric arteries.

in the lesser splanchnic nerve. Referred pain from abdominal organs localizes to the dermatome supplied by the spinal cord segment where the pain afferents synapse.

Rectum and anal canal

The retroperitoneal terminal section of the intestine (the upper third being covered on its anterior and lateral sides), the *rectum* runs from the end of the sigmoid colon anterior to S3, anterior to the sacrum and coccyx to end as the rectal ampulla, a distensible structure that stores faeces in advance of defecation. The bladder and the recto-urine or rectovesicle pouch (the Pouch of Douglas, an extension of the peritoneal cavity between the rectum and back wall of the uterus or bladder) sit anterior to the rectum. The middle sacral artery and lower sacral nerves are found to the posterior, with levator ani and coccygeus found laterally.

At the level of the pelvic floor, situated anterior to the tip of the coccyx, the anorectal junction marks a point at which the bowel narrows and turns sharply to the posterior. This point is characterized by the merging of the taenia coli to form a continuous layer of muscle. Puborectalis, comprising muscle fibres arising from the pubic symphysis, forms a sling around the anorectal junction and is continuous with the external anal sphincter.

Anal canal

The anal canal is the final structure in the alimentary tract. Its upper end is characterized by anal columns, longitudinal ridges that define furrows (sinuses) and in which are found terminal branches of the superior rectal arteries (Fig. 14.6). Anal valves, formed by folds of mucous membrane, join the distal ends of the columns. Just above the valves lies the dentate (pectineal) line, a demarcation of different embryological origins (endoderm to ectoderm). The morphology of the epithelial lining changes from columnar to stratified squamous epithelium through a region of transitional epithelium called the pecten. The columnar epithelium possesses submucosal glands that secrete mucus.

Circular muscle layers of involuntary smooth muscle and voluntary skeletal muscle, respectively, make up the internal and external anal sphincters. The intersphincteric groove, apparent as an indentation in the wall of anal canal, marks the boundary between the two sphincters.

Rectum

The rectum is supplied with blood by the superior rectal artery, which arises from the inferior mesenteric artery and the middle rectal artery (from the internal iliac artery). The superior rectal artery also supplies the anal canal above the dentate line, with that below the boundary supplied by the inferior rectal artery (from the internal pudendal artery that arises from the internal iliac artery). Anastomoses exist between the superior and inferior mesenteric arteries via the marginal artery and between the inferior mesenteric pudendal arteries. Venous drainage occurs through the rectal venous plexus, which envelops the rectum and comprises an internal plexus in the submucosa and an external plexus outside the muscularis. Free exchange between the portal and systemic venous systems is established by anastomoses between these two structures. The superior part of the internal plexus drains the anal canal above the dentate line to the superior rectal vein, which also receives blood from the superior part of the external plexus. The superior rectal vein continues upwards as the inferior mesenteric vein, which returns blood to the portal system. The inferior rectal veins, which feed the internal pudendal vein, receive blood from the inferior part of the external and internal plexus and drain blood from the anal canal below the dentate line. The middle part of the external plexus drains via the middle rectal vein to the internal iliac vein. The internal pudendal and iliac veins drain to the systemic circulation. Anastomoses exist between the superior, middle, and inferior rectal veins. Thick masses of highly vascularized submucosa possessing arteriovenous anastomoses, the anal cushions are situated around the anal canal at the 3, 7, and 11 o'clock positions. The cushions assist with the continence mechanism. Disruption and prolapse of the cushions result in haemorrhoids. Lymph drains from the rectum and anal canal in vessels that accompany blood vessels. The upper rectum drains to para-aortic nodes, while the lower rectum drains to inguinal nodes. Above the dentate line lymph from the anal canal drains to the internal iliac nodes, while that from below the dentate line passes to the superficial inguinal nodes. Parasympathetic innervation of the rectum and anal canal is derived from S2–4. Sympathetic supply is from fibres that synapse in the inferior mesenteric plexus. Both supplies run in the splanchnic nerves and are distributed via the pelvic (inferior hypogastric) plexus. Parasympathetic innervation to the anal canal relaxes the internal sphincter, whereas sympathetic innervation contracts it. The external sphincter is innervated by the inferior branch of the somatic pudendal nerve (S2), which also conveys sensation from regions of the canal below the dentate line.

Physiology

Secretion

Saliva

This comprises water, ions, and digestive enzymes. Its function is to lubricate the mouth, form a protective coating, and begin the digestion of starch. At rest, saliva secretion is 0.5 mL/min, but rises to 5 mL/min after stimulation. Salivary secretions can be serous (watery—these contain α amylase) or mucous (more viscous—these contain mucin). There are three main types of salivary glands—parotid, submandibular, and sublingual glands. Each are made up of secretory units, called lobules, formed by an acinus of epithelial cells defining an intercalated duct. This drains via intralobular ducts and interlobular ducts to a salivary duct. The parotid gland secretions are mainly serous and are secreted via Stensen's ducts into the oral cavity. The submandibular gland is responsible for about 70% of salivary secretions and produces a mixture of both serous fluid and mucus, which enters the oral cavity via Wharton's ducts. The sublingual glands also produce mixed secretions, although they are mainly mucus in nature. They are located beneath the tongue, anterior to the submandibular glands.

The primary secretion from acinar cells is isotonic NaCl. Na^+-K^+-$2Cl^-$ cotransport transports Cl^- ions across the basolateral membrane, which then diffuses out of the cell via channels in the apical membrane. Na^+ ions, attracted by the potential difference arising from the Cl^- flux, diffuse into the intercalated duct via the paracellular pathway and water follows by osmosis.

There are a number of similarities between the salivary glands and the exocrine pancreas.

There is secondary modification by cells lining the ducts (Fig. 14.7). Na^+ is exchanged for K^+, while Cl^- is replaced by HCO_3^-. More ions exit than enter the duct: the low water permeability of the duct cells means that the fluid becomes hypotonic. At high flow rates, secondary modification is curtailed.

Acinar cells also synthesize, and secrete α amylase, lingual lipase, mucin, antimicrobial factors (for example, lysozymes), and kallikreins (which catalyse the generation of bradykinin).

Post-ganglionic autonomic fibres innervate the acinar cells. Parasympathetic fibres in cranial nerves V and VII release acetylcholine, which binds M3 receptors and stimulates primary secretion by activating the apical Cl^- channel and by inducing exocytosis of secretory vesicles containing proteins. Sympathetic fibres release noradrenaline, which acts on α and β receptors to enhance secretion. This is an unusual exception to the rest and digest/fight or flight distinction of the autonomic nervous system divisions.

Gastric juice

This is secreted by gastric glands, which are invaginations of the epithelial cell lining. Glands possess a base, neck, and pit, with the latter opening into the stomach lumen. Different types of epithelial cell are present; parietal cells secrete HCl and intrinsic factor; chief cells secrete pepsinogen; mucous cells in the neck secrete mucus; superficial cells alkalinize the mucus. Endocrine cells at the base of the gland secrete gastrin (G cells) and somatostatin (D cells) into the bloodstream.

Secretion of gastric juice occurs in three phases:

- Cephalic (thought, sight, smell, taste).
- Gastric (stomach distension, protein digestion products in the stomach).
- Intestinal (protein digestion products, luminal pH in intestine).

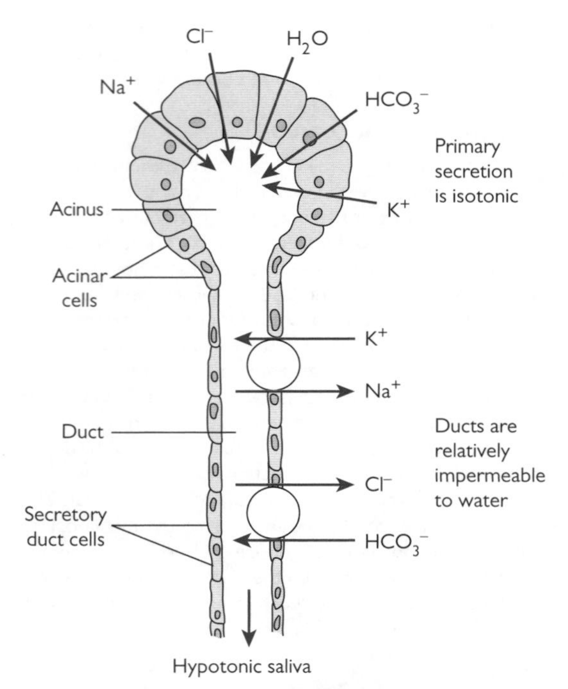

Fig. 14.7 Water and electrolyte transport leading to the formation of saliva by acinar and ductal cells of a salivary gland. This primary secretion is subsequently modified as fluid passes along the ducts.

Reproduced from G Pocock and CD Richards, *Human Physiology: The Basis of Medicine, Third Edition*, 2006, Figure 18.7, p. 384, by permission of Oxford University Press

The gastric phase is the dominant one (Fig. 14.8).

The luminal membrane of parietal cells displays deep infolds, which define a secretory canaliculus into which HCl is secreted (Fig. 14.9). H^+ and HCO_3^- ions are generated by the intracellular hydration of CO_2 catalysed by carbonic anydrase. H^+ secretion is mediated by H^+/K^+ ATPase proteins (inhibited by proton pump inhibitors such as omeprazole), which are activated when tubulovesicles possessing them are united with the luminal membrane. K^+ is taken up in exchange for H^+ and is recycled out of the cell via a channel. Cl^- ions enter the cell at the contraluminal membrane in exchange for HCO_3^- ions (which produce an 'alkaline tide' in the blood), and exit the cell via a channel in the luminal membrane.

Fusion of tubulovesicles with the luminal membrane is induced by acetylcholine (M_3 receptors) from the vagus nerve, gastrin (Cholecystokinin (CCK) $_B$ receptors) from G cells and histamine (H_2 receptors) from enterochromaffin-like (ECL) cells. Histamine release is also promoted by ACh and gastrin, and therefore acts a final 'common mediator' on the parietal cell. Pancreatic neuroendocrine gastrin-secreting tumours can cause gastric ulceration through excess gastric acid secretion, as well as diarrhoea. This is known

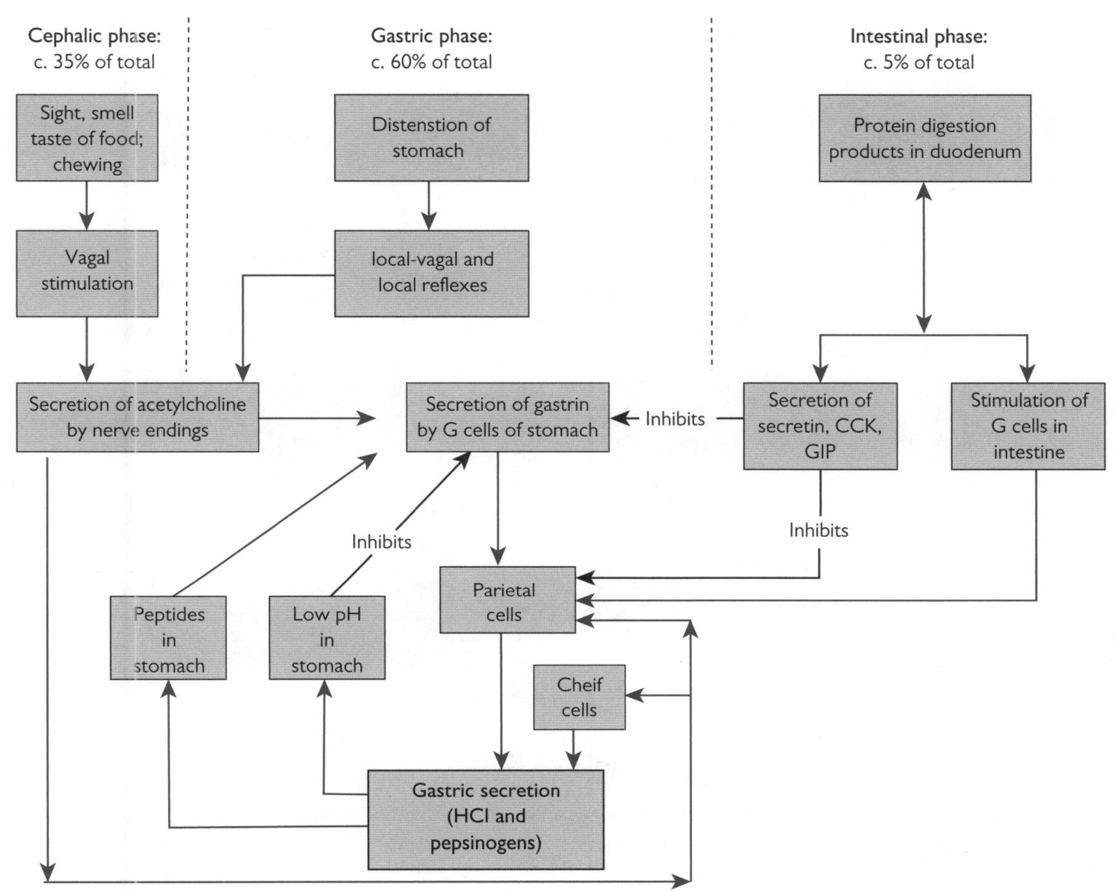

Fig. 14.8 The major factors involved in the regulation of gastric secretion. Secretin, CCK, and GIP are secreted by entero-endocrine cells in the epithelium of the upper small intestine and have an inhibitory action on gastrin secretion, as does a low pH in the lumen of the stomach. The stimulatory action of gastrin on mucus and enzyme secretion is omitted for clarity.

as Zollinger–Ellison syndrome, and such tumours may occur sporadically or as part of the autosomal dominant syndrome multiple endocrine neoplasia type 1 (MEN 1). Conversely, somatostatin (via ST_2 receptors) reduces HCl secretion—release of somatostatin from D cells is inhibited by *Helicobacter pylori*, which predisposes to gastric and duodenal ulceration.

Protein digestion

This is initiated by pepsins, secreted as inactive pepsinogens from secretory granules by chief cells. The acidic environment triggers spontaneous activation through proteolytic cleavage. Secretion is regulated by acetylcholine (M_3 receptors), by CCK and gastrin (CCK_B receptors), and by secretin.

A viscous mucus lining up to 200 μm thick is secreted by mucous cells and alkalinized by HCO_3^- secreted by superficial cells. Secretion is stimulated by acetylcholine (M_3 receptors). This lining presents a barrier to H^+ ion diffusion and neutralizes H^+ ions that penetrate it. The barrier can be disrupted by anti-inflammatory drugs and by alcohol.

Pancreatic juice

This is an alkaline protein-rich secretion of the exocrine pancreas that neutralizes stomach acid and continues digestion. The pancreas secretes up to 1.5 L/day of pancreatic juice. The exocrine glands are similar in structure to the salivary glands, and the mechanism of primary secretion by acinar cells is comparable with that in salivary glands. The primary secretion is an isotonic saline that acts as a vehicle in which to dissolve digestive enzymes—proteases, amylase, lipase, nucleases. Proteins can be secreted as zymogens (inactive precursors) or as already active forms. Duct cells

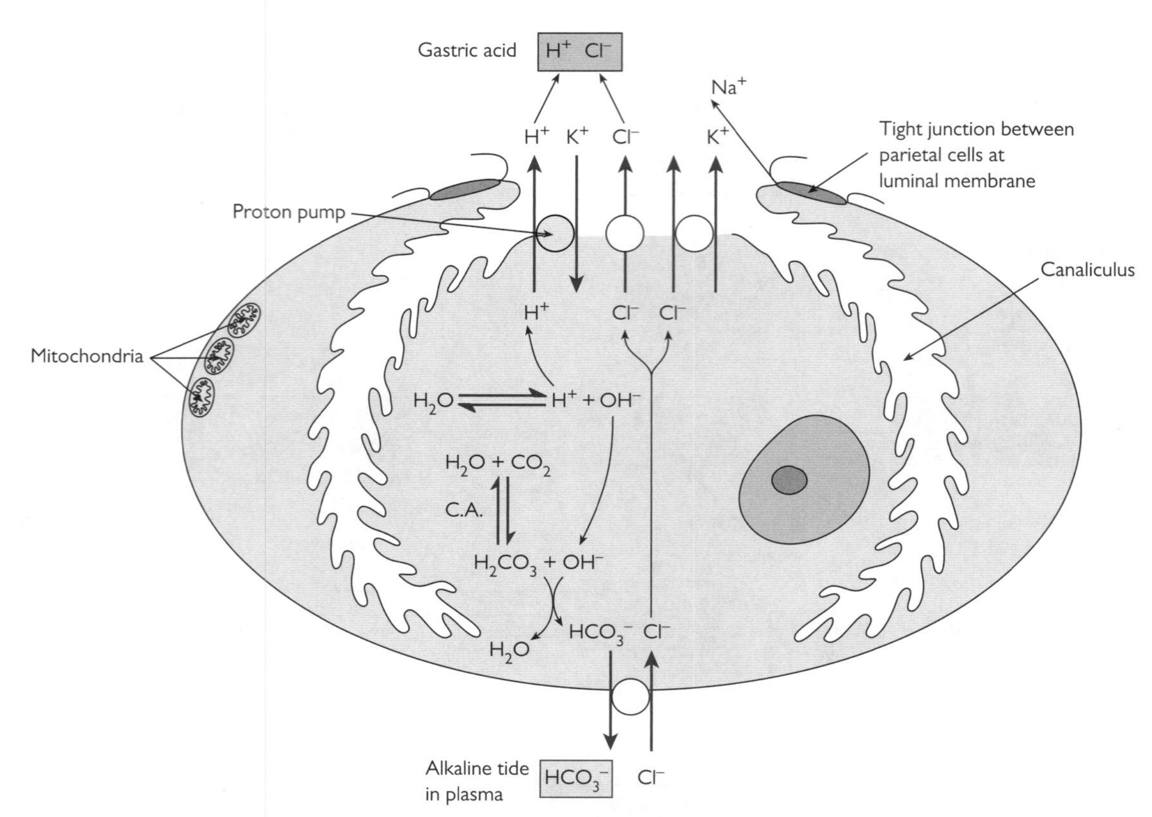

Fig. 14.9 The steps involved in the secretion of gastric acid by a parietal cell. C.A. carbonic anhydrase.

perform secondary modification to generate a hypotonic, HCO_3^--rich secretion. In cystic fibrosis, mutations in the apical Cl^- channel (the cystic fibrosis transmembrane conductance regulator, CFTR) compromise secondary modification leading to more viscous secretions. Like gastric secretion, pancreatic secretion exhibits three phases. Secretion is regulated by acetylcholine (cephalic phase) acting via M_3 receptors, by CCK and gastrin (gastric phase) acting through CCK_A receptors and by secretin (intestinal phase).

Bile

This is an alkaline secretion, the base components of which are similar to those of pancreatic juice. The secretion is supplemented by bile acids (to facilitate lipid digestion and absorption), and components destined for excretion including bilirubin, lecithin, and cholesterol. Catabolism of haem from senescent erythrocytes by reticulo-endothelial cells in the spleen yields bilverdin, which reduces to bilirubin. Bilirubin binds to albumin and is transported to the liver, where glucuronyl transferase catalyses its conjugation to glucuronic acid to generate a water-soluble form, which can be excreted in bile. Hepatocytes line a canaliculus into which bile is secreted, and which drains via ductules and ducts to the common hepatic duct. The cells synthesize bile acids (for example, cholic acid) from cholesterol, which are then conjugated to glycine and choline, and can exist as salts compounded to sodium or potassium ions (for example, sodium taurocholate). The bile acids are pumped into the canaliculus by ATP-binding cassette (ABC) transporters and water follows by osmosis. Cholangiocytes lining bile ducts supplement bile salt-dependent secretion with a dilute, HCO_3^--rich solution using a mechanism similar to that in the pancreas. This secretion is stimulated by secretin, glucagon, and VIP.

Deconjugation and dehydroxylation of primary bile acids by bacteria in the intestine yields secondary bile acids (for example, deoxycholic acid), which can be absorbed bound to albumin by the ileum and returned to the liver in the portal vein (enterohepatic circulation). Secondary acids are taken up from the blood by hepatocytes, reconjugated, and secreted again. This cycle may repeat up to three times during digestion of a meal. Water-soluble conjugated bilirubin secreted in bile can be similarly reabsorbed in the intestine and returned to the liver via the enterohepatic circulation. Intestinal enzymes metabolize residual bilirubin to urobilinogen, which can oxidize to yield stercobilinogen that gives faeces its characteristic brown colour. Some urobilinogen is reabsorbed, filtered by the kidneys, and lost in urine, giving urine its characteristic yellow colour.

- *Pre-hepatic jaundice:* arises from increased haemolysis, for example, in sickle cell anaemia, spherocytosis, and thalassemia. Increased haem catabolism results in an elevated serum level of unconjugated (insoluble) bilirubin and elevated levels of conjugated urobilinogen with unchanged urinary bilirubin in the urine. A congenital defect in glucuronyltransferase (Gilbert's syndrome) limits conjugation of bilirubin and subsequent excretion in bile, and results in a jaundice characterized by elevated serum levels of unconjugated bilirubin with no conjugated bilirubin or urobilinogen in urine.
- *Hepatic (hepatocellular) jaundice:* can arise from acute or chronic hepatitis, cirrhosis, alcoholic liver disease, and drug-induced toxicity. There is impairment of bilirubin excretion, characterized by elevated serum and urinary levels of conjugated bilirubin and normal or raised levels of urobilinogen in the urine.
- *Post-hepatic (obstructive) jaundice:* is the result of obstruction of the biliary system (by gallstones or cancer of the head of the pancreas). Elevated levels of conjugated bilirubin are observed in the serum and urine, while urinary urobilinogen levels are reduced.

Bile stored in the gall bladder during the fasting state is concentrated by reabsorption of isotonic NaCl by the epithelial cell lining: release is triggered by relaxation of the sphincter of Oddi by CCK (CCK_A receptor).

Enterocytes lining the villi and crypts of the small intestine also secrete an *isotonic solution of NaCl*, which acts as a vehicle for enzymes (for example, sucrase and maltase). The mechanism of secretion mirrors that for saliva and pancreatic juice. The cells are normally net absorbers of electrolytes and water—secretion is outweighed by absorptive processes. However, a number of bacterial enterotoxins (for example, cholera toxin) disrupt adenyl cyclase activity to activate CFTR and increase secretion, leading to production of large volumes of watery diarrhoea.

Absorption of nutrients

The small intestine is the site of entry of carbohydrates, proteins, fats, vitamins, and minerals (notably iron) into the body.

Carbohydrates

Starch constitutes the primary source of *carbohydrates* and is digested by amylases to generate disaccharides, trisaccharides, and α-limit dextrins. Enzymes (sucrase, maltase, lactase) expressed on the luminal membrane of enterocytes, work along with secreted forms to liberate the monosaccharides glucose, fructose, and galactose. Glucose and galactose are absorbed into enterocytes using the Na^+-dependent carrier, SGLT-1, whereas fructose is absorbed by the Na^+-independent carrier, GLUT5. All three monosaccharides leave the cell on GLUT2 and are taken up by the blood. Lactose intolerance results from lactase deficiency.

Proteins

The digestion of *proteins* is initiated in the stomach by the acidic secretions containing pepsin. Peptidases from the pancreas continue the digestion, generating peptides and amino acids, with enzymes expressed on the luminal membrane of enterocytes also digesting peptides to yield amino acids. Amino acids are absorbed into enterocytes using Na^+-dependent and -independent carriers, with specific carriers for neutral, cationic and anionic amino acids. Di- and tripeptides can also be absorbed using the H^+-dependent carrier PepT1 and digested by peptidases within the cell. Amino acids leave the cell on Na^+-independent carriers and are taken up by the blood (Fig. 14.10).

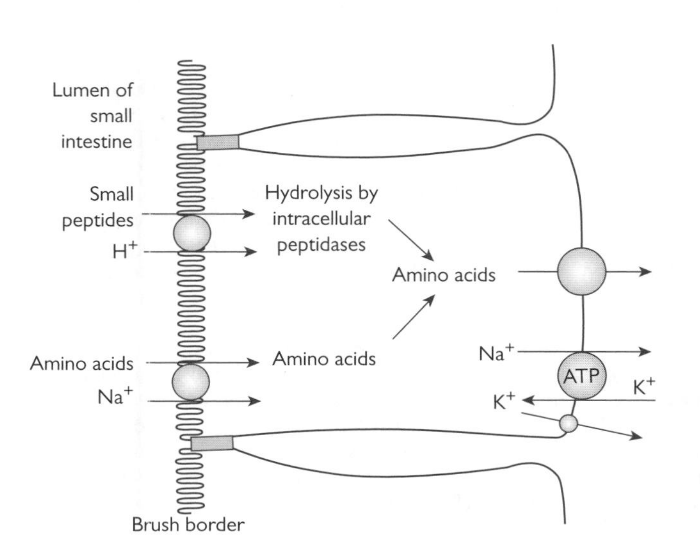

Fig. 14.10 The mechanisms by which amino acids and small peptides are absorbed in the small intestine.

Reproduced from G Pocock and CD Richards, *Human Physiology: The Basis of Medicine, Third Edition,* 2006, Figure 18.34, p. 409, by permission of Oxford University Press

Fats

Lingual lipase initiates the digestion of *fats* (the principal form of which is triglycerides), with muscular contractions of the stomach encouraging the formation of an emulsion of oil droplets in water. Pancreatic lipase, assisted by colipase, continues the digestion in the small intestine, generating monoglycerides and free fatty acids. Amphipathic bile acids facilitate the formation of small micelles that incorporate monoglycerides and free fatty acids for trafficking to epithelial cells. An unstirred, acidic layer adjacent to the luminal membrane promotes the dissociation of micelles and the presentation of components for diffusion into the cell. Within the cell, triglyceride is reassembled in the smooth ER and combined with apoproteins to generate chylomicrons that are exported by the Golgi apparatus and pass into lymphatic capillaries.

Vitamins

Fat-soluble *vitamins* (A, D, E, K) are presented for absorption in bile acid micelles and leave the cell in chylomicrons. Water-soluble vitamins (thiamine B_1, riboflavin B_2, folic acid B_9, B_{12}, C) are absorbed using carrier proteins (for example, vitamin C can be absorbed by GLUT1). Most fat and water-soluble vitamins are absorbed in the jejunum. However, vitamin B_{12} forms a complex with intrinsic factor secreted by the stomach, and binds to receptors in the luminal membrane, particularly of the terminal ileum.

Iron

Iron is absorbed in the form of Fe^{2+} using a H^+-driven carrier mainly in the duodenum. Fe^{3+} is converted to Fe^{2+} by a membrane-bound reductase. Within the cell, Fe^{2+} is converted to Fe^{3+} by an intracellular oxidase and either stored within the cell bound to ferritin or exported using a carrier before binding to transferrin in the plasma (which is usually about a third saturated). Iron stored in the enterocytes is lost when cells are shed: the balance between storage and export regulates iron levels in the body (the 'iron curtain hypothesis'). Transferrin bound iron can also be stored as ferritin in the plasma, liver, spleen, and bone marrow. There are several difficulties and pitfalls when trying to assess whether whole body iron is low and causing anaemia. Serum iron measurements by themselves do not give an accurate picture of whole body iron, and while plasma ferritin levels are decreased in iron deficiency anaemia, ferritin is also an acute phase protein and plasma levels are increased during infection in order to deny iron from the infective agent. A high total iron binding capacity (TIBC) of the plasma, or low plasma transferrin saturation (serum iron/TIBC × 100) are, therefore, more informative.

Absorption of electrolytes and water

Of the 9 L of fluid that enters the GI tract each day (7 L of secretions, 2 L ingested), only 100 mL is excreted in the stools. The small intestine absorbs up to 8.5 L, with the residual absorbed mostly by the proximal colon. Absorption of water (in large part through the cells via membrane aquaporins) is secondary to the absorption of electrolytes (principally Na^+) and nutrients. Na^+ absorption across the luminal membrane is coupled to glucose and amino acid absorption in the duodenum and jejunum, and with Cl^- absorption directly (by co-transport) or indirectly (by parallel exchangers) in the ileum and colon. In the colon and rectum, Na^+ ions also move through channels (ENaC), with Cl^- absorption taking place in exchange for HCO_3^- ions. ENaC is subject to regulation by the steroid hormone aldosterone. The gradient to energize Na^+ movement into the cell is maintained by Na^+ extrusion by the Na^+/K^+-ATPase on the contraluminal membrane. K^+ can be absorbed passively between cells in the small intestine and actively by H^+/K^+-ATPase in the colon. Alternatively, when aldosterone stimulates Na^+ absorption through ENaC, the resulting increase in intracellular $[K^+]$ (from increased Na^+/K^+-ATPase activity) may promote its loss to the faeces through channels in the luminal membrane.

Gastrointestinal motility

Circular and longitudinal layers of smooth muscle and the sphincters that separate different segments allow the contents of the gastrointestinal tract to be mixed and propelled in a staged fashion along its length. Apart from the oesophageal and the external anal sphincters, which are formed of striated muscle and under voluntary control, the sphincters and layers of smooth muscle can function without extrinsic regulation under the influence of the enteric nervous system. Activity is coordinated through reflex arcs that originate in chemoreceptors (for H^+ and digestion products) and mechanoreceptors with cell bodies in the submucosal plexus: interneurons then link to effector neurons with cell bodies in the myenteric plexus, which release one or more transmitters to modulate muscular activity. Mediators released include acetylcholine, CCK, NO, serotonin, somatostatin, substance P, and VIP. The arcs receive modulatory input from parasympathetic preganglionic fibres and sympathetic post-ganglionic fibres.

Swallowing and peristalsis

Swallowing is controlled by the medulla, through cranial nerves V, IX, and X. Food is first moved to the rear of the mouth by the tongue (oral phase). Pharyngeal muscles then contract to propel the bolus towards the oesophagus. The epiglottis closes and the upper oesophageal sphincter transiently relaxes to receive the food (pharyngeal phase). Peristalsis propels the bolus down the oesophagus and into the stomach as the lower oesophageal sphincter transiently relaxes (oesophageal phase); failure of this phase results in achalasia.

Within the stomach, waves of smooth muscle depolarization originating in the middle of the greater curvature generate peristalsis, propelling the bolus towards the antrum, where contractions mix the contents and advance them towards the pylorus. Transient relaxation of the pyloric sphincter allows small particles to progress to the small intestine; retropulsion forces larger particles back towards the antrum for further mixing and digestion. Emptying depends on the consistency, volume and particle size of the chyme and is influenced by the activity and contents of the duodenum. In the interdigestive state, migrating motor complexes (MMC; long periods of electrical inactivity, followed by increased activity building to a sustained peak which subsequently subsides) initiated by motilin sweep residual stomach contents into and along the small intestine.

Slow waves of depolarization, arising from suppression of enteric inhibitory transmitter release, initiate contraction of the circular smooth muscle of the small intestine. Isolated regions of contraction of the circular muscle cause segmentation and churning, with peristalsis propelling the bolus. MMC pulses propel the contents in the interdigestive state.

In response to a diverse array of stimuli, the medulla can initiate vomiting by reverse peristalsis of the small intestine smooth muscle and relaxation of the pyloric sphincter to return material to the stomach. From there, contraction of abdominal muscles and relaxation of the oesophageal sphincters leads to eject the contents.

Food progresses from the small to large intestines when the ileocaecal sphincter relaxes in response to distension of the ileum.

Slow wave depolarization of circular smooth muscle continues in the large intestine, increasing in frequency along the length of the colon and resulting in segmentation. Segmental contraction of haustra creates pendular movements, whereas concerted contraction moves the contents along. Mass movements—large peristaltic propulsions of up to 20 cm—occur up to three times each day. Distension of the stomach (the gastrocolic reflex) and standing (the orthocolic reflex) initiate these mass movements. In the distal colon, non-propulsive segmentation retards movement of faeces.

The rectum also displays segmental contraction with its distension initiating the rectosphincteric reflex by which the internal anal sphincter transiently relaxes. If required, contraction of the external anal sphincter, under voluntary control, can override the reflex. Evacuation upon relaxation of the external anal sphincter results from propulsion of the faeces through the anal canal, and voluntary contraction of abdominal wall muscles and the diaphragm to increase intra-abdominal pressure.

Drugs used in the treatment of gastroenterological disorders

For drugs used in the treatment of gastroenterological disorders, see Table 14.1. See Table 14.2 for common drug-induced gastrointestinal reactions.

Table 14.1 Drugs used in the treatment of gastroenterological disorders

Drug	Mechanism of action	Cautions/ contraindications	Side effects	Interactions
Acid suppressants				
Proton pump inhibitors, e g. omeprazole	Inhibits the H^+/K^+ ATPase on gastric parietal cells	May mask symptoms of malignancy	Diarrhoea, headache, dizziness. Interstitial nephritis (rarely). Altered LFTs. May increase risk of GI infections (e.g. *C. difficile*)	Minor degree of inhibition of cytochrome P450 system—may therefore enhance the effect of some drugs metabolized by this pathway
H_2 antagonists, e.g. ranitidine	Antagonist at H_2 receptors on parietal cells in the gastric mucosa	May mask symptoms of malignancy	Diarrhoea, headache, dizziness. Altered LFTs. Cimetidine can cause gynaecomastia	Cimetidine inhibits cytochrome P450 and, therefore, alters plasma concentration of drugs metabolized by this pathway
Prostaglandin analogues, e.g. misoprostol	Analogue of PGE_1 that acts directly on gastric parietal cell and inhibits secretion of acid. It also increase mucus and bicarbonate secretion	Pregnancy. Women of child-bearing age	Diarrhoea. Abdominal pain. Abnormal vaginal bleeding	

(*continued*)

Table 14.1 Drugs used in the treatment of gastroenterological disorders (*continued*)

Drug	Mechanism of action	Cautions/ contraindications	Side effects	Interactions
Anti-emetics				
Anti-histamines, e.g. cyclizine	Antagonist at H_1 receptors in the vestibular nuclei	Prostatic hypertrophy. Susceptibility to angle closure glaucoma	Anti-muscarinic side effects (e.g. urinary retention, dry mouth, blurred vision, constipation). Drowsiness	
Dopamine antagonists, e.g. metoclopramide	Antagonist at central dopamine (D_2) receptors in the chemoreceptor trigger zone. Also acts peripherally to stimulate cholinergic and antagonize dopaminergic receptors in the GI tract increasing GI motility	GI obstruction. Phaeochromocytoma. Parkinson's disease	Extrapyramidal effects (e.g. acute dystonic reactions, akathisa, Parkinsonism). Hyperprolactinaemia (e.g. gynaecomastia, galactorrhoea, impotence)	Increased rate of absorption of paracetamol and aspirin. Effect antagonized by opioids and anti-muscarinics Antagonizes effects of bromocriptine and cabergoline.
Dopamine antagonists, e.g. domperidone	Antagonist at central dopamine (D_2) receptors in the chemoreceptor trigger zone. Also acts peripherally increasing GI motility	GI obstruction	Rarely EPSEs (penetrates blood–brain barrier poorly)	Effect antagonized by opioids and anti-muscarinics
Dopamine antagonists, e.g. phenothiazines such as prochlorperazine	Antagonist at central dopamine (D_2) receptors in the chemoreceptor trigger zone	Parkinson's disease. Susceptibility to angle closure glaucoma	Extrapyramidal effects (as above). Neuroleptic malignant syndrome (hyperthermia, autonomic disturbance, muscle rigidity). Anti-muscarinic symptoms (as above). Hyperprolactinaemia (as above). Impaired temperature regulation	Avoid with other drugs that prolong the QT interval. Hypotensive effect of some anti-hypertensives increased. Antagonizes effects of bromocriptine and cabergoline
$5HT_3$ antagonists, e.g. ondansetron	Antagonist at $5HT_3$ receptor in the chemoreceptor trigger zone. Also acts peripherally on $5HT_3$ receptors in the GI tract reducing peristalsis	Hepatic impairment	Headache. Constipation. Flushing	Avoid with drugs that prolong QT interval
Antispasmodics				
Anti-muscarinics, e.g. Hyoscine butylbromide	Act on GI muscarinic receptors to inhibit parasympathetic activity	Myasthenia gravis. Paralytic ileus. Prostatic hypertrophy. Susceptibility to angle closure glaucoma	Anti-muscarinic effects (e.g. constipation, urinary retention, dry mouth, bradycardia)	Avoid with other agents with anti-muscarinic activity. Antagonizes effect of metoclopramide and domperidone
Mebeverine	Direct effect on GI smooth muscle. Receptors action unknown	Paralytic ileus	No serious adverse effects	

Table 14.2 Drug-induced gastrointestinal reactions

Gastrointestinal reaction	Drug
Oesophageal ulceration	Bisphosphonates. NSAIDs. Steroids
Nausea and vomiting	Antibiotics. Cytotoxics. Digoxin. Opiates
Gastric ulceration	Bisphosphonates. NSAIDs. Steroids
Pancreatitis	Azathioprine. Amiodarone. Oestrogens. Simvastatin. Sodium valproate. Steroids. Tetracycline
Acute hepatitis	Amiodarone. Atenolol. Enalapril. Halothane. Isoniazid. Ketoconazole. Methyldopa Nifedipine. Rifampicin. Verapamil
Cholestasis	Azathioprine. Cimetidine. Chlorpromazine. Cyclosporin. Erythromycin. Haloperidol. Imipramine. Nitrofuratoin. Oestrogens. Ranitidine
Constipation	Anticholinergics. Aluminium hydroxide. Iron. Opiate analgesics
Diarrhoea	Magnesium hydroxide. Antibiotics. Cimetidine. Digoxin. Laxatives. NSAIDS. PPIs. Propanolol

Multiple choice questions

1. Which of the following drugs increases gastrointestinal motility?

A. Erythromycin.
B. Ferrous sulphate.
C. Hyoscine butylbromide.
D. Loperamide.
E. Aluminium hydroxide-based antacids.

2. Which of the following anti-emetics are thought to act mainly through antagonism of 5HT3 receptors?

A. Metoclopramide.
B. Cyclizine.
C. Domperidone.
D. Granisetron.
E. Promethazine.

3. Children with cystic fibrosis are most likely to be deficient in which of the following vitamins, if left untreated?

A. Vitamin C.
B. Vitamin B12.
C. Vitamin B9.
D. Vitamin B6.
E. Vitamin A.

4. A 70-year-old man with a history of polymyalgia rheumatica and previous myocardial infarction presents with a 3-month history of lethargy and weakness. Blood results demonstrate the following: Hb = 7.5 g/dL, serum iron = 12 μmol/L (normal range: 11.6–31.7 μmol/L), ferritin=100 μg/L (normal range 20–250 μg/L), TIBC = 80 μmol/L (normal range: 45–66 μmol/L). Which of the following statements, based on these results, is correct?

A. He does not have an iron deficiency anaemia.
B. Transferrin saturation is 15%.
C. Iron is transported as Fe^{2+}
D. Transferrin saturation cannot be calculated without knowing the plasma transferrin concentration.
E. The iron deficiency anaemia most likely arises from lower GI blood loss.

5. Which of the following reduces gastric acid secretion?

A. Gastrin.
B. Histamine.
C. Somatastatin.
D. Acetylcholine.
E. NSAIDS.

6. Which of the following statements regarding cell types within the gastric mucosa is correct?

A. Parietal cells secrete intrinsic factor.
B. Chief cells secrete histamine.
C. Mucous cells secrete pepsinogen.
D. Enterochromaffin-like cells secrete gastrin.
E. G cells secrete mucus.

7. Which of the following statements regarding salivary glands is correct?

A. The parotid gland secretes the majority of saliva.
B. Submandibular gland secretion are mainly serous.
C. Secretions from the sub-lingual glad enter the oral cavity mainly via Wharton's ducts.
D. Serous salivary secretions contain α-amylase.
E. Parotid gland secretions are mainly mucinous.

8. The coeliac artery/trunk:

A. Supplies all parts of the duodenum.
B. Arises from the aorta at the level of the 3rd lumbar vertebra.
C. Indirectly supplies the gallbladder.
D. Is accompanied by the coeliac vein.
E. Supplies the greater curvature of the stomach via the left gastric artery.

9. Dietary fat:

A. Can only be absorbed as free fatty acids.
B. Is ingested predominantly as cholesterol.
C. Increases small intestinal transit time.
D. Absorption is reduced by bile salts.
E. Stimulates cholecystokinin release from the small intestine.

10. Folic acid:

A. Is also known as vitamin B2.
B. Is absorbed predominantly in the jejunum.
C. Is a fat soluble vitamin.
D. Requires binding to intrinsic factor for absorption.
E. Is effective treatment for alcohol-induced macrocytosis.

For answers, please see Appendix: Answers to multiple choice questions, page 313.

CHAPTER 15

Endocrinology

General principles

Through the release of hormones, the endocrine system helps coordinate internal homeostasis and orchestrate the organism's response to an altered external environment. It also regulates development, growth, and reproduction.

Hormones are chemical messengers released either by cells in specialized glands or diffuse endocrine tissue within an organ. They can also be directly released into the bloodstream via neurons (the neuroendocrine system). Hormones can influence the activity of distant cells, act locally (paracrine), or even on the same cell (autocrine) via a receptor. Hormones are normally present in *very low concentrations* (10^{-7}–10^{-13} mol/L) in the blood and/or extracellular fluid.

Characteristics of the main classes of hormones

- *Proteins /peptides/glycopeptides (hydrophilic):* translated on rough endoplasmic reticulum, they can be stored in large amounts in intracellular granules so secretion can be regulated (e.g. insulin, prolactin) or are constitutively released (cytokines, growth factors). The translated prohormone is usually proteolytically cleaved to yield the active hormone(s).
- *Steroids (hydrophobic, e.g. oestrogen):* synthesized rapidly on demand (not stored) from cholesterol via enzymes in the mitochondria and smooth endoplasmic reticulum. They act on intracellular receptors to alter gene expression over several hours to days. More recently, non-classical rapid actions of steroids have been identified that are dependent on membrane-bound receptors coupled to second messenger pathways.
- *Bioactive amines (hydrophilic, e.g. adrenaline):* produced from tyrosine via intracellular enzymes, stored in large amounts in intracellular granules.
- *Thyroid hormones (hydrophilic e.g. thyroxine):* produced by iodination and coupling of the tyrosyl residues of thyroglobulin. Large amounts of iodinated thyroglobulin, the precursor for thyroid hormone synthesis, are stored in the thyroid and released into the blood, which contains a large protein bound reservoir. Iodothyronines are then released by proteolysis of thyrogloblin.

Thyroid

Synthesis

See Fig. 15.1.

- *Epithelial cells of the thyroid* (follicular cells) are arranged into follicles around a lumen filled with colloid. The cuboidal follicular cells synthesize thyroglobulin, which is released into the colloid.
- *Production requires iodide:* a sodium/iodide symporter, on the basal membrane of follicular cells, traps and pumps in iodide from the plasma.
- *A thyroid peroxidase enzyme on the apical plasmalemma* oxidizes the iodide to iodine, iodinates tyrosyl residues in the thyroglobulin, and couples tyrosyl residues to produce the thyroid hormones T4 (thyroxine) and T3 (triiodothyronine) still bound in the thyroglobulin, which is inactive and stored in the colloid.
- *The glycoprotein thyroid-stimulating hormone (TSH)* stimulates endocytosis of colloid and its digestion by lysosomes, to free T4 and T3.
- *Iodine deficiency* can prevent formation of T4 and T3, whereas excess iodine inhibits thyroid activity.
- The *main thyroid product (T4)* is not the metabolically active hormone. Metabolism of T4 to produce active T3 occurs primarily in the liver by Type I (5')-deiodinase.

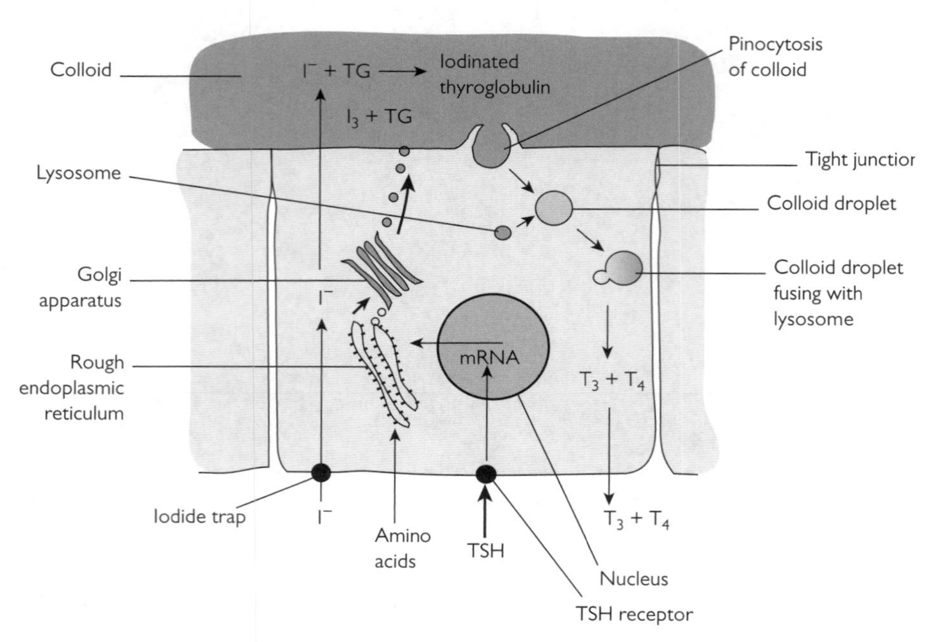

Fig. 15.1 The cellular processes involved in the synthesis and subsequent release of the thyroid hormones. Note that TSH stimulates both the synthesis of thyroglobulin (TG) and the secretion of T3 and T4.

Reproduced from G Pocock and CD Richards, *Human Physiology: The Basis of Medicine, Third Edition,* 2006, Figure 12.15, p. 205, by permission of Oxford University Press

- T4 and T3 are carried in the blood mainly by the thyroxine-binding globulin (TBG), but also by thyroid-binding pre-albumin and albumin. Levels of TBG can be increased in pregnancy and when using the contraceptive pill. Conversely, levels are low during thyrotoxicosis and nephrotic syndrome.

Mechanism of action of thyroid hormones

Thyroid hormones are transported into cells and T3 acts on nuclear receptors (TR). This interaction results in stimulation or inhibition of the production of many different proteins. Sensitivity to T3 is regulated via the number of TR.

Effects of thyroid hormones

- Increases metabolic rate of almost every tissue of the body.
- Stimulates normal development and maturation.
- Potentiates insulin effects increasing glycogenesis and glucose usage. Potentiates β adrenoceptor effects on glycogenolysis and gluconeogenesis.
- Hyperthyroidism increases hepatic gluconeogenesis, glycogenolysis, and intestinal glucose absorption, and can worsen glycaemic control in diabetic patients.
- Lowers circulating cholesterol. Stimulates cholesterol breakdown and synthesis, and increases the number of low-density lipoprotein (LDL) receptors on the cell surface and enhances lipolysis.
- Potentiates cardiac adrenergic drive, and has positive inotropic and chronotropic effects on the heart. Stimulates production of β adrenergic receptors and amplifies catecholamine action at a post-receptor site.
- Stimulates gut motility.
- Stimulates bone turnover (breakdown > synthesis).
- Increases speed of muscle contraction.

Thyroid axis pathology

- *Goitre (diffuse or multinodular):* common causes:
  - Iodine deficiency.
  - *Graves' disease*—the gland is enlarged because of the antibody-mediated over-activation of the TSH receptor.
- *Thyroid nodule:* may be functioning or non-functioning.

Thyrotoxicosis

Patients with thyrotoxicosis have raised metabolic rates, and hence weight loss, sweating, and heat intolerance, as well as increased sympathetic drive, causing tachycardia and often atrial fibrillation, tremor, nervousness, tiredness, and diarrhoea, as well as eye signs (lid retraction and lid lag). They can also have osteoporosis (if thyrotoxicosis is long term and untreated) and thyroid acropachy (very rare).

Causes

Graves' disease is an autoimmune aetiology caused by antibodies stimulating the TSH receptor, and is more common

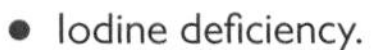

in females. It is the most common cause of hyperthyroidism and may also be associated with ophthalmopathy and dermopathy (pretibial myxoedema).

- Functioning solitary adenoma or multinodular goitre.
- Thyroiditis (e.g. post-partum, drug-induced, or secondary to viral infection; 'De Quervains's thyroiditis').
- Thyrotoxicosis facticia.
- *Rare forms:* ovarian stroma, metastatic thyroid carcinoma (follicular), hydatidiform mole, TSH-secreting pituitary tumour, pituitary resistance to T3 and T4.

Hypothyroidism

In the neonate, cretinism leads to gross deficits in CNS myelination and stunting of postnatal growth. In the adult, it can present as weight gain, constipation, cold peripheries, proximal myopathy, and bradycardia.

Causes

- *Hashimoto's thyroiditis:* autoimmune inflammation of the thyroid.
- Iodine deficiency.
- Post-thyroidectomy or after administration of I^{131}.
- Thyroiditis (usually transient).
- Inborn errors of thyroid hormone synthesis.
- Secondary to TSH or thyrotrophin-releasing hormone (TRH) deficiency from pituitary or hypothalamic damage
- Peripheral resistance to the action of thyroid hormones

Anterior pituitary

The anterior pituitary (adenohypophysis) consists of various types of cells classified (by using immunocytochemical and electron microscopic techniques) according to their specific secretory products: somatotrophs (growth hormone [GH]-secreting cells), lactotrophs (prolactin [PRL]-secreting cells), thyrotrophs (cells secreting thyroid-stimulating hormone [thyrotropin; TSH]), corticotrophs (cells secreting ACTH [corticotropin] and related peptides), and gonadotrophs (luteinizing hormone [LH] and follicle-stimulating hormone [FSH]-secreting cells). Secretion is controlled by hormones from the hypophyseal tract (see Fig. 15.2). Feedback

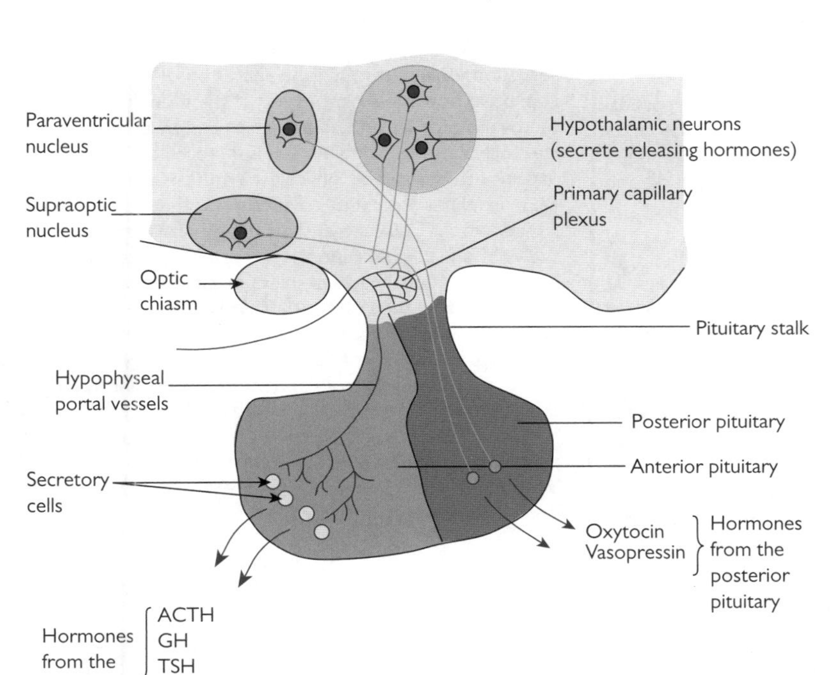

Fig. 15.2 The relationship between the hypothalamus and the pituitary gland. Note the prominent portal system that links the hypothalamus to the anterior pituitary gland. The anterior pituitary has no direct neural connection with the hypothalamus. In contrast, nerve fibers from the paraventricular and supraoptic nuclei pass directly to the posterior pituitary where they secrete the hormones they contain into the blood stream.

inhibition of secretion originates from either the hormone released by the target organ or the releasing/inhibiting hypophyseal hormone.

Thyroid stimulating hormone (TSH)

- *Actions:* Stimulates T3 and T4 production and increases iodine uptake by the thyroid. Stimulates thyroid growth.
- *Control:* TSH release is stimulated by TRH from the hypothalamus and is inhibited by T3 and T4 negative feedback. Secretion of TRH is stimulated via the CNS in response to stress and cold.

Adrenocorticotrophic hormone (ACTH)

Polypeptide cleaved from the prohormone, pro-opiomelanocortin (POMC).

- *Actions:* stimulates the secretion of glucocorticoids, mineralocorticoids, and androgens from the adrenal cortex.
- *Control:* ACTH release is stimulated by corticotrophin-releasing hormone (CRH) from the hypothalamus and inhibited by glucocorticoid negative feedback. Secretion varies in a diurnal rhythm (peaking first thing in the morning and being at its lowest at midnight), as well as in response to stress.

Gonadotrophins

Gonadotrophins include luteinizing hormone (LH) and follicle-stimulating hormone (FSH).

Actions

The gonadotrophins are responsible for the gonadal sex-steroid production by the Leydig cells of the testis and the ovarian follicles, secondary sexual development, the maintenance of secondary sexual characteristics, and fertility.

Control

During childhood LH and FSH rise gradually. In males, at puberty, LH and FSH are secreted by the anterior pituitary gland in response to hypothalamic gonadotrophin releasing hormone (GnRH). A failure of formation of GnRH producing neurons causing failure to enter puberty is found in Kallman's syndrome. LH acts on the Leydig cells to stimulate androgen production leading to the development of secondary sexual characteristics. Androgens also pass into the seminiferous tubules to affect spermatogenesis. FSH acts on Sertoli cells to stimulate spermatogenesis. Testosterone exerts a negative feedback on LH and FSH, while inhibin, a peptide secreted by the Sertoli cells exert a negative feedback on FSH.

In females, prior to menarche, pulsatile release of LH and FSH is established and pulses of secretion occur during sleep. This results in increased oestrogen secretion from the ovary, which triggers breast development, and the development of secondary sexual characteristics. The trigger for menstruation is not understood, but is thought to include increased ovarian sensitivity to LH and FSH, and an increased pituitary sensitivity of positive feedback effects of oestrogens.

Cyclical variations in LH and FSH in the menstrual cycle

In women, LH levels rise slightly during the follicular phase, they peak at the time of the mid-cycle surge and decline during the luteal phase (see Fig. 15.3). The FSH levels start rising during the late luteal phase, increase during the early follicular phase of the next cycle and decline just before the mid-cycle FSH surge. During the luteal phase, the FSH levels show a reduction and increase again prior the next menses. During the follicular phase, the LH pulses are followed by a release of oestrogens from the ovary, whereas in the mid- and late-luteal phase, the LH pulses induce progesterone secretion. In the follicular phase there is enhanced release of oestradiol, which induces the large discharge of LH responsible for ovulation. During this surge, LH levels remain increased for 36–48 hr and ovulation occurs. The post-ovulatory follicle becomes a corpus luteum under the influence of LH and secretes progesterone, as well as oestrogen, which prepare the uterus to receive and support an early embryo. In the absence of fertilization, the corpus luteum degenerates around days 24–28 and steroid production stops. As progesterone concentrations fall, the endometrium built up during the cycle is shed, together with blood from spiral arteries. This process is menstruation and marks the start of another menstrual cycle. The ovary exerts a negative feedback on FSH secretion, mainly through the secretion of inhibin, a glycoprotein hormone synthesized in the granulosa cells of the ovarian follicle and counterbalanced by activin. In the late follicular phase, inhibin levels increase and, in combination with oestradiol, inhibit the synthesis and release of FSH, an inhibition that it is overcome at the pre-ovulatory gonadotrophin discharge. The hypothalamic control of the FSH and LH secretion is very sensitive to environmental conditions, such as stress or changes in nutrition. Stress activates the CRH pathways, which may inhibit the GnRH neurones. Reduction in the daily food intake leads to a reduction in the GnRH secretion translated into a reduced and non-pulsatile secretion of FSH and LH into the circulation.

During menopause, few oocytes are left in the ovaries, the ovarian responsiveness to LH and FSH decreases and as levels of LH and FSH rise. Cycles become anovulatory and irregular before ceasing altogether.

Prolactin (PRL)

Actions

PRL stimulates the development and growth of secretory alveoli in the breast and milk production, and inhibits ovulation at the level of the ovaries and pituitary (causing 'lactational amenorrhoea' in women postpartum).

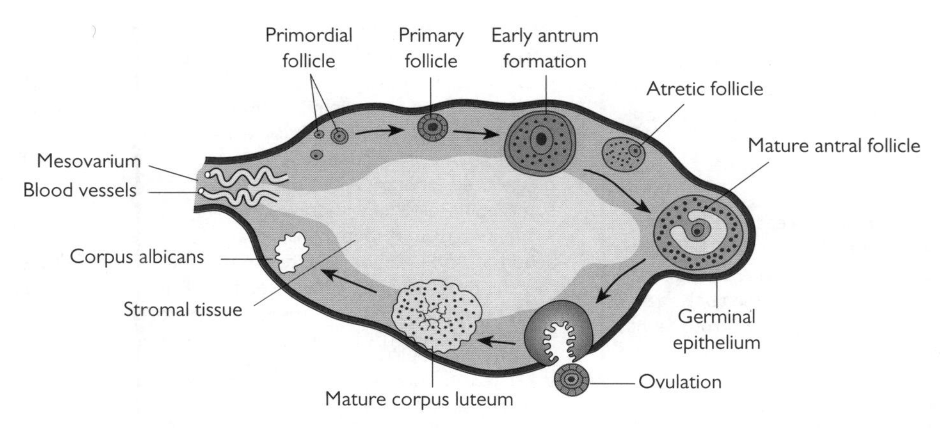

Fig. 15.3A The internal structure of the ovary showing the stages of follicular development, ovulation, the formation of the corpus luteum, and its subsequent regression. In reality, not all stages would be seen at the same time.

Reproduced from G Pocock and CD Richards, *Human Physiology: The Basis of Medicine, Third Edition,* 2006, Figure 20.9, p. 439, by permission of Oxford University Press

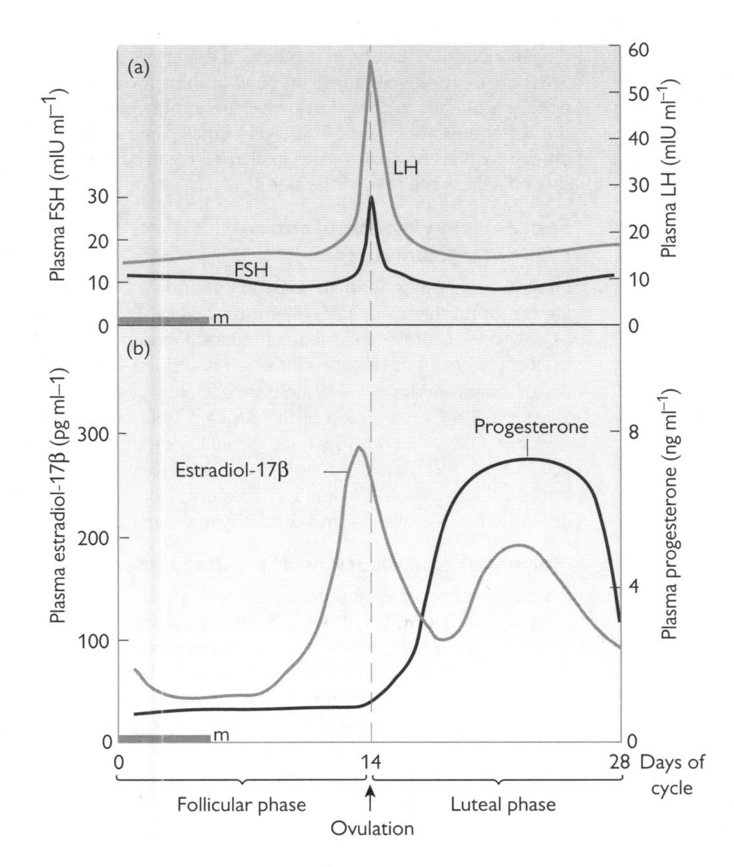

Fig. 15.3B The changes in hormone levels during the menstrual cycle. (a) The pattern of secretion shown by the gonadotrophins (FSH and LH); (b) the changes in the plasma levels of estradiol-17ᴸ and progesterone. The solid bar marked 'm' represents the period of menstruation.

Reproduced from G Pocock and CD Richards, *Human Physiology: The Basis of Medicine, Third Edition,* 2006, Figure 20.12, p. 441, by permission of Oxford University Press

Control

PRL release is inhibited by dopamine from the hypothalamus. Oestrogens induce hyperplasia of the lactotroph cells and enhance PRL secretion. Suckling increases secretion.

Growth hormone (GH)

Actions

Mediated either directly or mainly indirectly via the production of insulin-like growth factor (IGF)-I on the liver, bones, and other types of tissues. Promotes skeletal growth, mainly on long bones and regulation of several metabolic actions. Enhances the incorporation of amino-acids and protein synthesis in the muscles and free fatty acid release in adipose tissue.

Control

Secretion is increased via release of growth hormone-releasing hormone (GHRH) from the hypothalamus. Amino-acids (e.g. arginine, leucine), sleep, exercise, stress, hypoglycaemia, poorly-controlled diabetes mellitus type 1, hepatic cirrhosis, and anorexia nervosa enhance GH secretion. GH release is inhibited by somatostatin, as well as by negative feedback by IGF-I and GH itself.

Posterior pituitary

The posterior pituitary (neurohypophysis) is formed by the axons and nerve terminals of magnocellular neurosecretory neurons originating in the paraventricular (mainly oxytocin) and supraoptic (mainly anti-diuretic hormone (ADH)) nuclei of the hypothalamus. The posterior pituitary hormones are synthesized in these nuclei, packaged into secretory vesicles, transported down the axons and released by exocytosis into the systemic veins (see Fig. 15.2). Pituicytes (a type of glial cell) surround and support the terminals.

Anti-diuretic hormone (ADH)

Actions

Nonapeptide that increases water reabsorption at the collecting ducts of the nephron via V2 receptors and cAMP-dependent increased aquaporin 2 water channel expression. Also stimulates the production of clotting factor VIII via V2 receptors, vasoconstricts peripheral arterioles and veins via V1 receptors. Via V_3, a third type of receptor on the anterior pituitary, it regulates the secretion of ACTH.

Control

Release is stimulated by a 1–2% fall in plasma osmolality from 290 mOsm/L (sensed by anterior hypothalamic osmoreceptors) or a 10–15% fall in blood volume (sensed by baro/volume receptors).

Pathology

Lack of ADH as a result of damage to the neurohyphyseal system (e.g. by tumours, trauma, surgery, infiltrative diseases) can lead to central diabetes insipidus with polyuria and polydypsia. Alcohol can also inhibit the release of ADH.

Conversely, high levels of ADH can lead to low plasma Na with low plasma. The syndrome of inappropriate ADH release (SIADH—characterized by decreased osmolality; inappropriate concentration of the urine; clinical euvolaemia; increased urinary sodium excretion; and absence of other causes of euvolaemic hypo-osmolality, as hypothyroidism, adrenal insufficiency, or diuretic use) can be from ectopic ADH production (e.g. lung tumours and infection) or elevated pituitary ADH release (e.g. secondary to carbamazepine, alcohol withdrawal, meningitis).

Nephrogenic diabetes insipidus or resistance to the action of ADH, can be acquired (often due to hypercalcaemia, or drugs such as lithium) or hereditary with 90% of cases being linked to mutations in the gene for the V2 receptor (*AVPR2*) and 10% to the gene encoding the aquaporin 2 protein (*AQP2*)

Oxytocin

Actions

Nonapeptide that causes contraction of uterine myometrium in childbirth and causes contraction of breast myoepithelium to eject milk.

Control

Stretch of cervix/vagina during parturition (the Ferguson reflex), as well as stimulation of the nipple during suckling causes the milk ejection reflex.

Pituitary pathology

Pituitary tumours can have mechanical effects due to compression of local structures, as well as hormonal effects, either secondary to compression or due to hormone secretion of the tumour itself. Thus, very small tumours in the pituitary, only a few millimetres in diameter, can have extensive effects on the rest of the body.

Space-occupying complications of pituitary tumours

Pituitary adenomas tend to expand superiorly compressing the optic chiasm or laterally in the cavernous sinus(es) as the gland is confined in the sella turcica. Pressure atrophy of the chiasm classically produces a bitemporal hemianopia or quadrantinopia visual field defect (see Chapter 12, 'Neurology'). Compression of the pituitary stalk can lead to a modest rise in PRL as dopaminergic inhibition of its secretion is removed. Pituitary tumours also lead to deficiencies in the release of other pituitary hormones, due to direct compression within the gland or the hypothalamus.

Hormonal complications of pituitary adenomas

Pituitary adenomas arise predominantly in the anterior pituitary, which constitutes about 80% of the pituitary volume. Non-functioning pituitary adenomas often cause panhypopituitarism due to direct compression of the surrounding gland. Such patients can be hypoadrenal (see section on *Adrenal insufficiency*), hypothyroid, and/or hypogonadal. Bleeding within a pituitary tumour can lead to dangerous sudden hypopituitarism (apoplexy) and a similar presentation can arise from pituitary infarction post-partum (Sheehan's syndrome).

However, as the pituitary gland is composed almost entirely of cells that make hormones, an adenoma, will often make the same hormone as its cell of origin, but with loss of hypothalamic control over secretion leading to high circulating levels of the hormone. Adenomas of GH-producing cells present as pituitary gigantism if occurring before puberty, when the epiphyseal plates are still open and long bones can grow. Later in life, they present as acromegaly with disproportionate growth of the bones in the jaw, hands, and feet, sweating, organomegaly, and often diabetes. Acromegaly is biochemically diagnosed by an oral glucose tolerance test (the gold standard), which may also diagnose concurrent diabetes mellitus, and by measuring the IGF-I levels. Adenomas of ACTH-producing cells produce Cushing's disease (see section on *Cushing's syndrome*). Prolactinomas often present as amenorrhea, lack of testosterone in males, infertility, loss of libido, and galactorrhoea, while adenomas of TSH-producing cells are a rare (1%) cause of hyperthyroidism.

Functioning adenomas of the other hormone-producing cells (such as FSH and LH-producing cells) in the anterior pituitary can occur, but they are much less common.

Adrenal gland

The adrenal glands are located just medial to the upper pole of each kidney. The glands comprise an inner catecholamine secreting medulla, which is made up of sympathetic post-ganglionic chromaffin cells, and an outer cortex that synthesizes and secretes steroid hormones. The adrenal cortex is made up of sheets of cells surrounded by capillaries and arranged in three zones:

- The outer zona glomerulosa, which makes aldosterone (C21 steroid).
- Middle zona fasciculate, which makes cortisol (C21 steroid).
- Inner zona reticularis, which makes small amounts of androgens (C19 steroids), oestradiol (C18 steroid), and progestogens (C21 steroid).

The synthesis of all cortical steroid hormones originates from cholesterol, the rate-limiting step being its conversion to pregnenolone.

Aldosterone

Actions

In the distal tubules and collecting ducts of nephrons, aldosterone stimulates reabsorption of Na^+ in exchange for secretion of K^+, H^+, NH_3^+. This is achieved via Mineralocorticoid receptors (MR), which stimulate transcription of the Na/K ATPase protein and increase its expression on the basolateral membrane. In salivary and sweat glands aldosterone also regulates ion transport to retain sodium.

Control

Aldosterone release is stimulated by Angiotensin II in response to reduced renal perfusion pressure (see Chapter 10, 'Cardiology' and Chapter 16, 'Nephrology').

Conn's syndrome

Hyperaldosteronism leads to increased sodium and water retention causing hypertension. Increased sodium reabsorption at the distal convoluted tubule and collecting ducts leads to H^+ excretion via Na/H exchange and potassium loss due to increased Na/K ATPase activity. This causes a hypokalaemic metabolic alkalosis. In primary hyperaldosteronism (Conn's syndrome) due to an adrenal cortical adenoma or primary adrenal cortical hyperplasia, renin levels will be low (useful in the diagnostic process). Secondary hyperaldosteronism is in response to activation of the renin-angiotensin system due to decreased renal perfusion, for example, during congestive heart failure or renal artery stenosis.

Pseudohyperaldosteronism also produces hypertension with a hypokalaemic metabolic alkalosis and low rennin activity, but surprisingly with low aldosterone levels. This can be due to inhibition of 11-beta hydroxysteroid dehydrogenase by excess liquorice ingestion resulting in inappropriate stimulation of the mineralocorticoid receptor by cortisol, or secondary to genetic conditions, such as Liddle's syndrome. This autosomal dominant condition is due to increased activity of renal sodium channels (ENaC).

Cortisol

Actions

Provides protection of the body as part of the stress response. Glucocorticoid receptors (GR) are present in the cytoplasm of almost all cells and migrate to the nucleus to regulate gene transcription when cortisol binds. The effects of cortisol are, therefore, widespread and include:

- *Metabolic:* stimulates gluconeogenesis and opposes the action of insulin. Stimulates lipolysis and ketogenesis (results in redistribution of fat to trunk).
- *Cardiovascular:* in high concentrations maintains plasma volume via an action at mineralocorticoid receptors to promote Na and water retention and K^+ excretion. Also increases myocardial contraction and vascular tone.
- *Skeletal muscle:* maintains ability to give sustained contractile responses.
- *Immune system:* immunosuppressive actions by inhibiting leukocyte translocation from blood to sites of tissue damage or infection, and stimulating lymphocyte destruction.
- *CNS:* varied effects on mood and behaviour. High doses of exogenous corticosteroids can cause steroid psychosis.
- *Haemopoiesis:* when in excess it can increase red blood cell production via ACTH overproduction of androgens to enhancing oxygen carrying capacity of blood.

Control

See section on *Adrenocorticotrophic hormone (ACTH)*. 90% of plasma cortisol is not physiologically active, but bound mainly to cortisol-binding globulin and albumin.

Cushings's syndrome

Excess glucocorticoid hormones in the body can arise from:

- Pituitary ACTH-secreting adenoma (Cushing's Disease).
- Adrenal cortisol-secreting ademona, which has become autonomous from the pituitary-adrenal feedback loop.
- Ectopic ACTH produced, for example, by a small cell lung tumour.
- Excess exogenous glucocorticoids (e.g. long-term prednisolone). This is the commonest mechanism as steroids are powerful drugs that could control severe allergic and inflammatory conditions.

The complications of Cushing's syndrome include truncal obesity, hirsutism, proximal muscle weakness, depression, diabetes mellitus, decreased immunity to infections, thin skin, easy bruising, and osteoporosis.

In patients not taking exogenous steroids, it can be difficult to diagnose and often several methods are used, including measuring 24-hr urinary-free cortisol, overnight or low-dose dexamethasone suppression tests, and midnight cortisol levels. Once the biochemical diagnosis has been made, further tests are required to localize the tumour (such as high dose dexamethasone supression test, CRH test, and inferior petrosal sinus sampling and imaging).

Adrenal insufficiency

Adrenal failure can be caused by:

- Addison's disease or primary autoimmune adrenal destruction, which is often associated with other autoimmune diseases, such as vitiligo, Graves' disease, pernicious anaemia, and diabetes mellitus type 1.
- Infective infiltration, e.g. by TB or fungi.
- Infiltrative disorders, e.g.
  - Metastatic disease.
  - Infarction, e.g. in meningococcal septicaemia (Waterhouse-Friderichsen syndrome).
- Secondary to loss of anterior pituitary ACTH secretion

Lack of aldosterone and cortisol results in sodium and water loss, hypotension, and hyperkalaemia. In primary adrenal insufficiency, the high ACTH release from the anterior pituitary causes hyperpigmentation particularly of the skin creases, lips and mouth, and surgical scars. Diagnosis is via a failure of plasma cortisol to rise beyond 550 nmol/L at 30 min after injection of synthetic ACTH (the short synacthen test) or in any other dynamic test, as the insulin-induced hypoglycaemia.

Adrenal androgens

These are mainly dehydroepiandrosterone/androstenedione (DHEA) and are produced from pregnenolone in the adrenal cortex zona reticularis. They have minimal intrinsic androgenic activity, and they contribute to androgenicity by their peripheral conversion to the more potent androgens testosterone and dihydrotestosterone. High levels can be found in congenital adrenal hyperplasia. This is a group of autosomal recessive disorders in the synthesis of cortisol and aldosterone, which lead to precursors being channelled down a different pathway to produce excess sex steroids. Manifestations can range from ambiguous genitalia at birth to adult onset female hirsutism, acne, and virilization, similar to polycystic ovarian syndrome. The most common of these is 21-hydroxylase deficiency (90% of cases). 21-hydroxylase catalyses the conversion of 17-hydroxyprogesterone to 11-deoxycortisol from which corticosteroids and aldosterone are synthesized (see Fig. 15.4). In the most severe forms, it can present at birth with Addisonian crises in addition to female virilization. Neonatal screening is carried out by measuring levels of 17-hydroxyprogesterone, which are raised in congenital adrenal hyperplasia.

Adrenal medulla

Actions

The adrenal medulla contributes 10% of the total sympathetic nervous system response to stress.

Receptors

Adrenaline and noradrenaline act at alpha and beta-adrenergic receptors .

Stimuli

Any stressful stimuli that activates the sympathetic nervous system, e.g. hypotension, haemorrhage, pain, hypoglycaemia, and surgery.

Pathology

Catecholamine-secreting medullary tumours (phaeochromocytomas) can present with episodic hypertension, palpitations, tremor, headaches, pallor or flushing, and anxiety. They are often familial or present as *de novo* mutations, such as in the *RET* oncogene (causing the multiple endocrine neoplasia (MEN) type 2 syndrome) or *VHL* tumour suppressor gene (causing haemangioblastomas and renal cell carcinoma found in Von Hippel–Lindau disease). They are also seen in neurofibromatosis type 1 and succinate dehydrogenase subunit (*SDHB*, *SDHD*, and *SDHC*) gene mutations. Tumours of chromaffin tissue outside the adrenal gland (paragangliomas) can present with identical symptoms.

Pancreas

Whilst exocrine secretions are produced in the pancreatic acini and discharged into the ducts of the pancreas, the islets of Langerhans are diffusely distributed throughout the pancreas. They are highly vascular and innervated by the autonomic nervous system. They comprise of ß cells (insulin producing), α cells (glucagon producing), δ cells (somatostatin producing) and F cells (which produce pancreatic polypeptide). The endocrine pancreas regulates the availability of metabolic substrates.

Insulin

Synthesis

Proinsulin is cleaved to the 31 amino acid C peptide and the soluble 51 amino acid insulin in secretory granules. Insulin comprises an α and β chain linked by two disulphide; stored with zinc in granules.

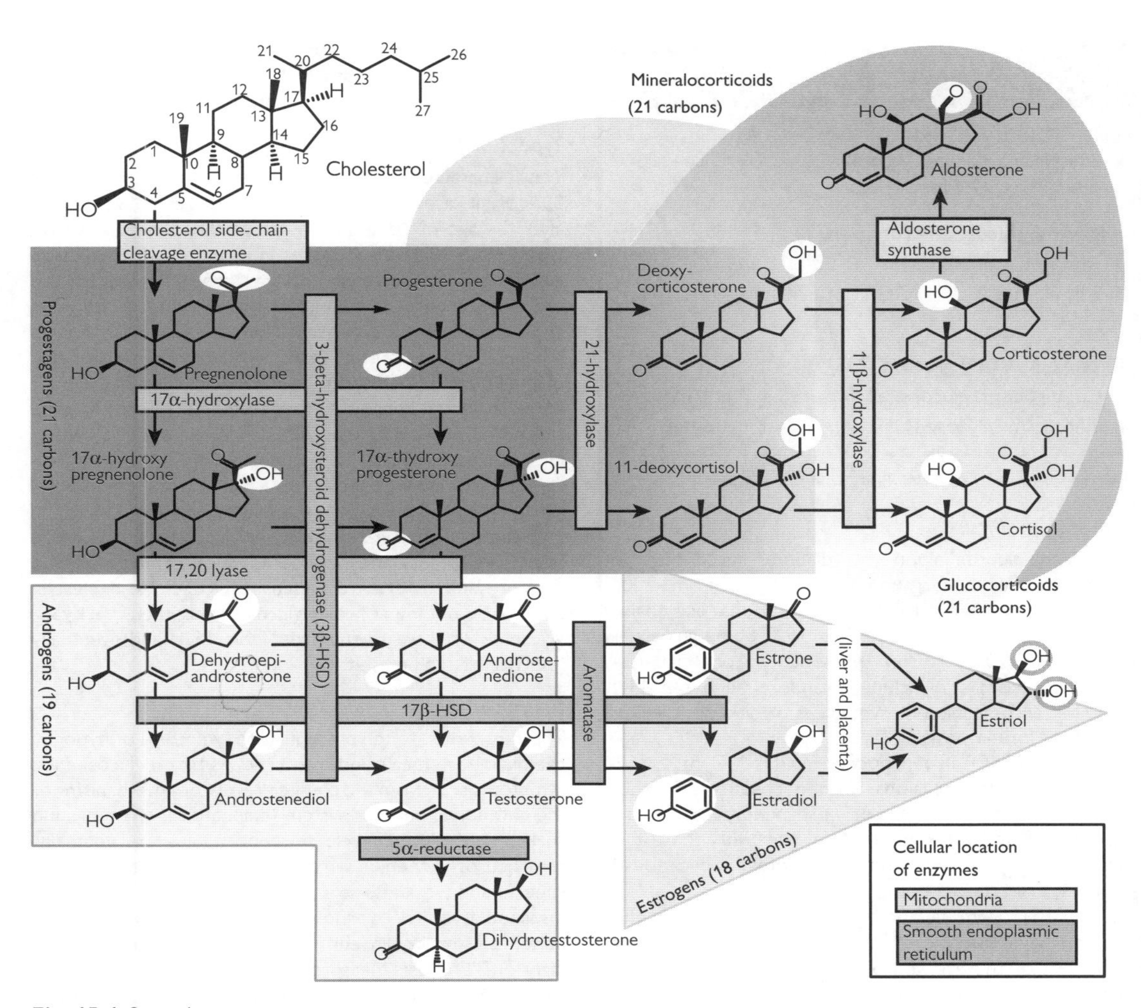

Fig. 15.4 Steroidogenesis.

Secretion

Insulin secretion is stimulated by plasma glucose, fatty acids, and ketone bodies, vagal nerve stimulation, amino acids (e.g. arginine and leucine), and gut hormones, such as gastrin, secretin, glucagon, CCK, and GIP. Secretion is inhibited by the alpha adrenergic effect of catecholamines, and somatostatin.

In response to elevated plasma glucose, diffusion into the β cells is facilitated by the glucose transporter 2 (GLUT 2) and its metabolism produces ATP. ATP closes ATP-dependent potassium channels present in the β cell membrane which, in turn, depolarizes the cell. This causes entry of calcium via voltage-gated calcium channels and stimulates the exocytosis of insulin-containing vesicles. Sulphonylurea drugs block the ATP-dependent K^+ channels and promote insulin release.

Mechanism of action

The insulin receptor is a tyrosine kinase-linked receptor, which phosphorylates insulin-receptor substrate (IRS) proteins and activates intracellular signalling cascades.

Insulin promotes anabolism. It acts to lower elevated plasma glucose by promoting uptake especially into liver, muscles, and adipose tissue. In liver it promotes glycogen synthesis, and inhibits gluconeogenesis and glucogenolysis, while in adipose tissue it promotes fatty acid synthesis and inhibits lipolysis. In muscle, it promotes glycogen synthesis, while increasing amino acid uptake and protein synthesis.

BOX 15.1 DIAGNOSTIC DEFINITION OF DIABETES MELLITUS

- Fasting plasma glucose: ≥7.0 mmol/L *or*
- 2 hr plasma glucose (via oral glucose tolerance test, OGTT*): ≥ 11.1 mmol/L.

Impaired glucose tolerance (IGT)

- Fasting plasma glucose: <7.0 mmol/L *and*
- 2 hr plasma glucose (OGTT*): ≥7.8 and <11.1 mmol/L.

Impaired fasting glucose (IfG)

- Fasting plasma glucose: ≥6.1 and ≤6.9 mmol/L *and*
- 2 hr plasma glucose (OGTT*): <7.8 (if measured).

*Venous plasma glucose 2 hr after ingestion of 75 g oral glucose load.

Diabetes mellitus

The diagnostic definition of diabetes according to the World Health Organization guidelines from 2006 (http://www.who.int/diabetes/publications/diagnosis_diabetes2006/en/) is shown in Box 15.1. Some guidelines (e.g. ADA, 2010, http://www.diabetes.org/diabetes-basics/diagnosis/) also include a random glucose ≥ 11.1 mmol/L if accompanied by symptoms of diabetes mellitus as sufficient for diagnosis.

In 2011, WHO also proposed an HbA_1C of ≥6.5% on two separate occasions (in the absence of anaemia, haemaglobinopathy, or pregnancy) as being diagnostic of diabetes mellitus in line with the ADA guidelines (http://www.who.int/diabetes/publications/diagnosis_diabetes2011/en/).

In the short term, fluctuating high levels of plasma glucose can have osmotic effects, such as causing swelling of the lens of the eye and blurred vision. Above plasma concentrations of 10 mmol/L, the reuptake of filtered glucose in nephrons becomes saturated and glucose can appear in the urine, trapping water with it, and so leading to polyuria and, subsequently, thirst and polydypsia. High levels of plasma and urinary glucose can also pre-dispose to infection.

In the long term, major complications can arise from persistent hyperglycaemia. Damage to the microvasculature in the retina, kidneys, and blood vessel around nerves (vaso nervosum) can cause retinopathy, blindness, proteinuria, and renal failure, as well as peripheral neuropathy. Macrovascular complications include coronary artery disease, ischaemic stroke, and peripheral vascular disease.

Type 1 diabetes mellitus

This is characterized by autoimmune destruction of the ß cells. Anti-islet cell antibodies are found in 60–90% at diagnosis, while anti-glutamic acid dehydrogenase (GAD) and/or anti-islet-associated antigen 2 (IA2) antibodies are found in 70–80%. Type 1 diabetes generally presents before the age of 40 years old with 25% presenting acutely as diabetic ketoacidosis. Treatment is via exogenous sc insulin. Secondary type 1 diabetes mellitus can arise in conditions, such as pancreatitis and haemochromatosis.

Type 2 diabetes mellitus

This is characterized by insulin resistance and accounts for 85% of all cases of diabetes mellitus. It generally presents after the age of 40 and has a far greater genetic link than type 1 with concordance rates in identical twin studies up to 90%. Some patients who have a strong family history can present with onset of the disease under the age of 25 years and are often found to have autosomal dominant single gene defects. Sixty per cent of cases of maturity onset diabetes of the young (MODY), can be linked to defects in the transcription factor hepatic nuclear factor 1α (*HNF-1A*) gene (MODY3), while a further 20% are linked to gene defects in glucokinase (MODY2). Secondary type 2 diabetes mellitus can arise during conditions such as Cushing's syndrome, acromegaly, and polycystic ovarian syndrome.

Treatment of type 2 diabetes initially rests with a change in diet, weight loss, and exercise, as well as controlling blood pressure and other cardiovascular risk factors. If lifestyle changes do not lower fasting glucose levels, then oral hypoglycaemic drug treatments (see Table 15.1) and eventually insulin itself can be used.

Insulinoma

This rare tumour often presents with symptoms of hypoglycaemia before meals and overnight. As blood glucose falls, symptoms arise from the counter-regulatory mechanisms of the autonomic nervous system (palpitations, sweating, and shaking) and glucagon release (hunger, nausea). Eventually, the neuroglycopenic symptoms of confusion, slurred speech, and weakness set in before seizures and/or coma. Insulinomas can be diagnosed biochemically by measuring paired plasma insulin and glucose levels during an overnight or 72 hr fast. Measures of plasma sulphonylureas are also taken to exclude factitious hypoglycaemia. In case of hypoglycaemias, hypoadrenalism should also be excluded. Insulinomas can form part of the multiple endocrine neoplasia (MEN) Type 1 syndrome arising secondary to mutation in the menin tumour suppressor gene *(MEN1)*.

Glucagon

Synthesis

29 amino acid hormone produced from cleavage of proglucagon in secretory granules of α cells.

Secretion

Increased in response to low plasma glucose, β adrenergic stimulation, exercise, and hormones, such as gastrin, cholecystokinin, and cortisol. Release is inhibited by glucose, somatostatin, insulin, and ketones. The mechanism of release is poorly understood.

Actions

Glucagon is a catabolic hormone that protects against a lack of metabolic substrates. Its actions are virtually all in the liver (via G_s, cAMP). Low levels of glucagon stimulate glycogenolysis, while medium levels stimulate gluconeogenesis. High levels of glucagon stimulate lipolysis, fatty acid oxidation, and ketogenesis.

Note its synergism with other hormones involved in metabolic control—catecholamines, glucocorticoids, and growth hormone, which all stimulate liver conversion of glycogen to glucose.

Somatostatin

Synthesized in the δ cells of the pancreas via cleavage of a large precursor molecule to form somatostatin 14 and 28.

Actions

Inhibits the secretion of insulin and glucagons (paracrine action). It also acts to inhibit the release of thyrotrophin and growth hormone from the anterior pituitary.

Calcium homeostasis

Ca^{2+} has very important effects on excitable tissues, as a cofactor in coagulation, and as an essential component of bones and teeth.

Hypocalcaemia

- Increases neuronal membrane excitability by increasing sodium permeability causing tetany (exacerbated by tapping on the facial nerve—'Chvostek's sign', or inflation of a sphygmomanometer—'Trousseau's sign') and eventually neuropsychiatric symptoms and seizures.
- QT prolongation is observed on the ECG, which predisposes to arrhythmias.

Hypercalcaemia

- Decreases neuron excitability causing muscle weakness, constipation, lethargy, and depression.
- Calcium salts are insoluble, so renal calculi can form, as well as calcification of other tissues.
- High calcium can make the kidneys unresponsive to ADH, thereby causing polyuria (nephrogenic diabetes insipidus).

A *fall* in plasma Ca^{2+} is *more dangerous* short term than a rise; endocrine control mechanisms reflect this.

Amounts of calcium and phosphate in the body

Of total body calcium approximately 99% is stored in bone, and 1% in teeth and soft tissues. Of the calcium in bone, 1% is rapidly exchangeable, whereas 99% is hydroxyapatite bound to collagen and is slowly exchangeable. Interstitial fluid calcium is freely exchangeable with plasma calcium.

Plasma contains approximately 2.5 mM total calcium (2.4–2.6 mM) of which 50% is ionized. The main controlled parameter is plasma ionized Ca^{2+} –1.2 mmol/L.

Of total body phosphate, 85% is stored in bone as hydroxyapatite and 15% in soft tissues. Plasma phosphate varies depending on age, sex, and diet, but is maintained between 0.8 and 1.4 mM.

Hormonal control of calcium and phosphate: Parathyroid hormone (PTH)

Secretion

Eighty-four amino acid hormone secreted from the parathyroid glands in response to minute by minute levels of plasma Ca^{2+}. Falling plasma Ca^{2+} causes an increase in PTH release, which restores plasma Ca^{2+} to normal and increases phosphate loss.

Mechanism of action

- *Intestine:* increased renal production of the intestinally active vitamin D metabolite $1,25(OH)_2D$ results in increased calcium absorption in the intestine.
- *Kidney*: *PTH* has direct effects on the tubular reabsorption of calcium and phosphate. Although the bulk of calcium is resorbed from tubule fluid together with sodium in the proximal convoluted tubule, the fine-tuning of calcium excretion occurs in the distal nephron, where PTH increases significantly the reabsorption of calcium (predominantly in the distal convoluted tubule—the precise nature of the transport mechanism is not clear). PTH inhibits the reabsorption of phosphate in the renal proximal tubule.
- *Bone*: Enhances the release of calcium from the bones through indirect stimulation of osteoclasts (binds to osteoblasts, and results in formation of osteoclasts and bone resorption.

Pathology

- *Hypoparathyroidism:* a rare cause of hypocalcaemia, this is caused by surgical removal following removal of parathyroid adenoma's or post-thyroidectomy, autoimmune destruction (polyglandular failure type 1), or congenitally in DiGeorge's syndrome. Pseudohypoparathyroidism arises from a G protein abnormality causing a resistance to PTH and, therefore, low plasma calcium with high compensatory levels of PTH, and is often accompanied by short stature and short 4th and 5th metacarpals (Albrights's hereditary osteodystrophy).
- *Hyperparathyroidism*
  - *Primary*—a common cause of hypercalcaemia secondary to be parathyroid adenoma or hyperplasia.
  - *Secondary*—as an appropriate response to maintain plasma Ca^{2+}, for example, in $1,25(OH)_2$ vit D_3 deficiency in chronic renal failure.
  - *Tertiary*—inappropriate autonomous release of PTH in chronic hypocalcaemia, for example, in end-stage renal failure.
  - *Ectopic*—due to the release of a parathyroid-related peptide from some tumours (e.g. squamous cell carcinoma of the lung and some breast cancers), which shares a similar functional N terminal sequence to PTH.

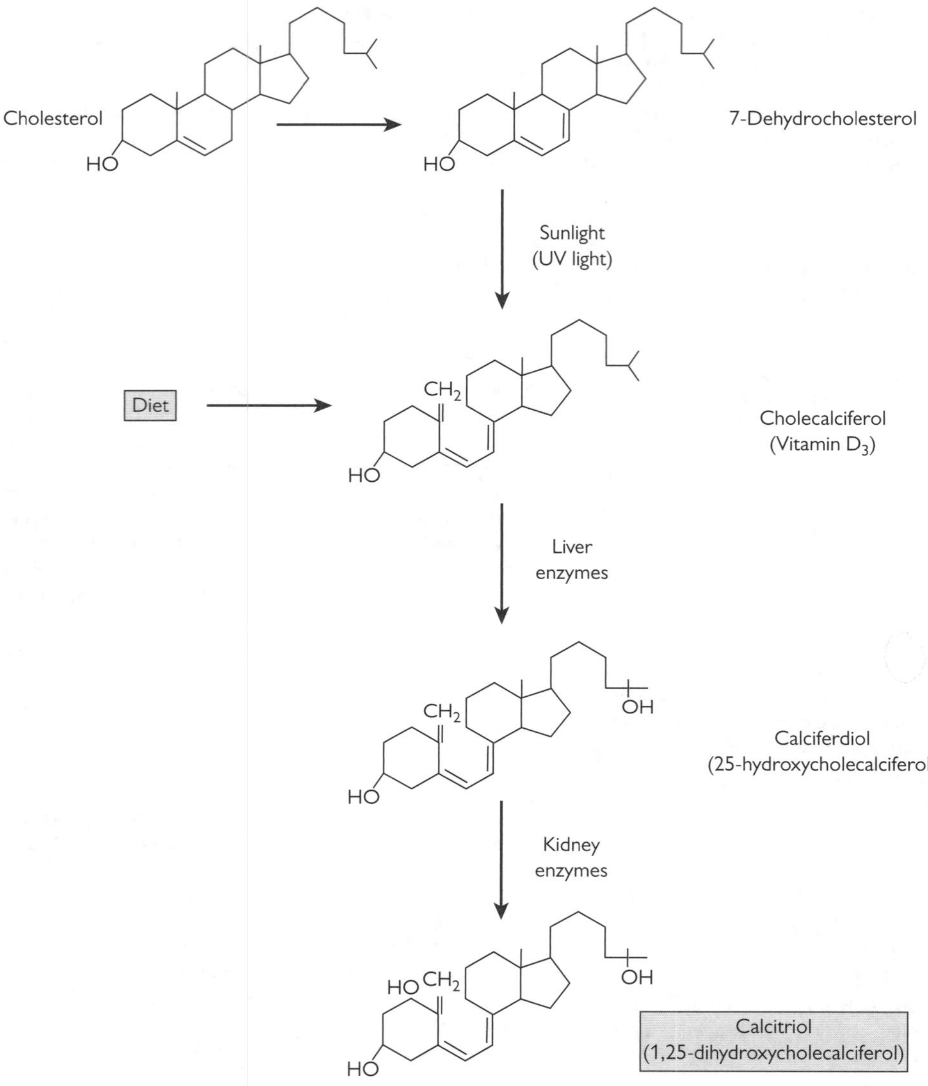

Cholesterol
HO
7-Dehydrocholesterol
HO
Sunlight
(UV light)
Diet
CH_2
HO
Cholecalciferol
(Vitamin D_3)
Liver
enzymes
CH_2
OH
HO
Calciferdiol
(25-hydroxycholecalciferol)
Kidney
enzymes
HO CH_2
OH
HO
Calcitriol
(1,25-dihydroxycholecalciferol)

Fig. 15.5 The synthesis of 1,25-dihydroxycholecalciferol from vitamin D.

Hormonal control of calcium and phosphate: 1,25(OH)$_2$ vitamin D3 (calcitriol)

Synthesis

UV light converts a cholesterol derivative in the skin to cholecalciferol or vitamin D_3. In the liver 25-hydroxylase produces 25-OH vit D_3. In kidney 1α-hydroxylase converts 25-OH vit D_3 to 1,25(OH)$_2$ vit D_3 (see Fig. 15.5). There is also some dietary intake of vitamin D_3 (egg yolks, fish oils).

Mechanism of action

Acts via nuclear receptors to regulate transcription and ultimately increase plasma calcium.

- *Intestine:* increases uptake of Ca^{2+} via synthesis of the calcium-binding protein, calbindin.
- *Kidney:* facilitates conservation of calcium and phosphate.
- *Bone:* necessary for the action of PTH. It regulates bone formation and resorption, and it promotes the differentiation of osteoblasts.

Pathology

Deficiency due to either dietary deficiency, malabsorption, lack of sunlight, lack of 25 hydroxylation (liver disease or phenytoin), or lack of 1α-hydroxylation (chronic renal failure) leads to an inadequate mineralization of osteoid. In adults this leads to osteomalacia, while in children this leads to rickets. Rickets can also be caused by 1α-hydroxylase deficiency (type 1), vit D3 receptor defect (type 2 vitamin D-dependent rickets) or X-linked hypophosphataemic rickets (vitamin D-resistant rickets).

Hormonal control of calcium and phosphate: Calcitonin

Secretion

Thirty-two amino acid polypeptide produced by the parafollicular C cells of thyroid and secreted in response to elevated plasma Ca^{2+}.

Mechanism of action

Debatable physiological importance in everyday control of plasma Ca^{2+}, but may help reduce hypercalcaemia by inhibiting calcium release from bone via decreasing the activity of osteoclasts (especially in the young) and helping to control rise in plasma Ca^{2+} with absorption from each meal via inhibiting gut absorption.

Pathology

Medullary thyroid cancer secretes calcitonin. It forms part of the multiple endocrine neoplasia (MEN) type 2 syndrome.

Drugs used in the treatment of endocrine disorders

For drugs used in the treatment of endocrine disorders (see Table 15.1). See Box 15.2 for common drug-induced endocrine reactions.

Table 15.1 Drugs used in the treatment of endocrine disorders

Oral hypoglycaemic drugs			
Drug	Mechanism of action	Side effects	Interactions
Sulphonylureas: e.g. glicazide	Increase insulin release via blocking β cell K_{ATP} channels	Hypoglycaemia, weight gain	Increases hypoglycaemia: alcohol, NSAIDS, warfarin, monoamine oxidase inhibitors and chloramphenicol. *Increases hyperglycaemia:* corticosteroids, thiazides, oral contraceptive pill, phenothiazines, lithium, (liver enzyme inducers) phenytoin, carbamazepine, barbiturates, rifampacin, chronic excess alcohol, sulphonylureas
Biguanides: e.g. metformin	Reduce insulin resistance and hepatic glucose production via activation of AMP-activated protein kinase (AMPK)	Lactic acidosis, nausea, vitamin B12 malabsorption	
Glitazones: e.g. rosiglitazone, pioglitazone	Reduce insulin resistance via activation of intracellular peroxisome proliferator activated receptors (PPAR-γ)	Fluid retention and exacerbation of heart failure. Hepatitis	
Glucagon like peptide (GLP-1) analogs: (e.g. liraglutide) and agonists (e.g. exenatide)	Act as an incretin and binds to the GLP-1 receptor on the β cells to increase the amount of insulin released	Indigestion, diarrhoea, nausea, headache, sulphonylurea hypoglycaemia. Possibly pancreatitis (exenatide)	
Gliptins: e.g. sitagliptin	Inhibit dipeptidyl peptidase-4, thereby preventing the breakdown of the insulin secretagogues GLP-1 and incretin	Nasopharyngitis, headache, nausea, hypersensitivity and skin reactions, pancreatitis	
α-Glucosidase inhibitors: e.g. acarbose	Delay absorption of sugars by inhibiting intestinal α-glucosidase	Diarrhoea, flatulence	

(*continued*)

Table 15.1 Drugs used in the treatment of endocrine disorders (*continued*)

Insulins			
Kinetics (peak/duration of action)	**Preparation examples**	**Peak action (hr)**	**Duration of action (hr)**
Rapid	Novarapid®, Humalog®	1.5	5
Short	Actrapid®, Humulin S®	<3	8–12
Intermediate	Insulatard®, Humulin I®	4–8	<24
Biphasic	Mixtard 30®, Humalog Mix25®	2–4	<24
Long	Glargine®, Detemir®	Little or no peak	24 hr
Anti-obesity drugs (BMI>30 or >28 with cardiovascular risk factors, continue beyond 3 months only if 5% or more weight loss)			
Drug	**Mechanism of action**	**Side effects**	**Interactions**
Orlistat	Inhibitor of gastric and pancreatic lipases to limit fat absorption	Steatorrhoea, flatulence, incontinence, malabsorption of fat soluble vitamins (A, D, E, K)	Impairs absorption of amiodarone and cyclosporin
Corticosteroid			
Drug	**Glucocorticoid/mineralocorticoid activity**	**Side effects**	**Interactions**
Cortisol	1.0/1.0	*General:* weight gain, truncal obesity, purpura and striae. *Metabolic:* Na retention/K loss, hypertension, hyperglycaemia, adrenal atrophy. *Musculoskeletal:* proximal myopathy, osteoporosis. *GI:* gastritis/ulceration. Immunosuppression, delayed wound healing. Steroid psychosis	*Reduces effect:* (liver enzyme inducers) phenytoin, carbamazepine, barbiturates, rifampacin, chronic excess EtOH, sulphonylureas
Hydrocortisone	0.7:1.0		
Prednisolone	4:1		
Dexamethasone	25:0		
Fludrocortisone	10:125		
Aldosterone	0.3:3000		
Hyperthyroidism			
Drug	**Mechanism of action**	**Side effects**	**Interactions**
Carbimazole	Inhibits thyroid peroxidase	*Common:* rash. *Rare:* agranulocytosis, aplastic anaemia, hepatitis, fever, arthritis, vasculitis	
Propylthiouracil	Inhibits thyroid peroxidase and 5'-deiodinase		Preferred drug in pregnancy
Oral contraceptives/HRT			
Drug	**Contraindications**	**Side effects**	**Interactions**
Combined oral contraceptive pill (COCP)	*Absolute:* previous DVT/PE, CVA, breast/uterine Ca, liver disease, undiagnosed breakthrough bleeding. *Relative:* hypertension, cardiac failure. *Caution:* DM, migraine with aura, >35 years old	DVT/PE (reduced hepatic antithrombin and increased fibrinogen production) hypertension, hyperlipidaemia, loss of libido, impaired glucose tolerance, cholestatic jaundice, increased thyroid binding, globulin, and altered TFTs. Changes in menstrual flow, breast tenderness/enlargement, acne. Increased risk of cervical and breast cancer, protective against ovarian and endometrial cancer. In addition to those of POP	*Reduced efficacy:* liver enzyme inducers. Phenytoin, carbamazepine, barbiturates, rifampacin, chronic excess EtOH, sulphonylureas
Progesterone only pill (POP)		Weight gain, nausea, breast discomfort, breakthrough bleeding	

Table 15.1 Drugs used in the treatment of endocrine disorders (*continued*)

Drug	Contraindications	Side effects	Interactions
Hormone replacement therapy (HRT)	*Absolute:* pregnancy, previous DVT/PE, coronary artery disease, severe liver disease, undiagnosed vaginal bleeding, endometrial cancer	DVT/PE and as for COCP Increased risk of cervical and breast cancer, protective against ovarian and endometrial cancer	
Miscellaneous			
Drug	**Mechanism of action**	**Side effects**	**Interactions**
Octreotide	Somatostatin analogue, which inhibits the release of many hormones, including GH, hence its use in the treatment of acromegaly	*Common:* diarrhoea, nausea, bradycardia. *Rare:* pancreatitis, hepatitis, QT prolongation on the ECG	Insulin/oral hypoglycaemics (inhibits secretion of insulin and glucagon), decreases cyclosporin levels, bradycardia with β-blockers, prolonged QT with Class III antiarrhythmics
Bromocriptine/cabergoline	Dopamine agonists used in treatment of prolactinomas and acromegaly	Anticholinergic (nausea, constipation, dry mouth). Fibrotic reactions (pulmonary fibrosis, pleurisy, pericarditis). Hypotension, arrhythmias, valvular heart disease (high doses for Parkinson's disease). *CNS reactions:* sleep disturbance, vertigo, depression	Dopamine antagonists, such as metocloramide, and neuroleptics
Metyrapone	Inhibits 11β-hydroxylase and ∴ cortisol synthesis. Used in the treatments of Cushing's syndrome	Dehydration, hypotension, nausea, hyperkalaemia	
Desmopressin	Synthetic analogue of ADH/vasopressin used to treat diabetes insipidus	Hyponatraemia, fluid overload	

Reproduced from *Definition and Diagnosis of Diabetes Mellitus and Immediate Hyperglycemia: Report of a WHO/IDF Consultation*, World Health Organization, 2006, Table in recommendation 7, http://www.who.int/diabetes/publications/Definition%20and%20diagnosis%20of%20diabetes_new.pdf. Accessed 16th April 2014

BOX 15.2 DRUG-INDUCED ENDOCRINE REACTIONS

- *SIADH:* carbamazepine, phenytoin, cytotoxic agents.
- *Nephrogenic diabetes insipidus:* lithium.
- *Hyperprolactinaemia:* dopamine antagonists (metaclopramide, neuroleptics), oestrogens, cimetidine.
- *Gynaecomastia:* spiranolactone, digoxin, oestrogens, cimetidine.
- *Hypothyroidism:* amiodarone (and hyperthyroidism), lithium, carbimazole, propylthiouracil.
- *Hyperglycaemia:* corticosteroids, thiazide diuretics, combined oral contraceptive pill.
- *Hypoglycaemia:* EtOH, beta-blockers.
- *Hypercalcaemia:* thiazides, vitamin D.
- *Osteoporosis:* glucocorticoids, levothyroxine excess, anticonvulsants, cyclosporin, tacrolimus.

Multiple choice questions

1. A 50-year-old female undergoes a standard 75-g glucose tolerance test. Initial plasma glucose = 5.9 and at 2 hr = 7.7. This diagnosis is:

A. Diabetes mellitus.
B. Impaired fasting glucose.
C. Normal result.
D. Impaired glucose tolerance.
E. Impaired random glucose.

2. Which of the following is not a cause of cranial diabetes insipidus?

A. Pituitary surgery.
B. Lithium.
C. Histiocytosis X.
D. Craniopharyngioma.
E. Head injury.

3. A 40-year-old man presents with polydipsia and is found to have a normal plasma calcium, potassium, and fasting glucose. He undergoes a water deprivation test. Initial plasma osmolarity is 288 mOsm/L, final plasma osmolarity is 315mOsm/L and final urine osmolarity is 162 mOsm/L. Post-desmopressin (DDAVP) urine osmolarity rises to 850 mOsm/L. The diagnosis is:

A. SIADH.
B. Nephrogenic diabetes insipidus.
C. Psychogenic polydipsia.
D. Cranial diabetes insipidus.
E. Pseudopseudohypoparathyroidism.

4. A 42-year-old women presents to accident and emergency with abdominal pain and vomiting. On initial assessment her T = 37.6°C, blood pressure (BP) = 100/50 P110, BM=3.3. Initial blood tests show Na = 130 mmol/L K = 5.5 mmol/L Ur = 16.0 mmol/L, Creat = 120. Which of the following is most appropriate initial treatment?

A. Ceftriaxone and metronidazole.
B. Propranolol.
C. Glucagon.
D. Levothyroxine.
E. Hydrocortisone.

5. A 25-year-old man presents with sweating, deep voice, spade-like hands, and is found to have a bitemporal hemianopia. The most useful diagnostic test would be:

A. Early morning growth hormone.
B. Insulin tolerance test.
C. Oral glucose tolerance test.
D. IGF-1.
E. Short synacthen test.

6. The best investigation to diagnose an insulinoma is:

A. Supervised fast.
B. Insulin tolerance test.
C. Early morning C-peptide.
D. Oral glucose tolerance test.
E. Glucagon stimulation test.

7. A 40-year-old women presents with neck swelling and fever, and has the following biochemical tests: TSH < 0.1, T4 = 188, WCC = 6.4 ESR = 75. The most likely diagnosis is:

A. Hashimotos thyroiditis.
B. Multinodular goitre.
C. De Quervains's disease.
D. Sick euthyroid.
E. Graves' disease.

8. Cushing's Disease can present with:

A. Hypokalaemic metabolic acidosis.
B. Hyperkalaemic metabolic alkalosis.
C. Hypocalcaemic metabolic acidosis.
D. Hypokalaemic metabolic alkalosis.
E. Hyperkalaemic metabolic acidosis.

9. Which of the following are associated with pseudohypoparathyroidism?

A. Short stature.
B. Short 4th and 5th metacarpals.
C. Low parathyroid hormone levels.
D. Hypocalcaemia.
E. Low IQ.

10. A 15-year-old girl presents with sweating and dizziness, and a reduced level of consciousness. Her father who is diabetic is concerned as she has had several similar episodes over the last week. Initial blood tests show: plasma glucose 1.9 mmol/L, insulin = 20 (NR: 6–10 mg/mL), Proinsulin = 20% (NR: 22–24%), C-peptide = 0.10 (NR: 0.2–0.4 nmol/L). The diagnosis is:

A. Insulin overdose.
B. Insulinoma.
C. Diabetes mellitus.
D. Oral hypoglycaemic abuse.
E. Addison's disease.

For answers, please see Appendix: Answers to multiple choice questions, page 313.

CHAPTER 16

Nephrology

Anatomy

The kidney

The kidneys lie in a retroperitoneal position, bilaterally to the vertebral column at T12–L3. The upper pole of the kidney is capped by the adrenal gland. Superiorly, the kidneys are separated from the pleura and 12th rib by the diaphragm. The posterior anatomical relations are quadratus lumborum, transversus abdominis, and psoas, along with the iliohypogastric, ilioinguinal, and subcostal nerves, and vessels. The liver, second part of the duodenum, and ascending colon lie anterior to the right kidney. The spleen, jejenum, pancreas, stomach, and descending colon lie anterior to the left kidney. The right lobe of the liver displaces the right kidney such that it sits slightly lower than its counterpart on the left.

Four coverings surround the kidney—a fibrous capsule almost entirely envelops it, with a layer of perirenal fat separating the capsule from the fibrous fascia, outside of which sits a layer of pararenal fat.

On the medial aspect, the renal hilum contains (moving posteriorly) the renal vein and artery, the renal pelvis and a subsidiary branch of the renal artery, together with nerves and lymphatic vessels, the position of which is less well defined. The left hilum is found at the level of the transpyloric plane, with the right being a little lower.

Structure

The kidney is made up of an outer cortex and an inner medulla, which is lighter in colour. The medulla is made up of a number (typically seven) of renal pyramids. The apex of the pyramid feeds into minor calyx. The medulla is characterized by striations, termed medullary rays that fan out from the apex and represent straight segments of renal tubules. The cortex constitutes the outer tissue of the kidney and renal columns, which dip between pyramids (Fig. 16.1).

Each pyramid drains urine into a renal papilla, the point at which renal tubules unite that, in turn, feeds a minor calyx. Two or three minor calyces drain into a major calyx, of which again there are two or three (Fig. 16.2). Major calyces drain into the renal pelvis (which may be intra- or extrarenal), the funnel-shaped proximal portion of the ureter.

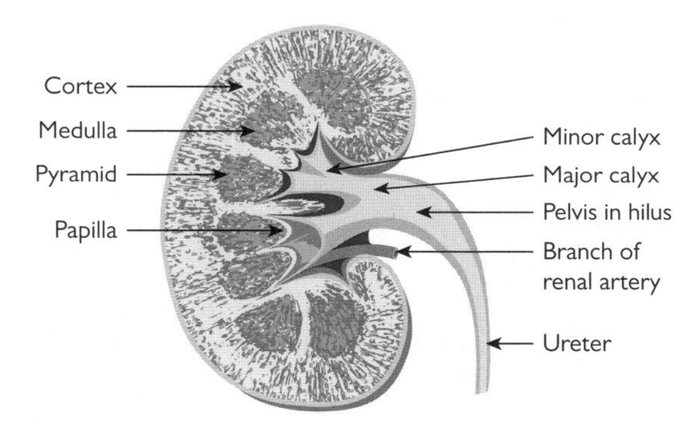

Fig. 16.1 Diagram of hemisected kidney to show its component parts.

Reproduced from P MacKinnon and J Morris, *Oxford Textbook of Functional Anatomy: Volume 2 Thorax and Abdomen*, 2005, Figure 6.7.3a, p. 172, by permission of Oxford University Press

Blood supply

The renal arteries arise from the abdominal aorta at L1–2. The longer right artery passes posterior to the inferior vena cava as it crosses to the right side. Segmental arteries, arising from division of the renal artery close to the hilum, supply segments of the kidney, giving rise to lobar arteries for each pyramid. Lobar arteries, in turn, give off two or three interlobar arteries, which penetrate the renal columns between the pyramids. At the boundary of the medulla and cortex, arcuate arteries arise that curve over the base of the pyramids. Interlobular arteries branch from the arcuate arteries and radiate through the cortex, giving rise to afferent arteries, which supply the glomerulus, a capillary knot. Efferent arterioles drain the glomerulus and progress to supply the renal tubules. Juxtamedullary efferent arterioles supply the vasa recta. Venous drainage parallels the arterial arrangement, with the longer left renal vein passing anterior to the abdominal aorta. Lymphatic drainage occurs through the para-aortic and lumbar lymph nodes. A renal plexus, derived from thoracic splanchnic nerves, contains autonomic vasomotor nerves.

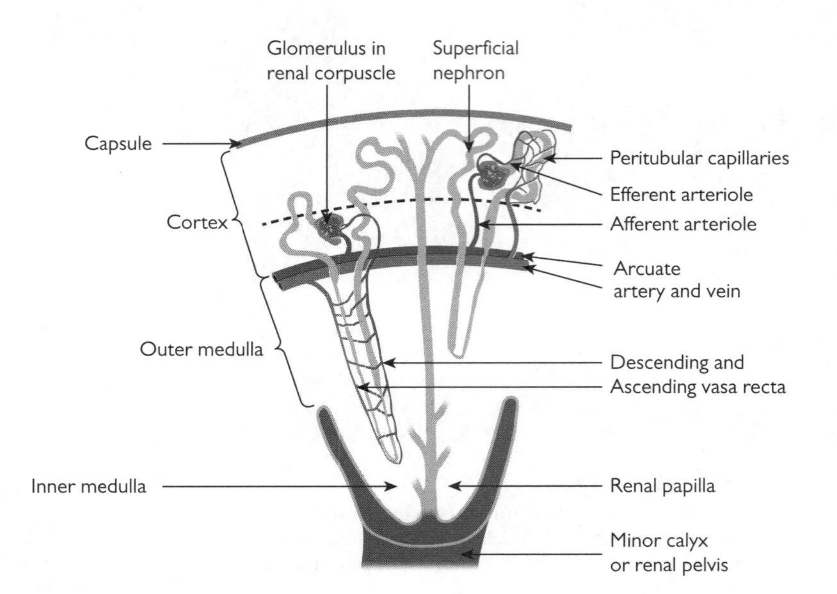

Fig. 16.2 Arrangement of kidney microvasculature.

Reproduced from P MacKinnon and J Morris, *Oxford Textbook of Functional Anatomy: Volume 2 Thorax and Abdomen*, 2005, Figure 6.7.3b, p. 172, by permission of Oxford University Press

The ureter

The ureter is a retroperitoneal distensible muscular tube, approximately 25cm in length, which conveys urine by peristalsis from the kidney to the bladder. The broad renal pelvis draining the major calyces narrows to become, sequentially, the abdominal, pelvic, and intravesicle segments of the ureter. The posterior peritoneum is anterior to the right ureter, which lies lateral to the inferior vena cava. The pelvis is also covered anteriorly by the second part of the duodenum. The right colic artery, gonadal artery, and ileocolic artery cross the right ureter. The left ureter runs behind the mesosigmoid and sigmoid colon, along the medial border of psoas. The left colic artery and gonadal artery cross the left ureter.

The pelvic segment of the ureter starts at the point at which it crosses the pelvic brim, close to the bifurcation of the common iliac artery. The ureter then runs along the lateral wall of the pelvis, turning medially to reach the bladder. The final intravesicle segment passes obliquely through the bladder wall. Constrictions of the ureter at the narrowing of the renal pelvis, at the pelvic brim and during its passage through the bladder wall are common sites of kidney stones.

Blood supply

The blood supply to different segments of the ureter arises from renal, gonadal, vesical, or internal iliac arteries, with venous drainage to the gonadal veins. Lymphatic drainage is to the lumbar and iliac lymph nodes. The adjacent renal and hypogastric plexuses innervate the ureter. Ureteric obstruction by a calculus results in distension and colic, with pain referred to the lumbar or hypogastric regions, or to the external genitalia depending on the site of obstruction.

The bladder

The bladder, a balloon-like retroperitoneal structure, is largely surrounded by peritoneal fat. It stores and excretes urine, which enters from the ureters and exits to the urethra via the internal meatus at the neck. Urine is excreted from the bladder under the voluntary control of the internal urethral sphincter.

The bladder lies behind the pubic symphysis and is bounded laterally by obturatus internus and levator ani. The rectum, seminal vesicles, and terminal vas deferens surround the bladder to the posterior in the male; the vagina and supravaginal cervix sit to the posterior in the female, while the uterus may lie against the postero-superior aspect. Peritoneum covers the superior aspect, above which is found the sigmoid colon and coils of small intestine. The pubovesical or puboprostatic ligaments anchor the bladder at the neck. In females, the neck rests on the pelvic fascia surrounding the urethra, whereas in males the bladder neck unites with the prostate.

Structure

The bladder varies in size, shape, and position dependent on the volume of urine that it contains. In adults, a bladder that is perceived to be full contains around 250 mL of urine. Although never completely empty, after voiding the bladder adopts a pyramidal shape, with an apex formed by the bladder wall posterior to the pubic symphysis and the base is formed by the fundus, its postero-inferior aspect. When empty, the bladder is located almost entirely within the pelvis, and lies on the pubis and pelvic floor. With filling, it can expand into the abdomen, lifting the peritoneum upwards from the anterior abdominal wall, and potentially reaching the level of the umbilicus. In children younger than 3 years old, the restricted size of the pelvis means that the bladder is an intra-abdominal, extraperitoneal organ.

The trigone, a smooth-walled triangular area defined by the ureteric orifices and the internal meatus (with an internal urethral sphincter formed from smooth muscle fibres), adheres to underlying smooth muscle. The interureteric ridge is a fold created by muscles fibres that run between the two ureteric orifices. The uvula, a fold found behind the internal meatus is formed by muscle fibres and/or the middle lobe of the prostate, can become more pronounced with increasing age. Elsewhere, the tissue loosely adheres to the underlying detrusor muscle, resulting in rugae (folds) of mucosa when the bladder is empty. Striated muscle from the urogential diaphragm (derived from skeletal muscles of the pelvic floor under cortical control and located in the pelvic arch), forms the external urethral sphincter. The urethra ends at the external meatus. In males the urethra is longer, comprising prostatic, membranous, and penile segments.

Blood supply

The superior and inferior vesicle branches of the internal iliac artery supply the bladder, with the superior vesicle artery supplying the antero-superior portion and, in males, the fundus; the vaginal arteries supply the fundus in females. Venous drainage is through the vesicle venous plexus. The plexus links with the prostatic venous plexus in males and with the vaginal venous plexus (and dorsal vein of the clitoris) in females to drain via the internal vesicle vein into the internal iliac vein. Lymphatic drainage is to the iliac and para-aortic lymph nodes.

Nerve supply

Autonomic innervation is received from the inferior hypogastric plexus, which contains sympathetic postganglionic fibres (L1–2) and parasympathetic preganglionic fibres from the splanchnic nerve (S2–4), which synapse with post-ganglionic fibres within the plexus. Sensory afferent fibres are conveyed to the CNS through the plexus or in the pelvic splanchnic nerve.

Voiding of the bladder

Micturition is a combination of autonomic spinal cord reflexes and voluntary control, achieved by contraction of detrusor, the bladder wall smooth muscle, accompanied by relaxation of the urethral sphincters. Stretch receptors in the bladder wall detect increases in tension, which are more marked at filling volumes greater than 250 mL, leading to a sensation of bladder fullness. The pontine micturition centre in the brainstem integrates impulses from sensory afferents to initiate the micturition reflex, which induces parasympathetic-mediated contraction of detrusor. The increased intravesicle pressure promotes opening of the internal urethral sphincter at the neck and expulsion of urine. Urine flow is sensed by urethral sensory receptors, which feedback to the micturition centre to enhance the reflex. Abdominal and pelvic muscle contraction promotes micturition by increasing pressure on the bladder wall.

The striated muscle of the external urethral sphincter underpins voluntary bladder control. Voluntary relaxation initiates the flow of urine during micturition. In addition, inhibitory inputs to the micturition centre from cortical and suprapontine centres, along with sympthatic fibres from the hypogastric plexus that inhibit contraction of detrusor, can suppress the reflex when micturition is inappropriate. Voluntary initiation of the reflex by higher centres can be effected in the absence of stretch receptor input when the bladder is not full. Damage to descending spinal pathways can lead to the loss of voluntary control and incontinence.

Physiology

Structural features of nephron segments and their functional roles

The glomerulus, a capillary knot at which blood is filtered, is supplied by an afferent arteriole and drained by an efferent arteriole (Fig. 16.3). There are around one million glomeruli in the kidney, each associated with a single renal tubule, the epithelial cells of which envelop the knot to form the Bowman's capsule and define the Bowman's space, which drains into the renal tubule. The glomerulus and its related structures are termed the renal corpuscle. The corpuscle, together with the tubule, forms the functional unit of the kidney, the nephron.

The structures of the renal corpuscle comprise the afferent and efferent arterioles, the capillaries formed from endothelial cell wall of the capillary knot, podocytes, intra- and extraglomerular mesangial cells, granular cells, and a portion of the distal convoluted loop of Henle that folds back to make close contact with the Bowman's capsule. The last three structures together constitute the juxtaglomerular apparatus. The endothelial cell wall and its basement membrane, along with podocytes, which wrap finger-like processes around the capillaries, make up the filtration barrier. The juxtaglomerular apparatus monitors and initiates adjustments to plasma sodium content, which determines plasma volume.

Structure

The renal tubule arises from the Bowman's capsule and receives the filtrate from Bowman's space (Fig. 16.4). The first segment is the *proximal tubule*, which runs from the outer cortex towards the medulla and has a convoluted appearance for the first two-thirds of its length before adopting a straighter configuration. The tubule is formed from cuboidal epithelial cells with an apical brush border membrane formed by microvilli and basolateral cell membranes with deep in-foldings to enhance the surface area

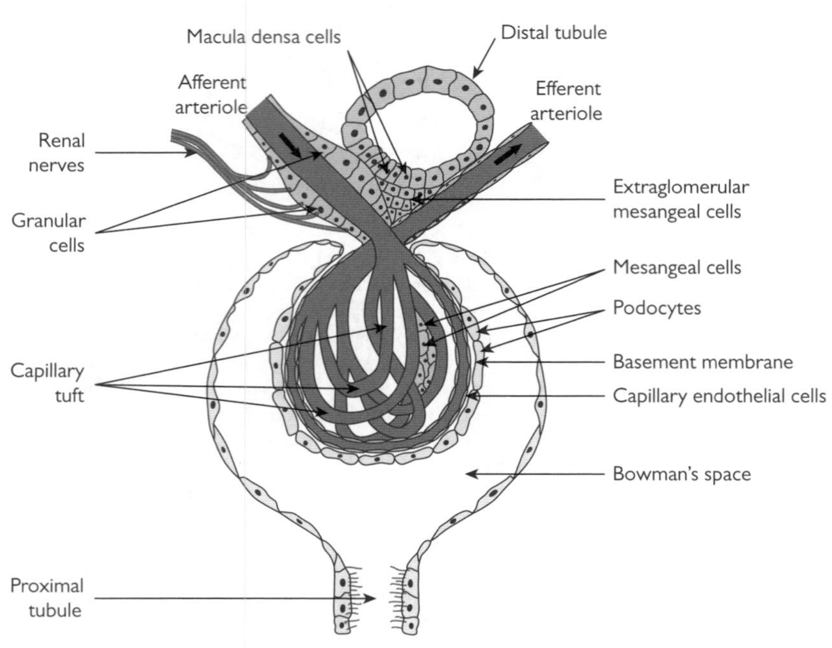

Fig. 16.3 The principal features of a renal glomerulus and the juxtaglomerular apparatus. The wall of the afferent arteriole is thickened close to the point of contact with the distal tubule where the juxtaglomerular cells are located. The cells secrete the enzyme renin in response to low sodium in the distal tubule.

Reproduced from G Pocock and CD Richards, *Human Physiology: The Basis of Medicine, Third Edition,* 2006, Figure 17.3, p. 349, by permission of Oxford University Press

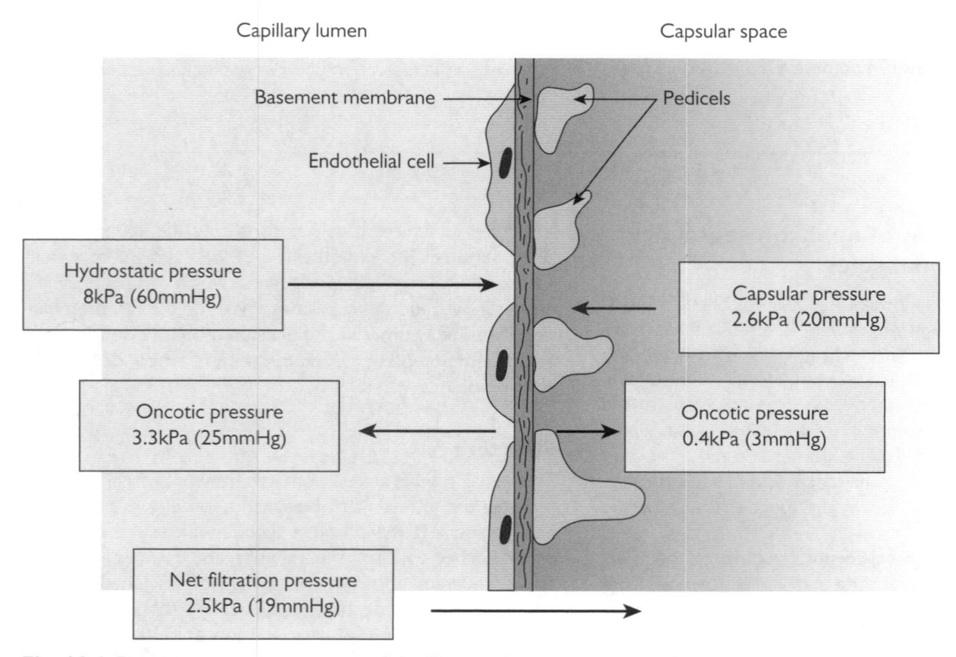

Fig. 16.4 Diagrammatic representation of the filtration barrier in the glomerulus and the hydrodynamic forces that determine the rate of ultrafiltration.

Reproduced from G Pocock and CD Richards, *Human Physiology: The Basis of Medicine, Third Edition,* 2006, Figure 17.11, p. 355, by permission of Oxford University Press

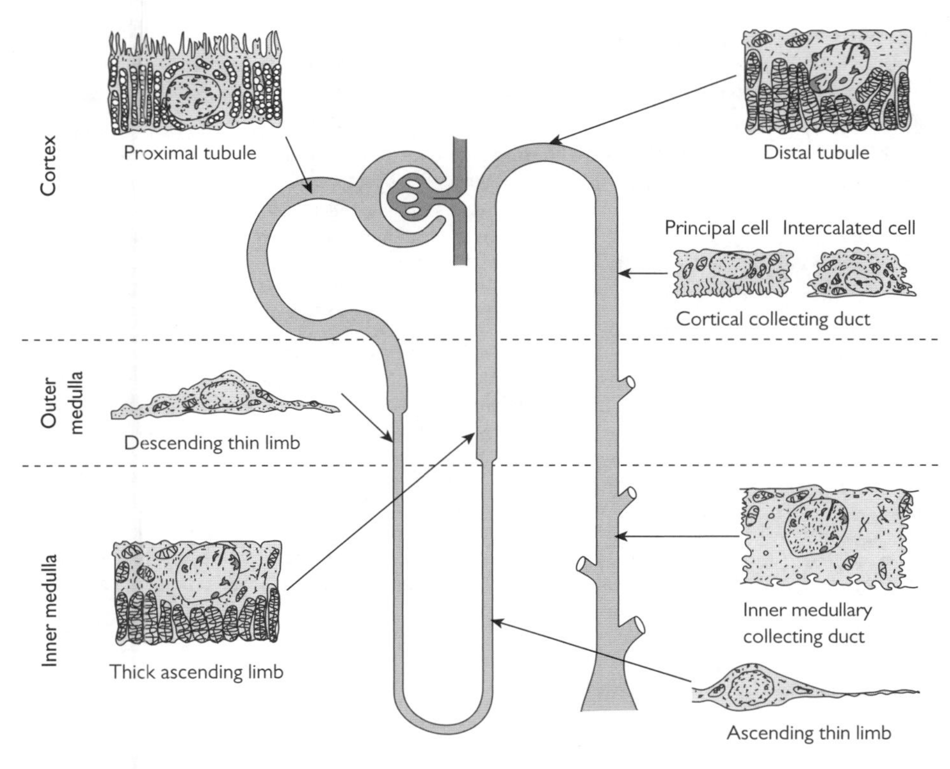

Fig. 16.5 The ultrastructure of the cells that constitute a nephron.

for solute and water transfer (Fig. 16.5). The cells are rich in mitochondria, reflecting the role of this segment in bulk reabsorption of important components of the filtered load, including organic solutes, salts, and water.

The proximal tubule gives way to the *descending limb of the loop of Henle*, characterized by thin, flattened squamous epithelial cells with few mitochondria, which provide a water-permeable lining that allows osmotic equilibration between the luminal fluid and the surrounding interstitial fluid. At the hairpin loop, the tubule turns through 180°C and becomes the *thin ascending limb*, the cells of which are similar in appearance to those in its descending counterpart, but which form a water-tight barrier. As the limb ascends, there is a transition to cuboidal cells, which lack a brush border. The cells of this *thick ascending limb* are rich in mitochondria, reflecting their role in active absorption of NaCl from the tubular fluid. Loops are variable in length, with the hairpin of superficial nephrons located in the cortex or outer medulla, and that of juxtamedullary nephrons found deep within the inner medulla. Interactions between these two types of nephrons facilitate urinary concentration by the hyperosmotic interstitial fluid that surrounds the renal tubules.

The ascending loop of Henle leads on to the *distal tubule*, also convoluted in structure, with cells of similar in appearance to those of the thick limb. The cells defining the tubule at the start of the distal tubule make contact with the structures of the juxtaglomerular apparatus and monitor the composition of the tubular fluid delivered from the ascending limb.

A short *connecting tubule* leads from the distal tubule to the *collecting tubule*, with several collecting tubules draining into a *collecting duct* in the cortex, which then descends into the medulla. Within the medulla, the collecting duct is divided into an outer and inner portion. Hormones such as ADH can differentially regulate the absorptive properties of the different segments of the collecting duct. Inner medullary collecting ducts give rise to papillary ducts that drain into a minor calyx. The collecting duct epithelium is characterized by two cell types, both cuboidal in appearance. Principal cells perform hormone-regulated absorption of NaCl and water, while intercalated cells secrete or absorb acid equivalents to maintain plasma acid-base balance.

Glomerular filtration

Ultrafiltration of blood takes place at the renal corpuscle, with the kidneys receiving around one-fifth of the cardiac output. With a typical haematocrit of 40%, renal plasma flow (RPF) in a young adult is approximately 625 mL/min. The filtration fraction is one-fifth, such that glomerular filtration rate (GFR) in a young adult is approximately 125 mL/min.

The filter in the renal corpuscle is only a barrier to cells and proteins, so the filtrate has the same composition as protein-free plasma. The filter has three components:

- The fenestrated endothelial cells of the capillary wall, which block the passage of cells.
- The negatively charged basement membrane of the endothelium, which exclude proteins.
- The interdigitating finger-like processes (pedicels) of visceral epithelial cells, called podocytes, which encircle the capillaries.

Negatively-charged molecules of the transmembrane protein nephrin protrude from the pedicel membrane and interdigitate to create slit pores. These negatively-lined pores provide a further barrier to proteins, and are responsible for the size and shape restrictions that the filter presents. Nephrotic syndrome, resulting from damage to the basement membrane or mutations in nephrin, leads to filtration of proteins and proteinuria.

Ultrafiltration across the capillary wall is driven by the difference between hydrostatic and osmotic pressures in the capillary and in the Bowman's space ('Starling forces': Fig. 16.5). Given that, with the exception of proteins, the composition of plasma and filtrate are identical, the osmotic pressure difference reflects the difference in osmotic pressure exerted by protein (the colloid osmotic pressure Π) either side of the barrier.

Hydrostatic pressure within the capillary (HP_{cap}) and the oncotic pressure within Bowman's space (Π_{BS}) drive filtration, whereas hydrostatic pressure in Bowman's space (HP_{BS}) and the oncotic pressure in the capillary (Π_{cap}) oppose filtration. Since proteins are effectively excluded from the Bowman's space, Π_{BS} is essentially zero.

Therefore, the net filtration pressure,

$$P_{uf} = HP_{cap} - (HP_{BS} + \Pi_{cap}),$$

and $GFR = K_f \times P_{uf}$, where the filtration coefficient, K_f = surface area × permeability.

Differential smooth muscle tone of afferent and efferent arterioles means that HP_{cap} is high (45 mmHg) and falls only slightly as blood is filtered along the length of the capillary. As proteins are left behind in the capillary and become concentrated, Π_{cap} increases. The tubule acts as a sink: as blood is filtered, HP_{cap} falls only slightly, but Π_{cap} rises as (protein) increases. HP_{BS} is around 10 mmHg, but does not appreciably increase with filtration, because the tubule drains the filtrate. Filtration equilibrium (where $HP_{cap} = (HP_{BS} + \Pi_{cap})$) is achieved late along capillary length, if at all.

GFR can be regulated through changes to arteriolar tone, with afferent arteriole dilation, increasing P_{GC} and hence GFR, and efferent arteriole dilation having the opposite effect. The contractile mesangial cells, which respond to angiotensin may alter the surface area available for filtration and, hence, K_f.

GFR is stabilized, such that it alters far less than would be predicted for arterial BP changes in the range 75–150 mmHg. This stabilization is called autoregulation and is also seen for RPF. Autoregulation reflects altered smooth muscle tone in afferent arterioles, arising from two responses:

- A myogenic mechanism, whereby increases in the pressure difference across the arteriole wall induces increased muscle contraction to reduce the lumen diameter.
- A flow-dependent mechanism (tubulo-glomerular feedback), in which increases in the amount of NaCl reaching (and being absorbed across) the macula densa trigger the release of adenosine from the macula densa cells, which induces arteriole constriction.

GFR and RPF are assessed from clearance measurements. Renal clearance (*C*) is the hypothetical volume of plasma from which a marker, X, is completely removed each minute to yield the amount of X excreted in the urine. In reality, no volume of blood is entirely swept of a substance: most substances are incompletely filtered from a larger volume. *C* can be calculated if the concentration of X in plasma (*P*) and urine (*U*), and urine flow rate (*V*) are known. Since the amount that disappears from the blood per minute is equivalent to the amount that appears in the urine per minute,

$$P \times C = U \times V$$

so

$$C = (U \times V)/P$$

For a marker that is freely filtered, not absorbed from, or secreted into, the tubule, and not metabolized or synthesized by the kidney, *C* will be equivalent to GFR. The infused polysaccharide marker inulin is the gold standard for clearance measurements of GRF. Creatinine is commonly used for clinical measurements, although it does not entirely conform to this ideal behaviour, since it is secreted into the tubule, leading to overestimates of GFR.

For substances (for example, the organic anion para-aminohippurate, PAH) which are totally removed from the blood during its passage through the kidney (by active secretion into the tubule), C will be equivalent to RPF.

The proximal tubule: reabsorption of the filtered load

Structure

The renal tubule obeys the Ussing dual membrane paradigm of epithelial transport, with cells possessing apical membranes that have specialized channels and carriers to mediate absorptive (and secretory) processes, and basolateral membranes that have housekeeper proteins for cellular homeostasis and hormone receptors. Tight junctions, which separate apical and basolateral membranes, exhibit varying degrees of leakiness, with the tubule becoming increasingly tight along its length. The early tubule recovers filtered essentials (ions, glucose), whereas the later, more regulated segments adjust urine composition for body fluid homeostasis.

The first nephron segment, the proximal tubule, is a leaky epithelium that is relatively unregulated and performs bulk reabsorption in an apparently 'isotonic' fashion. For water to move there must, in fact, be an osmotic gradient, but the very high water permeability exhibited by these cells, which reflects abundant expression of water channels (aquaporins), rather than the leaky nature of the tight junctions. This means that small, almost indiscernible, osmotic gradients can drive large fluxes of water.

Absorption

Organic solutes (glucose, amino acids) and around two-thirds of the filtered Na^+, K^+, Cl, HCO_3^- and water are reabsorbed by the proximal tubule. These absorptive processes are ultimately dependent on transepithelial Na^+ absorption, powered by the basolateral Na^+, K^+ ATPase, with transport of Na^+ being associated with the movement of other solutes.

Glucose

This is absorbed across the apical membrane by secondary active Na^+-glucose cotransporters (principally by the low affinity, high capacity SGLT2 protein, with the high affinity, low capacity SGLT1 protein scavenging glucose in the later proximal tubule); glucose exits to the interstitial fluid and so to the blood on passive GLUT1 and 2 proteins in the basolateral membrane. Carrier-mediated transport processes saturate, so renal tubules exhibit transport maxima for solutes such as glucose, with 'overspill' into the urine when plasma (and, hence, tubular fluid) concentrations rise above levels that can be fully absorbed.

Amino acids

These are transported using a similar template for secondary active, Na^+-driven accumulation across the apical membrane and passive efflux across the basolateral membrane. Specific systems for cationic, basic, and neutral amino acids have been described.

Bicarbonates

An apical Na^+-H^+ exchange is responsible for reabsorption of HCO_3^- ions (Fig. 16.6). The NHE3 variant of this secondary active transporter moves H^+ ions into the lumen, where they combine with HCO_3^- ions to form CO_2 and H_2O, catalysed by carbonic anhydrase. These species diffuse into the cell, where the reverse carbonic anhydrase-catalysed reaction occurs to reform H^+ and HCO_3^-. H^+ recycles on NHE3, and HCO_3^- leaves the cell across the basolateral membrane on a Na^+-HCO_3^- cotransporter (NBC), with $3HCO_3^-$ ions providing the driving force to move one Na^+ ion against its electrochemical gradient. Mutations in NHE3 and NBC give rise to proximal renal tubular acidosis.

Chlorine

Cl^- ions are also in part reabsorbed through the action of NHE3. H^+ ions in the lumen can combine with organic anions, such as formate ($HCOO^-$) to produce uncharged species that can cross the apical membrane. Inside the cell, the uncharged species dissociates to the H^+ ion, which recycles on NHE, and the anion, which moves down its electrochemical gradient back into the lumen on a passive carrier in exchange for Cl^- ions. Cl^- ions may also be absorbed using a Na^+-Cl^- cotransporter (NCC).

A large fraction of the Cl^- reabsorption, however, occurs in the later proximal tubule through paracellular pathways (across the tight junctions), after electrical and chemical gradients have been established by the preceding movement of other solutes and associated water.

Phosphate

Phosphate species are reabsorbed across the apical membrane by a secondary active Na^+-phosphate cotransporter (NaPi). The transported species can be HPO_4^{2-}, energized by the movement of $3Na^+$ ions, or $H_2PO_4^-$, energized by the movement of 2 Na^+ ions.

Calcium

Ca^{2+} ions are reabsorbed transcellularly and paracellularly. Ca^{2+} enters the cell through apical epithelial Ca^{2+} channels (ECaC), and is extruded across the basolateral membrane by Ca^{2+}-ATPase, $Na^+ \times Ca^{2+}$ exchange; these processes can be stimulated by PTH. Alternatively, the paracellular absorption of Cl^- ions in the later proximal tubule can establish a lumen positive potential difference that can drive paracellular Ca^{2+} movement. K^+ ions can similarly be reabsorbed through the paracellular pathway.

Secretion

Secretion of organic anions such as para-aminohippurate (PAH) also occurs. Organic anions are accumulated inside the cell by basolateral exchange for divalent cations, such as α-ketoglutarate. Efflux of α-ketoglutarate from the cell energizes this process, using an electrochemical gradient established by basolateral Na^+-dependent accumulation of the cation. PAH then exits to the lumen on an apical anion exchanger.

Glomerulotubular balance

This ensures that the proximal tubule continues to reabsorb around two-thirds of the filtered load if GFR should increase. Increased delivery of solutes stimulates carrier-mediated transport, and increased filtration reduces the hydrostatic pressure, while increasing the oncotic pressure in the peritubular capillary to promote greater uptake into capillaries.

The loop of Henle

After the wide range of absorptive activities seen in the proximal tubule, other parts of the nephron display increasingly specialized and limited function. The loop of Henle absorbs about 20% of the filtered load. The descending limb of the loop of Henle is essentially permeable only to water, which moves through aquaporin 1, and there is little solute transport. In contrast, the ascending limb of the loop of Henle lacks aquaporins, and so is water impermeable,

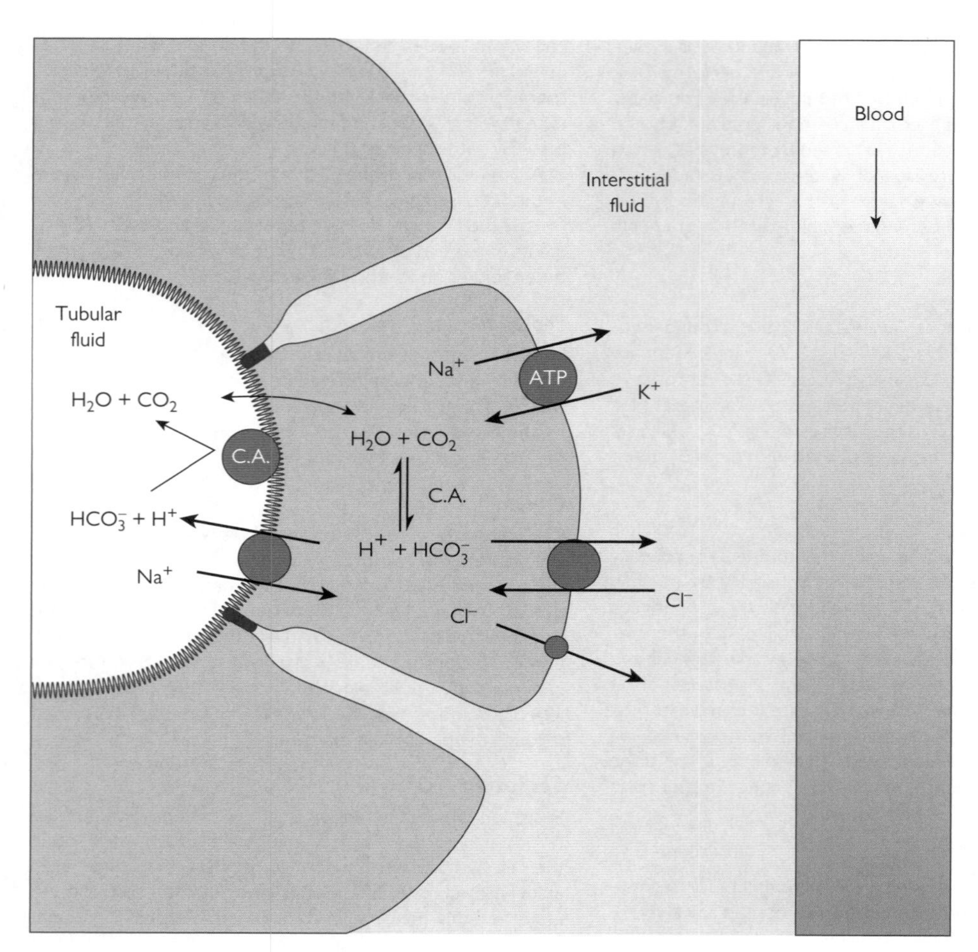

Fig. 16.6 Schematic representation of bicarbonate reabsorption in the proximal tubule.

Reproduced from G Pocock and CD Richards, *Human Physiology: The Basis of Medicine, Third Edition,* 2006, Figure 17.14, p. 361, by permission of Oxford University Press

but absorbs NaCl passively in the thin segment and actively in the thick segment using apical Na^+-K^+-$2Cl^-$ cotransport (NKCC2).

This difference in permeability properties makes the two limbs of the loop of Henle, with their opposite directions of flow, a counter-current multiplication system, which can concentrate the interstitial fluid surrounding the renal tubule (Fig. 16.7). The hyperosmotic environment that results can be used, when required, to extract large quantities of water by osmosis from the collecting duct. Therefore, the kidney has the capacity to produce dilute or concentrated urines, according to water balance, with the default being to produce dilute urine.

Comparison of the length of loops of Henle of different species shows that the longer the loop, the more concentrated the urine produced can be, since greater counter-current multiplication of interstitial osmolarity can be achieved.

Absorption of NaCl

Tubular fluid entering the loop of Henle from the proximal tubule is iso-osmotic. The central process in counter-current multiplication is the active absorption of NaCl by NKCC in the water-tight thick ascending limb (termed the 'single effect'). Loop diuretics, such as furosemide, target this process. The absorption of NaCl concentrates the interstitial fluid surrounding the tubule and this hypertonic environment draws water by osmosis from the descending limb. The osmotic equilibration of the tubular fluid in the descending limb with the interstitium concentrates Na^+ in the tubule, such that at the hairpin loop the fluid is hyperosmotic. The delivery of tubular fluid with a high [Na^+] promotes further NaCl absorption in the ascending limb. In the thin ascending limb, which lacks Na^+, K^+ ATPases, the high concentration of Na^+ established in this way encourages passive diffusion of Na^+ into the interstitium. The increased absorption from the

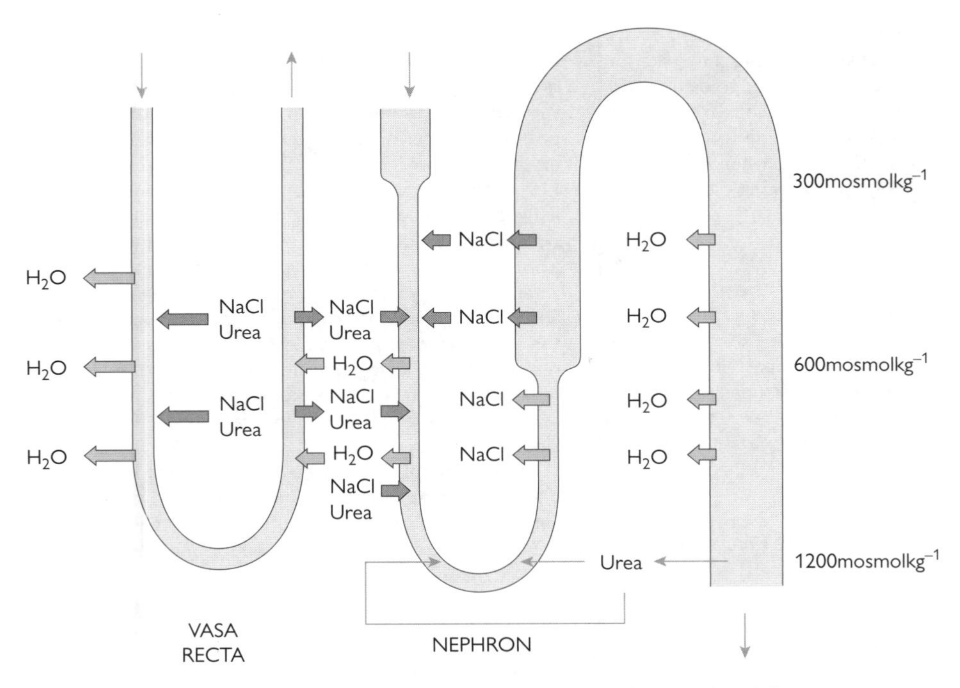

Fig. 16.7 Schematic representation of the countercurrent multiplier of the renal medulla.

Reproduced from G Pocock and CD Richards, *Human Physiology: The Basis of Medicine, Third Edition*, 2006, Figure 17.24, p. 369, by permission of Oxford University Press

ascending limb further concentrates the interstitium, extracting even more water from the descending limb and raising its [Na^+] yet further. As fluid continues to flow around the hairpin this ever-increasing luminal [Na^+] drives further NaCl efflux and creates an increasingly hypertonic interstitium.

Vasa recta

The vasa recta deliver nutrients and O_2 to tubule cells, and remove excess solutes and water from the medulla. These hairpin capillaries arise from efferent arterioles, and run parallel to the limbs of the loop of Henle. Their configuration allows them to act as a counter-current exchange system to minimize the washout of interstitial hypertonicity. Water is extracted from the vasa recta by osmosis and Na^+ enters down its gradient as blood passes down the descending limb, with the reverse processes occurring as blood flows up the ascending limb.

Mutations in NKCC2 give rise to Bartter's syndrome—the primary genetic defect of Bartter's syndrome, leading to excess Na^+, K^+, and water loss in the urine.

Distal tubule and collecting duct

The separation of water and solute movements in the distal tubule and collecting duct is essential for body fluid homeostasis. Maintenance of extracellular osmolarity and volume by the kidney requires that the delivery of tubular fluid to the tight hormone-regulated epithelium of these distal sections is kept steady.

Sodium and chlorine reabsorption

Na^+ and Cl^- reabsorption continues in the distal tubule, with about 7% of the load absorbed in this segment, mediated by an apical Na^+-Cl^- cotransport protein (NCC). Mutations in NCC give rise to Gitelman's syndrome, which is characterized by hypokalaemia.

Principal cells in the collecting duct absorb about 5% of the filtered using apical Na^+ channels (ENaC); Cl^- ions move paracellularly down their electrochemical gradient or are reabsorbed by type B intercalated cells, in exchange for HCO_3^- ions. K^+ secretion by principal cells through apical K^+ channels also occurs in the collecting duct.

NaCl absorption from the ascending limb means that the fluid that moves from the loop to the distal tubule is hypotonic. When water intake is sufficient, water is not reabsorbed from the dilute tubular fluid, since the apical membrane in distal tubule and collecting duct cells lacks a constitutive permeability to water. Large volumes of hypotonic urine are therefore produced.

Antidiuresis

The tight collecting duct is a heavily regulated site, that 'fine-tunes' urine composition. In antidiuresis, circulating ADH, a 9-amino acid hormone released from the posterior pituitary in response to elevated plasma osmolarity (2% change), induces the insertion of aquaporin 2 water channels into the apical membrane (basolateral membranes possess constitutive aquaporin 3 and 4). The channels are embedded in the membrane of vesicles, which fuse with the apical membrane. Now, the axial hypertonic gradient established by the loop of Henle can extract water as fluid flows along the tubule and small volumes of hypertonic urine are produced. Diabetes insipidus (DI) results when ADH secretion fails (central DI) or when renal responses to ADH are absent (nephrogenic DI).

Urea

Urea also contributes to the interstitial hypertonicity that extracts water from the collecting duct. Urea is concentrated as tubular fluid is reabsorbed along the nephron. In the presence of ADH, which activates passive urea carriers (UT), it is reabsorbed from the last (inner medullary) portion of the collecting duct. Up to 50% of the osmotic potential in the inner medulla can be contributed by urea, which has been reabsorbed in this way.

Plasma osmolarity

This is very tightly regulated, so effective circulating volume (the volume of plasma perfusing the tissues) is determined by plasma NaCl content, since changes in NaCl will alter the volume of water in which the salt must be dissolved. Reduced effective circulating volume induces the renin-angiotensin-aldosterone cascade to increase NaCl absorption and, hence, water retention. Systemic baroreceptors detect low pressure and induce sympathetic discharge to the kidney that elicits release of renin from granular cells in the renal corpuscle. Reduced afferent arteriole distension and reduced tubuloglomerular feedback (reduced adenosine release from the macula densa in response to reduced GFR) also enhance renin release. Renin converts angiotensinogen to angiotensin I, which is in turn converted to angiotensin II by a converting enzyme found in vascular endothelium, notably the lungs. Angiotensin is a potent vasoconstrictor and stimulates Na^+ absorption in the proximal tubule by increasing NHE3 activity. It also induces release of the steroid hormone aldosterone from the adrenal cortex. Aldosterone acts through genomic (and non-genomic) pathways to promote Na^+ (and, hence, Cl^-) absorption from the collecting duct. It stimulates transcription of ENaC and of the Na^+, K^+ ATPase. The increased exchange of Na^+ for K^+ by the ATPase results in enhanced secretion of K^+. Drugs that act to inhibit Na^+ absorption in earlier segments of the nephron, or mutations in the transport proteins that perform the absorption, increase Na^+ delivery to the collecting duct. The enhanced absorption of Na^+ at this site also increases K^+ secretion and can result in hypokalaemia. Excessive aldosterone production, termed primary hyperaldosteronism (Conn's syndrome) can arise from adrenal hyperplasia or adrenal adenoma. It is characterized by hypertension, hypokalaemia, and alkalosis. Secondary hyperaldosteronism arises from over-activity of the renin-angiotensin system, for example, as a result of a renin-producing juxtaglomerular cell tumour or in cases of renal artery stenosis. Constitutive activation of ENaC by mutations can lead to pseudohyperaldosteronism, called Liddle's disease.

Atrial natriuretic peptide, a 28-amino acid hormone, is released from atrial myocytes in response to distension. It antagonizes the actions of the renin-angiotensin-aldosterone cascade to reduce NaCl absorption and, hence, the volume of water in which the salt is dissolved, thereby reducing the effective circulating volume.

Plasma acid-base homeostasis

The collecting duct also plays a role in plasma acid-base homeostasis. Intercalated cells in the collecting duct secrete acid (type A) or base (type B) into the lumen. Type A cells possess apical H^+-ATPases and basolateral anion exchangers that move H^+ and HCO_3^- (produced by carbonic anhydrase-catalysed hydration of CO_2 within the cell) into the lumen and blood, respectively. The secreted H^+ is predominantly buffered in the lumen by NH_3 synthesized by proximal tubule cells. Type B cells have the reverse configuration and secrete base. In normal circumstances, metabolic reactions lead to a daily non-volatile acid load to the plasma of around 70 mmol, so acid secreting type A cells predominate. In alkalosis, type B cells become more prevalent. Acid-base disorders are often associated with disturbances of K^+ balance—acidosis induces hyperkalaemia through inhibition of K^+ secretion, while hyperkalaemia inhibits ammoniagenesis and causes acidosis.

Pharmacology

Diuretics

Diuretics (Table 16.1) promote Na^+ excretion (natriuresis) and hence diuresis by inhibiting reabsorptive processes in the renal tubule. Diuretics are used in cases of fluid retention where the effective circulating volume is compromised by cardiac, hepatic, or renal dysfunction, and to treat hypertension. Diuretics are classified by their action and often have deleterious effects on electrolyte balance, notably K^+ homeostasis. Most diuretics act proximal to the site of K^+ secretion in the collecting duct. The increased delivery of Na^+ to the collecting duct induced by these drugs promotes K^+ secretion and hypokalaemia.

Carbonic anhydrase inhibitors

Carbonic anhydrase inhibitors, such as acetazolamide are commonly used to treat glaucoma and mountain sickness. They inhibit the generation of H^+ for NHE3-mediated Na^+ absorption in the proximal tubule. Their use can induce a metabolic acidosis (because they impair HCO_3^- absorption) and K^+ depletion.

Table 16.1 Diuretic drugs

Drug	Mechanism of action	Cautions/ Contraindications	Side effects	Interactions
Loop diuretics, e.g. furosemide, bumetanide	Inhibit Na^+ reabsorption by inhibiting Na^+, K^+, $2Cl^-$ transporter in the thick segment of ascending loop of Henle	Avoid if disturbance of electrolytes. Avoid if history of gout	Hypokalaemia, natremia, calcaemia, magnesia. Metabolic alkalosis. Hyperuricaemia and gout. Hypotension	Enhanced hypotensive effect with ACE-I, β- blockers and nitrates. Increased risk of cardiotoxicity with digoxin. Reduced excretion of lithium. Theophylline increases risk of hypokalaemia
Thiazide diuretics, e.g. bendroflumethiazide, metolazone	Inhibit Na^+ reabsorption by Na^+, Cl^- co-transporter in the distal convoluted tubule (DCT)	Avoid if disturbance of electrolytes. Avoid if history of gout. Avoid if poorly controlled diabetes mellitus	Hypokalaemia, natremia, calcaemia, magnesia. Metabolic alkalosis. Hyperuricaemia and gout. Hypotension. Hyperglycaemia. Lipid disturbance	Enhanced hypotensive effect with ACEI, β-blockers and nitrates. Increased risk of cardiotoxicity with digoxin. Reduced excretion of lithium. Theophylline increases risk of hypokalaemia
Potassium sparing diuretics, e.g. spironalactone, eplerenone	Aldosterone antagonist, inhibiting Na^+ reabsorption in the collecting duct	Avoid if at risk of hyperkalaemia. Addison's disease	Hyperkalaemia. Hyponatraemia. Gynaecomastia. Impotence. Menstrual irregularities	Increased risk of hyperkalaemia with ACE inhibitors, heparin, K^+ supplements NSAIDs and tacrolimus. Decreased excretion of lithium. Increased concentration of digoxin
Potassium sparing diuretics, e.g. amiloride	Inhibit Na^+ channels to reduce Na^+ reabsorption in the collecting duct	Avoid if at risk of hyperkalaemia	Hyperkalaemia. Hyponatremia	Increased risk of hyperkalaemia with ACE inhibitors, heparin, K^+ supplements, NSAIDs and tacrolimus
Osmotic diuretics, e.g. mannitol	Filtered in the glomerulus, but not reabsorbed. Exert an osmotic effect and reduce water reabsorption (used in treatment of cerebral oedema)		Hyponatraemia. Chills, fevers	
Carbonic anhydrase inhibitors, e.g. acetazolamide	Increase HCO_3^- excretion	Avoid if disturbance of electrolytes	GI disturbance. Taste disturbance. Flushing and headache. Thirst and polyuria. Rashes, including Stevens Johnson syndrome. Blood dyscrasia	Electrolyte disturbance including increased risk of hypokalaemia when given with other diuretics. Metabolic acidosis. Increased risk of cardiotoxicity with digoxin. Increased concentration of carbamazepine. Increased excretion lithium

Loop diuretics

Loop diuretics such as furosemide and bumetanide are used to treat acute and chronic fluid retention associated with heart failure. They inhibit NKCC2 in the thick ascending limb of the loop of Henle, which reduces Na^+ reabsorption and compromises the hypertonic environment of the interstitial fluid that is used to extract water from the collecting duct. Loop diuretics can cause excessive depletion of plasma volume, K^+ depletion, and alkalosis (by augmented acid secretion and ammoniagenesis).

Thiazaide diuretics

Thiazaide diuretics, such as bendroflumethiazide, are used to treat hypertension and metolazone can be added to a loop diuretic to treat resistant fluid overload in heart failure. They inhibit NCC in the distal tubule to reduce NaCl absorption; K^+ depletion and Ca^{2+} retention (through potentiation of the effects of PTH) can result.

Potassium-sparing diuretics

Potassium-sparing diuretics, such as amiloride, spironolactone, and eplerenone, may be used as an adjunct to K^+-wasting diuretics or to offset mild hypokalaemia. Amiloride inhibits ENaC in the collecting duct, whereas spironolactone and eplerenone are aldosterone receptor antagonists. Both act to reduce absorption of Na^+ (and secretion of K^+) in the collecting duct. The K^+ retention associated with these drugs can initiate a subsequent acidosis.

Osmotic diuretics

Osmotic diuretics, such as mannitol, may be used to treat increased intracranial or intraocular pressure, or to force a diuresis in cases of overdose. These drugs are trapped in the lumen, where their osmotic potential traps water in the tubule. Osmotic diuretics can cause a high degree of Na^+ washout in the urine.

Drug-induced renal reactions

Table 16.2 summarises drug-induced renal reactions.

Table 16.2 Drug-induced renal reactions

Acute tubular necrosis	ACE inhibitors. Amphotericin B. Aminoglycosides. NSAIDs. Tetracyclines
Interstitial nephritis	Allopurinol. Amphotericin. Analgesics. Antibiotics: • Cephalosporins, penicillins, rifampicin, sulphonamides. Cimetidine. Cisplatin. Cyclosporin. Diuretics. Furosemide, thiazide. NSAIDs. Omeprazole. Phenytoin. Phenindione
Renal tubular acidosis[1]	*Type I (Distal):* amphotericin, lead, lithium, NSAIDs.*Type II (Proximal):* acetazolamide, heavy metals, sulphonamides, expired tetracyclines. *Type IV (hypoaldosterone-related):* ACE-i/A2A, NSAIDs, spironolactone
Nephrotic syndrome	*Membranous Nephropathy*[2]: captopril, gold, NSAIDs, penicillamine, probenecid
Hyponatraemia	*Renal loss:* diuretics. *SIADH related:* • Anti-depressants (e.g. SSRIs), anti-psychotics, carbamazepine, NMDA, opiates, vincristine and other cytotoxics. *Enhancement of ADH activity:* certain sulphonylureas.*ADH like activity:* desmopressin
Hyperkalaemia	ACE inhibitors, heparin, K^+ sparing diuretics (e.g. spironalactone), K^+ therapy, NSAIDs, suxamethonium, tacrolimus
Hypokalaemia	*Increased K^+ excretion:* corticosteroids, diuretics, carbenoxolone, RTA drug-induced causes (as above). *Increased Na^+, K^+ ATPase activity at the cellular level:* beta-agonists, insulin

Table 16.2 Drug-induced renal reactions (*continued*)

Metabolic acidosis	*Increased anion gap*[3]: biguanides (lactic acidosis), ethylene glycol and methanol poisoning, salicylates. *Normal anion gap:* acetazolamide, RTA drug-induced causes (as above)
Urinary retention	Anticholinergics

[1]Renal tubular acidosis (RTA) is a metabolic acidosis that is caused by a decreased excretion of acid by the kidneys. There are four types of RTA that are categorized according to the underlying cause.
[2]Membranous nephropathy is a type of glomerulonephritis. It often presents with nephrotic syndrome, characterized by proteinuria, hypoalbuminaemia, oedema and hyperlipidaemia.
[3]The anion gap is the difference between measured anions and cations:

$$([Na^+]+[K^+])-([Cl^-]+[HCO_3^-])$$

The normal anion gap in plasma is usually between 10 and– 16 mmol/L. A change in the production of unmeasured ions will increase the anion gap.

Multiple choice questions

1. Which of the following statements regarding glomerular filtration rate is correct?

A. Net filtration pressure is around 50 mmHg.
B. Filtration favours positively charged ions.
C. Filtration fraction is around 40%.
D. Daily filtration volume is around 360 L.
E. Filtration is reduced by efferent arteriole constriction.

2. Renal clearance:

A. Can be defined as the volume of blood completely cleared of a substance per minute.
B. Of a compound that is freely filtered and not secreted or reabsorbed is equal to renal plasma flow.
C. Of creatinine as an estimate glomerular filtration rate produces an underestimation of the actual value.
D. Of a substance can be calculated from plasma concentration, urinary concentration, and filtration fraction.
E. Of glucose is similar to glomerular filtration rate as it is freely filtered.

3. The loop of Henle:

A. Acts as a counter-current exchanger.
B. Has a descending limb which is impermeable to water.
C. Generates a hypotonic medullary interstitium.
D. Is longer in camels compared with humans.
E. Is the main mechanistic site for the protein defect that gives rise to Gitelman's syndrome.

4. Renin:

A. Converts angiotensin I to angiotensin II.
B. Is released in response to renal parasympathetic stimulation.
C. Is released from granular cells of the juxtaglomerular apparatus.
D. Is released in response to efferent arteriole distension.
E. Activity in the plasma of Afro-Caribbean's tends to be higher than in Caucasians.

5. Which of the following drugs is most likely to cause a metabolic acidosis?

A. Metolazone.
B. Bumetanide.
C. Mannitol.
D. Bendroflumethiazide.
E. Acetazolamide.

6. Which of the following will result in an increase in urinary sodium excretion?

A. Reduced renal sympathetic stimulation.
B. Conn's disease.
C. Increased plasma protein concentration.
D. A sustained fall in arterial pressure.
E. Cushing's disease.

7. Which of the following drugs is most likely to cause hyperkalaemia?

A. Corticosteroids.
B. Acetazolamide.
C. Insulin.
D. Lithium.
E. Heparin.

8. Sodium reabsorption in the nephron occurs mainly at the:

A. Proximal convoluted tubule.
B. Descending limb of the loop of Henle.
C. Ascending limb of the loop of Henle.
D. Distal convoluted tubule.
E. Collecting duct.

9. Which of the following is a genetic disease that may involve the kidney?

A. Noonan's syndrome.
B. Angelman's syndrome.
C. Systemic lupus erythematosus.
D. von Hippel–Lindau disease.
E. Brugada syndrome.

10. Which of the following is the least likely place for a urinary calculus to cause obstruction?

A. Pelviureteric junction.
B. Abdominal ureter.
C. Vesicoureteric junction.
D. Trigone.
E. Prostatic urethra.

For answers, please see Appendix: Answers to multiple choice questions, page 313.

CHAPTER 17

Dermatology

Structure and function

Skin protects the body from the external environment providing a barrier against dehydration, sunlight and infection and plays an important immunological role. It also plays a key role in thermoregulation and detection of sensory stimuli. Skin is comprised of a specialized epithelium, incorporating sweat and sebaceous glands, and hair follicles with associated supporting tissues. It is arranged as a number of layers, the relative thickness and structure of which is dependent on the area of the body and its' required function. These layers include the epidermis (outermost layer), dermis, and sc tissue (hypodermis; see Fig. 17.1).

Epidermis

The epidermis consists of stratified epithelium with a tough keratinized upper layer. Deep layer keratinocytes form keratin plaques/squames when they die and these are constantly being shed. There is, therefore, a constant need to replenish the epidermis. Turnover of cells from basal cells to desquamated keratin varies from 25 days with the soles of the feet to 45 days with the back. The turnover and shedding of keratinocytes gives the epidermis several distinct layers from deep to superficial (see Fig. 17.2).

Stratum germinativum/basale

This layer is responsible for keratinocyte production and sits on the basement membrane, separating the dermis from the epidermis. There are no blood vessels in the epidermis, but there are capillaries in the upper layer of the dermis. Keratinocytes are cuboidal or columnar and are continually undergoing mitosis throughout a lifetime. They contain abundant ribosomes and mitochondria to enable rapid cell turnover and protein synthesis. Melananocytes synthesize melanin in cytoplasmic membrane-bound granules in this layer. This is responsible for skin colouring and reduces damage caused by ultraviolet radiation. Granules advance along cytoplasmic processes into the cytoplasm of basal and prickle layer keratinocytes. Fingernails and toenails are hard plates of keratinized epithelium, which originate from this layer.

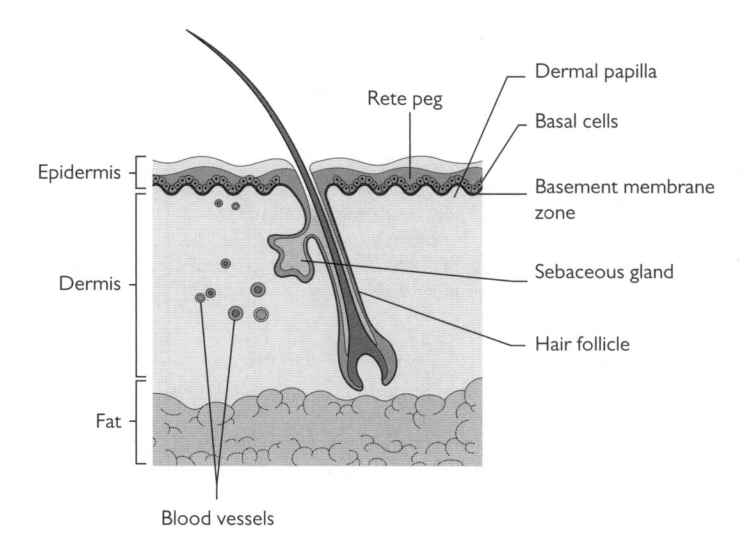

Fig. 17.1 Diagram of skin: epidermis, dermis, and fat.

Reproduced from S Burge and D Wallis, *Oxford Handbook of Medical Dermatology*, 2010, Figure 1.1, p. 5, by permission of Oxford University Press

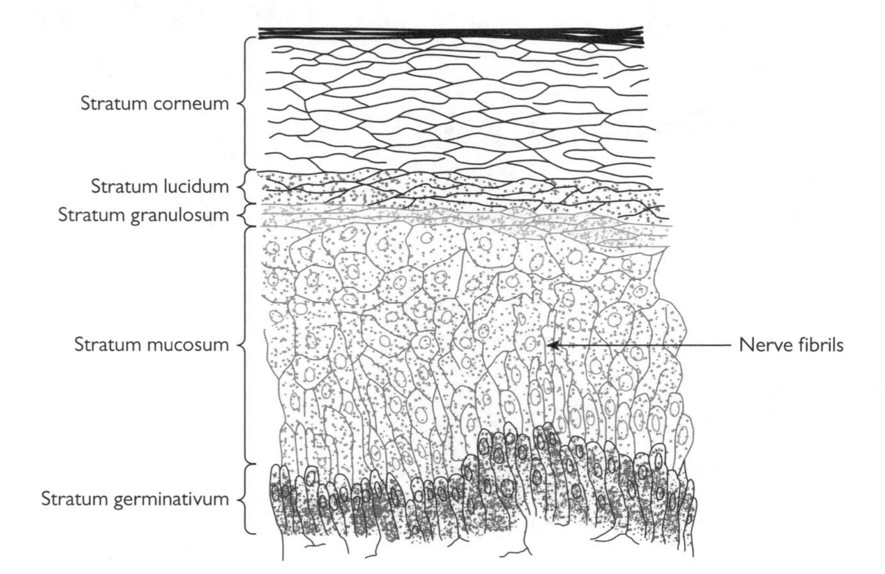

Fig. 17.2 The distinct layers of the epidermis from deep to superficial.

This figure was published in Gray, *Anatomy of the Human Body*, Twentieth edition, throughly revised and re-edited by Warren H. Lewis, plate 941, Elsevier. Copyright the editors, 1918.

Stratum spinosum/mucosum

This layer is known as the spinous or prickle cell layer as its polyhedral cells possess cytoplasmic projections between cells, which terminate as desmosomal junctions. Langerhans cells are most frequently seen in the prickle layer of the skin. They present phagocytosed antigenic material to lymphocytes and in inflamed skin the number of their cytoplasmic processes increases, especially during autoimmune or allergy related skin disorders.

Stratum granulosum

This is a thin layer in which the cells contain abundant keratohyaline granules that promote hydration and cross-linking of keratin. At the transition between this layer and the stratum corneum, cells secrete lamellar bodies (containing lipids and proteins) into the extracellular space, which results in the formation of a hydrophobic lipid envelope responsible for the skin's barrier properties.

Stratum lucidum

This thin, translucent layer merges with the upper layers of the stratum granulosum and is most noticeable in areas of thick skin, particularly on the palms of the hands and the soles of the feet. It consists of flattened cells with no organelles or nuclei, as the granular cells become non-viable corneocytes.

Stratum corneum

The uppermost layer of the epidermis in which keratin plaques are formed from dead cells. This layer is also thickest on the palms of the hands and soles of the feet. Here, the cell membrane is replaced by a layer of ceramides covalently linked to an envelope of structural proteins, and corneodesmosomes facilitate cellular adhesion by linking adjacent cells. This linking is responsible for the stretchy mechanical properties of skin. Corneodesmosomes are degraded by proteases permitting cells to be shed at the surface. Disruption of the serine protease inhibitor lympho-epithelial Kazal-type-related inhibitor (LEKTI) due to autosomal recessive mutations in the *SPINK5* gene leads to excessive desquamation in Netherton syndrome. This layer also provides waterproofing, but dead keratin cells can also absorb water, as shown by the wrinkling of the skin of the hands after extended exposure to water.

The basement membrane

This comprises three layers and separates the epidermal layer from the underlying dermis. Basal cells are attached to the outermost layer, the lamina densa and, from here, anchoring proteins cross to the lamina lucida. Fibronectin is abundant in the zone below the lamina densa (fibroreticular lamina). The lower surface of the lamina densa is attached to collagen fibres in the papillary dermis by fibrils made of type VII collagen.

Dermo-epidermal junction

The dermo-epidermal junction binds the dermis and the epidermis together. Tethering fibres pass between the two layers and the intervening basement membrane. The rete system is a series of down-growths of the epidermis into the dermis, which increases the area of attachment between the two layers. This attachment is minimal over the back, and more extensive over the fingertips and soles, where shearing forces are increased. Abnormalities generated in this area can give rise to blistering (although blisters may also arise within the epidermis if desmosomal adhesions fail).

Dermis

The dermis contains blood vessels, lymphatics, nerves, hair follicles, sebaceous gland, and eccrine sweat glands. These are embedded in a connective tissue stroma, which is produced by fibroblasts, the main cell type of this layer. The dermis consists of two layers.

Superficial papillary dermis

A thin layer of loosely-arranged collagen and elastin fibres, containing small capillary-sized blood vessels, fine nerves, and nerve endings.

Deep reticular dermis

The reticular dermis is thicker, forming the bulk of the dermis, and is made up of dense bands of collagen, and long thick fibres of elastin running in parallel with the skin. The reticular dermis contains the secretory part of eccrine sweat glands with ducts running through the epidermis to communicating with the exterior. The bulb of hair follicles, and their associated erector pili muscle and sebaceous glands can also be found in the reticular dermis. There are also deep vascular plexi in the reticular dermis, one superficial, the other deep. Variations in blood flow are controlled by many arteriovenous anastomoses within the dermis to allow the skin to participate in thermoregulation.

Subcutaneous tissue

The subcutis or hypodermis is the deepest layer of skin and varies in size over the body. It attaches skin to underlying bone and muscle, as well as supplying it with blood vessels and nerves. It consists of loose connective tissue and elastin, but adipose tissue forms the majority of this layer, making up 50% of body fat and serving as padding and insulation.

The nerve supply of the skin

There are four major specialized nerve endings detecting cutaneous sensation in skin:

- Free nerve endings detect pain, itch and temperature and can be myelinated A-δ fibres or unmyelinated C fibres.
- Meissner's corpuscles detect touch, are found mainly on the hands and feet, and have ordered nerve endings, which are confined to dermal papillae.
- Merkel's cells are slow adapting touch receptors.
- Pacinian corpuscles detect pressure and vibration, and are encapsulated nerve endings with a characteristic structure. They are found mainly in deep dermis, and sc fat on palms and soles.

The nerve supply to the skin also consists of a sympathetic supply of unmyelinated nerves, which control skin appendages (for example, sweat glands) and vascular flow.

Patterns of skin disease

Skin can display a vast range of signs and reaction patterns that can give clues to systemic disease, as well as primary dermatological conditions. Diagnostic clues can be obtained from the nature of the lesions and its growth pattern, their distribution, and associated symptoms. Biopsy and histological examination of the tissue can help determine the underlying pathology. A range of different pathologies can produce similar dermatological phenomena and the aim of this section is to provide some common examples of these.

Pruritus

Many chemical, mechanical, and thermal stimuli can produce itching, which is sensed by nociceptors in the basal epidermal and superficial papillary dermis and carried by unmyelinated C-fibres and some A-δ fibres. These nociceptors respond to histamine released by a type I hypersensitivity reaction, or neuronal, chemical, or mechanical stimulation, and can be sensitized by a range of inflammatory mediators. They all produce the common sensation of itching and the reflex scratching response that accompanies it. For causes see Box 17.1.

Plaques

A localized epidermal proliferation or oedematous inflammation may result in a plaque (see Fig. 17.3). This is defined as a broad plateau-like lesion greater in width than depth (usually more than 1 cm in diameter). For causes see Box 17.2.

Nodules

A nodule is a raised lesion greater than 1 cm in width and depth that tend to originate in the dermis or sc fat (see Fig. 17.4). For causes see Box 17.3.

BOX 17.1 CAUSES OF PRURITUS

- Contact dermatitis
- Eczema
- Psoriasis
- Urticaria
- Infections and infestations (viral, parasitic)
- Xerosis/dry skin
- Trauma/healing
- Iron deficiency or polycythaemia
- Uraemia
- Malignancy
- Drugs (see later)
- Endocrine (Diabetes Mellitus, hypo/hyperthyroidism)

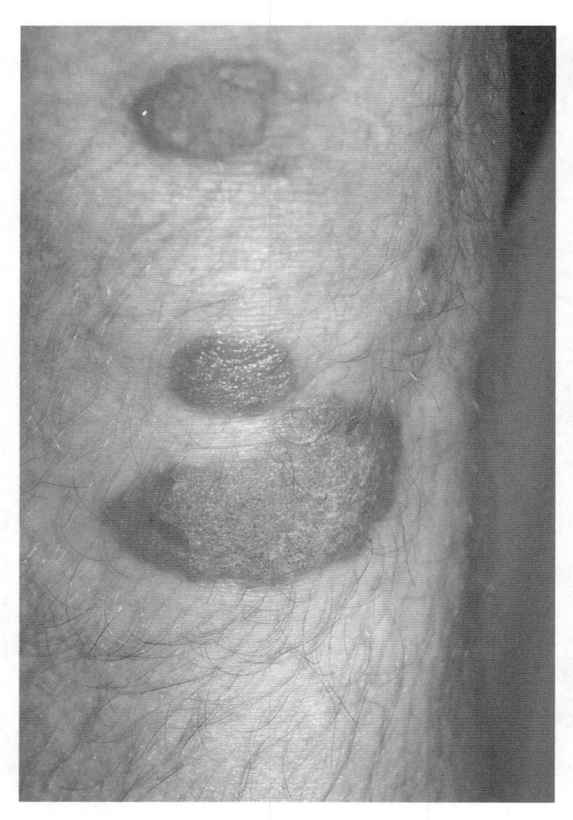

Fig. 17.3 Plaque.

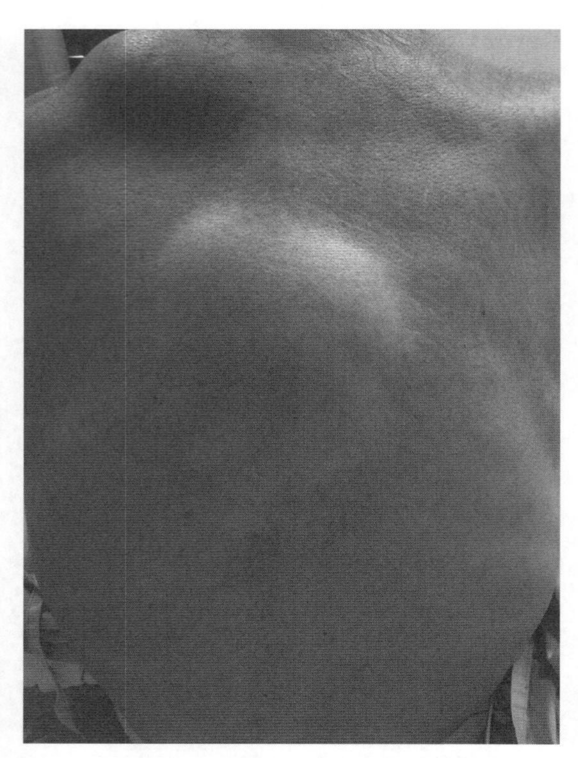

Fig. 17.4 Nodule.

BOX 17.2 CAUSES OF CUTANEOUS PLAQUES

- Psoriasis
- Eczema
- Urticaria
- Tinea corporis
- Necrobiosis lipoidica (Diabetes mellitus, rheumatoid arthritis)
- Sarcoidosis
- Granuloma annulare (Diabetes Mellitis, thyroid disease, SLE, HIV)
- Kaposi's sarcoma

BOX 17.3 CAUSES OF CUTANEOUS NODULES

- Infections: *Staphylococcus aureus*, scabies, tinea corporis, secondary syphilis, cutaneous leishmaniasis.
- Lipomas.
- Skin tumours.
- Rheumatoid nodules.
- Xanthelasma.
- *Erythema nodosum:* idiopathic, infections, sarcoidosis, inflammatory bowel disease, malignancy.
- Cutaneous lymphoma.
- Cutaneous sarcoidosis.
- *Neutrophilic dermatitis:* Sweet's syndrome.
- *Granuloma annulare:* Diabetes mellitis, thyroid disease, SLE, HIV.
- *Genetic:* tuberous sclerosis, neurofibromatosis.

Purpura

Bleeding underneath the skin can produce small petechiae (less than 3 mm) and/or ecchymosis (greater than 1 cm). Lesions between 0.3 and 1 cm are known as purpuric lesions (see Fig. 17.5) and they can result from blood vessel inflammation, or disorders of platelets and clotting (see Box 17.4).

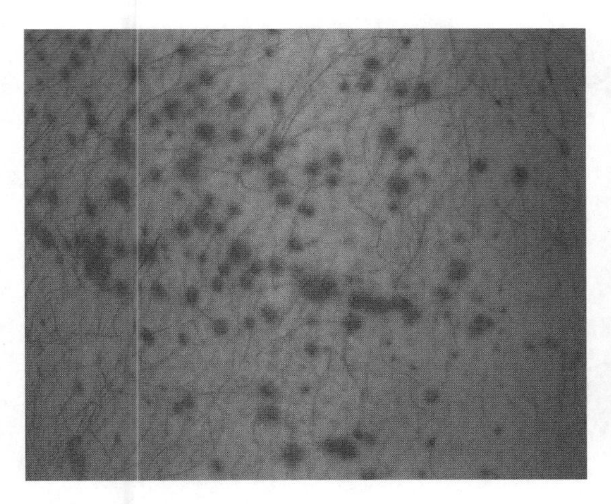

Fig. 17.5 Purpuric lesions.

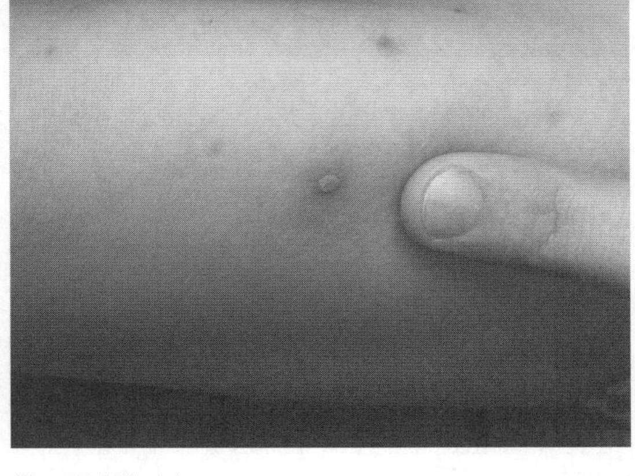

Fig. 17.6 Vesicle.

BOX 17.4 CAUSES OF A PURPURIC RASH

- Meningococcal septicaemia.
- Vasculitis (Henoch–Schonlein purpura, Wegener's disease, polyarteritis nodosum, senile purpura).
- Platelet disorders (idiopathic thrombocytopenic purpura, thrombotic thrombocytopenic purpura).
- Coagulation disorders (disseminated intravascular coagulopathy).

BOX 17.5 CAUSES OF A VESICULAR RASH

- *Infections:*
  - *Viruses:* herpes, Coxsackie, poxviruses.
  - *Bacteria:* staphylococcal, rickettsia.
  - *Fungal:* scabies.
- Acute contact dermatitis.
- *Autoimmune:* dermatitis herpetiformis, pemphigus/pemphigoid, toxic epidermal necrolysis.
- *Metabolic:* porphyria cutanea tarda.

Vesicles

Vesicles are fluid filled epidermal elevation less than 1 cm in diameter as shown in Fig. 17.6. Causes of a vesicular rash can be found in Box 17.5.

Bullae

Large fluid-filled elevations greater than 1 cm in diameter are known as bullae). The 1 cm cut-off for the definition of a vesicle and bullae is somewhat arbitrary, and there will be some cross-over in terms of aetiology of the two manifestations. Bullae can be differentiated from cysts, which are located in the epidermis, are epithelial lined and can contain solid, or semi-solid material, rather than just fluid. If the cavity contains purulent necrotic inflammatory material then it is known as a pustule. Bullae usually form at the dermo-epidermal junction and can arise from sheer stress due to trauma, as is the case with blisters that arise on the feet from ill-fitting shoes. They can also arise from IgG autoantibodies against the type XVII collagen component of hemidesmosomes in bullous pemphigoid, or IgA and C3 deposition in linear IgA dermatosis (Box 17.6). In pemphigoid, autoantibodies are directed against desmogleins between squamous cells of the epidermis, whereas dermatitis herpetiformis blister formation is in the lamina lucida of the basement membrane with granular IgA deposits leading to sub-epidermal separation.

BOX 17.6 CAUSES OF BULLOUS ERUPTIONS

- *Trauma-induced blisters:* including thermal burns, sunburn, and insect bites.
- *Infections:* staphylococcal scalded skin syndrome.
- *Drugs:* see 'Stevens–Johnson syndrome/toxic epidermal necrolysis'
- *Immune:* pemphigus/pemphigoid, dermatitis herpetiformis.
- *Metabolic:* porphyria cutanea tarda.

BOX 17.7 CAUSES OF PHOTOSENSITIVITY

- Drugs (see 'Drug-induced photosensitivity') and phytophotodermatitis.
- Polymorphic light eruption.
- Autoimmune (SLE).
- Genetic (porphyria cutanea tarda).

Photosensitivity

Phototoxic reactions occur because of the damaging effects of light-activated compounds (such as uroporphyrinogen in porphyria cutanea tarda), whereas photoallergic reactions are cell-mediated immune responses to a light-activated compound (Box 17.7). Phototoxic reactions develop in most individuals if they are exposed to sufficient amounts of light and drug. Photoallergic reactions require multiple exposures and resemble allergic contact dermatitis, with a distribution limited to sun-exposed areas of the body. However, when the reactions are severe or prolonged, they may extend into covered areas of skin. Drugs responsible for these two types of reactions are listed in the following section.

Pigmentation

Hyperpigmentation can arise from deposition in the dermis or epidermis (e.g. iron in haemochromotosis or heavy metal drugs such as gold), stimulation of melanocytes (e.g. chloroquine or the oral contraceptive pill, which are reversible, or by ACTH/melanocyte stimulating hormone in Nelson's syndrome), or post-inflammatory changes in the skin (e.g. chemotherapy agents; see Box 17.8). Other mechanisms are more complex, including photosensitivity reactions (e.g. amiodarone). Proliferation of melanocytes can also be genetic (as in Peutz–Jeghers syndrome with mutation in *STK11* tumour suppressor gene on chromosome 19), or malignant (as in melanoma). However, melanoma and seborrhoeic warts produce highly localized, rather than generalized pigmentation.

BOX 17.8 CAUSES OF HYPERPIGMENTATION (LOCALIZED AND GENERALIZED)

- Seborrhoeic keratosis.
- Melanoma.
- *Endocrine:* Addison's, Cushing's, Nelson's disease, pregnancy.
- *Drugs:* heavy metals, chloroquine, oral contraceptive pill, amiodarone.
- *Metabolic:* haemochromatosis, cirrhosis, porphyrias.
- *Genetic:* Peutz–Jeghers syndrome, Albright's syndrome, neurofibromatosis.
- Malnutrition.

BOX 17.9 CAUSES OF HYPOPIGMENTATION

- *Infections:* pityriasis versicolor.
- *Autoimmune:* vitiligo.
- *Drugs*: chloroquine, Imatinib mesylate
- *Genetic:* phenylketonuria, tuberous sclerosis, albinism.

Conversely, hypopigmentation can result from a direct toxic effect on melanocytes (e.g. via autoimmune vitiligo), inhibition of melanogenesis (e.g. corticosteroids) or a decrease in tyrosine, which melanocytes use to make melanin (e.g. from dicarboxylic acids from Tinea versicolor, which inhibit tyrosine kinase; see Box 17.9).

Alopecia

Hair growth occurs in cycles consisting of a long growing phase of 2–3 years (anagen), followed by an involution phase of 2–3 weeks (catagen) and then a resting phase of 3–4 months (telogen), after which hairs falls out (exogen). New hair growth then starts in the follicle. At any time the vast majority of follicles are, therefore, in their anagen phase.

The histological diagnosis of alopecia is based on whether there is evidence of scarring or not (Box 17.10). Scarring alopecia displays loss of follicular ostia or atrophy with clinically apparent inflammation. Often a particular cell type, such as lymphocytes or neutrophils may predominate, and point to a particular group of causes. Non-scarring alopecia has preserved follicular ostia without clinical evidence of inflammation. Examples include telogen effluvium where extensive loss of hair occurs in the growing phase secondary to illness or metabolic stress. Alopecia areata is an autoimmune T cell mediated non-scarring form of hair loss associated with other autoimmune diseases (such as vitiligo), whereas chemotherapy agents cause Anagen effluvium (see 'Drug-induced alopecia'). Many alopecia types are biphasic. Androgenic alopecia eventually results in loss of ostia and, thus, may eventually appear like a scarring alopecia.

Hirsuitism/hypertrichosis

Hirsuitism can arise from an increase in the levels of androgen like hormones or an increase in the sensitivity of hair

BOX 17.10 CAUSES OF ALOPECIA

- *Scarring:* hereditary, infections (TB, syphilis, fungal), injury (burns, radiotherapy), autoimmune (SLE and lichen planus, rarely sarcoidosis and pemphigoid).
- *Non-scarring:* autoimmune (alopecia areata associated with vitiligo), androgenic, endorine (hypopituitarism, hypothyroid, hypoparathyroid, pregnancy), drugs (see 'Drug-induced alopecia').

BOX 17.11 CAUSES OF HIRSUITISM

- *Ovarian:* polycystic ovarian syndrome, ovarian tumours.
- *Adrenal:* congenital adrenal hyperplasia, Cushings.
- Androgen therapy.

BOX 17.12 CAUSES OF HYPERTRICHOSIS

- Congenital.
- *Endocrine:* hypo/hyperthyroidism.
- *Drugs:* see 'Drug-induced hirsuitism/hypertrichosis'.

follicles to androgens (Box 17.11). In contrast, hypertrichosis involves excessive hair growth in areas that are not normally androgen sensitive and can occur through transformation of soft fine vellous hair into larger terminal hair, or an increased anagen phase of hair follicles (Box 17.12).

BOX 17.13 TYPES OF NAIL DISORDERS

- *Onycholysis:* psoriasis, dermatitis, fungal infection, hypo/hyperthyroidism.
- *Koilonychia:* concave deformity associated with iron deficiency.
- *Beau's lines:* transverse depressions due to temporary cessation of growth with severe illness.
- *Yellow nail syndrome:* associated with recurrent pleural effusions, bronchiectasis, nephrotic syndrome, and hypothyroidism.
- *Half-and-half nails:* white proximal bed and darker distal bed associated with renal failure and rheumatoid arthritis.

Nail disorders

Many systemic disorders as well as dermatological conditions can influence the growth of nail beds. Examples are listed in Box 17.13.

Drug-induced skin reactions

Maculopapular erythema

Can occur with almost any drug. Common examples include antibiotics, thiazides, allopurinol, and carbamazepine.

Fixed drug eruption

These occur in a localized site each time a drug is administered. Common precipitants include antibiotics, salicylates, and phenytoin.

Erythema multiforme

Erythema multiforme is a type III hypersensitivity reaction with IgM immune complexes present in the microvasculature of the skin and oral mucous membranes. It can be triggered by infection (such as herpes simplex), and drugs such as antibiotics, salicylates, thiazides, phenytoin, and carbamazepine.

Stevens--Johnson syndrome/toxic epidermal necrolysis

A life-threatening condition whereby a type IV hypersensitivity reaction causes separation of the dermis and epidermis in the skin and the mucous membranes. This lichenoid (or interface) reaction is characterized by an inflammatory infiltrate composed of mononuclear cells with basal cell degeneration and apoptosis in the lower part of the epidermis or in the dermis. The reaction can also produce pigment 'incontinence' with melanin granules appearing in the dermis, and within dermal macrophages due to damage of basal keratinocytes and melanocytes. Drugs such as penicillin, phenytoin, and barbiturates are known triggers.

Urticaria

Urticaria is characterized by itchy wheals and hives due to the release of histamine from cutaneous mast cells. Although 95% of cases of urticaria are idiopathic, it can be precipitated by antibiotics (especially penicillins, cephalosporins), opiates, salicylates, and angiotensin convertin enzyme (ACE) inhibitors.

Drug-induced photosensitivity

Drugs causing phototoxic reaction include antibiotics, NSAIDs, amiodarone, thiazides, sulphonylureas, and retinoids. Photoallergic reactions are more common with sulphonylureas, statins, oral contraceptives, sunscreens, and fragrances.

Drug-induced lupus

A predisposing factor to drug-induced lupus is deficiency in N-acetyltransferase, which is associated with HLA DR4 ('slow acetylators'). This presents with arthralgia, pleuritic, or pericarditic inflammation, a photosensitive butterfly rash with positive antibodies to histones and double-stranded DNA. The most common drugs to cause this are hydralazine and procainamide.

Drug-induced hyper/hypopigmentation

See 'Pigmentation'.

Drug-induced hirsuitism/hypertrichosis

Drugs that induce hirsuitism by their androgenic actions include thigh dose oral contraceptive pills, testosterone, danazol, and high dose corticosteroids. Drug-induced hypertrichosis causes uniform hair growth in areas of the body that are not usually androgen dependent and the mechanism by which drugs act on hair follicles to cause this is not known. Examples of drugs causing this include phenytoin, cyclosporine, minoxidil, diazoxide, psoralen, and penicillamine.

Drug-induced alopecia

Medications can lead to two types of non-scarring hair loss, the most severe of which is Anagen effluvium. This is commonly seen within a few days to weeks of taking cytotoxic drugs, which cause hair loss during the anagen phase of the hair cycle preventing matrix cells from dividing and producing new hair. It generally leads to total body hair loss. Telogen effluvium is the most common form of drug-induced hair loss and can occur within a few months of withdrawal of the oral contraceptive pill, or from administration of heparin, l-dopa, carbimazole, tricyclic antidepressants, lithium, β-blockers, cimetidine, and retinoids. In this condition, hair follicles to go into their resting (telogen) phase and fall out early.

Multiple choice questions

1. The layer of the epidermis responsible for keratinocyte production is the:

A. Stratum corneum.
B. Stratum lucidum.
C. Stratum granulosum.
D. Stratum spinosum.
E. Stratum germinativum.

2. The layer of the epidermis that provides waterproofing is the:

A. Stratum corneum.
B. Stratum lucidum.
C. Stratum granulosum.
D. Stratum spinosum.
E. Stratum germinativum.

3. The layer of the skin that contains vascular plexi with arteriovenous anastomoses to control thermoregulation is:

A. Superficial papillary dermis.
B. Reticular dermis.
C. Lamina densa.
D. Stratum germinativum.
E. Hypodermis.

4. A broad plateau-like lesion greater in width than depth due to localized epidermal proliferation or oedematous inflammation is known as a:

A. Bullae.
B. Nodule.
C. Plaque.
D. Pupuric lesion.
E. Vesicle.

5. Which of the following is an example of a scarring alopecia?

A. Androgenic alopecia.
B. Alopecia areata.
C. Telogen effluvium.
D. Lichen planus.
E. Anagen effluvium.

6. Which of the following is *not* associated with hirsuitism?

A. Minoxidil.
B. Congenital adrenal hyperplasia.
C. Systemic lupus erythematosis.
D. Cushing's disease.
E. Polycystic ovarian syndrome.

7. Which of the following is most likely to cause a bullous eruption?

A. Tinea corpis.
B. Pityriasis versicolor.
C. *Neisseria meningitidis*.
D. *Staphylococcus aureus*.
E. *Borrelia burgdorferi*.

8. Which of the following is correct regarding urticarial rashes?

A. The precipitant is identified in the majority of cases.
B. Most are induced by type 3 hypersensitivity reactions.
C. Most are non-pruritic.
D. They are not induced by drugs.
E. They are characterized by wheals and hives.

9. A 55-year-old man with a history of epilepsy presents with a fever, and widespread blistering rash over his body and in the oral cavity having changed his anticonvulsant medication. Slight rubbing of the skin results in exfoliation of the outermost layer (Nikolsky's sign). The most likely diagnosis is:

A. Bullous pemphigoid.
B. Stevens–Johnson syndrome/toxic epidermal necrolysis.
C. Dermatitis herpetiformis.
D. Drug-induced lupus.
E. Porphyria cutanea tada.

10. Excessive desquamation due to autosomal recessive mutations in the *SPINK5* gene and disruption of the serine protease inhibitor lympho-epithelial Kazal-type-related inhibitor (LEKTI) is known as:

A. Netherton syndrome.
B. Nelson's syndrome.
C. Peutz–Jeghers syndrome.
D. Albright's syndrome.
E. von Recklinghausen disease.

For answers, please see Appendix: Answers to multiple choice questions, page 313.

Appendix: Answers to multiple choice questions

Chapter 1

1. A. 2. E. 3. D. 4. B. 5. A. 6. B. 7. A. 8. C. 9. D. 10. E.

Chapter 2

1. E. 2. B. 3. C. 4. C. 5. E. 6. D. 7. A. 8. B. 9. D. 10. A.

Chapter 3

1. A. 2. B. 3. D. 4. C. 5. B. 6. A. 7. C. 8. D. 9. A. 10. C.

Chapter 4

1. B. 2. C. 3. C. 4. C. 5. B. 6. A. 7. D. 8. E. 9. B. 10. D.

Chapter 5

1. C. 2. B. 3. E. 4. D. 5. B. 6. A. 7. E. 8. A. 9. D. 10. C.

Chapter 6

1. C. 2. D. 3. A. 4. B. 5. C. 6. D. 7. E. 8. B. 9. E. 10. A.

Chapter 7

1. E. 2. C. 3. A. 4. B. 5. D. 6. A. 7. E. 8. C. 9. B. 10. D.

Chapter 8

1. C. 2. D. 3. A. 4. E. 5. B. 6. B. 7. D. 8. A. 9. C. 10. E.

Chapter 9

1. D. 2. A. 3. C. 4. B. 5. D. 6. D. 7. D. 8. B. 9. C. 10. E.

Chapter 10

1. D. 2. A. 3. E. 4. B. 5. C. 6. C. 7. D. 8. A. 9. B. 10. E.

Chapter 11

1. B. 2. B. 3. C. 4. A. 5. D. 6. E. 7. A. 8. C. 9. D.. 10. A.

Chapter 12

1. B. 2. D. 3. A. 4. C. 5. E. 6. C. 7. D. 8. B. 9. A. 10. E.

Chapter 13

1. A. 2. D. 3. E. 4. B. 5. D. 6. C. 7. A. 8. E. 9. B. 10. B.

Chapter 14

1. A. 2. D. 3. E. 4. B. 5. C. 6. A. 7. D. 8. C. 9. E. 10. B.

Chapter 15

1. C. 2. B. 3. D. 4. E. 5. C. 6. A. 7. C. 8. D. 9. B. 10. A.

Chapter 16

1. B. 2. A. 3. D. 4. C. 5. E. 6. A. 7. E. 8. A. 9. D. 10. D.

Chapter 17

1. E. 2. A. 3. B. 4. C. 5. D. 6. C. 7. D. 8. E. 9. B. 10. A.

Index

Notes
vs. indicates a comparison or differential diagnosis
Page numbers suffixed with *f* indicate material in figure, *t* in tables and *b* in boxes.

B

C

D

E

F

G

H

I

N

T

U

V

W

X

Y

Z